Practical Guides in Radiation Oncology

Series Editors
Nancy Y. Lee, Department of Radiation Oncology, Memorial Sloan-Kettering Cancer Center, New York, NY, USA
Jiade J. Lu, Department of Radiation Oncology, Shanghai Proton and Heavy Ion Center, Shanghai, China

The series Practical Guides in Radiation Oncology is designed to assist radiation oncology residents and practicing radiation oncologists in the application of current techniques in radiation oncology and day-to-day management in clinical practice, i.e., treatment planning. Individual volumes offer clear guidance on contouring in different cancers and present treatment recommendations, including with regard to advanced options such as intensity-modulated radiation therapy (IMRT) and stereotactic body radiation therapy (SBRT). Each volume addresses one particular area of practice and is edited by experts with an outstanding international reputation. Readers will find the series to be an ideal source of up-to-date information on when to apply the various available technologies and how to perform safe treatment planning.

Chelsea Pinnix • Yolanda D. Tseng
Sarah A. Milgrom • Stephanie Terezakis
Editors

Target Volume Delineation in Hematologic Malignancies

Springer

Editors
Chelsea Pinnix
Department of Radiation Oncology
The University of Texas MD
Anderson Cancer
Houston, TX, USA

Sarah A. Milgrom
Univ. of Colorado School of Medicine
Department of Radiation Oncology
Aurora, CO, USA

Yolanda D. Tseng
Department of Radiation Oncology
University of Washington
Seattle, WA, USA

Stephanie Terezakis
Department of Radiation Oncology
University of Minnesota
Minneapolis, MN, USA

ISSN 2522-5715 ISSN 2522-5723 (electronic)
Practical Guides in Radiation Oncology
ISBN 978-3-031-67721-2 ISBN 978-3-031-67722-9 (eBook)
https://doi.org/10.1007/978-3-031-67722-9

This Springer imprint is published by the registered company Springer Nature Switzerland AG
The registered company address is: Gewerbestrasse 11, 6330 Cham, Switzerland

Contents

Target Volume Delineation for Early-Stage Adult Hodgkin Lymphoma

1

Lena Specht, Danijela Dejanovic, and Anne Kiil Berthelsen

Contents

L. Specht (✉)
Department of Oncology, Rigshospitalet, University of Copenhagen, Copenhagen, Denmark
e-mail: lena.specht@regionh.dk

D. Dejanovic
Department of Nuclear Medicine and PET, Rigshospitalet, University of Copenhagen, Copenhagen, Denmark

A. K. Berthelsen
Department of Oncology, Rigshospitalet, University of Copenhagen, Copenhagen, Denmark

Department of Nuclear Medicine and PET, Rigshospitalet, University of Copenhagen, Copenhagen, Denmark
e-mail: anne.kiil.berthelsen@regionh.dk

C. Pinnix et al. (eds.), *Target Volume Delineation in Hematologic Malignancies*, Practical Guides in Radiation Oncology,
https://doi.org/10.1007/978-3-031-67722-9_1

Part 1: Background and Epidemiology

- Hodgkin lymphoma (HL) in adults is a relatively rare disease with an annual worldwide incidence of 1.4 per 100,000 in males and 1.1 per 100,000 in females. However, there are distinct geographical variations. The incidence in Europe is 3.3 per 100,000 in males and 2.6 per 100,000 in females; in North America, the corresponding figures are 3.7 and 2.8; in Australia and New Zealand, 4.0 and 2.6; in South America, 2.3 and 1.6; in Africa, 1.2 and 0.87; and in Asia, 0.86 and 0.59 [1].
- The age-specific incidence is bimodal, with a peak in young adults and a second peak after 60 years of age. HL is about equally common in young adult women and men, whereas it is more common in older men than older women [1].
- The nodular sclerosis subtype is associated with high socioeconomic status [2]. The mixed cellularity subtype is more frequent in developing countries and in patients with HIV, and it is associated with Epstein-Barr virus infection [3, 4].
- Approximately 90% of HL cases are classic HL (CHL). CHL is a CD30-positive B-cell neoplasm that is composed of multinucleated Reed–Sternberg cells and mononuclear Hodgkin cells in a background of non-neoplastic reactive immune cells [5]. CHL is divided into four subtypes:
  - Nodular sclerosis (NS), which accounts for about 70% of all CHL cases in Europe and North America, but a lower percentage in less affluent societies. Its incidence peaks at 15–35 years of age, and the incidence is similar in males and females.
  - Lymphocyte-rich (LR), which accounts for about 5% of all CHL cases, occurs most commonly in the 30–50-year-old age group, and most often in males.
  - Mixed cellularity (MC), which accounts for about 20–25% of all CHL cases, occurs more frequently in developing countries and in patients with HIV infection. Its incidence peaks in older patients, and most patients are male.
  - Lymphocyte-depleted (LD), which accounts for less than 1% of all CHL cases in the Western World, but it may be more common in developing countries, occurs in older adults, males, and patients with HIV infection.
- The remaining 10% of HL cases are nodular lymphocyte predominant (NLP). NLPHL is a CD20-positive B-cell neoplasm that is composed of "popcorn cells" in a background of small lymphocytes and histiocytes. Like LRCHL, it is most common in the 30–50-year-old age group and in males.
- The most common presentation of CHL is a young adult with an enlarged, non-tender lymph node in the neck or supraclavicular fossa, or less commonly in the axilla or inguino-femoral region. In other cases, a mediastinal mass is discovered on imaging [6]. However, with the changing demographics in Western countries, an increasing number of patients are being diagnosed at older ages; in these patients, mediastinal involvement is less common. About 40% of patients have B symptoms (unexplained fever, night sweats, and/or unexplained weight loss of more than 10% of the usual body weight in the 6 months prior to diagnosis).
- Most patients with NLPHL present with enlarged peripheral lymph nodes, typically in the neck, axilla, or inguinal region.

Part 2: Management of Early-Stage Adult Hodgkin Lymphoma

Baseline Evaluation and Imaging

- The current staging system for HL is the Ann Arbor classification [7], with the modifications included in the Lugano classification [8, 9]. The initial work-up includes a history and physical examination, blood counts, and routine laboratory tests (erythroid sedimentation rate (ESR), lactate dehydrogenase (LDH), alkaline phosphatase, albumin, liver function, and virology), and imaging with a 2-[18F]fluoro-2-deoxy-D-glucose (FDG)-positron emission tomography (PET)/computed tomography (CT). A CT scan with intravenous and oral contrast is important to differentiate lymph nodes from vessels and bowel, respectively. A bone marrow biopsy is no longer recommended if an FDG-PET/CT scan has been performed, unless patients have unexplained cytopenia [10].
- The initial staging FDG-PET/CT scan images are important for planning consolidative radiation therapy (RT) after the completion of systemic treatment in CHL and for planning upfront definitive RT in NLPHL. At the time of treatment planning, this PET/CT scan is fused with the simulation CT scan to delineate the sites of involvement. Therefore, ideally, the initial FDG-PET/CT scan is performed in the position that will be used for RT, thus allowing for optimal image fusion [27]. Furthermore, in patients with mediastinal disease, RT in deep inspiration breath hold (DIBH) significantly reduces radiation dose to the heart and the lungs [28, 29]. Thus, if possible, in patients with mediastinal disease, the staging FDG-PET/CT scan should also be performed in DIBH, as described below, to allow for optimal image fusion with the post-chemotherapy DIBH simulation CT scan. However, obtaining the initial PET/CT in the RT treatment position and in DIBH is not possible in many clinical settings.
  - An FDG-PET may be obtained in DIBH according to the following steps. First, a whole body FDG-PET/CT scan is performed in free breathing. Then, a limited FDG-PET/CT scan encompassing the mediastinal region is acquired in DIBH (one bed position). The patient performs six repeated breath holds of 20 seconds each. The six DIBH FDG-PET scans are post-processed into a summed static FDG-PET dataset comparable to a full 120 second scan. The technical details as implemented at present at the University of Copenhagen are summarized in Table 1.1.
  - In the future, the procedure to obtain an FDG-PET in DIBH may be simplified due to several technical improvements. At present, the axial field of view (FOV) of the 5-ring Siemens CT scanner is 25 cm, so it will typically cover only a part of the lungs. Next generation scanners from several vendors (Siemens Vision 600, GE Discovery IQ) will have an increased FOV of 30 cm allowing for better coverage. Furthermore, the new digital scanners have an increased sensitivity, in part driven by FDG-PET Time of Flight reconstructions, that should reduce the number of DIBH FDG-PET repetitions that are required for each patient. The Siemens Vision FDG-PET/CT scanner can also use continuous bed motion, with no defined fixed bed size, so the full thorax

Table 1.1 Technical details for whole body FDG-PET/CT scan with intravenous (IV) contrast and deep inspiration breath hold (DIBH), as implemented at Rigshospitalet, Copenhagen, Denmark, with a Siemens Biograph CT scanner

• CT Topogram: 120 kV, 35 mA. Assess the attenuation • CT Pre-Monitoring: Identify and mark the aorta on the appropriate slice • CT Monitoring: After IV contrast has been injected, measure the Hounsfield units (HU) in the marked aorta. When this value exceeds 80 HU, initiate the whole-body CT • Whole-Body CT: – Quality reference mAs: 200 mAs (automatically adjusted according to the attenuation data from the topogram with the care dose technology) – 120 kV (automatically optimized for soft tissue contrast with the care kV technology) – Collimation: 0.6 mm * 64 – Reconstructed slice thickness: 2.0 mm – Pitch of spiral CT: 0.8 – Rotation time: 0.5 s • Whole body 2-[18F]fluoro-2-deoxy-D-glucose (FDG)-PET: Performed 1 h after injection of 4 MBq/kg FDG; 1.5 min/bed position, adjusted according to the patient's body mass index (BMI). • DIBH CT: Select the appropriate region. Ask the patient to inspire and hold his/her breath. The CT scan of the lungs is performed with the following parameters: – Quality reference mAs: 226 mAs (Care Dose technology is used) – 120 kV (Care kV technology is activated and optimized for low noise) – Collimation: 0.6 mm * 64 – Reconstructed slice thickness: 2.0 mm – Pitch of spiral CT: 1.4 – Rotation time: 0.5 s • Acquire DIBH FDG-PET recordings by asking the patient to inspire and hold his/her breath for 20 seconds, repeated six times. The DIBH CT and DIBH FDG-PET must match, because the DIBH CT is used for FDG-PET attenuation correction • The six individual DIBH FDG-PET recordings are decay corrected to the first acquisition and averaged to produce to final DIBH FDG-PET image

can be covered with each repetition. Finally, novel artificial intelligence (AI)-based image reconstruction and noise reduction may allow the full DIBH FDG-PET to be performed with just one scan.

- In addition to tumor imaging, tests of pulmonary and cardiac function are typically performed before chemotherapy is given.

Principles of Management

- Standard treatment in patients with early-stage CHL is combined modality treatment. Randomized trials have demonstrated that radiation therapy (RT) cannot be omitted for patients with a complete metabolic response after a short course of Adriamycin, bleomycin, vinblastine, dacarbazine (ABVD) without a loss of local tumor control [11–14].
- In the combined modality setting, RT should start as soon as the patient has recovered from the last cycle of chemotherapy, ideally within 3–4 weeks. However, this timing may be difficult to achieve if the results of a post-

chemotherapy FDG-PET/CT scan are needed to decide further treatment, since the FDG-PET/CT scan must be performed at an interval after the last chemotherapy to reduce the risk of rebound phenomena and false positive findings. It is generally agreed that RT should start no later than 6 weeks after the last chemotherapy.

- The overall treatment approach is modified according to risk factors. Trials underlying these regimens were carried out by the German Hodgkin Study Group (GHSG) [15, 17], and therefore the risk factors separating patients into favorable and unfavorable categories are often those used by the German group, i.e., large mediastinal mass, extranodal disease, ESR ≥ 50 if no B-symptoms and ESR ≥ 30 if B-symptoms present, and ≥3 involved areas. Note that the areas defined by the GHSG are not the same as the regions defined in the Ann Arbor classification (Fig. 1.1).
  - In patients without risk factors according to the GHSG criteria, a standard treatment is 2 cycles of ABVD, followed by involved site radiotherapy (ISRT) to a total dose of 20 Gy at 2 Gy per fraction [15, 16].
  - In patients with one or more risk factors according to the GHSG criteria, a standard treatment is 4 cycles of ABVD followed by ISRT to a total dose of 30 Gy at 1.8–2 Gy per fraction [17].

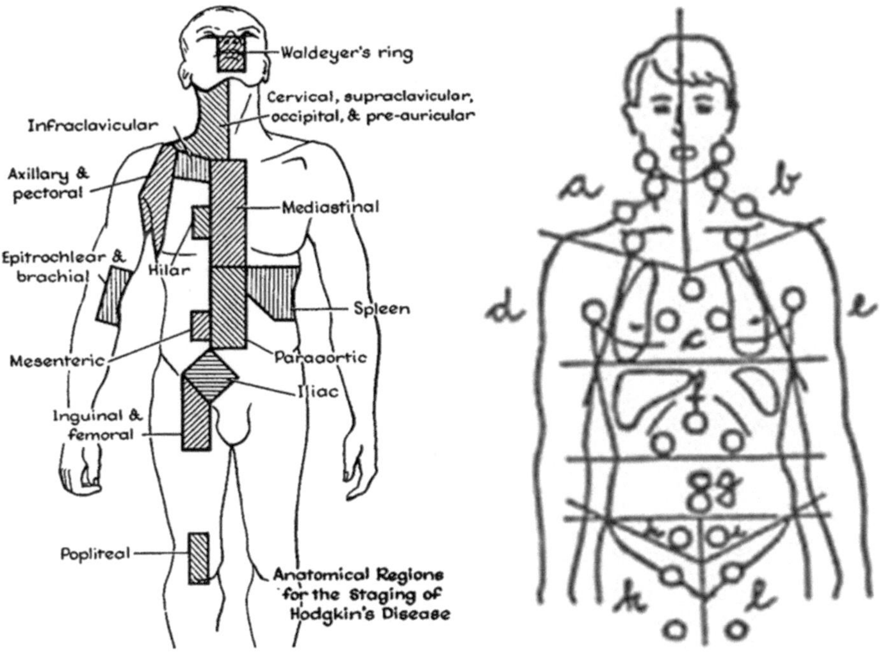

Fig. 1.1 Lymph node regions defined in the Ann Arbor classification (left) and lymph node areas defined by the German Hodgkin Study Group (right)

- Substitution of bleomycin in the ABVD regimen with brentuximab vedotin or a checkpoint inhibitor may be an even more effective combination [18, 19], but there are no data to show that RT can be omitted.
- For patients with early-stage CHL whose disease remains FDG-PET-positive after 2 cycles of ABVD, escalation to the more intensive chemotherapy regimen of bleomycin, etoposide, Adriamycin, cyclophosphamide, vincristine, procarbazine, prednisolone (BEACOPP) followed by ISRT to a total dose of 30 Gy has been shown to improve progression-free survival [11], and this is considered one standard for patients who are able to tolerate this regimen.
- Recently, the GHSG HD17 trial demonstrated that in patients with early-stage unfavorable CHL who achieved a complete metabolic response after 2 cycles of escalated BEACOPP followed by 2 cycles of ABVD, RT could be omitted with no deterioration in 5-year progression-free survival [48]. However, this finding is relevant only for young, fit patients who can tolerate escalated BEACOPP. Moreover, many clinicians would hesitate to treat early-stage CHL with such an intensive regimen, unless the patient had particularly poor prognostic characteristics.
- Management is controversial for stage IIB CHL with a large mediastinal mass and/or extranodal disease. The German group classifies such cases as advanced-stage disease and treats these patients accordingly. However, the European Organization for Research and Treatment of Cancer (EORTC) Lymphoma Group treats all patients with stage IIB HL, even if they have these risk factors, using an early-stage disease approach, and they have reported excellent results.
- Patients with early-stage NLPHL usually have small volume, peripherally located disease. NLPHL has indolent behavior and excellent overall survival, but frequent relapses occurring years after the primary treatment [20–22].
- Standard treatment for localized early-stage NLPHL (i.e., stage I and stage II in contiguous areas) in adults is ISRT to 30 Gy [16], with more generous margins to include adjacent lymph nodes in that site. Although there are no randomized trials due to the rarity of the disease, it is clear from large registry studies that RT is an essential component of the treatment of early-stage NLPHL [30, 31]. No advantage for more extensive treatment fields has been demonstrated [23–25], and the addition of systemic treatment to RT does not improve outcomes [20, 26]. Regarding contiguous stage II disease, it must be remembered that the lymphatic system is continuous throughout the body and that divisions into regions or areas are artificial and arbitrary. Hence, disease that happens to be localized in two adjacent regions may be biologically equivalent to disease located in just one area.
- For the rare patients with NLPHL involving two or more non-contiguous areas, e.g., in both axillae, the disease is more advanced. Such cases should be treated like CHL with combined modality treatment.

General Considerations for Radiotherapy

- Radiation should encompass the clinical target volume (CTV) which is "the gross target volume (GTV) and/or a volume containing subclinical malignant disease with a certain probability of occurrence considered relevant for therapy" as stated in the ICRU83 guidelines [32].
- The goal is to irradiate the smallest effective volume, thus maintaining a high local control rate while minimizing the irradiation of normal tissues.
- If RT is given after effective chemotherapy, then it targets the pre-chemotherapy sites of disease and any residual post-chemotherapy GTV. The aim is to irradiate the tissue volume that contained macroscopic lymphoma before chemotherapy, since these sites are at the highest risk of harboring residual microscopic disease after chemotherapy [16, 33, 34].
- If RT is given as the only modality, then all evident sites (GTV) plus an adequate margin to encompass potential adjacent subclinical disease should be treated [16, 34].
- Patients should be immobilized and simulated as appropriate for different anatomical target locations. It is useful to implement departmental standard protocols to ensure that the staff knows how to position patients correctly for each site.
- In general, the pre-chemotherapy FDG-PET/CT scan is used for target delineation. Optimal image fusion allows the strictest form of ISRT, defined as involved node radiation therapy (INRT) [16, 35, 36]. For INRT, pre-chemotherapy imaging must be performed in the radiation treatment position. Even if this is not possible, the pre-chemotherapy FDG-PET/CT scan is used as a visual guide for contouring the CTV for ISRT. Therefore, a general rule is to immobilize and treat the patient in the same position that was used for the staging FDG-PET/CT scan, which is usually done with the patient in the arms-up position. However, if the target is solely in the neck, it is best to immobilize patients with the arms down, since this will not change the position of the target significantly, and it will enable the use of a thermoplastic head-and-neck mask. If the target, as is often the case, includes the chest, then a change in arm position will lead to significant changes in the position of the target compared to the pre-chemotherapy FDG-PET/CT scan; hence, to allow optimal image fusion, the patient should typically be immobilized with the arms up. With the arms up, it is not possible to use a thermoplastic head-and-neck mask; instead, if head immobilization is required, it may be accomplished with a bite block or shorter thermoplastic face mask. For mediastinal sites, DIBH should be used whenever possible to reduce dose to the lungs and heart; a visual feedback system can be useful to improve breath-hold position reproducibility (Fig. 1.2). For infra-diaphragmatic targets, reproducible immobilization can be achieved with knee- and footrests (Fig. 1.3). The arms may be down, but should be positioned so they are not included in the irradiated area.
- Axial CT images of the immobilized patient that encompass the area that is to be irradiated should be acquired with a slice thickness of 2–3 mm to enable good 3D reconstructions. For targets in the chest, the CT scan should be acquired in DIBH

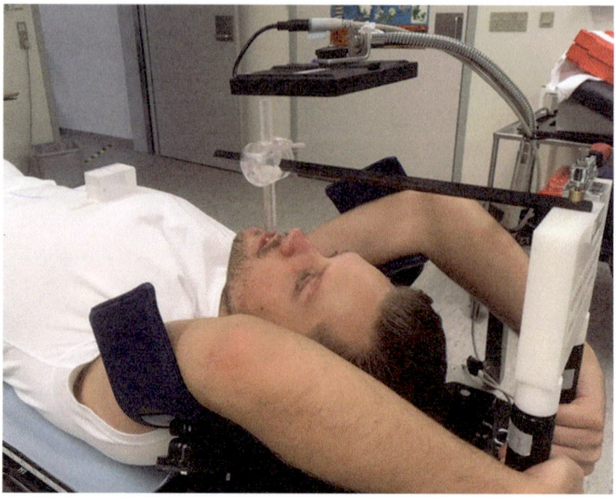

Fig. 1.2 Immobilization with the arms up for treatment of mediastinal lymphoma. The head is immobilized with a bite block. The box on the patient's chest measures the movement of the thorax during breathing. Visual feedback is provided on a screen, so the patient can reproduce the breath holds for treatment using a DIBH technique

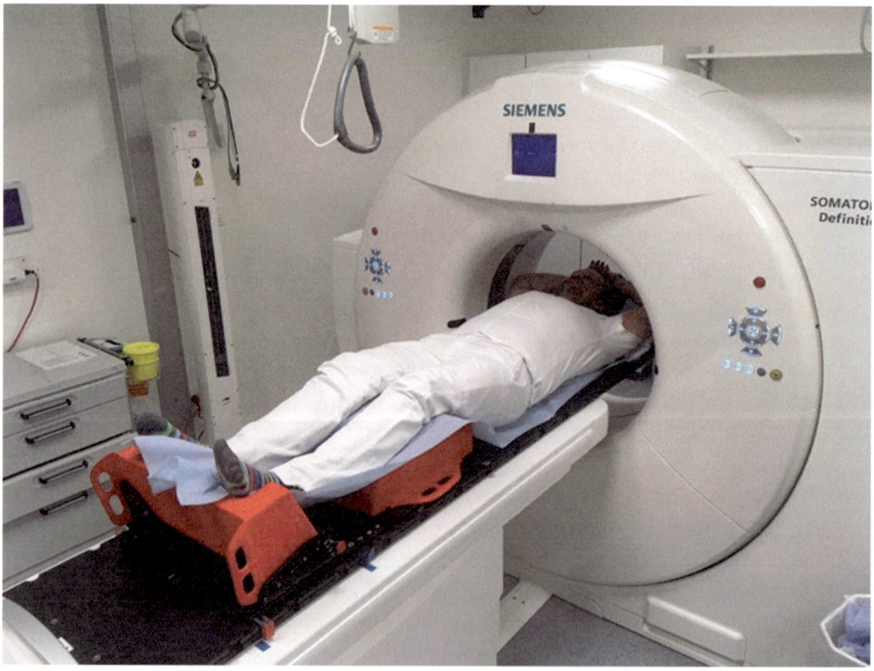

Fig. 1.3 Immobilization using knee- and footrests for treatment of targets in the lower body

to allow optimal planning of RT using a DIBH technique. Intravenous contrast is recommended, unless contraindicated, to help distinguish blood vessels from lymph nodes. For the abdomen and pelvis, oral contrast is recommended to help distinguish bowel from lymph nodes.

- Equipment and algorithms for MR simulation and treatment planning are being developed. At some centers, MR accelerators are now in clinical use and allow direct monitoring of target movement during treatment. This may further improve motion management, for example, for mediastinal lymphomas.
- Generally, four target volumes, as defined in the ICRU83 guidelines [32], are relevant for treatment planning in early-stage HL:
  - The gross tumor volume (GTV) is the macroscopic lymphoma. In patients treated with combined modality, there may be two GTVs. There is always a pre-chemotherapy GTV. If residual lymphoma remains after chemotherapy, then there should also be a post-chemotherapy GTV.
  - The clinical target volume (CTV) is the GTV (at the time of RT) and/or subclinical lymphoma with a high enough probability to require RT. In patients treated with combined modality therapy, the CTV includes any post-chemotherapy GTV, as well as the tissue volume that contained the pre-chemotherapy GTV accounting for changes in anatomy that have occurred with chemotherapy. If effective chemotherapy was administered, then it has treated subclinical disease that was present initially; therefore, no margin is added to cover possible subclinical disease at presentation. However, margins may be needed to compensate for uncertainties due to suboptimal image fusion, for example due to differences in patient positioning for images obtained before and after chemotherapy. In patients treated with RT alone, and in patients treated with chemotherapy with uncertain efficacy, the CTV must also include volumes with a high likelihood of harboring subclinical disease at presentation.
  - The internal target volume (ITV) was defined in the ICRU62 guidelines [37] as the CTV plus a margin taking into account uncertainties in size, shape, and position of the CTV within the patient. This volume includes an internal margin to account for target movement within the patient. The ITV is optional for mobile targets; some radiation oncologists may prefer to include the internal margin in the delineation of the PTV. Either way, it is important to consider internal motion, in particular for targets in the chest and upper abdomen, where respiratory motion may add uncertainties.
  - The planning target volume (PTV) is a geometrical concept introduced to shape the absorbed dose distribution so that the prescribed dose is delivered to all parts of the CTV. It incorporates the setup uncertainties in patient positioning and beam alignment. The size of the PTV margin depends on the equipment, immobilization, and treatment protocol at each individual institution. Immobilization should be performed carefully with equipment suitable for the body region being irradiated, and it will often allow for smaller margins; for example, in the head-and-neck region, face masks provide excellent control of movement. Daily imaging, particularly with cone beam CT scans, may allow further reduction in the PTV margins. Appropriate PTV margins must be determined by individual institutions, based on these factors.
- The organs-at-risk (OARs) include normal structures that are at risk of RT-related toxicity and that must be considered during treatment planning. For supra-

diaphragmatic HL, OARs include the heart, lungs, breasts in young females, thyroid, spinal cord, salivary glands, and potentially other structures in the head-and-neck area if they are near the treated volume. Emerging data suggest that cardiac substructures, such as the valves and the coronary arteries, are important OARs, although the optimal dose constraints for these substructures are yet to be defined. It is important that consensus is reached for contouring cardiac substructures to ensure standardized reporting of dose and to allow accurate investigations into dose-toxicity relationships [38]. For infra-diaphragmatic HL, the kidneys and ovaries in young women are particularly important OARs. Most other organs below the diaphragm have tolerances well above the modest radiation doses that are normally prescribed for lymphomas; nonetheless, OAR doses should always be kept as low as possible to minimize the risk of second malignancies.

- Delivery of the prescribed dose may be achieved with different techniques including 3-dimensional (3D) conformal radiotherapy, intensity modulated radiotherapy (IMRT) [39, 40], volumetric arc therapy (VMAT) [41], helical tomotherapy, or proton therapy [42]. The preferred technique in each case depends upon the location of the lymphoma, the surrounding normal structures, and patient characteristics such as age, sex, and comorbidities. There is no single best technique that should be used for all early-stage HL patients [43–45].
- For targets in the chest, treatment in DIBH will often offer significant sparing of the heart and lungs [28, 29, 43]. Additionally, a "butterfly" beam arrangement can reduce dose to the breast and lung tissue [40].

Part 3: Cases

Case 1

A 20-year-old woman was diagnosed with stage IIA CHL, nodular sclerosis subtype, with involvement of the bilateral lower neck, mediastinum, left hilum, and left axilla. There was no disease bulk. Her ESR level was 13. She was classified as having early-stage, unfavorable disease according to the GHSG criteria (due to three or more involved regions). She was treated with 4 cycles of ABVD followed by INRT, 1.8 Gy × 17 fractions, with 5 fractions per week.

The patient had an initial staging FDG-PET/CT scan that was performed in DIBH (see above for technical details), as shown in Figs. 1.4 and 1.5. After chemotherapy, a planning simulation CT scan was performed in DIBH with the patient in the same position as for the pre-chemotherapy FDG-PET/CT scan, enabling optimal image fusion. The pre-chemotherapy GTV was contoured on the initial PET/CT scan, taking care to include both FDG-PET-positive and FDG-PET-negative sites of disease and to exclude normal tissues with physiologic FDG uptake. Then, the pre-chemotherapy GTV was transferred to the planning CT scan. This volume was modified to account for anatomic changes that occurred with chemotherapy; specifically, the volume was adjusted to exclude normal structures, such as the

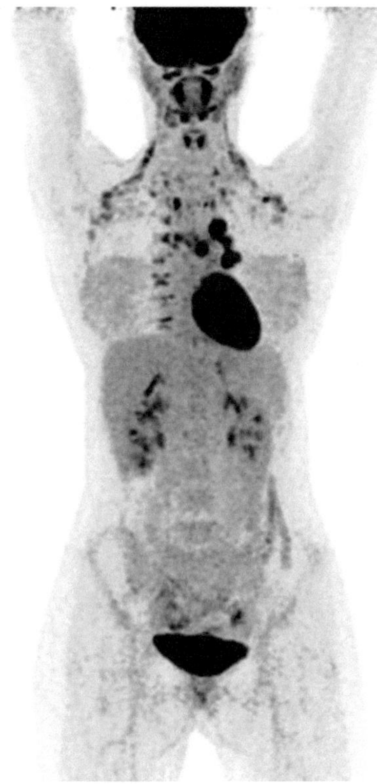

Fig. 1.4 Initial staging FDG-PET/CT scan for patient 1. Maximal intensity projection image

lungs, that were displaced by, but not invaded by, lymphoma initially. This volume is the CTV that includes the tissue that was initially involved by HL, as shown in Fig. 1.6.

An appropriate PTV margin was added, and a treatment plan was created. In this case, VMAT was used with constraints on heart, lung, breast, and thyroid doses (Fig. 1.7). Because the prescribed doses for lymphomas are relatively low, the constraints used for solid tumors cannot be applied. Doses to normal structures should always be kept as low as reasonably achievable (the ALARA principle). Acceptable OAR doses depend on the location and extent of the lymphoma, and on the patient's age, sex, and comorbidities. In this case, OAR doses were well below the dose constraints cited in the ILROG guidelines for proton therapy [42]. Currently, decision-support tools are being developed that quantify the risk of long-term effects of RT in the individual patient and may aid in treatment planning [46, 47].

Case 2

A 51-year-old male was diagnosed with stage IIB CHL, nodular sclerosis subtype, with involvement of right lower neck, right subpectoral area, mediastinum, and right hilum. There was no disease bulk. His ESR level was 56. He had drenching

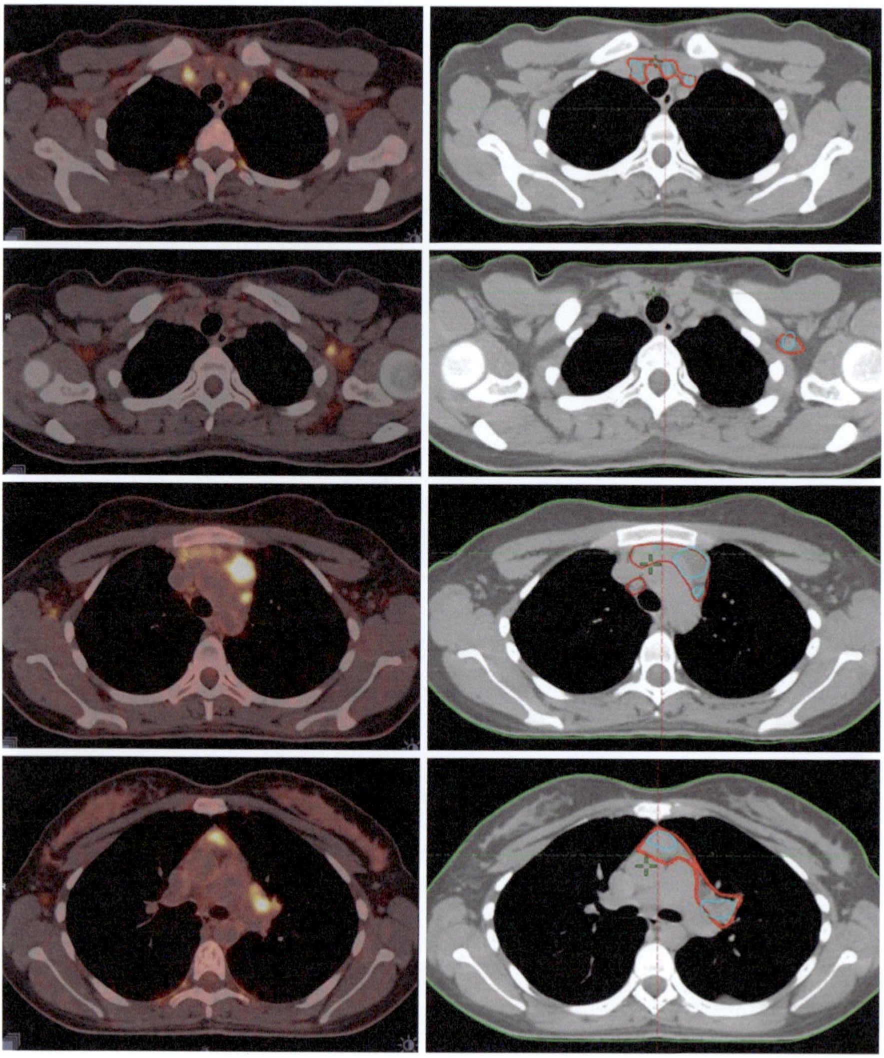

Fig. 1.5 The initial staging FDG-PET/CT scan for patient 1. Selected slices of the DIBH FDG-PET/CT scan are shown on the left, and the corresponding slices of the DIBH CT scan are shown on the right. The initially FDG-PET-positive volume is contoured in cyan blue. The entire initially involved site, including both FDG-avid and non-FDG-avid disease, is contoured in red (GTV)

night sweats, but no other B-symptoms. He was classified as having early-stage, unfavorable disease according to the GHSG criteria, so he was treated with 4 cycles of ABVD followed by INRT, 1.8 Gy × 17 fractions, with 5 fractions per week.

The patient had an initial staging FDG-PET/CT-scan in DIBH (see above for technical details), as shown in Figs. 1.8 and 1.9. After chemotherapy, a planning simulation CT scan was performed in DIBH. However, because the patient's body

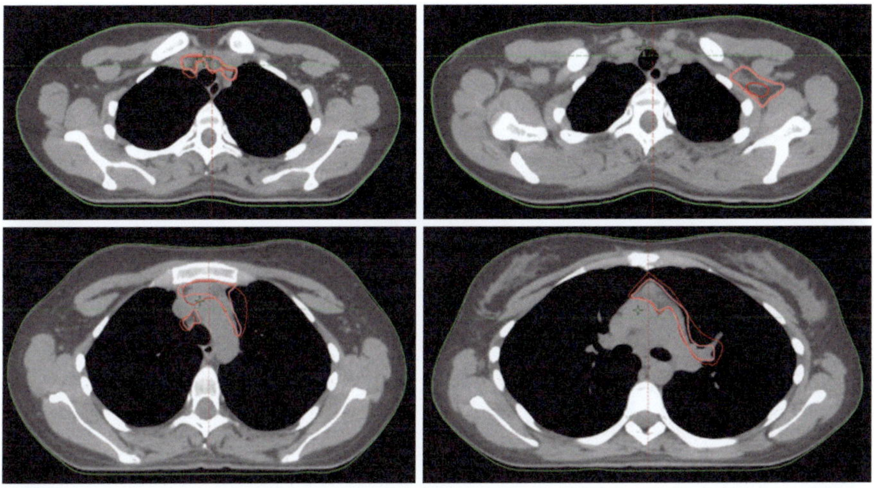

Fig. 1.6 The post-chemotherapy planning CT scan for patient 1, with slices at the same levels as shown in Fig. 1.5. The pre-chemotherapy GTV (red) is transferred from the pre-chemotherapy staging FDG-PET/CT scan to the post-chemotherapy planning CT scan. This volume is modified to account for anatomical changes that occurred during chemotherapy; for example, it is cropped out of the lung that was initially displaced by the mediastinal mass and has now moved back to its normal position. In addition, the volume is adjusted to allow for uncertainties if the fusion is not optimal. The resulting volume, shown in pink, encompasses the tissue that contained lymphoma initially (CTV)

position was not identical for imaging performed before and after chemotherapy, it was necessary to perform separate fusions for the neck and for the chest (focused on the sternum). The pre-chemotherapy GTV was contoured on the initial PET/CT scan, taking care to include both FDG-PET-positive and FDG-PET-negative sites of disease and to exclude normal tissues with physiologic FDG uptake. Then, the pre-chemotherapy GTV was transferred to the planning CT scan. This volume was modified to account for anatomic changes that occurred with chemotherapy and differences in patient positioning between scans. This volume was the CTV that encompassed the initially involved tissue (Fig. 1.10).

An appropriate PTV margin was added, and a treatment plan was created. A VMAT technique was used, with constraints on heart and lung doses (Fig. 1.11). The same considerations apply as for Case 1, and heart and lung doses should always be kept as low as reasonably achievable. Given the disease distribution in this case, OAR doses were higher than in Case 1 and were close to the constraints cited in the ILROG guidelines for proton therapy [42].

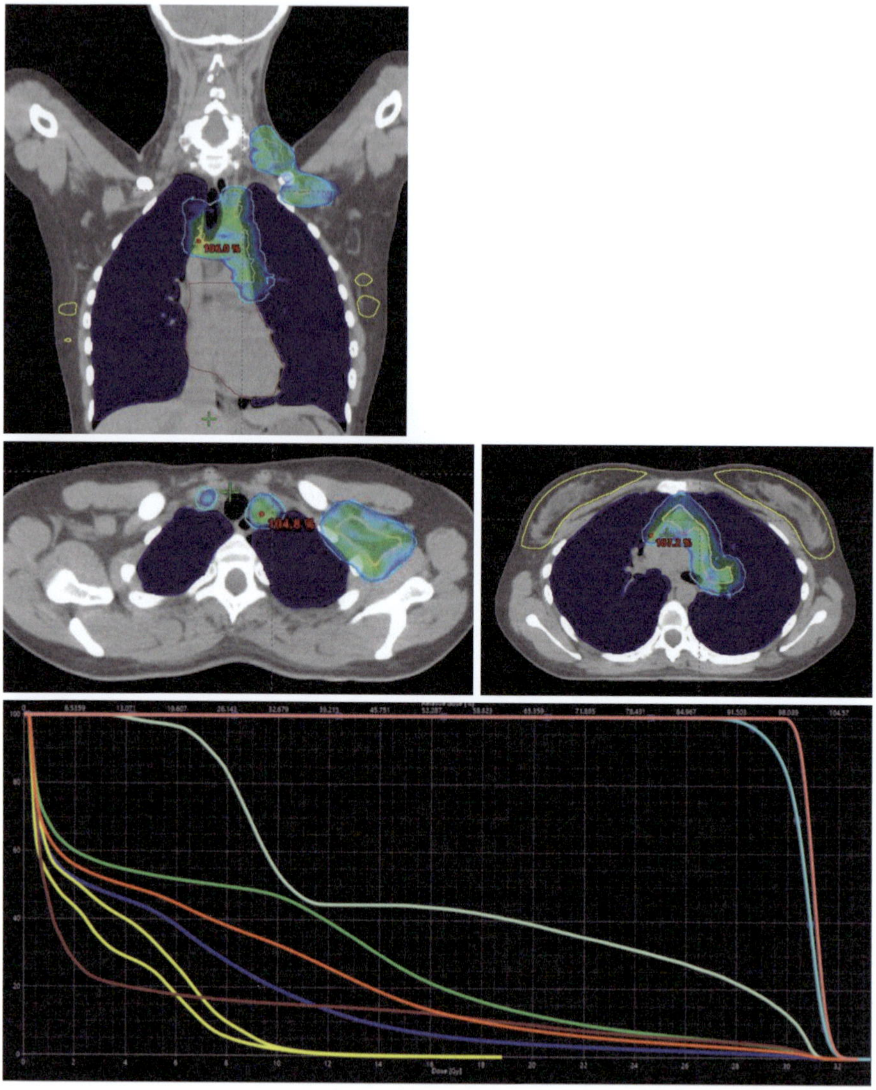

Fig. 1.7 Treatment plan for patient 1. Volumetric arc therapy (VMAT) was used with constraints on heart, lung, breast, and thyroid doses. A volume representing 95% of the prescription dose is shown. The mean heart dose was 4.5 Gy. The lung V5 was 48%, V20 was 8%, and mean dose was 7.2 Gy. Mean doses to the breast were 3.4 Gy (left) and 2.7 Gy (right). The thyroid V25 was 30%. Coronal slice (top), two axial slices (middle), and DVH (bottom; CTV pink, PTV cyan blue, thyroid light green, left lung green, right lung blue, both lungs together orange, left and right breast yellow, heart brown)

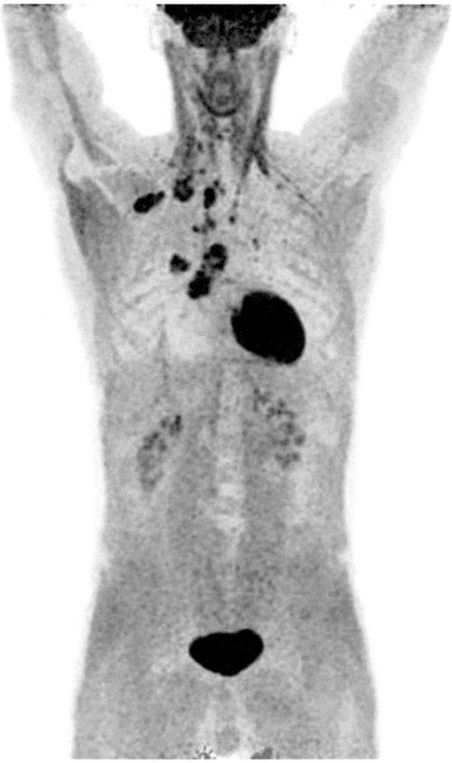

Fig. 1.8 Initial staging FDG-PET/CT scan for patient 2. Maximal intensity projection image

Case 3

A 48-year-old woman was diagnosed with stage IA NLPHL involving the right groin. There was no disease bulk. Her ESR was 3. She had no B-symptoms. She was treated with ISRT alone, 1.8 Gy × 17 fractions, with 5 fractions per week.

An excisional biopsy of a right groin lymph node confirmed the diagnosis, and then the patient had an initial FDG-PET/CT scan (Figs. 1.12 and 1.13). A planning CT scan was performed in the same position. The FDG-PET-positive lymphoma volume was contoured and transferred to the planning CT scan. On the planning CT scan, the macroscopically involved lymphoma volume (GTV) was contoured, and lymph nodes in the lower right iliac region of uncertain significance (i.e., reactive or involved by disease) were also included. The CTV was contoured to include the GTV and adjacent lymph node areas at high risk of harboring microscopic disease, since the patient was treated with RT alone.

An appropriate PTV margin was added, and a treatment plan was created using VMAT (Fig. 1.14). Given the modest prescribed dose, it was not difficult to keep the dose to the surrounding normal structures at a very acceptable level.

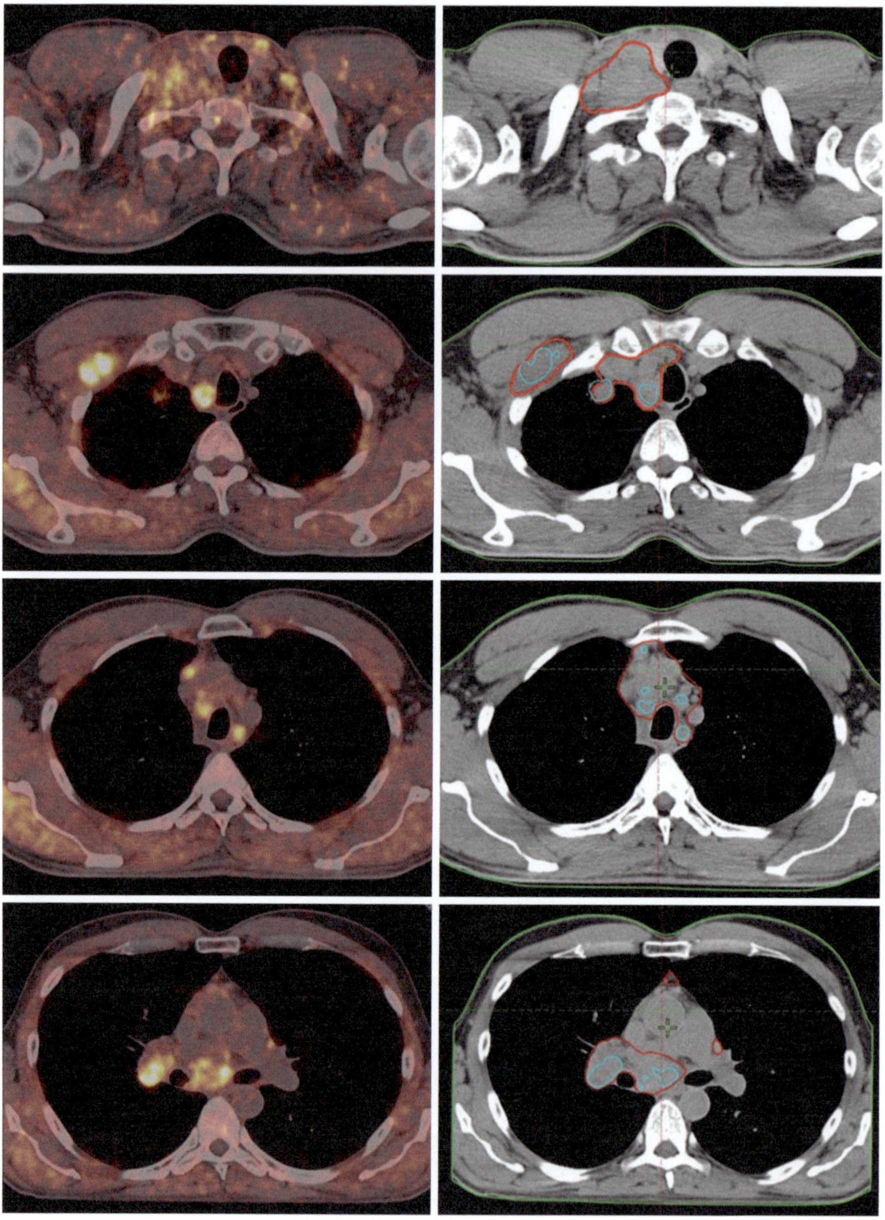

Fig. 1.9 The initial staging FDG-PET/CT scan for patient 2. Selected slices of the DIBH FDG-PET/CT scan are shown on the left, and the corresponding slices of the DIBH CT scan are shown on the right. The initially FDG-PET-positive volume is contoured in cyan blue. The entire initially involved site, including both FDG-avid and non-FDG-avid disease, is contoured in red (GTV). Note that a fairly large proportion of the lymphoma volume is not FDG-PET-positive

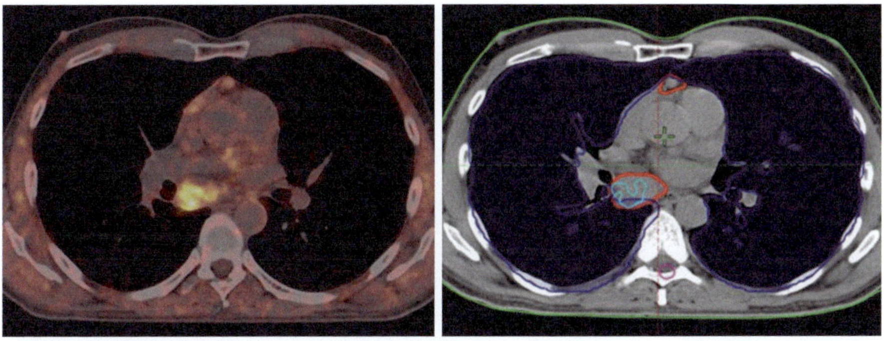

Fig. 1.9 (continued)

Part 4: Special Considerations

Contouring the CTV in early-stage HL can be challenging. FDG-PET scans facilitate detection of all sites of disease involvement; however, lymphomas may have variable FDG-avidity and areas of disease may be appreciable only on CT but not FDG-PET, as demonstrated in Case 2. Analyses of the patterns of relapse in HL have demonstrated that recurrences may occur in lymph nodes that were FDG-PET-negative initially [33]. Hence, it is important to pay attention to both the CT scan and the FDG-PET scan. Moreover, FDG-PET scans are not always easy to interpret. One challenge, particularly in younger patients, is brown fat that may limit interpretation of FDG-PET scans (Fig. 1.15). Premedication with a β-blocker reduces FDG uptake in brown fat and may be useful in patients with brown fat activity. Expert nuclear medicine input is important to achieve high quality images that enable the most accurate contouring for radiation treatment planning.

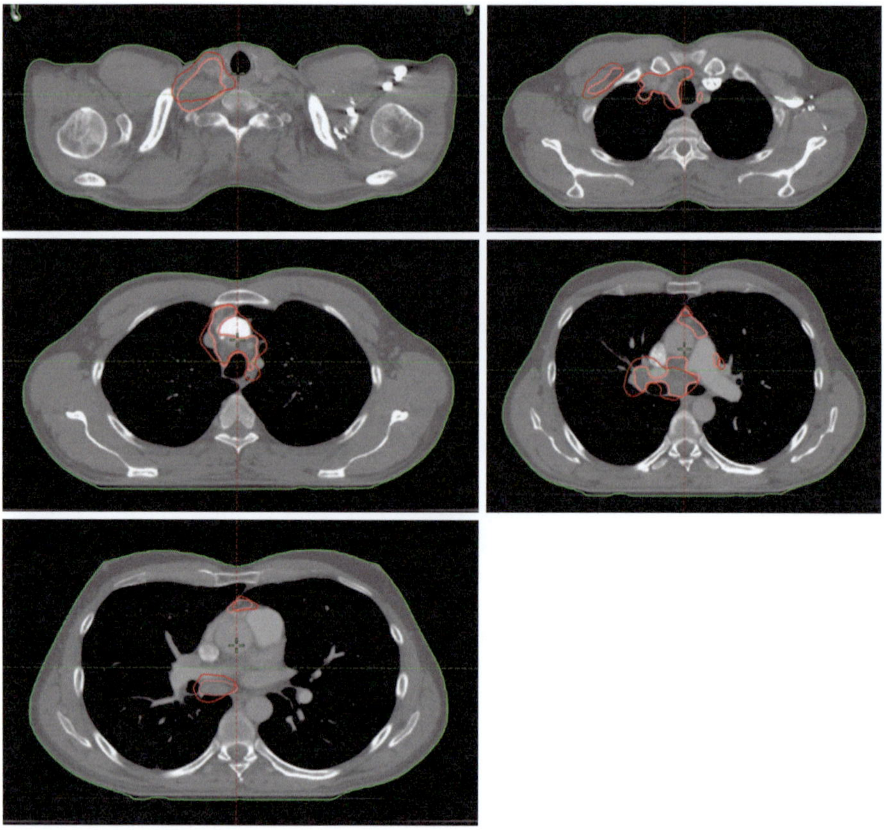

Fig. 1.10 The post-chemotherapy planning CT scan for patient 2, with slices at the same levels as in Fig. 1.9. The pre-chemotherapy GTV (red) is transferred from the pre-chemotherapy staging FDG-PET/CT scan to the post-chemotherapy planning CT scan. This volume is modified to account for anatomical changes that occurred during chemotherapy; for example, it is cropped out of the muscle and lung that were initially displaced by the lymphoma masses and have now moved back to their normal positions. In addition, the volume is adjusted to allow for uncertainties if the fusion is not optimal. The resulting volume, shown in pink, encompasses the tissue that contained lymphoma initially (CTV)

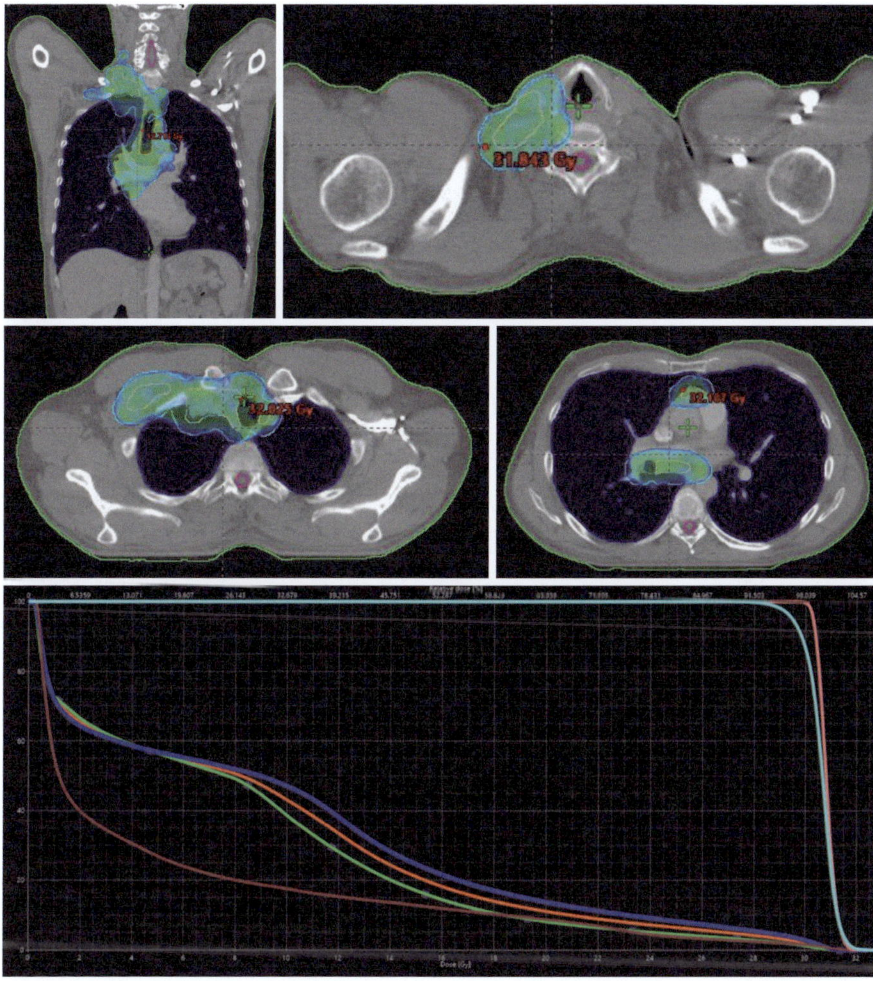

Fig. 1.11 Treatment plan for patient 2. Volumetric arc therapy (VMAT) was used with constraints on heart and lung doses. A volume representing 95% of the prescription dose is shown. The mean heart dose was 5.1 Gy. The lung V5 was 56%, V20 was 11%, and mean dose was 8.9 Gy. Coronal slice (upper left), three axial slices (upper right, middle left, and right), and DVH (bottom; CTV pink, PTV cyan blue, left lung green, right lung blue, both lungs together orange, heart brown)

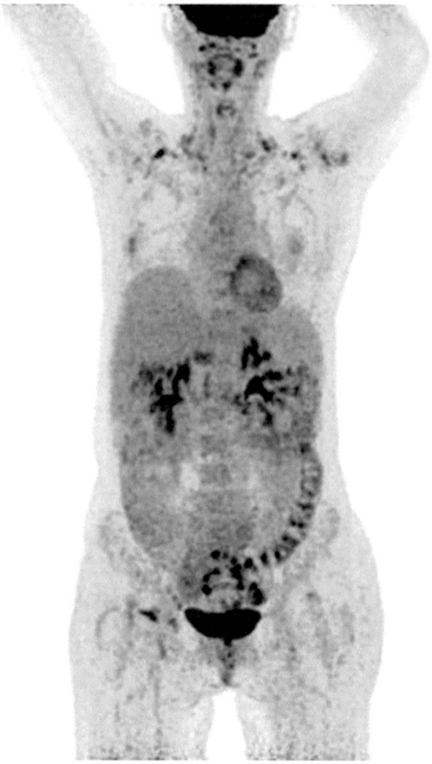

Fig. 1.12 Initial staging FDG-PET/CT-scan for patient 3. Maximal intensity projection image

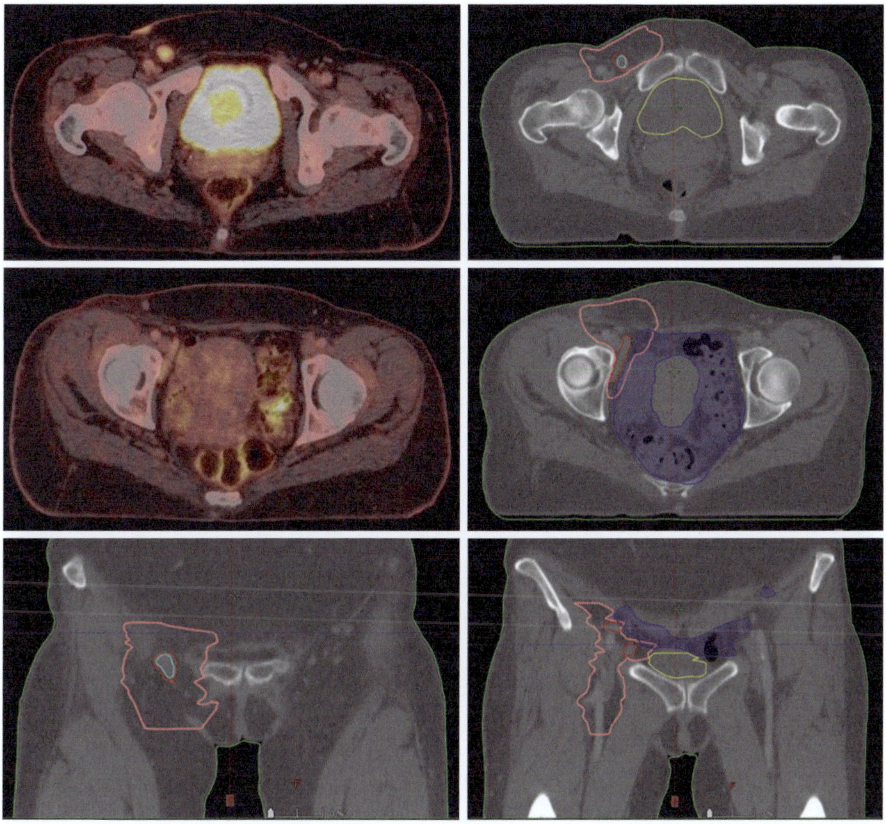

Fig. 1.13 The initial staging FDG-PET/CT scan and the planning CT scan for patient 3. Two selected axial slices of the FDG-PET/CT are shown on the left, and the corresponding slices of the planning CT scan are shown on the right. Below are two coronal slices of the planning CT-scan, demonstrating the extent of the CTV in the superior-inferior direction. The FDG-PET-positive volume is contoured in cyan blue. The entire involved site, including both FDG-avid and non-FDG-avid disease, is contoured in red (GTV). The GTV and the volume with a high risk of harboring microscopic disease in this patient who did not receive any systemic treatment is contoured in pink (CTV). The bladder is yellow, rectum is brown, and bowel is blue

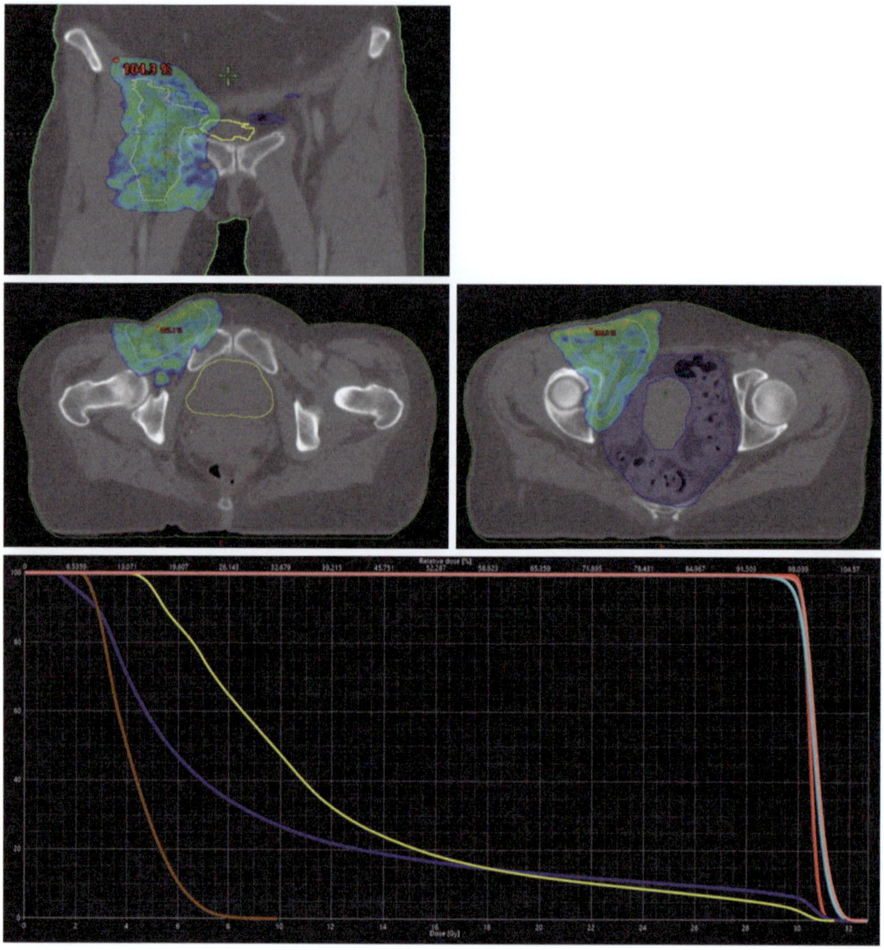

Fig. 1.14 Treatment plan for patient 3. Volumetric arc therapy (VMAT) was used. A colorwash representing 95% of the prescription dose is shown. The mean bladder dose was 11.7 Gy, mean rectum dose was 4.2 Gy, and the volume of bowel receiving 20 Gy or more was 129 cm^3. Coronal slice (top), two axial slices (middle), and DVH (bottom; GTV red, CTV pink, PTV cyan blue, bladder yellow, rectum brown, bowel blue)

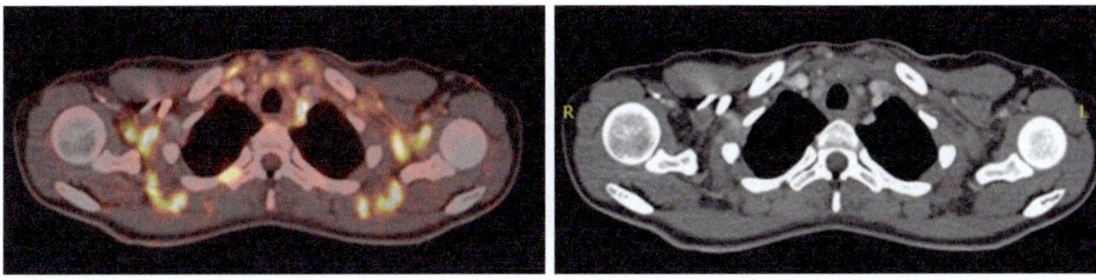

Fig. 1.15 Staging FDG-PET/CT scan for a 20-year-old woman with early-stage Hodgkin lymphoma demonstrating extensive brown fat that complicates interpretation of the imaging. The uptake in brown fat is distributed symmetrically on the FDG-PET scan (left) and has no anatomic correlate on the CT scan (right)

References

1. Ferlay J, Ervik M, Lam F, Colombet M, Mery L, Pineros M, Znaor A, Soerjomataram I, Bray F. Global cancer observatory. Cancer Today. 2018; https://gco.iarc.fr/today
2. Clarke CA, Glaser SL, Keegan TH, Stroup A. Neighborhood socioeconomic status and Hodgkin's lymphoma incidence in California. Cancer Epidemiol Biomarkers Prev. 2005;14:1441–7.
3. Glaser SL, Lin RJ, Stewart SL, Ambinder RF, Jarrett RF, Brousset P, Pallesen G, Gulley ML, Khan G, O'Grady J, Hummel M, Preciado MV, Knecht H, Chan JK, Claviez A. Epstein-Barr virus-associated Hodgkin's disease: epidemiologic characteristics in international data. Int J Cancer. 1997;70:375–82.
4. Sleckman BG, Mauch PM, Ambinder RF, Mann R, Pinkus GS, Kadin ME, Sherburne B, Perez-Atayde A, Thior I, Mueller N. Epstein-Barr virus in Hodgkin's disease: correlation of risk factors and disease characteristics with molecular evidence of viral infection. Cancer Epidemiol Biomarkers Prev. 1998;7:1117–21.
5. Jaffe ES, Stein H, Swerdlow SH. Classic Hodgkin lymphoma. I: Swerdlow SH, Campo E, Harris NL, Jaffe ES, Pileri SA, Stein H, eds. WHO classification of tumours of haematopoietic and lymphoid tissues. 4th ed. udg. Lyon: International Agency for Research on Cancer, 2017: 435-442.
6. Hodgson DC, Gospodarowicz MK. Clinical evaluation and staging of Hodgkin lymphoma. I. In: Hoppe RT, Mauch PM, Armitage JO, Diehl V, Weiss LM, editors. Hodgkin Lymphoma. 2nd ed. udg. Philadelphia: Lippincott Williams & Wilkins; 2007. p. 123–32.
7. Carbone PP, Kaplan HS, Musshoff K, Smithers DW, Tubiana M. Report of the committee on Hodgkin's disease staging classification. Cancer Res. 1971;31:1860–1.
8. Brierley JD, Gospodarowicz MK, Wittekind C. TNM classification of malignant Tumours. Oxford: John Wiley & Sons; 2017.
9. Cheson BD, Fisher RI, Barrington SF, Cavalli F, Schwartz LH, Zucca E, Lister TA. Recommendations for initial evaluation, staging, and response assessment of Hodgkin and non-Hodgkin lymphoma: the Lugano classification. J Clin Oncol. 2014;32:3059–68.
10. El-Galaly TC, D'Amore F, Mylam KJ, de Nully BP, Bogsted M, Bukh A, Specht L, Loft A, Iyer V, Hjorthaug K, Nielsen AL, Christiansen I, Madsen C, Johnsen HE, Hutchings M. Routine bone marrow biopsy has little or no therapeutic consequence for positron emission tomography/computed tomography-staged treatment-naive patients with Hodgkin lymphoma. J Clin Oncol. 2012;30:4508–14.
11. Andre MPE, Girinsky T, Federico M, Reman O, Fortpied C, Gotti M, Casasnovas O, Brice P, van der Maazen R, Re A, Edeline V, Ferme C, Van IG, Merli F, Bouabdallah R, Sebban C, Specht L, Stamatoullas A, Delarue R, Fiaccadori V, Bellei M, Raveloarivahy T, Versari A, Hutchings M, Meignan M, Raemaekers J. Early positron emission tomography response-

adapted treatment in stage I and II Hodgkin lymphoma: final results of the randomized EORTC/LYSA/FIL H10 trial. J Clin Oncol. 2017;35:1786–94.
12. Fuchs M, Goergen H, Kobe C, Kuhnert G, Lohri A, Greil R, Sasse S, Topp MS, Schafer E, Hertenstein B, Soekler M, Vogelhuber M, Zijlstra JM, Keller UB, Krause SW, Wilhelm M, Maschmeyer G, Thiemer J, Duhrsen U, Meissner J, Viardot A, Eich H, Baues C, Diehl V, Rosenwald A, von TB, Dietlein M, Borchmann P, Engert A. Positron emission tomography-guided treatment in early-stage favorable Hodgkin lymphoma: final results of the international, randomized phase III HD16 trial by the German Hodgkin study group. J Clin Oncol. 2019;37:2835–45.
13. Picardi M, De Renzo A, Pane F, Nicolai E, Pacelli R, Salvatore M, Rotoli B. Randomized comparison of consolidation radiation versus observation in bulky Hodgkin's lymphoma with post-chemotherapy negative positron emission tomography scans. Leuk Lymphoma. 2007;48:1721–7.
14. Radford J, Illidge T, Counsell N, Hancock B, Pettengell R, Johnson P, Wimperis J, Culligan D, Popova B, Smith P, McMillan A, Brownell A, Kruger A, Lister A, Hoskin P, O'Doherty M, Barrington S. Results of a trial of PET-directed therapy for early-stage Hodgkin's lymphoma. N Engl J Med. 2015;372:1598–607.
15. Engert A, Plutschow A, Eich HT, Lohri A, Dorken B, Borchmann P, Berger B, Greil R, Willborn KC, Wilhelm M, Debus J, Eble MJ, Sokler M, Ho A, Rank A, Ganser A, Trumper L, Bokemeyer C, Kirchner H, Schubert J, Kral Z, Fuchs M, Muller-Hermelink HK, Muller RP, Diehl V. Reduced treatment intensity in patients with early-stage Hodgkin's lymphoma. N Engl J Med. 2010;363:640–52.
16. Specht L, Yahalom J, Illidge T, Berthelsen AK, Constine LS, Eich HT, Girinsky T, Hoppe RT, Mauch P, Mikhaeel NG, Ng A. Modern radiation therapy for Hodgkin lymphoma: field and dose guidelines from the international lymphoma radiation oncology group (ILROG). Int J Radiat Oncol Biol Phys. 2014;89:854–62.
17. Eich HT, Diehl V, Gorgen H, Pabst T, Markova J, Debus J, Ho A, Dorken B, Rank A, Grosu AL, Wiegel T, Karstens JH, Greil R, Willich N, Schmidberger H, Dohner H, Borchmann P, Muller-Hermelink HK, Muller RP, Engert A. Intensified chemotherapy and dose-reduced involved-field radiotherapy in patients with early unfavorable Hodgkin's lymphoma: final analysis of the German Hodgkin Study Group HD11 trial. J Clin Oncol. 2010;28:4199–206.
18. Brockelmann PJ, Goergen H, Keller U, Meissner J, Ordemann R, Halbsguth TV, Sasse S, Sokler M, Kerkhoff A, Mathas S, Huttmann A, Bormann M, Zimmermann A, Mettler J, Fuchs M, Von TB, Baues C, Rosenwald A, Klapper W, Kobe C, Borchmann P, Engert A. Efficacy of Nivolumab and AVD in early-stage unfavorable classic Hodgkin lymphoma: the randomized phase 2 German Hodgkin Study Group NIVAHL Trial. JAMA Oncol. 2020;6:872–80.
19. Connors JM, Jurczak W, Straus DJ, Ansell SM, Kim WS, Gallamini A, Younes A, Alekseev S, Illes A, Picardi M, Lech-Maranda E, Oki Y, Feldman T, Smolewski P, Savage KJ, Bartlett NL, Walewski J, Chen R, Ramchandren R, Zinzani PL, Cunningham D, Rosta A, Josephson NC, Song E, Sachs J, Liu R, Jolin HA, Huebner D, Radford J. Brentuximab Vedotin with chemotherapy for stage III or IV Hodgkin's lymphoma. N Engl J Med. 2018;378:331–44.
20. Chen RC, Mauch PM. Management of lymphocyte predominant Hodgkin lymphoma. I. In: Specht L, Yahalom J, editors. Radiotherapy for Hodgkin lymphoma. Heidelberg: Springer; 2011. p. 53–66.
21. Diehl V, Sextro M, Franklin J, Hansmann ML, Harris N, Jaffe E, Poppema S, Harris M, Franssila K, van Krieken J, Marafioti T, Anagnostopoulos I, Stein H. Clinical presentation, course, and prognostic factors in lymphocyte-predominant Hodgkin's disease and lymphocyte-rich classical Hodgkin's disease: report from the European Task Force on Lymphoma Project on Lymphocyte-Predominant Hodgkin's Disease. J Clin Oncol. 1999;17:776–83.
22. Nogova L, Reineke T, Brillant C, Sieniawski M, Rudiger T, Josting A, Bredenfeld H, Skripnitchenko R, Muller RP, Muller-Hermelink HK, Diehl V, Engert A. Lymphocyte-predominant and classical Hodgkin's lymphoma: a comprehensive analysis from the German Hodgkin Study Group. J Clin Oncol. 2008;26:434–9.

23. Bodis S, Kraus MD, Pinkus G, Silver B, Kadin ME, Canellos GP, Shulman LN, Tarbell NJ, Mauch PM. Clinical presentation and outcome in lymphocyte-predominant Hodgkin's disease. J Clin Oncol. 1997;15:3060–6.
24. Nogova L, Reineke T, Eich HT, Josting A, Muller-Hermelink HK, Wingbermuhle K, Brillant C, Gossmann A, Oertel J, Bollen MV, Muller RP, Diehl V, Engert A. Extended field radiotherapy, combined modality treatment or involved field radiotherapy for patients with stage IA lymphocyte-predominant Hodgkin's lymphoma: a retrospective analysis from the German Hodgkin Study Group (GHSG). Ann Oncol. 2005;16:1683–7.
25. Wirth A, Yuen K, Barton M, Roos D, Gogna K, Pratt G, Macleod C, Bydder S, Morgan G, Christie D. Long-term outcome after radiotherapy alone for lymphocyte-predominant Hodgkin lymphoma: a retrospective multicenter study of the Australasian Radiation Oncology Lymphoma Group. Cancer. 2005;104:1221–9.
26. Binkley MS, Rauf MS, Milgrom SA, Pinnix CC, Tsang R, Dickinson M, Ng AK, Roberts KB, Gao S, Balogh A, Ricardi U, Levis M, Casulo C, Stolten M, Specht L, Plastaras JP, Wright C, Kelsey CR, Brady JL, Mikhaeel NG, Hoppe BS, Terezakis SA, Picardi M, Della PR, Kirova Y, Akhtar S, Maghfoor I, Koenig JL, Jackson C, Song E, Sehgal S, Advani RH, Natkunam Y, Constine LS, Eich HT, Wirth A, Hoppe RT. Stage I-II nodular lymphocyte-predominant Hodgkin lymphoma: a multi-institutional study of adult patients by ILROG. Blood. 2020;135:2365–74.
27. Specht L, Berthelsen AK. PET/CT in radiation therapy planning. Semin Nucl Med. 2018;48:67–75.
28. Paumier A, Ghalibafian M, Gilmore J, Beaudre A, Blanchard P, El NM, Azoury F, Al HH, Lefkopoulos D, Girinsky T. Dosimetric benefits of intensity-modulated radiotherapy combined with the deep-inspiration breath-hold technique in patients with mediastinal Hodgkin's lymphoma. Int J Radiat Oncol Biol Phys. 2012;82:1522–7.
29. Petersen PM, Aznar MC, Berthelsen AK, Loft A, Schut DA, Maraldo M, Josipovic M, Klausen TL, Andersen FL, Specht L. Prospective phase II trial of image-guided radiotherapy in Hodgkin lymphoma: benefit of deep inspiration breath-hold. Acta Oncol. 2015;54:60–6.
30. Alonso C, Dutta SW, Mitra N, Landsburg DJ, Zaorsky NG, Grover S, Peterson J, Trifiletti DM. Adult nodular lymphocyte-predominant Hodgkin lymphoma: treatment modality utilization and survival. Cancer Med. 2018;7:1118–26.
31. Parikh RR, Grossbard ML, Harrison LB, Yahalom J. Early-stage nodular lymphocyte-predominant Hodgkin lymphoma: the impact of radiotherapy on overall survival. Leuk Lymphoma. 2016;57:320–7.
32. DeLuca P, Jones D, Gahbauer R, Whitmore G, Wambersie A. Prescribing, recording, and reporting photon-beam intensity-modulated radiation therapy (IMRT). J ICRU. 2010;10:1–106.
33. Nielsen K, Maraldo MV, Berthelsen AK, Loft A, de Nully BP, Vogelius IR, Petersen PM, Specht L. Involved node radiation therapy in the combined modality treatment for early-stage Hodgkin lymphoma: analysis of relapse location and long-term outcome. Radiother Oncol. 2020;150:236–44.
34. Wirth A, Mikhaeel NG, Aleman BMP, Pinnix CC, Constine LS, Ricardi U, Illidge TM, Eich HT, Hoppe BS, Dabaja B, Ng AK, Kirova Y, Berthelsen AK, Dieckmann K, Yahalom J, Specht L. Involved site radiation therapy in adult lymphomas: an overview of international lymphoma radiation oncology group guidelines. Int J Radiat Oncol Biol Phys. 2020;107:909–33.
35. Girinsky T, van der Maazen R, Specht L, Aleman B, Poortmans P, Lievens Y, Meijnders P, Ghalibafian M, Meerwaldt J, Noordijk E. Involved-node radiotherapy (INRT) in patients with early Hodgkin lymphoma: concepts and guidelines. Radiother Oncol. 2006;79:270–7.
36. Girinsky T, Ghalibafian M, Specht L. Target definition for Hodgkin lymphoma: the involved node radiation field concept. In: Specht L, Yahalom J, editors. Radiotherapy for Hodgkin lymphoma. Heidelberg: Springer; 2011. p. 91–122.
37. ICRU. International Commission on Radiation Units and Measurements. Prescribing, recording, and reporting photon therapy. (Supplement to ICRU Report 50). ICRU Report 62. 1999.
38. Milo MLH, Offersen BV, Bechmann T, Diederichsen ACP, Hansen CR, Holtved E, Josipovic M, Lorincz T, Maraldo MV, Nielsen MH, Nordsmark M, Nystrom PW, Pohl M, Rose HK,

Schytte T, Yates ES, Lorenzen EL. Delineation of whole heart and substructures in thoracic radiation therapy: national guidelines and contouring atlas by the Danish Multidisciplinary Cancer Groups. Radiother Oncol. 2020;150:121–7.
39. Girinsky T, Pichenot C, Beaudre A, Ghalibafian M, Lefkopoulos D. Is intensity-modulated radiotherapy better than conventional radiation treatment and three-dimensional conformal radiotherapy for mediastinal masses in patients with Hodgkin's disease, and is there a role for beam orientation optimization and dose constraints assigned to virtual volumes? Int J Radiat Oncol Biol Phys. 2006;64:218–26.
40. Voong KR, McSpadden K, Pinnix CC, Shihadeh F, Reed V, Salehpour MR, Arzu I, Wang H, Hodgson D, Garcia J, Aristophanous M, Dabaja BS. Dosimetric advantages of a "butterfly" technique for intensity-modulated radiation therapy for young female patients with mediastinal Hodgkin's lymphoma. Radiat Oncol. 2014;9:94.
41. Filippi AR, Ragona R, Piva C, Scafa D, Fiandra C, Fusella M, Giglioli FR, Lohr F, Ricardi U. Optimized volumetric modulated arc therapy versus 3D-CRT for early stage mediastinal Hodgkin lymphoma without axillary involvement: a comparison of second cancers and heart disease risk. Int J Radiat Oncol Biol Phys. 2015;92:161–8.
42. Dabaja BS, Hoppe BS, Plastaras JP, Newhauser W, Rosolova K, Flampouri S, Mohan R, Mikhaeel NG, Kirova Y, Specht L, Yahalom J. Proton therapy for adults with mediastinal lymphomas: the International Lymphoma Radiation Oncology Group guidelines. Blood. 2018;132:1635–46.
43. Aznar MC, Maraldo MV, Schut DA, Lundemann M, Brodin NP, Vogelius IR, Berthelsen AK, Specht L, Petersen PM. Minimizing late effects for patients with mediastinal Hodgkin lymphoma: deep inspiration breath-hold, IMRT, or both? Int J Radiat Oncol Biol Phys. 2015;92:169–74.
44. Maraldo MV, Brodin NP, Aznar MC, Vogelius IR, Munck Af RP, Petersen PM, Specht L. Estimated risk of cardiovascular disease and secondary cancers with modern highly conformal radiotherapy for early-stage mediastinal Hodgkin lymphoma. Ann Oncol. 2013;24:2113–8.
45. Maraldo MV, Specht L. A decade of comparative dose planning studies for early-stage Hodgkin lymphoma: what can we learn? Int J Radiat Oncol Biol Phys. 2014;90:1126–35.
46. Brodin NP, Maraldo MV, Aznar MC, Vogelius IR, Petersen PM, Bentzen SM, Specht L. Interactive decision-support tool for risk-based radiation therapy plan comparison for Hodgkin lymphoma. Int J Radiat Oncol Biol Phys. 2014;88:433–45.
47. Rechner LA, Modiri A, Stick LB, Maraldo MV, Aznar MC, Rice SR, Sawant A, Bentzen SM, Vogelius IR, Specht L. Biological optimization for mediastinal lymphoma radiotherapy—a preliminary study. Acta Oncol. 2020;59:879–87.
48. Borchmann P, Plutschow A, Kobe C, et al. PET-guided omission of radiotherapy in early-stage unfavourable Hodgkin lymphoma (GHSG HD17): a multicentre, open-label, randomised, phase 3 trial. Lancet Oncol. 2021;22(2):223–34.

Further Reading

Dabaja BS, Hoppe BS, Plastaras JP, Newhauser W, Rosolova K, Flampouri S, Mohan R, Mikhaeel NG, Kirova Y, Specht L, Yahalom J. Proton therapy for adults with mediastinal lymphomas: the International Lymphoma Radiation Oncology Group Guidelines. Blood. 2018;132:1635–46.

Dabaja BS, Ng AK, Terezakis SA, Plastaras JP, Yunes M, Wilson LD, Specht L, Yahalom J. Making every single Gray count: involved site radiation therapy delineation guidelines for hematological malignancies. Int J Radiat Oncol Biol Phys. 2020;106:279–81.

Mikhaeel NG, Milgrom SA, Terezakis S, Berthelsen AK, Hodgson D, Eich HT, Dieckmann K, Qi S, Yahalom J, Specht L. The optimal use of imaging in radiation therapy for lymphoma—Guidelines from the International Lymphoma Radiation Oncology Group (ILROG). Int J Radiat Oncol Biol Phys. 2019;104:501–12.

Ricardi U, Specht L, Versari A, Berthelsen AK. FDG PET and radiotherapy in lymphoma. Clin Translat Imaging. 2015;3:321–30.

Specht L. Radiotherapy for Hodgkin lymphoma: reducing toxicity while maintaining efficacy. Cancer J. 2018;24:237–43.

Specht L, Berthelsen AK. PET/CT in radiation therapy planning. Semin Nucl Med. 2017;48:67–75.

Specht L, Yahalom J, editors. Radiotherapy for Hodgkin lymphoma. Berlin: Springer-Verlag; 2011.

Specht L, Yahalom J. The concept and evolution of involved site radiation therapy (ISRT) for lymphoma. Int J Clin Oncol. 2015;20:849–54.

Specht L, Yahalom J, Illidge T, Berthelsen AK, Constine LS, Eich HT, Girinsky T, Hoppe RT, Mauch P, Mikhaeel NG, Ng A, on behalf of ILROG. Modern radiation therapy for Hodgkin lymphoma: field and dose guidelines from the international lymphoma radiation oncology group (ILROG). Int J Radiat Oncol Biol Phys. 2014;89:854–62.

Terezakis S, Plastaras JP. Hodgkin lymphoma. In: Dabaja BS, Ng AK, editors. Radiation therapy in hematologic malignancies. Berlin: Springer-Verlag; 2017. p. 1–28.

Wirth A, Mikhaeel NG, Aleman BMP, Pinnix CC, Constine LS, Ricardi U, Illidge TM, Eich HT, Hoppe BS, Dabaja B, Ng AK, Kirova Y, Berthelsen AK, Dieckmann K, Yahalom J, Specht L. Involved site radiation therapy in adult lymphomas: an overview of international lymphoma radiation oncology group guidelines. Int J Radiat Oncol Biol Phys. 2020;107:909–33.

Target Volume Delineation for Adult Advanced Stage Hodgkin Lymphoma

2

Joanna Yang and Joachim Yahalom

Contents

J. Yang (✉)
Department of Radiation Oncology, Washington University School of Medicine in St. Louis, St. Louis, MO, USA
e-mail: jcyang@wustl.edu

J. Yahalom
Memorial Sloan Kettering Cancer Center, New York, NY, USA
e-mail: yahalomj@mskcc.org

C. Pinnix et al. (eds.), *Target Volume Delineation in Hematologic Malignancies*, Practical Guides in Radiation Oncology,
https://doi.org/10.1007/978-3-031-67722-9_2

Part 1: Background and Epidemiology

- Classical Hodgkin lymphoma (HL) is a rare disease with approximately 8000 new cases annually. The majority of patients present with early-stage disease but approximately 1/3 of newly diagnosed patients have advanced-stage disease [1].
- The disease most commonly affects young adults in their 20s and 30s, with a slight predilection for male gender [2].
- Classical HL is comprised of four histologic subtypes (nodular sclerosis, mixed cellularity, lymphocyte rich, and lymphocyte depleted), all of which feature the pathognomonic Reed-Sternberg cell. The disease has a characteristic pattern of CD15 and CD30 positivity and CD20 and CD45 negativity on immunohistochemistry [2].
- Patients most commonly present with painless lymphadenopathy and may exhibit B symptoms (>10% weight loss over 6 months, drenching night sweats, and/or fevers).
- Staging work-up generally consists of an excisional or core needle biopsy, a baseline set of labs including a complete blood count (CBC), comprehensive metabolic panel (CMP), erythrocyte sedimentation rate (ESR), and pregnancy test for women of childbearing age, and a PET-CT scan from base of skull to feet (with contrast, if possible). Accurate and complete staging is critical as treatment paradigms differ significantly for early-stage and advanced-stage disease.
- While early-stage patients are generally treated with combined modality therapy, the backbone of treatment for advanced stage disease is systemic therapy with radiation therapy (RT) used in specific clinical scenarios [3].

Pre-Radiotherapy Imaging and Evaluation

- Imaging obtained prior to RT is essential for radiation therapy planning.
- All patients should undergo a PET/CT scan *prior to the start of chemotherapy* to understand the extent of disease and to facilitate radiation therapy planning with involved-node (INRT) or involved-site (ISRT) technique. Often the PET-CT scan is performed with contrast. In certain scenarios, diagnostic CT imaging with contrast may also be helpful for disease assessment and particularly if the PET scan is performed sans contrast. It is ideal, if possible, to obtain these scans with immobilization in the treatment position.

Table 2.1 Definitions of advanced stage Hodgkin lymphoma

Organization	Definition
National Comprehensive Cancer Center (NCCN)	Ann Arbor Stage III or IV disease
European Organization for Research and Treatment (EORTC)	Ann Arbor Stage III or IV disease
Lymphoma Study Association (LYSA)	Ann Arbor Stage III or IV disease
German Hodgkin Study Group (GHSG)	Ann Arbor Stage IIB disease with bulk and/or extranodal disease Ann Arbor Stage III or IV disease

- All patient should also undergo a PET/CT scan *following completion of chemotherapy* to assess disease response to systemic therapy and to facilitate RT planning.
- An interim PET/CT scan after 2 cycles of chemotherapy is often performed. For patients with advanced stage HL, an interim negative PET may help identify patients in whom bleomycin can be omitted and/or define areas of disease that can be omitted from the treatment field or treated with a lower dose.
- RT should start within 6 weeks of completion of systemic therapy, most commonly doxorubicin, vinblastine, and dacarbazine (AVD) chemotherapy with either brentuximab vedotin (BV) or bleomycin (B).

Part 2: Management and Treatment of Adult Advanced Stage Hodgkin Lymphoma

Adult Advanced Stage Hodgkin Lymphoma: Principles of Management

- The mainstay of therapy for advanced stage Hodgkin lymphoma is systemic therapy, with RT reserved for use in specific clinical scenarios.
- In the pre-PET era, patients with advanced stage Hodgkin lymphoma who presented with *initial bulky disease* or who had a residual mass on CT imaging at the end of chemotherapy were given consolidation RT [4–6].
- In patients with advanced stage Hodgkin lymphoma who have a *partial response* on PET-CT imaging at the end of chemotherapy, higher RT doses of 36–40Gy can be used to treat the residual areas of PET-avid disease [7–10]. For patients with bulky disease who attain a complete metabolic response after 2 and 6 cycles of ABVD chemotherapy, consolidation RT may be deferred for the site of initial bulk [11, 12].

Advanced Stage Hodgkin Lymphoma: General Considerations for Radiotherapy

- Radiation therapy for advanced stage Hodgkin lymphoma is delivered to (1) areas of initial bulky disease or (2) areas of partial response to chemotherapy. Unlike RT for early-stage Hodgkin lymphoma, the goal is rarely to treat all pre-chemotherapy sites of disease involvement.
- The ideal simulation position and immobilization will depend on the area being treated. In general, for treatment of disease in the mediastinum, patients should be simulated supine in an alpha cradle. If deep inspiration breath hold (DIBH) technique is available, it should be used for treatment of disease in the mediastinum as it allows for better target immobilization and normal tissue sparing [13, 14].
- Axial CT images should be acquired in 3 mm or smaller increments.

- Post-chemotherapy PET-CT fusion with the CT simulation scan can be helpful in certain cases. However, given the differences in patient positioning, caution should be used when fusions are performed.
- The clinical target volume (CTV) and planning target volume (PTV) should be delineated. In some instances, creation of a pre-chemotherapy gross tumor volume (pre-chemo GTV) and post-chemotherapy gross tumor volume, if applicable (post-chemo GTV) can help guide target delineation. These volumes are further described in Table 2.2.
- Target volumes should be treated with planning techniques that permit maximal sparing of normal tissue. This often includes intensity modulated radiotherapy (IMRT), volumetric arc radiotherapy (VMAT), proton therapy, or 3D conformal radiation therapy (3D-CRT). Beam arrangements should be chosen to minimize dose to organs at risk [15, 16].
- Radiation dose is dependent on treatment intent. For consolidation of bulky disease after a 5PS response of 1–3 on PET-CT imaging, doses of 30 Gy in 1.8–2.0Gy daily fractions may be used. For the treatment of chemorefractory disease in patients with a partial response on PET-CT (5PS of 4–5), higher RT doses of 36–40Gy should be used.

Table 2.2 Planning target definitions for treatment of advanced stage Hodgkin lymphoma

Volume	Description	
Gross tumor volume (GTV)	**Pre-chemo GTV**	• Contains gross tumor volume as identified on diagnostic imaging, preferably PET-CT with or without CT c/a/p with IV contrast, prior to initiation of systemic therapy
	Post-chemo GTV (for patients with 5PS of 4–5)	• Contains gross tumor volume as identified on PET-CT (5PS of 4–5), after completion of systemic therapy
Clinical target volume (CTV)	– Should include the pre-chemo GTV and the post-chemo GTV with modifications to account for response to chemotherapy; should be shaved off of normal tissues such as the heart, lung, salivary glands, and thyroid gland – Should be modified to respect anatomic boundaries	
Planning target volume (PTV)	• Contains CTV plus a 0.3–0.7 cm margin to account for setup uncertainties associated with patient position and beam alignment • CTV-to-PTV expansions are patient- and institution-specific; any recommendations in this chapter or elsewhere must be adjusted to reflect factors unique to the patient and institution	
Organs at risk (OAR)	• Includes uninvolved normal structures at risk of RT-related toxicity for which RT planning or dose may be altered. • For treatment of disease in the mediastinum, these generally include the heart and its substructures, each lung, the thyroid gland, and in female patients, the bilateral breasts. The lung contour should include the entire lung and not the lung minus the PTV. For treatment of other sites of disease, nearby organs should be included.	

Part 3: Cases

Case 1

A 33-year-old woman presented with night sweats and was diagnosed with Hodgkin lymphoma involving the supraclavicular fossae, mediastinum, and cardiophrenic lymph nodes. She is considered to have advanced-stage Hodgkin lymphoma by German Hodgkin Study Group Criteria due to her Ann Arbor Stage IIB disease with bulky mediastinal involvement. However, by NCCN, EORTC, and LYSA criteria, she would have early-stage unfavorable Hodgkin lymphoma, stage IIB. As such, she was eligible for treatment with combined modality therapy. She received 4 cycles of ABVD chemotherapy with a PET-CT scan at the end of chemotherapy showing a Deauville 3 response. She received 30.6 Gy of consolidation ISRT in 17 daily fractions (Fig. 2.1).

Case 2

A 65-year-old man was diagnosed with advanced stage Hodgkin lymphoma involving the mediastinum with a separate biopsy-proven left upper lobe lung nodule at diagnosis. He received 6 cycles of ABVD chemotherapy with an end-of-chemotherapy PET-CT showing a Deauville 3 response with resolution of the lung nodule. He was referred for consideration of ISRT to consolidate his initial site of bulky disease. He received 30.6 Gy in 17 daily fractions to his mediastinum alone without treatment to the area where the lung nodule had been pre-chemotherapy (Fig. 2.2). *Note that based on more recent data, if the patient had achieved a complete metabolic response after 2 and 6 cycles of ABVD chemotherapy, another option would be to observe and defer radiation.*

Case 3

A 68-year-old gentleman was diagnosed with advanced stage Hodgkin lymphoma involving the neck, mediastinum, and pelvis. He received 6 cycles of ABVD chemotherapy with an end-of-chemotherapy PET-CT showing a partial response in the pelvis, 5PS of 5. He was referred for consideration of ISRT. He received 39.6Gy in 22 daily fractions to the site of involvement and residual disease in the pelvis (Fig. 2.3).

Case 4

A 36-year-old woman with multiply treated, chemorefractory advanced-stage Hodgkin lymphoma presents with right sided back spasms after progressing on a clinical trial. She was found to have biopsy proven relapsed Hodgkin lymphoma within the paraspinal musculature and is referred for palliative RT. She received 30Gy in 2 Gy daily fractions to the painful right paraspinal nodule (Fig. 2.4).

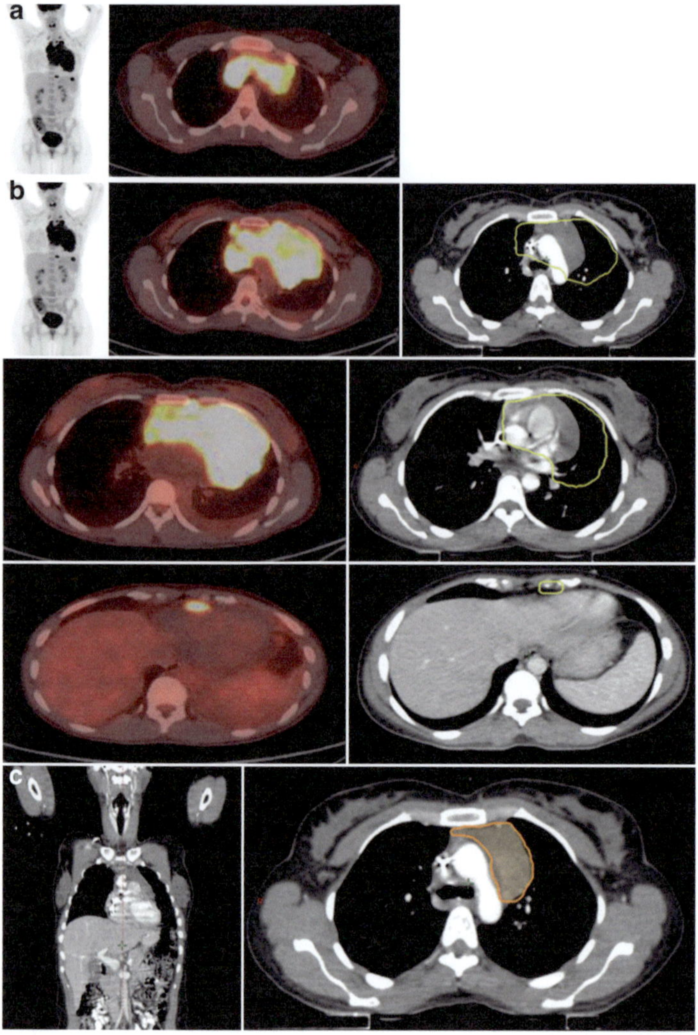

Fig. 2.1 (a–e) Consolidation ISRT planning for a patient with NCCN/EORTC/LYSA early-stage unfavorable Hodgkin lymphoma and GHSG advanced-stage Hodgkin lymphoma treated with combined modality therapy. As the pre-chemotherapy PET-CT scan was not performed in the treatment position, it was not fused with the CT simulation images. However, it was used as a reference to delineate the pre-chemotherapy GTV. (**a, b**) The prechemotherapy GTV was delineated in yellow on the planning CT scan (right). This volume was constructed based on the pre-chemotherapy PET-CT scan (left and middle). (**c**) The post-chemotherapy residual on CT (orange) was drawn from the most superior extent of disease to the most inferior extent of disease using the pre-chemotherapy PET-CT scan for guidance. (**d**) The pre-chemotherapy GTV (yellow) and the post-chemotherapy residual on CT (orange) were combined with a small margin to form an initial CTV (purple). This initial CTV was then adjusted by shaving off of normal tissues such as heart and lungs in order to create a final CTV (red). Please note that the initial CTV was added in this case in order to better show how the CTV in ISRT is shaved off of normal tissues like heart and lungs in cases where the initial disease has shrunken down after chemotherapy. Note that the final CTV in red may also further be trimmed off of lung and bone if these were not initially involved. (**e**) As this patient was treated with DIBH, a 0.5 cm margin on the CTV was added to create a PTV volume (blue)

(continued)

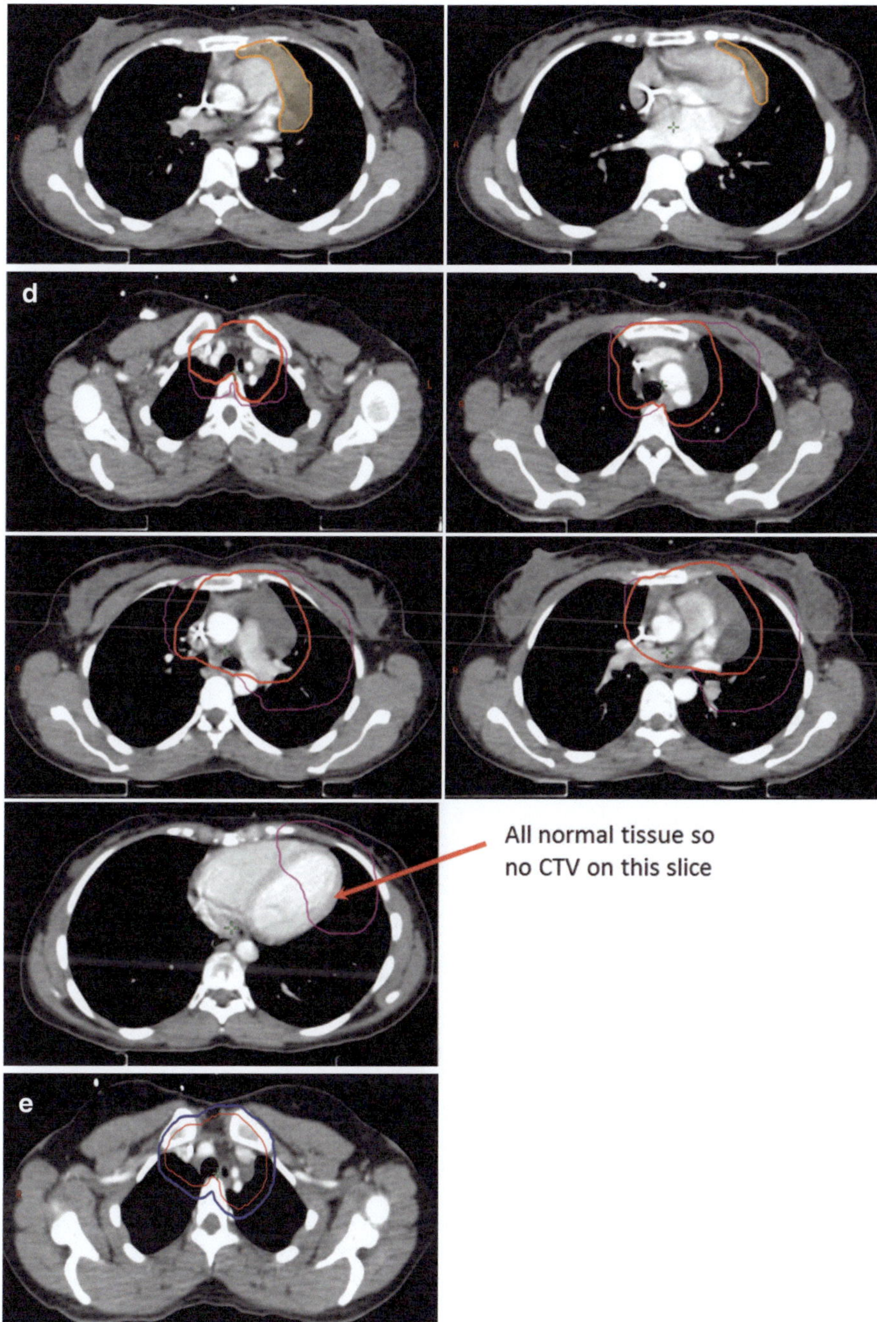

Fig. 2.1 (continued)

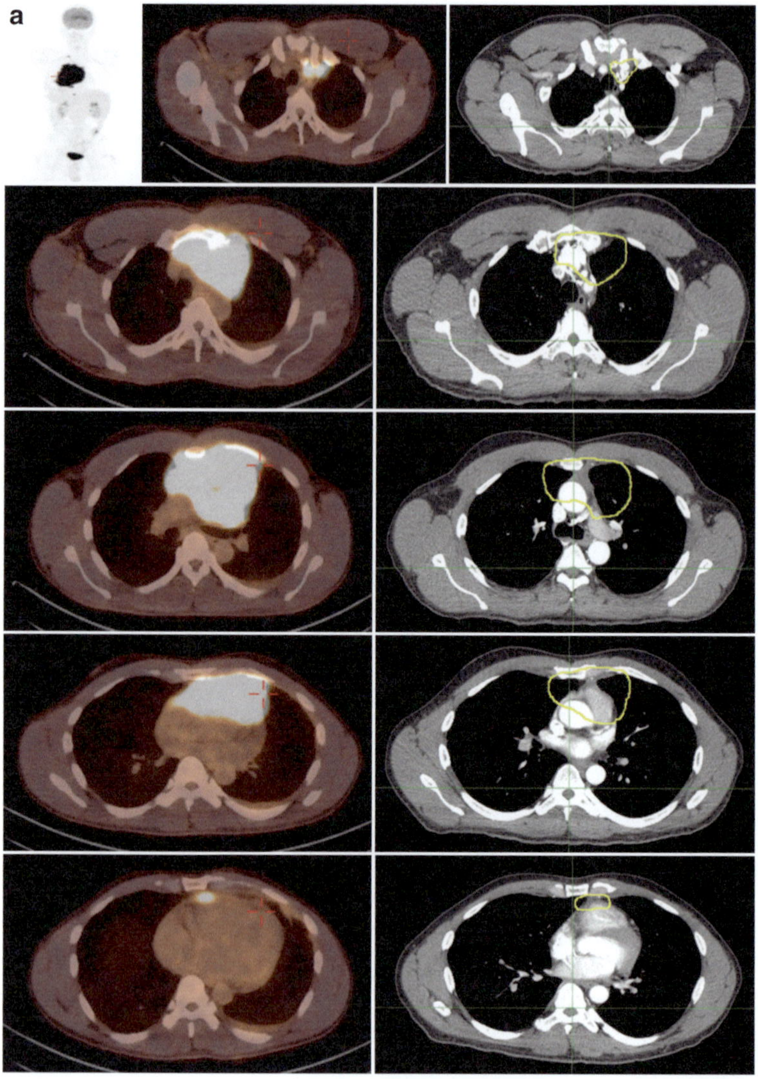

Fig. 2.2 (**a**–**d**) Consolidation ISRT planning to a site of pre-chemotherapy bulky mediastinal disease for a patient with advanced stage Hodgkin lymphoma treated with 6 cycles of ABVD chemotherapy. As the pre-chemotherapy PET-CT scan was not performed in the treatment position, it was not fused with the CT simulation images. However, it was used as a reference to delineate the CTV. (**a**) The pre-chemotherapy GTV was delineated in yellow on the planning CT scan (right). This volume was constructed based on the pre-chemotherapy PET-CT scan (left and middle) from the most superior extent of disease to the most inferior extent of disease. (**b**) The post-chemotherapy residual on CT was delineated in orange to include all areas of CT-based abnormalities on the planning CT scan. (**c**) The pre-chemotherapy GTV (yellow) and the post-chemotherapy residual on CT (orange) were combined to create a CTV (red). This CTV was adjusted by shaving it off of normal tissues such as lungs and heart. Of note, the CTV did not include all of the initial sites of disease in this patient and deliberately excluded the region where the patient had a biopsy-proven non-bulky left upper lobe lung nodule pre-chemotherapy with advanced stage HL. (**d**) A 0.5mm margin was added to the CTV to create a PTV (blue) As this patient was treated with DIBH, a 0.5 cm margin on the CTV was felt to be sufficient

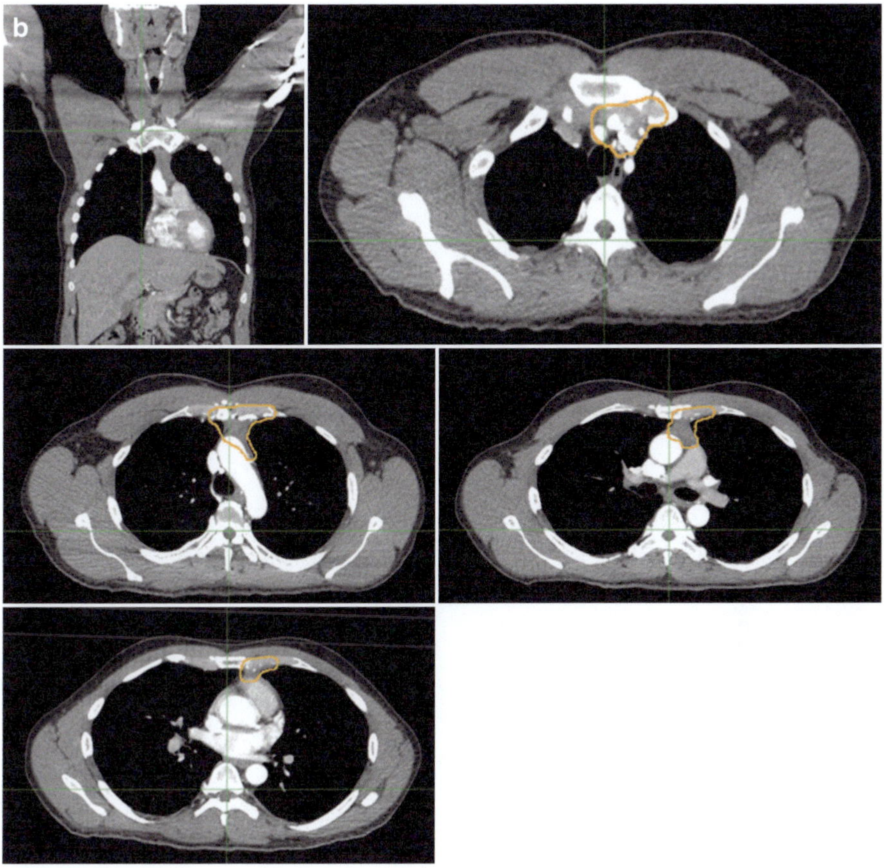

Fig. 2.2 (continued)

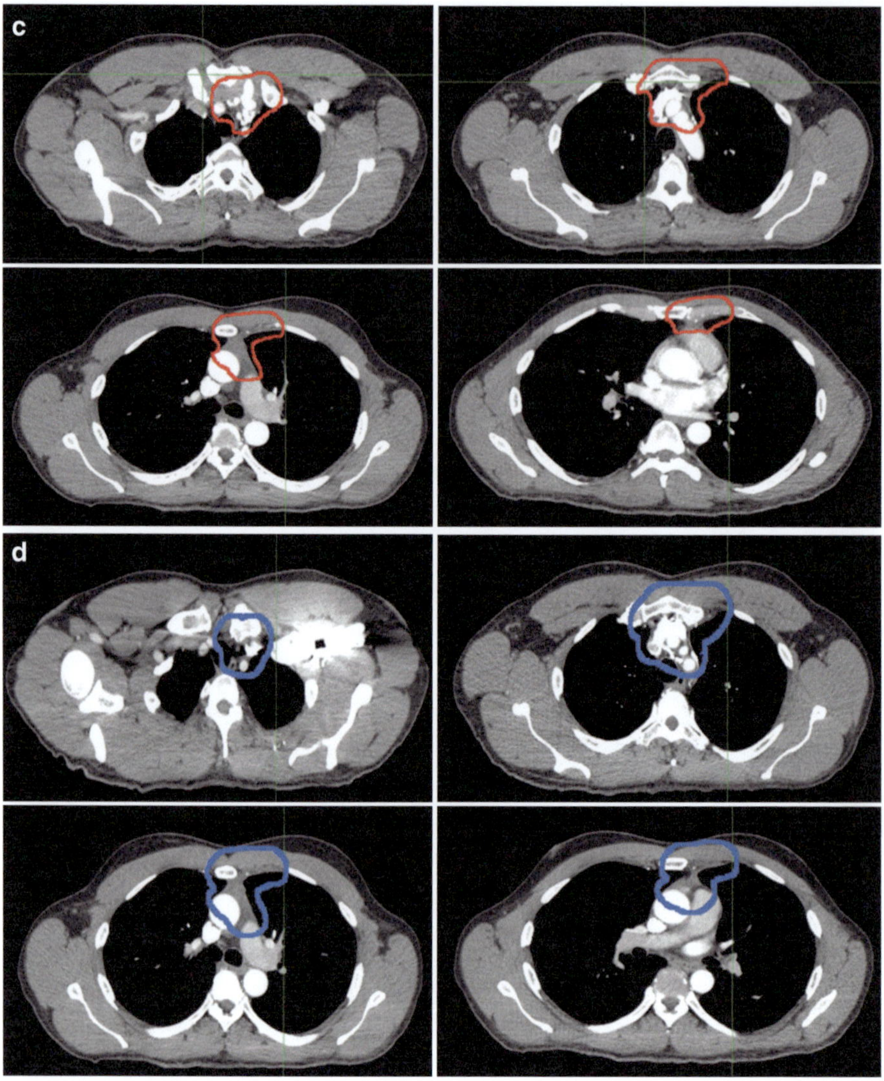

Fig. 2.2 (continued)

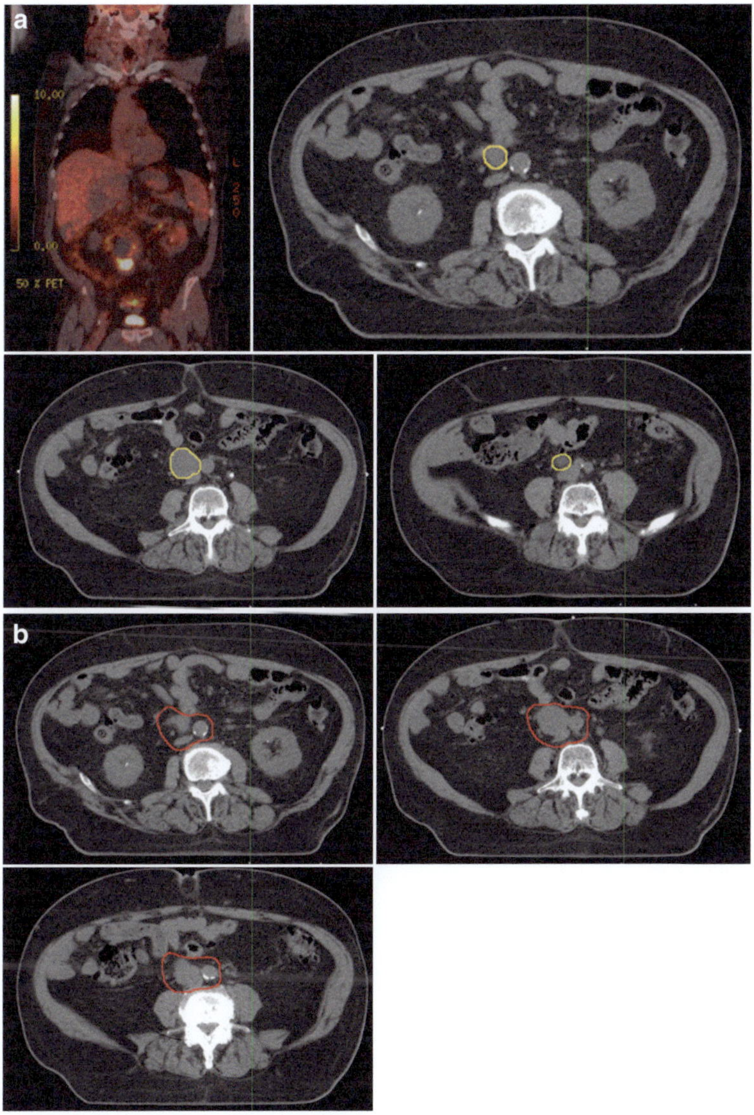

Fig. 2.3 (**a**–**d**) ISRT planning to the pelvis disease for a patient with advanced stage Hodgkin lymphoma treated with 6 cycles of ABVD chemotherapy with a partial response. (**a**) The post-chemotherapy GTV (orange) was then delineated based on the FDG-avid portion of the post-chemotherapy PET-CT scan as well as CT abnormalities visualized on the CT simulation images. (**b**) The pre-chemotherapy and post-chemotherapy extent of disease involvement was considered when creating the CTV (red). Of note, the final CTV was revised to include the surrounding vasculature and to exclude the normal bowel. (**c**) As this patient's disease had a partial response, a plan was created with the initial extent of disease (dark blue) receiving 30Gy in 15 fractions. The patient then received a conedown to the area that was still FDG-avid (light blue) using 5 additional fractions. While it is possible to treat both targets (e.g. 30 Gy initial, 40 Gy boost) simultaneously using a dose-painting plan, it is our preference to deliver the additional dose to the FDG-avid region using a conedown approach so that the dose per fraction remains consistent

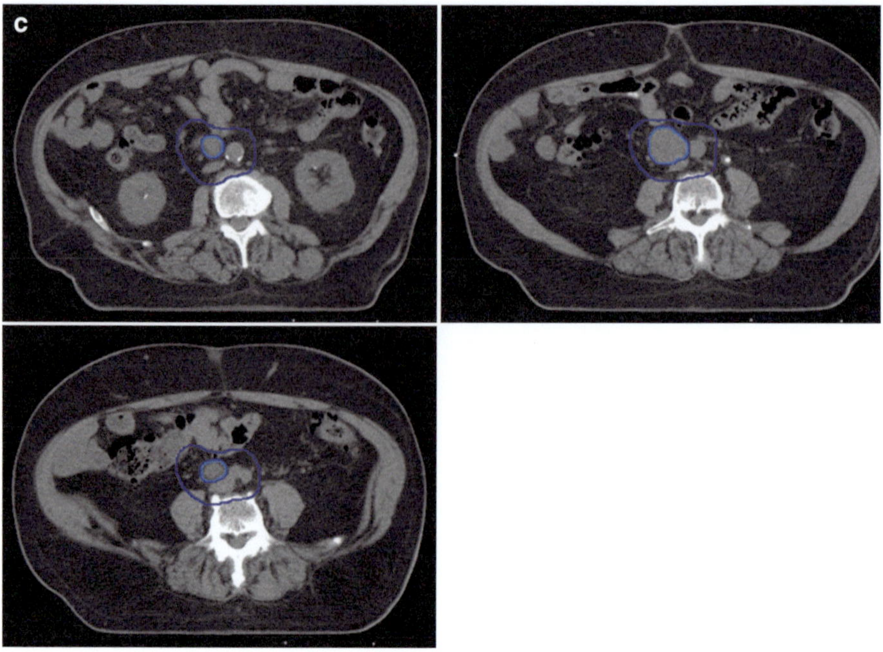

Fig. 2.3 (continued)

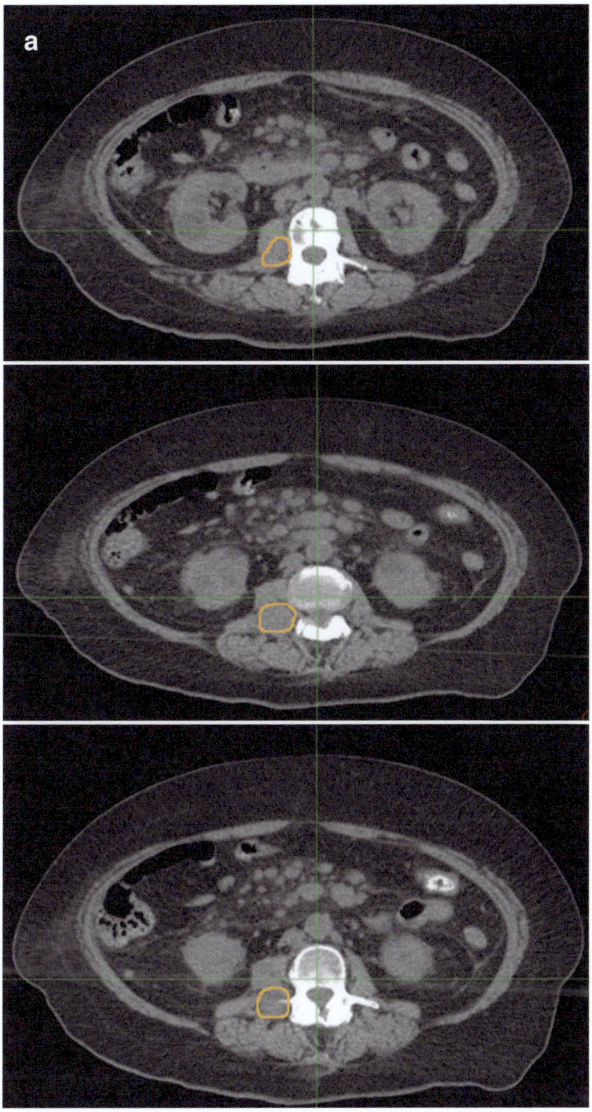

Fig. 2.4 (**a**–**c**) Palliative RT to the right paraspinal musculature for a patient with incurable advanced-stage Hodgkin lymphoma. As the treatment intent was palliative, no fusions were performed to the CT simulation images. (**a**) The GTV was delineated in orange on the planning CT scan (orange). (**b**) The GTV was then expanded by 1 cm to create an initial CTV, which was then edited to include all of the right paraspinal musculature and to spare the vertebral bodies and spinal cord. The final CTV appears in red. Note that the paraspinal musculature is fuller on the right than the left. (**c**) The CTV was then expanded 1 cm to create the PTV (blue). Caution was exercised during RT planning to limit dose to the right kidney

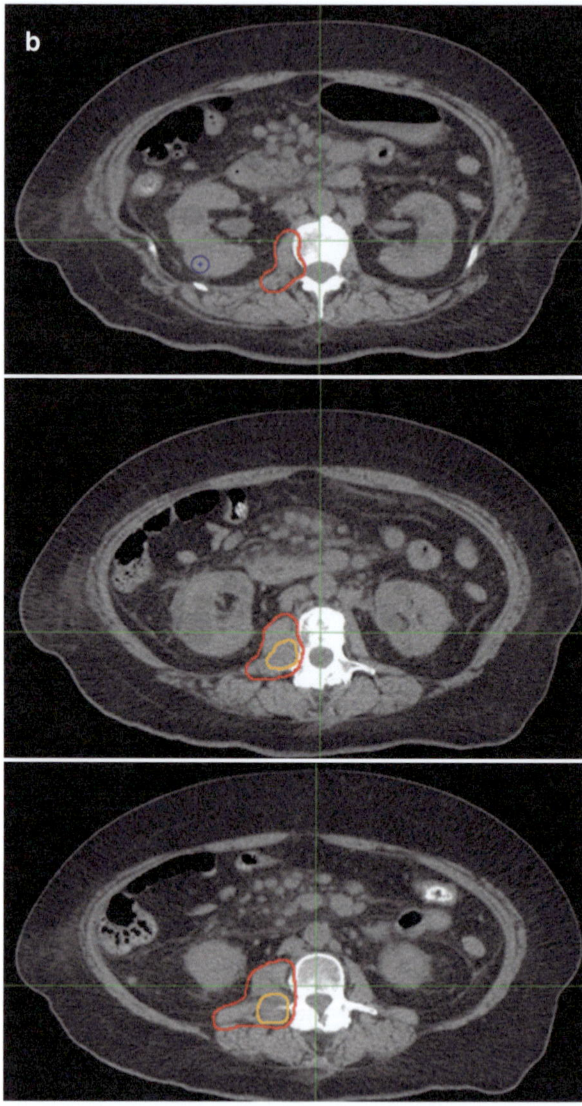

Fig. 2.4 (continued)

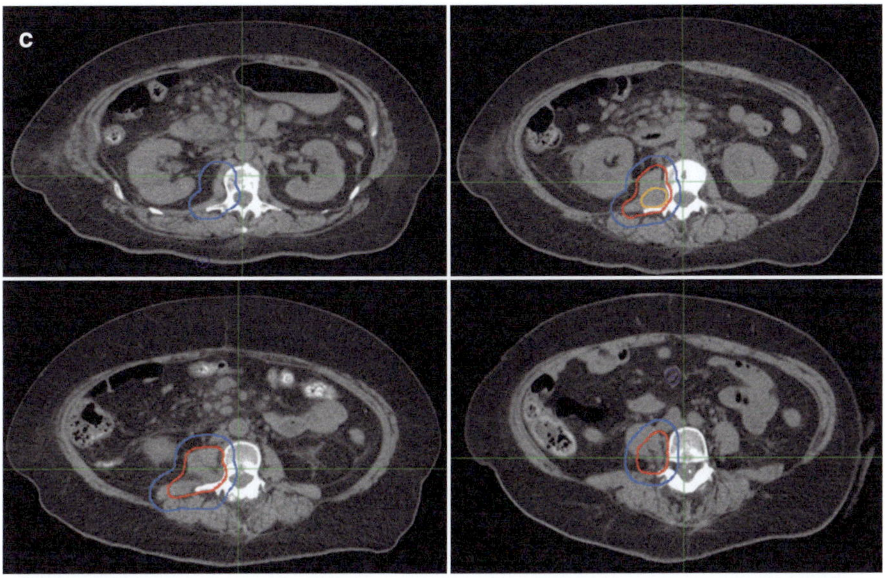

Fig. 2.4 (continued)

Part 4: Special Considerations

In this contemporary era, definitive radiation alone is infrequently used as a curative treatment for Hodgkin lymphoma. However, in the setting of chemotherapy intolerance or chemotherapy ineligibility, definitive radiation in the form of ISRT or total lymphoid irradiation (TLI) can still be considered a curative treatment option.

TLI may also be used as a component of conditioning prior to autologous stem cell transplant.

References

1. Siegel RL, Miller KD, Jemal A. Cancer statistics, 2019. CA Cancer J Clin. 2019;69:7–34.
2. Shanbhag S, Ambinder RF. Hodgkin lymphoma: a review and update on recent progress. CA Cancer J Clin. 2018;68:116–32.
3. National Comprehensive Cancer Network. Hodgkin lymphoma (Version 2.2020). https://www.nccn.org/professionals/physician_gls/pdf/hodgkins.pdf. Accessed 10 May 2020.
4. Johnson PW, Sydes MR, Hancock BW, et al. Consolidation radiotherapy in patients with advanced Hodgkin's lymphoma: survival data from the UKLG LY09 randomized controlled trial (ISRCTN97144519). J Clin Oncol. 2010;28:3352–9.
5. Aleman BM, Raemaekers JM, Tirelli U, et al. Involved-field radiotherapy for advanced Hodgkin's lymphoma. N Engl J Med. 2003;348:2396–406.
6. Gordon LI, Hong F, Fisher RI, et al. Randomized phase III trial of ABVD versus Stanford V with or without radiation therapy in locally extensive and advanced-stage Hodgkin lymphoma:

an intergroup study coordinated by the Eastern Cooperative Oncology Group (E2496). J Clin Oncol. 2013;31:684–91.
7. Engert A, Haverkamp H, Kobe C, et al. Reduced-intensity chemotherapy and PET-guided radiotherapy in patients with advanced stage Hodgkin's lymphoma (HD15 trial): a randomised, open-label, phase 3 non-inferiority trial. Lancet. 2012;379:1791–9.
8. Borchmann P, Goergen H, Kobe C, et al. PET-guided treatment in patients with advanced-stage Hodgkin's lymphoma (HD18): final results of an open-label, international, randomised phase 3 trial by the German Hodgkin Study Group. Lancet. 2018;390:2790–802.
9. Johnson P, Federico M, Kirkwood A, et al. Adapted treatment guided by interim PET-CT scan in advanced Hodgkin's lymphoma. N Engl J Med. 2016;374:2419–29.
10. Specht L, Yahalom J, Illidge T, et al. Modern radiation therapy for Hodgkin lymphoma: field and dose guidelines from the international lymphoma radiation oncology group (ILROG). Int J Radiat Oncol Biol Phys. 2014;89:854–62.
11. Ricardi U, Levis M, Evangelista A, et al. Role of radiotherapy to bulky sites of advanced Hodgkin lymphoma treated with ABVD: final results of FIL HD0801 trial. Blood Adv. 2021;5(21):4504–14.
12. Gallamini A, Rossi A, Patti C, et al. Consolidation radiotherapy could be safely omitted in advanced Hodgkin lymphoma with large nodal mass in complete metabolic response after ABVD: final analysis of the randomized GITIL/FIL HD0607 trial. J Clin Oncol. 2020;38(33):3905–13.
13. Charpentier AM, Conrad T, Sykes J, et al. Active breathing control for patients receiving mediastinal radiation therapy for lymphoma: impact on normal tissue dose. Pract Radiat Oncol. 2014;4(3):174–80.
14. Paumier A, Ghalibafian M, Gilmore J, et al. Dosimetric benefits of intensity-modulated radiotherapy combined with the deep-inspiration breath-hold technique in patients with mediastinal Hodgkin's lymphoma. Int J Radiat Oncol Biol Phys. 2012;82(4):1522–7.
15. Girinsky T, Pichenot C, Beaudre A, et al. Is intensity-modulated radiotherapy better than conventional radiation treatment and three-dimensional conformal radiotherapy for mediastinal masses in patients with Hodgkin's disease, and is there a role for beam orientation optimization and dose constraints assigned to virtual volumes? Int J Radiat Oncol Biol Phys. 2006;64(1):218–26.
16. Voong KR, McSpadden K, Pinnix CC, et al. Dosimetric advantages of a "butterfly" technique for intensity-modulated radiation therapy for young female patients with mediastinal Hodgkin's lymphoma. Radiat Oncol. 2014;9:94.

Further Reading

Specht L, Yahalom J, Illidge T, et al. Modern radiation therapy for Hodgkin lymphoma: field and dose guidelines from the international lymphoma radiation oncology group (ILROG). Int J Radiat Oncol Biol Phys. 2014;89:854–62.

Early-Stage Diffuse Large B-Cell Lymphoma

3

Sarah A. Milgrom and Chris R. Kelsey

Contents

S. A. Milgrom (✉)
Department of Radiation Oncology, University of Colorado, Aurora, CO, USA
e-mail: sarah.milgrom@cuanschutz.edu

C. R. Kelsey
Department of Radiation Oncology, Duke University, Durham, NC, USA
e-mail: christopher.kelsey@duke.edu

C. Pinnix et al. (eds.), *Target Volume Delineation in Hematologic Malignancies*, Practical Guides in Radiation Oncology,
https://doi.org/10.1007/978-3-031-67722-9_3

Part 1: Background and Epidemiology

- The World Health Organization (WHO) recognizes numerous large B-cell lymphomas, with diffuse large B-cell lymphoma (DLBCL) not otherwise specified being the most common. In the United States, there are 5.6 new cases of DLBCL per 100,000 people annually [1].
- DLBCL is most frequently diagnosed in middle-aged and elderly adults. The median age at diagnosis is 66 years [1]. There is a slightly higher incidence in men than women [1]. Immunosuppression is a significant risk factor [2, 3].
- DLBCL is CD20+, CD45+, and CD3−.
- Cell of origin phenotype, based on gene expression profiling, distinguishes cases as germinal center B-cell-like (GCB) or activated B-cell-like (ABC) DLBCL. Patients with the GCB subtype experience more favorable outcomes [4]. The Hans algorithm is a commonly used immunohistochemical surrogate for gene expression profiling to discriminate between GCB and non-GCB DLBCL [5].
- DLBCL/high-grade B-cell lymphoma with *MYC* and *BCL2* rearrangements is an aggressive large cell lymphoma [6]. "Double-hit" lymphoma has coexisting *MYC* and *BCL2* translocations. These translocations are identified by fluorescence in situ hybridization (FISH). Double-expressor DLBCL exhibits protein over-expression of MYC and BCL-2 that is identified by immunohistochemistry. These DLBCL subtypes are associated with inferior survival, and intensification of systemic therapy may be considered [7].
- The clinical presentation of DLBCL varies, based on the anatomical site of involvement. Patients may present with painless, palpable adenopathy. Symptoms may occur due to involvement of extranodal sites or compression of adjacent neurovascular structures or organs. Patients may have B symptoms (unexplained fevers, drenching night sweats, unintentional weight loss of >10% of body weight within the 6 months prior to diagnosis).
- The work-up includes an assessment for the presence of B symptoms, evaluation of performance status, and physical examination with special attention to the nodal regions, liver, and spleen. Laboratory evaluation should include a complete blood count (CBC) with differential, lactate dehydrogenase (LDH), comprehensive metabolic panel, and uric acid. Imaging studies should include a whole-body PET/CT scan +/− a contrast-enhanced CT scan of the neck/chest/abdomen/pelvis. A bone marrow biopsy should be performed in most cases but is not necessary if the PET/CT demonstrates bone disease. Hepatitis B testing is necessary prior to treatment with rituximab, and echocardiography is indicated prior to treatment with an anthracycline. Pregnancy testing should be performed as appropriate [8].
- DLBCL is staged according to the Ann Arbor system [9]. Bulky disease is variably defined, but a maximal diameter of ≥7–7.5 cm is a commonly used definition [8].
- The International Prognostic Index (IPI) score is associated with survival outcomes (Table 3.1). One point is assigned for each of the following risk factors:

Table 3.1 Overall survival after R-CHOP by IPI score [11]

International prognostic index score	3-Year overall survival
0–1	91.4%
2	80.9%
3	65.1%
4–5	59%

age > 60 years, Eastern Cooperative Oncology Group (ECOG) performance status 2–4, elevated serum LDH, >1 extranodal site of disease involvement, and Ann Arbor stage III–IV [10, 11].

- The standard chemotherapy for DLBCL is 3–6 cycles of R-CHOP (rituximab, cyclophosphamide, doxorubicin, vincristine, and prednisone). For patients with concerning features, such as double-hit lymphoma, chemotherapy may be escalated to dose-adjusted R-EPOCH (rituximab, etoposide, prednisone, vincristine, cyclophosphamide, and doxorubicin, with doses adjusted based on blood count nadirs).
- Involved site radiation therapy (ISRT) is used after 3 cycles and in some cases after 4–6 cycles of immuno-chemotherapy.

Pre-Radiotherapy Imaging and Evaluation

- A PET/CT scan should be obtained after chemotherapy and prior to ISRT to assess response to systemic therapy. A complete metabolic response is defined as a Deauville 5-point score of 1–3 [9, 12].
- Additional tests after chemotherapy and prior to ISRT may be useful depending upon the area to be irradiated (e.g. consider pulmonary function tests and an echocardiogram if irradiating the mediastinum; consider a differential renal function scan if irradiating the upper abdomen).
- RT is typically started by 4 weeks after the completion of chemotherapy, as long as the patient has recovered from the acute toxicity of systemic therapy.

Part 2: Management and Treatment of Early-Stage DLBCL

- In the pre-chemotherapy era, early-stage DLBCL was generally treated with radiation therapy (RT) alone. While complete response rates were relatively high (~80%), long-term progression-free survival (PFS) was modest (30–60%). Subsequent treatment strategies incorporated combination chemotherapy with improved rates of complete response (~90%) and PFS (70–85%) [13–16]. Rituximab further improved clinical outcomes [17–19].
- As systemic therapy has become more effective, the need for consolidation RT has logically come under scrutiny. Multiple randomized studies in early-stage DLBCL have been conducted comparing chemotherapy (most without rituximab), with a combined modality program (Table 3.2) [20–27]. Interpretation of

these trials can be challenging, given their individual peculiarities, but the following brief synopsis may be helpful:

- Two conclusions can be drawn from the Southwest Oncology Group (SWOG) S8736 study [23], along with the long-term update [27]. First, consolidation RT can replace cycles of chemotherapy. Second, late relapses distant from original sites of involvement are common in early-stage DLBCL, and giving only 3 cycles of systemic therapy may be inadequate for some patients [24].
- The trial, Eastern Cooperative Oncology Group (ECOG) 1484, demonstrated that consolidation RT can decrease the risk of relapse in higher-risk patients even when a full course (in this case, 8 cycles) of chemotherapy is administered [21].
- The Groupe d'Etude des Lymphomes de l'Adulte (GELA) 93-4 study demonstrated that older patients without adverse risk factors derive less benefit from consolidation RT [20]. If the risk of relapse is relatively low, or competing risks are significant (e.g., advanced age), the value of an adjuvant modality is less.

Table 3.2 Randomized trials of chemotherapy or combined modality therapy for early-stage DLBCL

Study	*N*	Disease characteristics	Randomization	Progression-free survival[a]	Comments
SWOG [23, 27]	401	I II (non-bulky)	CHOP × 8 CHOP × 3 + RT	64% 77% (p = 0.03)	No difference with long f/u
ECOG [21]	172	I (high-risk) II	CHOP × 8 CHOP × 8 + RT	56% 73%[b] ($p = 0.05$)	Only patients in CR by CT randomized
GELA 93–4 [20]	576	I–II without risk factors	CHOP × 4 CHOP × 4 + RT	61% 64% ($p = 0.6$)	Only patients ≥60 years old
GELA 93–1 [25]	647	I–II without risk factors	ACVBP × 3[c] CHOP × 3 + RT	82% 74% ($p < 0.01$)	Only patients ≤61 years old
IELSG [22]	44	I–II gastric DLBCL	CHOP[d] CHOP[d] + RT	82% 100% ($p = 0.04$)	Closed early due to poor accrual
LYSA/GOELAMS [26]	301	I–II non-bulky	R-CHOP X 4–6 R-CHOP X 4–6 + RT	89% 92% ($p = 0.18$)	In PET-CT CR

RT radiation therapy, *DLBCL* diffuse large B-cell lymphoma, *SWOG* Southwest Oncology Group, *CHOP* cyclophosphamide, adriamycin, vincristine, prednisone, *ECOG* Eastern Cooperative Oncology Group, *GELA* Groupe d'Étude des Lymphomas de l'Adulte, *ACVBP* doxorubicin, cyclophosphamide, vindesine, bleomycin, and prednisone, *IELSG* International Extranodal Lymphoma Study Group, *LYSA/GOELAMS* The Lymphoma Study Association/The French Acute Leukemia and Blood Diseases West-East Group, *CR* complete response

[a]5-year unless otherwise noted

[b]6-year

[c]Plus consolidation chemotherapy with methotrexate, etoposide, ifosfamide, and cytarabine

[d]CHOP or CHOP-like chemotherapy

- GELA 93-1 showed that aggressive chemotherapy regimens may be effective at controlling both systemic and local disease, thus eliminating the need for consolidation RT, but at the expense of significant toxicity and cost [25].
- The Lymphoma Study Association/The French Acute Leukemia and Blood Diseases West-East Group (LYSA/GOELAMS) and FLYER trials demonstrated that patients with low-risk (IPI 0-1), non-bulky disease, in complete response by PET-CT, have very good outcomes with R-CHOP alone [26, 28].

Management [29]

- For patients with favorable (IPI 0-1), stage I–II, non-bulky (<7–7.5 cm) DLBCL, 3 cycles of R-CHOP + RT (30 Gy) is a good treatment strategy for many patients. Alternatively, 4 cycles of R-CHOP alone are reasonable as per the LYSA/GOELAMS and FLYER trials. Both assume that the patient achieves a complete response (Deauville 1–3) by PET-CT to R-CHOP.
- For patients with non-bulky (<7–7.5 cm) stage I–II disease with multiple risk factors, either 3–4 cycles of R-CHOP + RT or 6 cycles of R-CHOP alone is reasonable.
- In the presence of bulky disease (≥7–7.5 cm), results from the RICOVER-60 [30] and UNFOLDER [31] trials, both of which enrolled patients with both early- and advanced-stage disease, suggest that RT should be incorporated into the treatment regimen. We generally favor 6 cycles of R-CHOP + consolidation RT (30 Gy).

Part 3: General Considerations for Radiotherapy

- A series of dose de-escalation studies have been conducted to identify the optimal radiation dose to be used as a part of combined modality therapy. A British National Lymphoma Investigation randomized study showed no difference in freedom from local progression, PFS, or overall survival (OS) between 30 Gy and 40–45 Gy [32]. Numerous other studies have shown high (~95%) rates of local control when ~30 Gy of RT is given after a complete response by CT or PET/CT to systemic therapy [16, 21, 33–36]. A phase II study from Duke University demonstrated a 5-year local control rate of 98% when 20 Gy was given after achievement of a complete response (Deauville 1–3) after at least 4 cycles of chemo-immunotherapy [37]. A confirmatory International Lymphoma Radiation Oncology Group (ILROG) study examined whether 20 Gy is sufficient after ≥3 cycles of a chemo-immunotherapy regimen (NCT03681535). This study has completed accrual.
- The recommended dose of RT in a combined modality treatment program for stage I–II disease is 30 Gy when a complete response (Deauville 1–3) has been achieved by PET/CT.

- For patients who only achieve a partial response to systemic therapy (Deauville 4), higher doses of consolidation RT are generally recommended (36–50 Gy) [33, 34].
- In the unusual circumstance when RT alone is pursued for patients with localized disease, a dose of ≥40 Gy is recommended.
- DLBCL can occur in any part of the body. Therefore, the choice of immobilization device (e.g., vacuum bag, thermoplastic head mask), utilization of other imaging modalities during the simulation or treatment planning process (e.g., MRI, PET/CT), utilization of respiratory control measures (e.g., 4D-CT, breath-hold), and radiation technique (e.g., 2D, 3D, intensity modulated radiation therapy [IMRT], protons) depends upon location of disease, proximity to normal tissues, and other clinical factors.
- Regarding field design, detailed guidelines from ILROG are available [38, 39]. These guidelines recommend treatment using "involved-site radiation therapy" (ISRT). ISRT is not formulaic but rather principle-based and utilizes the concepts of gross tumor volume (GTV), clinical target volume (CTV), and planning target volume (PTV) to design rational RT fields using CT-based treatment planning (Table 3.3).
- The CTV consists of the pre-chemotherapy extent of disease, adjusted to exclude uninvolved normal tissues after chemotherapy, and expanded to account for uncertainties in re-creating the pre-chemotherapy disease volume (anatomical changes, patient positioning differences between diagnostic PET-CT and planning CT scan, imaging uncertainties, etc.).
- A PTV is then created to account for setup variation and potential organ motion. The latter can also be incorporated into an internal target volume (ITV). For patients with localized disease (stage I–II), all sites of original involvement should generally be treated.
- In circumstances when RT alone is used as the definitive modality, the CTV may be expanded to include some degree of elective coverage in the immediate vicinity, since chemotherapy cannot be relied upon to eradicate microscopic disease. However, since DLBCL does not spread in a predictable, systematic fashion like Hodgkin lymphoma, elective coverage should be limited.

Part 3: Cases

Case 1

A 65-year-old female presented with nasal congestion that did not respond to conservative measures. CT of the sinuses demonstrated opacification of the left maxillary sinus with several areas of bone destruction and soft tissue extension into the left nasal cavity and left orbit. Biopsy showed DLBCL, non-germinal center subtype. Fluorescence in situ hybridization (FISH) was negative for *MYC*, *BCL2,* and *BCL6* translocations. Brain MRI showed a 6 cm mass centered in the left maxillary sinus with invasion of the orbit and bilateral nasal cavities (Fig. 3.1a). The mass was

Table 3.3 Planning target definitions for treatment of DLBCL

Volume	Description	
Gross tumor volume (GTV)	**Pre-chemotherapy GTV**	• Includes original extent of disease identified on diagnostic imaging (typically PET/CT), prior to initiation of treatment. • In rare circumstances when definitive RT is recommended, includes original extent of disease
	Post-chemotherapy GTV	• In the setting of a partial response (Deauville 4) or refractory disease, includes active disease after chemotherapy. In the setting of a residual soft tissue mass (even with a complete metabolic response), includes the disease remnant that is visualized on CT
Clinical target volume (CTV)	**CTV**	• Includes pre-chemotherapy GTV adjusted to: – Exclude uninvolved normal tissues (e.g., lung that was displaced and returns to its normal position when a mediastinal mass shrinks) – Include regions of potential subclinical disease in the immediate vicinity (if desired) – Account for uncertainties in recreating the original extent of disease (e.g., patient positioning differences between diagnostic PET/CT and planning CT scans, suboptimal pre-chemotherapy imaging, anatomical changes between scans, etc.)
	Boost CTV	• In the setting of a partial response (Deauville 4), includes the post-chemotherapy GTV adjusted to: – Include regions of potential subclinical disease in the immediate vicinity (if desired) – Account for uncertainties in delineating the post-chemotherapy GTV (e.g., patient positioning differences, etc.)

(continued)

Table 3.3 (continued)

Volume	Description
Internal target volume (ITV)	• Includes the CTV plus an internal margin that accounts for respiratory motion, typically assessed using a 4D planning CT scan. This is most pertinent for lymphomas involving the mediastinum and upper abdomen.
Planning target volume (PTV)	• Includes the CTV or ITV plus a margin to account for setup uncertainties associated with day-to-day patient positioning • CTV-to-PTV expansions are patient- and site-specific and must be individualized based on the clinical setting
Organs at risk (OAR)	• Includes uninvolved normal structures at risk of RT-related toxicities

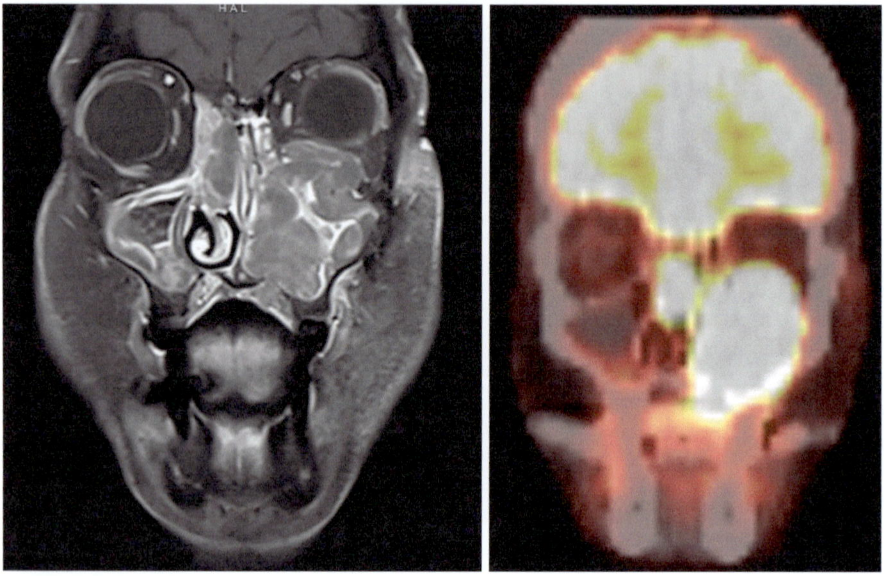

Fig. 3.1 Coronal MRI showing mass centered in the left maxillary sinus extending into the left orbit and bilateral nasal sinuses

18F-fluorodeoxyglucose (FDG)-avid on PET-CT with no other sites of disease (Fig. 3.1b). Bone marrow biopsy and lumbar puncture were negative. LDH was elevated at 450. She received 6 cycles of R-CHOP with central nervous system prophylaxis using intrathecal methotrexate. PET/CT at the completion of treatment showed a complete response (Deauville 1). Consolidation RT was pursued.

Simulation/Treatment Planning

A customized thermoplastic headholder was constructed with the patient's head in a neutral position. A planning CT was obtained using 3 mm slices. No IV or oral contrast was deemed necessary. Both the pre-chemotherapy PET/CT and MRI were fused with the planning CT scan, with the PET-CT proving more helpful for target delineation.

The original extent of disease was contoured on the fused PET-CT (Fig. 3.2a) as "PreChemoGTV". A clinical target volume (Fig. 3.2b—orange contour) was then designed that included the original extent of disease but adjusted to exclude normal uninvolved tissues (e.g., the left globe) and expanded to allow for uncertainties inherent in recreating the original extent of disease using fused baseline diagnostic imaging. This requires clinical judgment and depends on the quality and completeness of staging examinations, differences in head position between imaging studies, and confidence in the integrity of the image fusion. Lymphoma in the paranasal sinuses is often not well marginated on imaging. Therefore, in this case, the CTV was expanded in some areas to encompass immediately adjacent ethmoid sinuses and portions of the nasal cavity to ensure that all sites of original disease were adequately encompassed. In circumstances of greater uncertainty, larger CTV expansions are generally necessary to avoid a marginal miss.

Finally, a PTV was designed to encompass daily set-up error. With adequate immobilization of the head, and daily kV on-board imaging, a small (3 mm) PTV expansion was utilized. In Fig. 3.3, the pre-chemotherapy GTV, and post-chemotherapy CTV and PTV targets are demonstrated. Note, while a CTV expansion should not extend into uninvolved normal tissues, a PTV expansion may.

A volumetric modulated arc (VMAT) plan was generated to optimize target coverage but minimize dose, as much as possible, to the eyes, lacrimal glands, and brainstem (Fig. 3.4). A dose of 30 Gy in 2 Gy fractions was prescribed. Figure 3.4b shows the CTV and PTV contours as well as isodose lines.

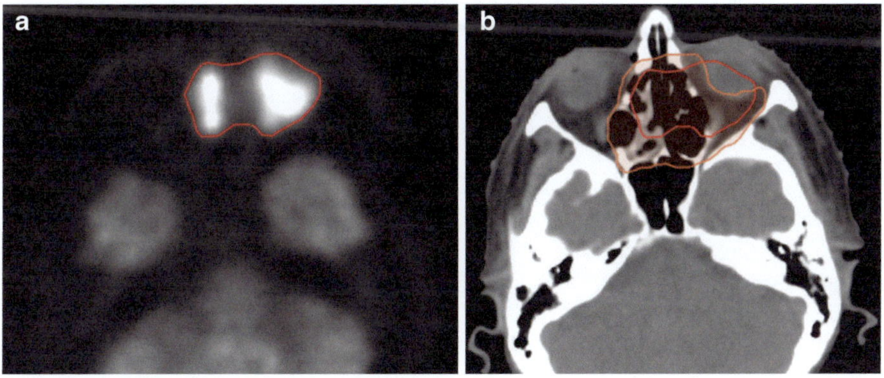

Fig. 3.2 Diagnostic PET with pre-chemotherapy extent of disease in the paranasal sinuses contoured in red (**a**) fused to the planning CT scan (**b**). A clinical target volume is shown in orange with the left eye removed from the target volume

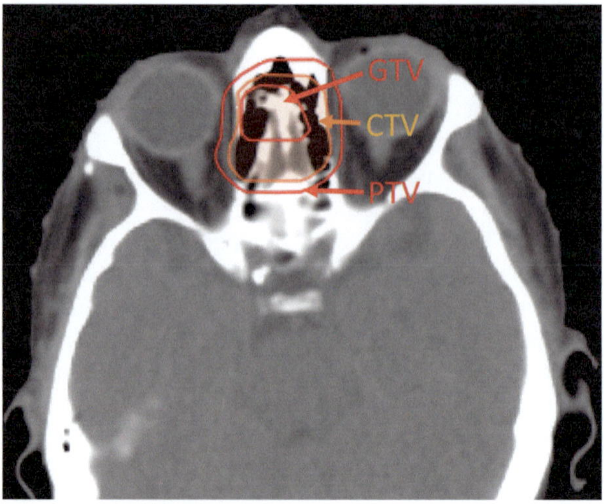

Fig. 3.3 Planning CT scan with GTV, CTV, and PTV contours delineated

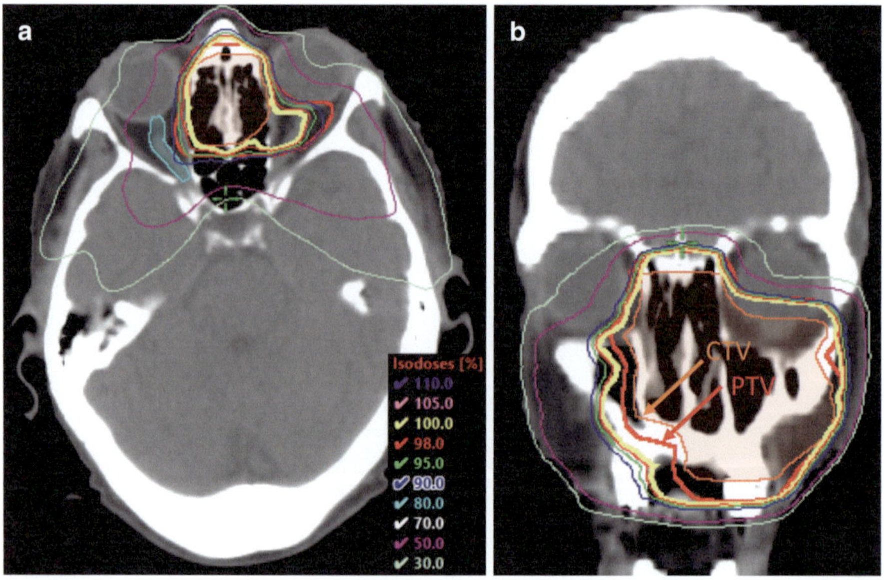

Fig. 3.4 Axial (**a**) and coronal (**b**) images showing CTV, PTV, and dose distribution for a patient with localized DLBCL involving the right maxillary sinus, left orbit, and bilateral nasal cavities

Case 2

A 66-year-old male with a 1-year history of peptic ulcer disease was found to have a mass in the distal stomach on upper endoscopy. Biopsy showed DLBCL, germinal center B-cell subtype. FISH studies did not show a *MYC*, *BCL2*, or *BCL6* translocation. PET-CT showed no disease involvement of the proximal stomach (Fig. 3.5a),

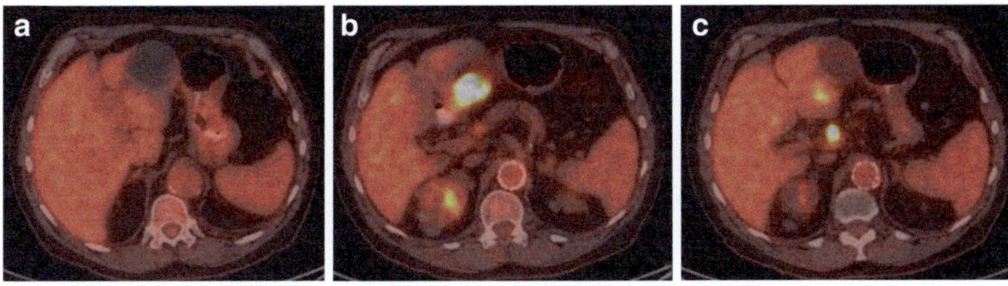

Fig. 3.5 Staging PET/CT scan of a patient with stage IIE DBCL of the distal stomach showing lack of involvement of the fundus and body (**a**), FDG-avid mass involving the gastric antrum (**b**), and involved peri-portal lymph node (**c**)

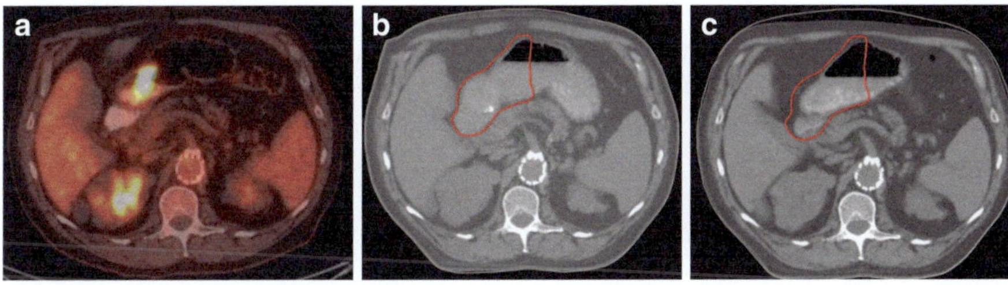

Fig. 3.6 Staging PET/CT showing disease of distal stomach (**a**) with a clinical target volume created to encompass the distal stomach as visualized on both maximum intensity projection (MIP) (**b**) and free-breathing datasets (**c**)

FDG-avid disease in the gastric antrum (Fig. 3.5b), as well as an involved peri-portal lymph node (Fig. 3.5c). Bone marrow biopsy was negative. He received four cycles of R-CHOP with a post-chemotherapy PET-CT showing a complete response (Deauville 1). A course of consolidation radiation therapy was pursued.

Simulation/Treatment Planning

The patient was instructed to fast for 3 h prior to his simulation appointment. He was immobilized supine in an indexed wing-board with his arms above his head. A small amount of barium sulfate (10 mL) was administered prior to a planning 4D CT scan to help delineate the stomach and identify the pyloric sphincter but avoid expanding the stomach unnecessarily. Intravenous contrast was not deemed necessary. On the 4D scan, the distal stomach was not found to move appreciably. A free-breathing CT was then obtained and exported, along with a maximum intensity projection (MIP) dataset, to the treatment planning software. The pre-chemotherapy PET-CT was fused to the planning CT scan.

In some circumstances, a pre-chemotherapy diagnostic imaging study cannot be easily used for target delineation. This was such a circumstance, since the shape and position of the stomach in the abdomen were quite different at the two time points. Therefore, a clinical target volume was generated manually. The FDG-avid mass within the antrum of the stomach at presentation is shown in Fig. 3.6a. On the planning CT scan, both the MIP dataset (b) and free-breathing dataset (c) were used to create a clinical target volume that takes organ motion into account. Further, since there was more uncertainty in regards to the original extent of disease, a larger CTV expansion was utilized—note the generous proximal margin to ensure adequate coverage. Since the disease was confirmed by both endoscopy and imaging to only involve the distal stomach, treatment of the entire organ was unnecessary.

A three-dimensional conformal plan was designed (Fig. 3.7). This utilized four fields to maximize conformality and avoid, as much as possible, surrounding normal tissues including the liver, kidney, and proximal stomach. The clinical target volume (inner contour) and planning target volume (outer contour) are shown in Fig. 3.7a. A larger CTV to PTV expansion was utilized in this case (1 cm) given the possibility of greater organ motion during treatment than was visualized during the planning 4D CT scan as well as the likelihood that the stomach will be in a slightly different position day to day. Further, daily cone-beam CT scans were performed on days 1–3 and then weekly to ensure that the fields were treating the distal stomach accurately. Figures 3.7b, c show the dose distribution in axial and coronal projections, respectively. A dose of 30.6 Gy in 1.8 Gy fractions was prescribed. When treating the entire stomach, prophylactic anti-emetics are often utilized. This is often not necessary when treating partial organ.

Case 3

A 49-year-old female presented with a palpable right neck mass. Core needle biopsy showed DLBCL, germinal center subtype, without gene rearrangements of *MYC*, *BCL2*, or *BCL6*. PET/CT showed multiple FDG-avid right cervical lymph nodes (Fig. 3.8). Bone marrow biopsy was negative, and her LDH was not elevated. For stage I DLBCL, she received 3 cycles of R-CHOP and achieved a complete metabolic response on PET/CT (Deauville 1). Consolidation radiation therapy was then pursued.

Simulation/Treatment Planning

The patient was immobilized supine, with the head in a neutral position and arms down, in a thermoplastic head holder. Intravenous (IV) contrast is often utilized to

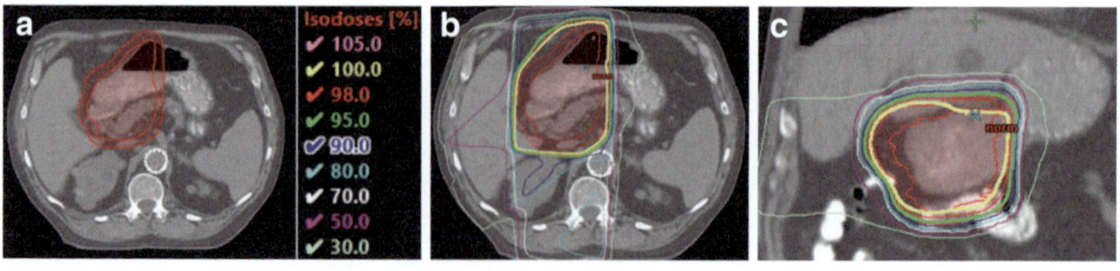

Fig. 3.7 Planning CT scan showing a clinical target volume (inner contour) and planning target volume (outer contour) (**a**) with a dose distribution from a four-field 3D conformal plan on axial (**b**) and coronal (**c**) projections

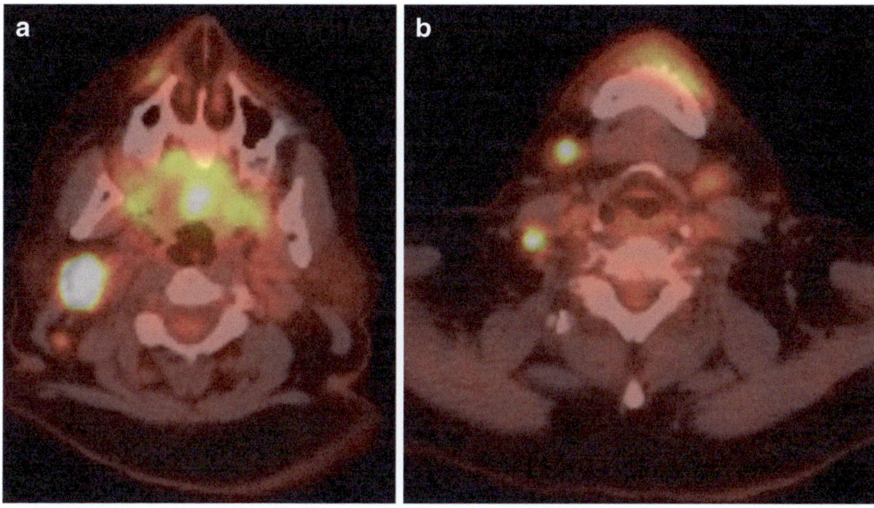

Fig. 3.8 Diagnostic PET/CT showing enlarged, FDG-avid right cervical lymph nodes in the upper (**a**) and mid (**b**) neck

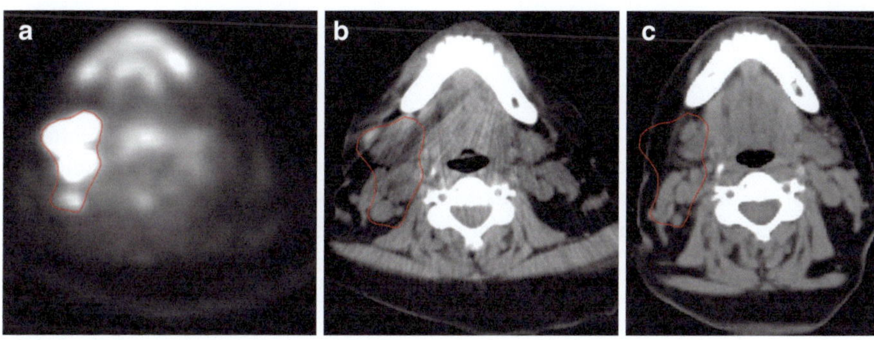

Fig. 3.9 Diagnostic PET/CT (**a**, **b**) with pre-chemotherapy extent of disease in the right neck contoured in red fused with the planning CT scan (**c**)

optimally delineate the vessels which correspond with lymph node chains, but it was not used in this case due to a contrast allergy. The pre-chemotherapy PET-CT was fused with the planning CT scan and the gross disease was contoured (Fig. 3.9a, b). Given slight differences in head position, tumor shrinkage, and weight loss, the pre-chemotherapy GTV extends outside the body and into normal structures (sternocleidomastoid muscle) (Fig. 3.9c). A CTV was then created which encompasses the original extent of disease but removing normal uninvolved structures (Fig. 3.10a) and confining the target volume to the body. The CTV should be enlarged to account for uncertainties in re-creating a target volume based on imaging performed at diagnosis. Finally, a PTV is designed with a margin that will account for daily setup error and organ motion if relevant, typically 3–5 mm in the head and neck region

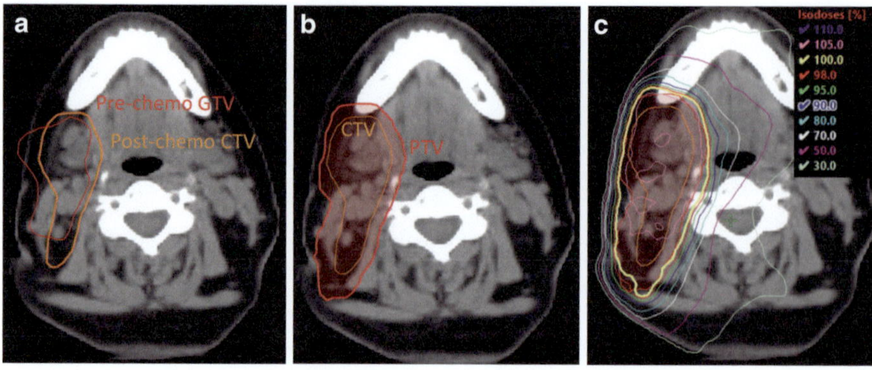

Fig. 3.10 Planning CT scan (**a**) showing pre-chemotherapy GTV (red) and a post-chemotherapy CTV (orange). In panel **b** an additional expansion is created to create a PTV (red contour). The dose distribution from a VMAT plan is shown in panel **c**

(Fig. 3.10b). A VMAT plan was designed, given the proximity of the PTV to the left parotid and submandibular glands. A dose of 30 Gy in 2 Gy fractions was prescribed (Fig. 3.10c).

Case 4

A 65-year-old man presented with a firm right axillary mass. A CT showed enlarged right axillary lymph nodes, the largest of which measured 3 cm. An excisional biopsy of the largest lymph node revealed a diagnosis of DLBCL, GCB subtype. FISH was positive for a rearrangement in *MYC*, but negative for rearrangements in *BCL2* and *BCL6*. A PET revealed several right axillary and infraclavicular lymph nodes measuring up to 2 cm, with a maximum standardized uptake value (SUV) of 15. There was no other evidence of disease. A bone marrow biopsy was negative for malignancy. The patient had an IPI score of 1 for age > 60 years. He was treated with 3 cycles of R-CHOP. A subsequent PET/CT scan showed a complete metabolic response (Deauville 5-point score of 1) with previously involved right axillary lymph nodal remnants measuring up to 1.8 cm. He received consolidative ISRT.

Simulation/Treatment Planning

The patient was positioned supine, with his right arm above his head. An alpha-cradle was used for immobilization. The pre-chemotherapy PET/CT was fused with the planning CT scan, and the pre-chemotherapy nodal disease was contoured (Fig. 3.11). A CTV (red contour) was created which encompassed all original nodal disease but excluded normal uninvolved structures, including the adjacent muscle (Fig. 3.12). A PTV (yellow contour) was created with a 5 mm margin (Fig. 3.12). A 3D conformal RT plan was designed. A dose of 30 Gy in 15 fractions was prescribed.

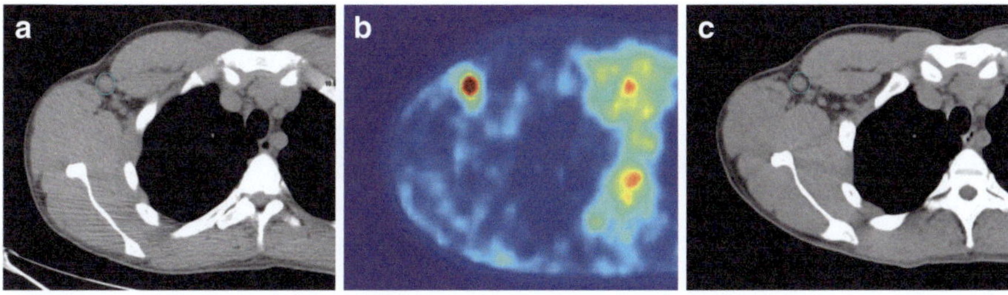

Fig. 3.11 The pre-chemotherapy CT scan (**a**) and PET scan (**b**) were fused with the planning CT scan (**c**), and the initially involved nodes were contoured as the pre-chemotherapy GTV (blue)

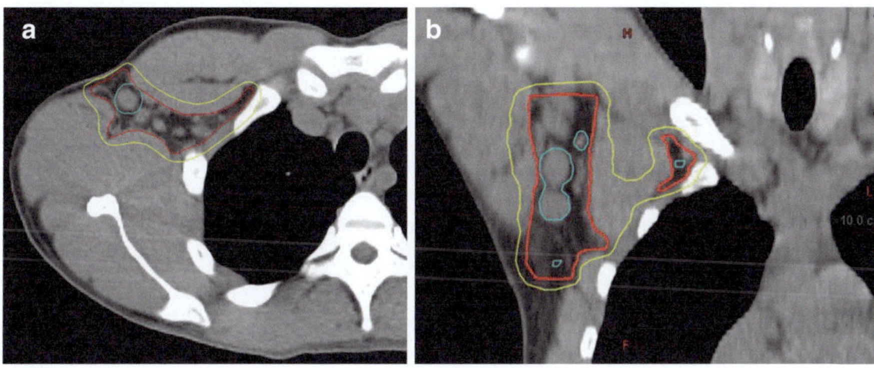

Fig. 3.12 Axial (**a**) and coronal (**b**) slices from the planning CT scan show that the CTV (red) encompassed the pre-chemotherapy GTV (blue), but excluded normal tissues that were not involved by disease, such as the adjacent muscle. The PTV was a 5 mm expansion of the CTV that was cropped so as not to extend outside the body

Case 5

A 55-year-old man presented with abdominal pain. He was found to have a 16 × 14 × 14 cm abdominal mass. A biopsy of the mass revealed a diagnosis of DLBCL, ABC subtype. FISH was negative for rearrangements in *MYC*, *BCL2*, and *BCL6*. A PET scan showed a large FDG-avid mass, with no other evidence of disease. A bone marrow biopsy was negative for malignancy. The patient had an IPI score of 1 for an elevated serum LDH. He was treated with 6 cycles of R-CHOP. A subsequent PET/CT scan showed a complete metabolic response (Deauville 5-point score of 2). There was a residual 9 × 7 × 5 cm abdominal soft tissue mass on CT. He was treated with consolidative ISRT to the initially bulky site of disease.

Simulation/Treatment Planning

The patient was positioned supine, with his arms above his head. An alpha-cradle was used for immobilization. A 4D-CT scan demonstrated negligible motion of the abdominal mass with respiration. The pre-chemotherapy PET/CT was fused with the planning CT scan and the pre-chemotherapy disease was contoured (Fig. 3.13). A CTV (red contour) was created that encompassed the original extent of disease but excluded normal uninvolved structures that were initially displaced by disease, such as the bowel (Fig. 3.14). A PTV (yellow contour) was created with an 8 mm margin (Fig. 3.14). An IMRT plan was designed. A dose of 30 Gy in 15 fractions was prescribed. On-board imaging with a daily cone-beam CT was used during treatment with alignment to the residual soft tissue mass.

Part 4: Special Considerations

DLBCL of the Testicle

Standard treatment of testicular lymphoma includes orchiectomy, immunochemotherapy including central nervous system (CNS)-directed therapy, and RT to the contralateral testis. Testicular RT is an important component of therapy that improves local disease control in the contralateral testis as well as overall survival [40, 41].

Several RT techniques are possible. One reasonable approach is a single electron field. CT-based planning may be useful for measurement of depth and selection of the appropriate electron energy. The patient should be positioned supine in a frog leg position. The penis should be immobilized superiorly on the abdomen. The entire testis, tunica albuginea, epididymis, and spermatic cord constitute the CTV. If the testis is elevated, for example, on a piece of Styrofoam, and a direct anterior beam is selected, there is minimal dose to the perineum (Fig. 3.15). However, if the beam is angled toward the pelvis, there may be perineal dose, in which case skin collimation may be useful. At the time of treatment, it is critical to confirm that the scrotum and testicle are encompassed within the light field. If skin collimation is used, care must be taken to ensure that the testicle does not retract behind it (for example, if the patient is cold). Typically, bolus is not necessary, because the electrons are of a high enough energy to give adequate superficial dose (i.e., ≥16 MeV). However, if lower energy electrons are used, bolus should be considered. Another alternative that also avoids dose to the internal pelvic anatomy is to treat with a superior anterior oblique photon field that is set up clinically using 1.5 cm bolus.

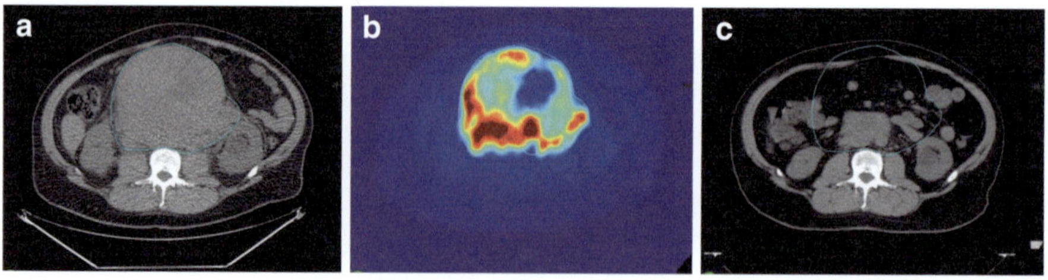

Fig. 3.13 Pre-chemotherapy CT scan (**a**) and PET scan (**b**) were fused with the planning CT scan (**c**), and the initial site of disease was contoured as the pre-chemotherapy GTV (blue)

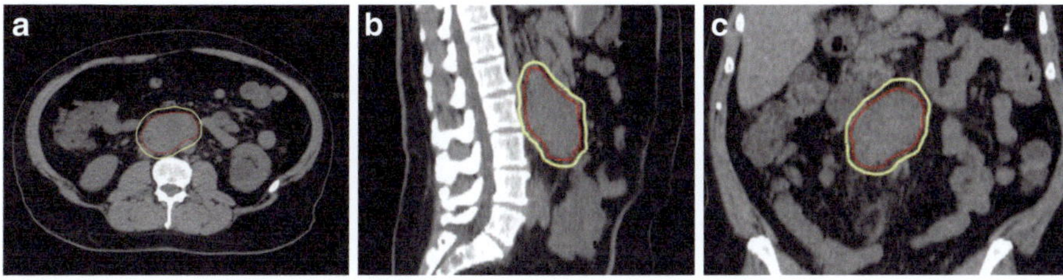

Fig. 3.14 Axial (**a**), sagittal (**b**), and coronal (**c**) slices from the planning CT scan showing the post-chemotherapy GTV = CTV (red), which encompassed the residual soft tissue mass (i.e., the pre-chemotherapy disease, excluding normal tissues that were initially displaced by the bulky mass, such as the bowel). The PTV was an 8 mm expansion of the CTV. A larger PTV margin was considered to be unnecessary, because a 4D-CT at the time of the simulation demonstrated negligible motion of the target, and a cone-beam CT scan was performed prior to RT daily with alignment to the mass

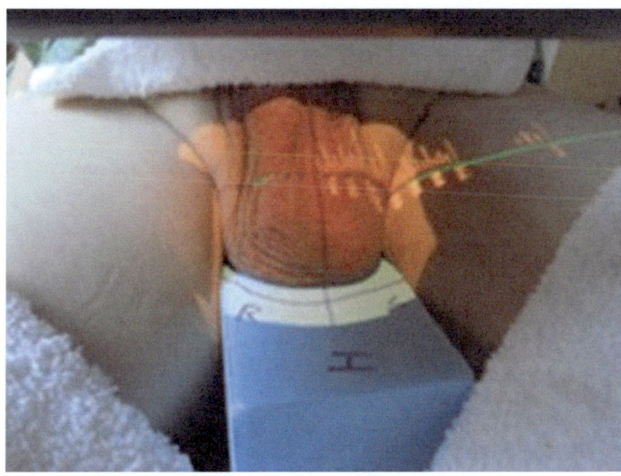

Fig. 3.15 Patient set-up for testicular RT. The penis was immobilized superiorly on the abdomen, and the testicle and scrotum were elevated on a Styrofoam block. The target was fully encompassed within the light field and was treated with a single AP electron beam

Primary DLBLC of the Breast

Approximately 40–50% of early-stage DLBCL cases involve extranodal sites. Involvement of the breast, however, is quite rare. Like primary testicular lymphoma, DLBCL of the breast is associated with a relatively high risk of failure in the contralateral organ (breast) and CNS [42, 43]. CNS prophylaxis is generally recommended. An International Extranodal Lymphoma Study Group (IELSG) retrospective study showed a benefit for consolidation RT in DLBCL of the breast [43]. Prophylaxis of the contralateral organ (e.g., breast), unlike for testicular DLBCL, is not generally pursued.

In most patients, the CTV should include the entire breast and any regional lymph nodes involved at diagnosis [38]. The disease is often relatively large (4 cm in the IELSG study) and often poorly defined. The original distribution of disease in the breast may be challenging to re-create on post-chemotherapy imaging. The risks of treating the entire breast with 30 Gy are small. However, under special circumstances, when the benefit of whole breast irradiation is felt to be outweighed by potential risks, the disease is well circumscribed, and the disease site can be re-created confidently, then partial organ irradiation is reasonable. Appropriate margins should be employed to avoid a marginal miss.

References

1. SEER. Cancer stat facts: diffuse large B-cell lymphoma. https://seer.cancer.gov/statfacts/html/dlbcl.html. Accessed April 2020.
2. Biggar RJ, Chaturvedi AK, Goedert JJ, Engels EA, Study HACM. AIDS-related cancer and severity of immunosuppression in persons with AIDS. J Natl Cancer Inst. 2007;99(12):962–72.
3. Gibson TM, Engels EA, Clarke CA, Lynch CF, Weisenburger DD, Morton LM. Risk of diffuse large B-cell lymphoma after solid organ transplantation in the United States. Am J Hematol. 2014;89(7):714–20.
4. Alizadeh AA, Eisen MB, Davis RE, et al. Distinct types of diffuse large B-cell lymphoma identified by gene expression profiling. Nature. 2000;403(6769):503–11.
5. Hans CP, Weisenburger DD, Greiner TC, et al. Confirmation of the molecular classification of diffuse large B-cell lymphoma by immunohistochemistry using a tissue microarray. Blood. 2004;103(1):275–82.
6. Alaggio R, Amador C, Anagnostopoulos I, et al. The 5th edition of the World Health Organization classification of haematolymphoid tumours: lymphoid neoplasms. Leukemia. 2022;36(7):1720–48.
7. Dunleavy K. Double-hit lymphomas: current paradigms and novel treatment approaches. Hematology Am Soc Hematol Educ Program. 2014;2014(1):107–12.
8. NCCN Guidelines, B-cell lymphoma. https://www.nccn.org/professionals/physician_gls/pdf/b-cell.pdf. Accessed April 2020.
9. Cheson BD, Fisher RI, Barrington SF, et al. Recommendations for initial evaluation, staging, and response assessment of Hodgkin and non-Hodgkin lymphoma: the Lugano classification. J Clin Oncol. 2014;32(27):3059–68.
10. International Non-Hodgkin's Lymphoma Prognostic Factors P. A predictive model for aggressive non-Hodgkin's lymphoma. N Engl J Med. 1993;329(14):987–94.
11. Ziepert M, Hasenclever D, Kuhnt E, et al. Standard International prognostic index remains a valid predictor of outcome for patients with aggressive CD20+ B-cell lymphoma in the rituximab era. J Clin Oncol. 2010;28(14):2373–80.
12. Barrington SF, Mikhaeel NG, Kostakoglu L, et al. Role of imaging in the staging and response assessment of lymphoma: consensus of the International Conference on Malignant Lymphomas Imaging Working Group. J Clin Oncol. 2014;32(27):3048–58.
13. Monfardini S, Banfi A, Bonadonna G, et al. Improved five year survival after combined radiotherapy-chemotherapy for stage I-II non-Hodgkin's lymphoma. Int J Radiat Oncol Biol Phys. 1980;6(2):125–34.
14. Nissen NI, Ersboll J, Hansen HS, et al. A randomized study of radiotherapy versus radiotherapy plus chemotherapy in stage I-II non-Hodgkin's lymphomas. Cancer. 1983;52(1):1–7.
15. Prestidge BR, Horning SJ, Hoppe RT. Combined modality therapy for stage I-II large cell lymphoma. Int J Radiat Oncol Biol Phys. 1988;15(3):633–9.
16. Shenkier TN, Voss N, Fairey R, et al. Brief chemotherapy and involved-region irradiation for limited-stage diffuse large-cell lymphoma: an 18-year experience from the British Columbia Cancer Agency. J Clin Oncol. 2002;20(1):197–204.
17. Feugier P, Van Hoof A, Sebban C, et al. Long-term results of the R-CHOP study in the treatment of elderly patients with diffuse large B-cell lymphoma: a study by the Groupe d'Etude des Lymphomes de l'Adulte. J Clin Oncol. 2005;23(18):4117–26.
18. Pfreundschuh M, Trumper L, Osterborg A, et al. CHOP-like chemotherapy plus rituximab versus CHOP-like chemotherapy alone in young patients with good-prognosis diffuse large-

B-cell lymphoma: a randomised controlled trial by the MabThera International Trial (MInT) Group. Lancet Oncol. 2006;7(5):379–91.
19. Habermann TM, Weller EA, Morrison VA, et al. Rituximab-CHOP versus CHOP alone or with maintenance rituximab in older patients with diffuse large B-cell lymphoma. J Clin Oncol. 2006;24(19):3121–7.
20. Bonnet C, Fillet G, Mounier N, et al. CHOP alone compared with CHOP plus radiotherapy for localized aggressive lymphoma in elderly patients: a study by the Groupe d'Etude des Lymphomes de l'Adulte. J Clin Oncol. 2007;25(7):787–92.
21. Horning SJ, Weller E, Kim K, et al. Chemotherapy with or without radiotherapy in limited-stage diffuse aggressive non-Hodgkin's lymphoma: Eastern Cooperative Oncology Group study 1484. J Clin Oncol. 2004;22(15):3032–8.
22. Martinelli G, Gigli F, Calabrese L, et al. Early stage gastric diffuse large B-cell lymphomas: results of a randomized trial comparing chemotherapy alone versus chemotherapy + involved field radiotherapy. (IELSG 4). [corrected]. Leuk Lymphoma. 2009;50(6):925–31.
23. Miller TP, Dahlberg S, Cassady JR, et al. Chemotherapy alone compared with chemotherapy plus radiotherapy for localized intermediate- and high-grade non-Hodgkin's lymphoma. N Engl J Med. 1998;339(1):21–6.
24. Miller TP, LeBlanc M, Spier C. CHOP alone compared to CHOP plus radiotherapy for early stage aggressive non-Hodgkin's lymphomas: update of the Southwest Oncology Group (SWOG) randomized trial. Blood. 2001;98:724a.
25. Reyes F, Lepage E, Ganem G, et al. ACVBP versus CHOP plus radiotherapy for localized aggressive lymphoma. N Engl J Med. 2005;352(12):1197–205.
26. Lamy T, Damaj G, Soubeyran P, et al. R-CHOP 14 with or without radiotherapy in nonbulky limited-stage diffuse large B-cell lymphoma. Blood. 2018;131(2):174–81.
27. Stephens DM, Li H, LeBlanc ML, et al. Continued risk of relapse independent of treatment modality in limited-stage diffuse large B-cell lymphoma: final and long-term analysis of southwest oncology group study S8736. J Clin Oncol. 2016;34(25):2997–3004.
28. Poeschel V, Held G, Ziepert M, et al. Four versus six cycles of CHOP chemotherapy in combination with six applications of rituximab in patients with aggressive B-cell lymphoma with favourable prognosis (FLYER): a randomised, phase 3, non-inferiority trial. Lancet. 2019;394(10216):2271–81.
29. NCCN (2020) Clinical practice guidelines in oncology- B-cell lymphomas. https://www.nccn.org/professionals/physician_gls/pdf/b-cell.pdf. Updated May 5, 2020. Accessed.
30. Held G, Murawski N, Ziepert M, et al. Role of radiotherapy to bulky disease in elderly patients with aggressive B-cell lymphoma. J Clin Oncol. 2014;32(11):1112–8.
31. Pfreundschuh M, Murawski N, Ziepert M, et al. Radiotherapy (RT) to bulky (B) and extra-lymphatic (E) disease in combination with 6XR-CHOP-14 or R-CHOP-21 in young good-prognosis DLBCL patients: results of the 2X2 randomized UNFOLDER trial DSHNHL/GLA. J Clin Oncol. 2018;36(15 supplement):7574.
32. Lowry L, Smith P, Qian W, et al. Reduced dose radiotherapy for local control in non-Hodgkin lymphoma: a randomised phase III trial. Radiother Oncol. 2011;100(1):86–92.
33. Dorth JA, Chino JP, Prosnitz LR, et al. The impact of radiation therapy in patients with diffuse large B-cell lymphoma with positive post-chemotherapy FDG-PET or gallium-67 scans. Ann Oncol. 2011;22(2):405–10.
34. Halasz LM, Jacene HA, Catalano PJ, et al. Combined modality treatment for PET-positive non-Hodgkin lymphoma: favorable outcomes of combined modality treatment for patients with non-Hodgkin lymphoma and positive interim or postchemotherapy FDG-PET. Int J Radiat Oncol Biol Phys. 2012;83(5):e647–54.
35. Phan J, Mazloom A, Medeiros J, et al. Benefit of consolidative radiation therapy in patients with diffuse large B-cell lymphoma treated with R-CHOP chemotherapy. J Clin Oncol. 2010;28(27):4170–6.
36. Krol AD, Berenschot HW, Doekharan D, Henzen-Logmans S, van der Holt B, van 't Veer MB. Cyclophosphamide, doxorubicin, vincristine and prednisone chemotherapy and radiotherapy for stage I intermediate or high grade non-Hodgkin's lymphomas: results of a strat-

egy that adapts radiotherapy dose to the response after chemotherapy. Radiother Oncol. 2001;58(3):251–5.
37. Kelsey CR, Broadwater G, James O, et al. Phase 2 study of dose-reduced consolidation radiation therapy in diffuse large B-cell lymphoma. Int J Radiat Oncol Biol Phys. 2019;105(1):96–101.
38. Yahalom J, Illidge T, Specht L, et al. Modern radiation therapy for extranodal lymphomas: field and dose guidelines from the International Lymphoma Radiation Oncology Group. Int J Radiat Oncol Biol Phys. 2015;92(1):11–31.
39. Illidge T, Specht L, Yahalom J, et al. Modern radiation therapy for nodal non-Hodgkin lymphoma-target definition and dose guidelines from the International Lymphoma Radiation Oncology Group. Int J Radiat Oncol Biol Phys. 2014;89(1):49–58.
40. Ho JC, Dabaja BS, Milgrom SA, et al. Radiation therapy improves survival in patients with testicular diffuse large B-cell lymphoma. Leuk Lymphoma. 2017;58(12):2833–44.
41. Zucca E, Conconi A, Mughal TI, et al. Patterns of outcome and prognostic factors in primary large-cell lymphoma of the testis in a survey by the International Extranodal Lymphoma Study Group. J Clin Oncol. 2003;21(1):20–7.
42. Ludmir EB, Milgrom SA, Pinnix CC, et al. Primary breast diffuse large B-cell lymphoma: treatment strategies and patterns of failure(*). Leuk Lymphoma. 2018;59(12):2896–903.
43. Ryan G, Martinelli G, Kuper-Hommel M, et al. Primary diffuse large B-cell lymphoma of the breast: prognostic factors and outcomes of a study by the International Extranodal Lymphoma Study Group. Ann Oncol. 2008;19(2):233–41.

Further Reading

ILROG Guidelines for Nodal Non-Hodgkin Lymphomas [ref. 38]
ILROG Guidelines for Extranodal Lymphomas [ref. 37]
NCCN Guidelines for B-cell Lymphomas [ref. 43]

Target Volume Delineation for Advanced Stage Diffuse Large B Cell Lymphoma

4

Hans Theodor Eich, Mario Levis, Michael Oertel, and Umberto Ricardi

Contents

Part 1: Introduction

Background, Epidemiology, and Treatment Overview

- Diffuse large B cell lymphoma (DLBCL) is the most common B cell lymphoma, accounting for approximately 30% of all new diagnosis of non-Hodgkin lymphomas (NHL) [1].
- The incidence is similar in USA and Europe, with 4–5 new cases per 100,000/year [2, 3]. The incidence increases with age, reaching a peak around the sixth–seventh decades.

H. T. Eich · M. Oertel
Department of Radiation Oncology, University Hospital Muenster, Muenster, Germany
e-mail: hans.eich@ukmuenster.de; Michael.Oertel@ukmuenster.de

M. Levis (✉) · U. Ricardi
Department of Oncology, University of Torino, Torino, Italy
e-mail: mario.levis@unito.it; umberto.ricardi@unito.it

C. Pinnix et al. (eds.), *Target Volume Delineation in Hematologic Malignancies*, Practical Guides in Radiation Oncology,
https://doi.org/10.1007/978-3-031-67722-9_4

- A family history of lymphoma, autoimmune disease, human immunodeficiency virus (HIV) infection, hepatitis C virus (HCV) seropositivity, a high body mass and some occupational exposures have been identified as risk factors for DLBCL [4].
- The majority of patients are diagnosed with an advanced stage disease [5]. Extranodal spread is very frequent with bone marrow involvement in almost one third of cases [6].
- For prognostic purposes, the International Prognostic Index (IPI) should be calculated. The score incorporates known risk factors including, age > 60 years, elevated serum lactate dehydrogenase (LDH), Stage III–IV, Eastern Cooperative Group performance status 2–4, and extranodal sites >1. Patients with more than 2 risk factors have a poorer outcome, with an overall survival (OS) rate <60% at 3 years [7].
- For newly diagnosed DLBCL, R-CHOP-21 (rituximab, cyclophosphamide, doxorubicin, vincristine, and prednisone given every 21 days) remains the cornerstone of therapy [8–12]. The number of cycles administered and the addition of consolidation RT is influenced by stage and the presence of bulky disease. Although initially many respond to this therapeutic approach, the 5-year OS rate is approximately 60% for advanced stage patients [8, 9, 12–16].
- Gene expression profiling has identified two main subgroups of DLBCL, based on the cell of origin, that include germinal center B-cell type (GCB) and non-GCB. A small amount of DLBCL (≈10%) with an immunophenotype that could not be put in either category is defined as unclassifiable [17].
- R-mini-CHOP (low dose) may be adopted to improve tolerability in frail and in elderly patients >80 years of age with comorbidities [18, 19].
- The 2017 World Health Organization (WHO) classification for lymphomas has included a new category of high-grade lymphomas with rearrangement of *MYC* and *BCL2* and/or *BCL6* (HGBL-DH/TH), previously referred to as double hit or triple hit lymphoma [20].
  - These very aggressive lymphomas, often present with intermediate features between DLBCL and Burkitt lymphoma.
  - HGBL-DH/TH tend to exist within the GCB subgroup.
  - They account for less than 10% of all DLBCL and have a poor prognosis.
  - It remains unclear if HGBL-DH/TH necessitate an intensified chemotherapy although several studies have advocated for this. Early consolidation with autologous stem cell transplant (ASCT) and intensive regimens as CODOX-M/IVAC (cyclophosphamide, vincristine, doxorubicin, high-dose methotrexate/ifosfamide, etoposide, high-dose cytarabine) and HyperCVAD/MA (hyperfractionated cyclophosphamide, vincristine, doxorubicin, and prednisolone/high dose methotrexate and cytarabine) were tested [21, 22], with limited benefit and elevated toxicity, particularly in elderly patients. Dose-adjusted (DA) EPOCH-R (etoposide, prednisone, vincristine, cyclophosphamide, doxorubicin, and rituximab) has conversely shown promising results in a prospective phase II study, with durable remission (event free survival [EFS]:

71% at 4 years) and lower toxicity compared to the other intensified regimens (including ASCT) [23].
  - It is important to discriminate these lymphomas from the larger family of Double-Expressor lymphoma (DEL), which are defined as DLBCL with protein overexpression of the c-MYC oncogene and BCL2 (assessed by immunohistochemistry, ≥40% and >50%, respectively). Most DEL have an ABC-DLBCL phenotype (rarely are unclassifiable) and mimic the same clinical behavior and outcome [24].
- Figure 4.1 shows the different subtypes of DLBCL.
- Response evaluation: Positron emission tomography computed tomography (PET/CT) is used for response evaluation, both during and at the end of systemic treatment, in patients with advanced DLBCL.
- Interim evaluation: Interim PET/CT (i-PET) can be used to guide treatment on the basis of the response to therapy, eventually offering an alternative approach to refractory patients [25]. The utility of i-PET is debated. In fact, a negative i-PET seems to predict improved progression-free survival (PFS), but not a better OS [26, 27]. Actually, International Guidelines discourage to change treatment regimen solely on the basis of the i-PET/CT, unless there is clear evidence of progression [18, 28, 29].
- Upon completion of frontline therapy (often with R-CHOP), restaging with positron emission tomography computed tomography (PET/CT) imaging is considered mandatory according to International guidelines [4, 30, 31]. PET-CT imaging may identify patients who may benefit from additional therapy, including consolidation RT [32]. Residual metabolic uptake at the end of chemotherapy is predictive of shorter PFS and worse survival [28, 29, 33–36].
- Response assessment by PET/CT should be done according to the Deauville 5-point scale (5-PS), [35, 37] with score 1–3 indicating a complete metabolic response (CMR) and score 4–5 being representative of a residual disease [37].
- An incomplete metabolic response (score 4–5) is predictive of shorter PFS [26] and worse survival [33, 34], particularly when patients are not candidates for

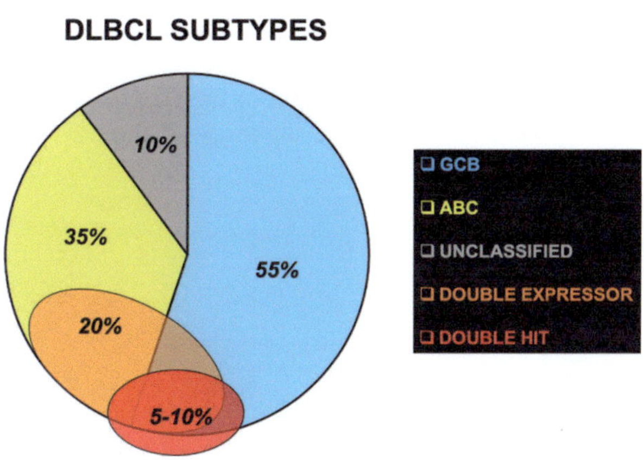

Fig. 4.1 Characterization of DLBCL based on WHO Grade (modified from Friedberg JW [24])

intensified therapies. When salvage treatment is being considered, a re-biopsy is recommended to confirm the presence of residual DLBCL [29].

- Patients with advanced DLBCL tend to relapse at sites of original involvement, particularly at sites of original bulky disease. After chemotherapy alone, the rate of local failure is higher. Consolidation RT is utilized based on a personalized risk-benefit evaluation taking into account initial risk factors but also response to systemic immunochemotherapy [38].
- In advanced stage DLBCL, after a CMR to frontline systemic therapy, RT may be offered as consolidation to sites at increased risk of local failure, including sites of bulky disease and osseous involvement [39].
- In instances of insufficient response to systemic therapy, with low burden residual PET positive disease, RT shall be offered [25, 40].
- The dominant pattern of failure after combined therapy is usually disseminated disease, with few patients relapsing in the field of radiation [41].
- The clinical cases presented in this chapter depict the most frequent scenarios to effectively integrate RT in the curative setting for patients with advanced stage DLBCL.

Pre-Radiotherapy Imaging and Evaluation

- Recommendations on pre-RT imaging are based on the guidelines by the International Lymphoma Radiation Oncology Group (ILROG) [32, 42]:
  - A planning computer tomography with or without intravenous contrast agent, acquired in 3–5 mm slice thickness forms the cornerstone and is mandatory for 3D planning.
  - Suitable immobilization devices such as thermoplastic masks or vacuum mattresses should be employed.
  - With functional imaging as PET-CT being used both in lymphoma staging and response evaluation, image transfer to and fusion within the treatment planning system are utilized, especially when positioning between the diagnostic PET-CT and RT treatment are similar. In some scenarios when there are significant differences in patient position between the PET-CT and CT simulation, the baseline PET-CT images will be used to guide target delineation without image fusion in the treatment planning system. Putative false-positive and -negative findings of the PET-scans have to be considered, respectively [43, 44].

Part 2: Management and Treatment of Advanced Stage DLBCL

Consolidation Radiotherapy of Bulky Disease

Management Principles

- RT has been traditionally used for consolidation after completion of chemotherapy in patients with bulky lymphoma, but this indication has been challenged in recent trials.
  - Studies in the pre-PET era defined varying sizes of lymphoma residues after chemotherapy as arbitrary cut-offs for consolidative radiation therapy (<5 cm, ≥6 cm, ≥7.5 cm) [13, 45, 46].
  - Application of RT for advanced stage DLBCL resulted in a superior local control, with no isolated in-field recurrences, and was accompanied by superior progression-free survival (PFS) and overall survival (OS) before the introduction of rituximab [45, 46].
  - Median doses varied between 30 and 40 Gy in conventional fractionation [45, 46].
- Modern clinical trials have adopted PET-guidance to evaluate RT indication for advanced-stage DLBCL and to achieve risk-adapted therapy de-escalation.
  - Analyses incorporating rituximab-containing regimens demonstrate a prognostic advantage of consolidative RT for stage III/IV DLBCL regarding local control (LC) and progression-free survival, with resulting 5-year values of >90% (LC) and 76–85% (PFS), respectively [47, 48].
  - In comparison, omission of RT resulted in a deterioration in LC, with in-field failure rates of 31–51% and a drop in 5-year PFS to 44–55% [47–49].
  - The impact of RT on overall survival is controversial, as some studies postulated a 5-year advantage of 20% [47, 48], whereas others failed to identify a prognostic benefit [49].
  - Bulky disease (≥5 cm, ≥7.5 cm) had no significant prognostic impact, although an association between tumor size and decreasing local/in-field control could be identified [49].
  - Preliminary results from the German UNFOLDER trial for young patients (18–60 years of age) reveal a deterioration in EFS by omission of RT for extranodal and bulky disease (68% vs 84% after 3 years), without effect on PFS and OS [50]. This study however did not incorporate PET-CT imaging for response assessment.
  - Correspondingly, the RICOVER-noRth trial for older patients (61–80 years of age) demonstrates a significant decrease in EFS if RT is omitted for bulky disease after R-CHOP immunochemotherapy (hazard ratio, 2.1; 95% confidence interval 1.3–3.5; $P = 0.005$) [51].
  - A retrospective study evaluating PET-guided radiation therapy for advanced DLBCL reported that patients with bulky DLBCL and a negative end of treatment PET for whom RT was omitted had outcomes similar to patients without bulky disease. PET positive patients on the other hand received RT and had outcomes that rivaled those of PET negative patients [40].

– Accordingly, the recent OPTIMAL trial by the German High-Grade Non-Hodgkin's Lymphoma group (DSHNHL) has abandoned the strategy of its predecessor RICOVER, by restricting post-chemotherapy RT to sites of residual PET-positive lymphoma [13, 52]. Preliminary data suggest equality in outcome regarding PFS and OS and a significant reduction in RT series [52].

General Considerations for Radiotherapy and Contouring

- Detailed contouring guidelines are provided by ILROG and encompass a careful multistep process [32, 42]. Pre-therapy PET-CT imaging must be utilized to guide target delineation. Image fusion with pre-chemotherapy CT and PET/CT scan is helpful if there is alignment between patient positioning for the pre-treatment PET-CT scan and the CT simulation scan (Table 4.1).
- **Dose:** An RT dose of 30–45 Gy is recommended, with 30 Gy as consolidation for patients that have a negative PET-CT upon completion of therapy (5PS of 1–3) 40–45 Gy for residual PET-CT positivity (5PS of 4–5).

Clinical Case 1: Abdominal Bulk in a 62-Year-Old Lady after 6 Cycles of R-CHOP Chemotherapy

A 62-year-old woman presented with nausea and epigastric pain. Initial CT imaging demonstrated bulky abdominal adenopathy as well as low burden adenopathy above the diaphragm. She was diagnosed with Ann Arbor stage IIIA DLBCL. With initial PET/CT-staging not performed, the patient was started on R-CHOP chemotherapy. After 6 cycles of chemotherapy, PET-CT imaging revealed 5PS of 2. She

Table 4.1 Planning target definitions of bulky lesions

Volume		Description
GTV (gross tumor volume)	**Pre-chemotherapy GTV**	Includes all lymphoma tissue of the bulky lesion on pre-therapy imaging
	Post-chemotherapy GTV	Will include residual morphological and metabolic positive abnormalities after completion of systemic therapy
CTV (clinical target volume)		Adaption of pre-chemotherapy GTV to patient anatomy at the time of CT simulation, uninvolved normal tissues should be removed from the CTV
ITV (internal target volume)		An expansion of the CTV that accounts for motion. The ITV can be created based on 4D-CT imaging, fluoroscopy, or serial deep inspiration breath hold (DIBH) images. Without these examinations, an expansion of 1.5–2 cm may be necessary. ITV is not required in locations with fixed shape and position of the tumor
PTV		Expansion of ITV or CTV to account for set-up variability. Expansion size depends on location, immobilization devices used, and the type of image guidance used for therapy

was referred for consolidation RT to the initial site of bulky disease in the abdomen (Figs. 4.2, 4.3, 4.4, 4.5, 4.6, 4.7, 4.8 and 4.9).

Consolidation Radiotherapy of Focal Residual PET/CT Uptake after Chemotherapy

Management Principles

General Considerations for Consolidation Radiotherapy for 5PS 4–5 on End of Treatment PET-CT Imaging

- Patients with advanced DLBCL and an incomplete metabolic response after chemotherapy with or without rituximab are at a higher risk of relapse compared with patients with a negative post-chemotherapy PET [27, 34, 36].
- Limited data are available regarding the role of consolidation RT in residual PET/CT positive disease after chemotherapy for aggressive NHL. The addition of IFRT improves the local control rate [43, 53, 54] and may affect the poor outcome of these patients. In fact, several retrospective studies have demonstrated that the omission of consolidation RT to areas of residual PET uptakes after chemotherapy is a strong predictor of subsequent treatment failure and local relapses in advanced DLBCL [55, 56].
- On the other hand, the addition of consolidation RT to focal residual uptake may offset the negative prognostic value of an interim or end-of-treatment positive PET/CT scan [43]. Two retrospective studies from MD Anderson Cancer Center

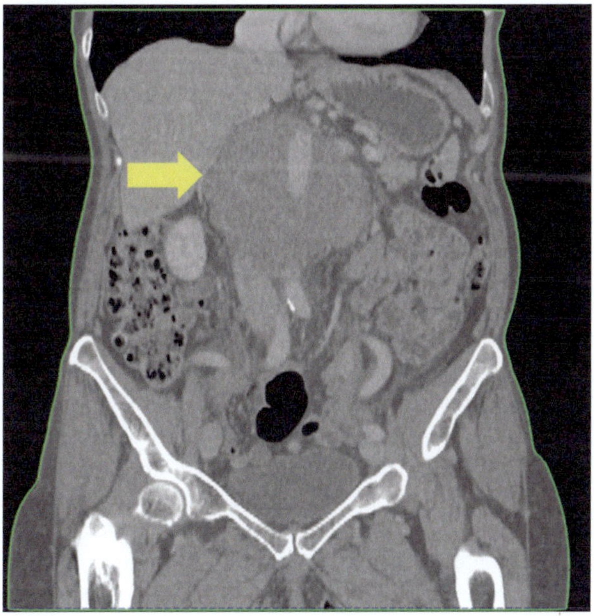

Fig. 4.2 Initial CT imaging in coronary view demonstrating bulky adenopathy (yellow arrow) beginning below the liver and extending to the renal hila. There was prominent encasing of the abdominal aorta and inferior vena cava

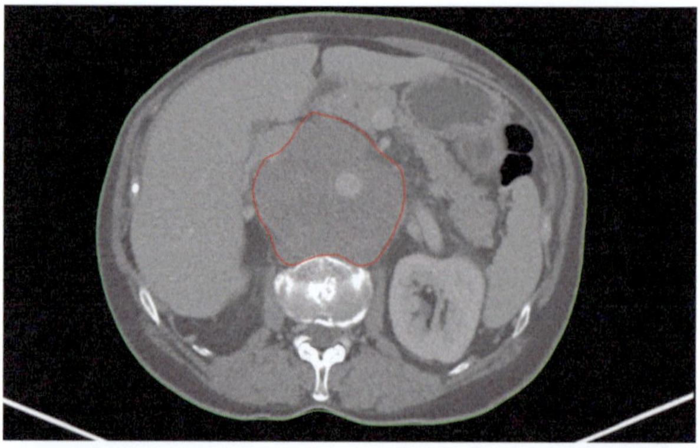

Fig. 4.3 Axial CT at baseline. Pre-chemotherapy GTV is contoured (red). Note encasing of the abdominal aorta and displacement of bowel

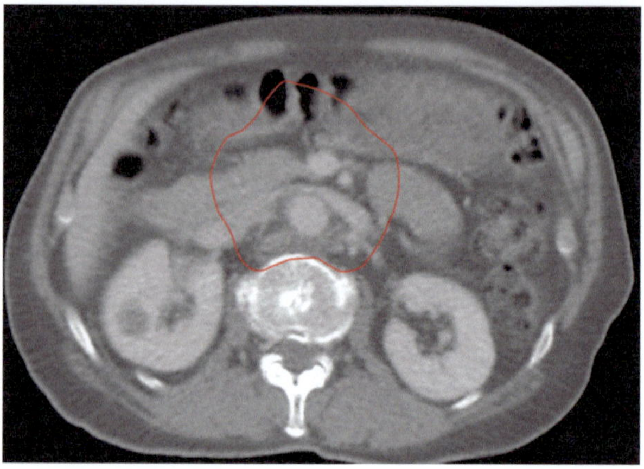

Fig. 4.4 Axial CT scan after completion of 6 cycles of R-CHOP. Transfer of pre-chemotherapy GTV to post-chemotherapy CT scan (red) covering large areas of previously displaced, but not involved, intestinal loops

[25] and Duke University [53] confirmed the role of consolidation RT in mitigating the negative prognostic value of residual metabolic uptake after chemotherapy, with a 5-year PFS above 60% in both studies for patients receiving radiation.

- For patients with persistent PET positive disease (DS 4–5), higher doses of consolidation RT may be required to achieve optimal local control (≥40 Gy) [43, 53]. ILROG Guidelines recommend a dose of 40–50 Gy delivered with conventional fractionation [32, 42].
- The target of treatment should be encompassed in respect to the "ISRT" principles, as described in the ILROG guidelines [32].
- The GTV is usually limited to sites of residual PET—avidity on post-chemotherapy imaging. If the PET positive lesion constitutes part of a residual mass on CT scan, the PET/CT negative residuum should also be included. The CTV is defined as residual mass containing PET-positive areas on the post-chemotherapy scan, with an adequate margin to accomplish all planning uncertainties (e.g., different positioning between diagnostic and planning imaging) [32].
- The contouring process should incorporate all information on pre- and post-chemotherapy imaging studies. Ideally, all diagnostic imaging studies (CT and

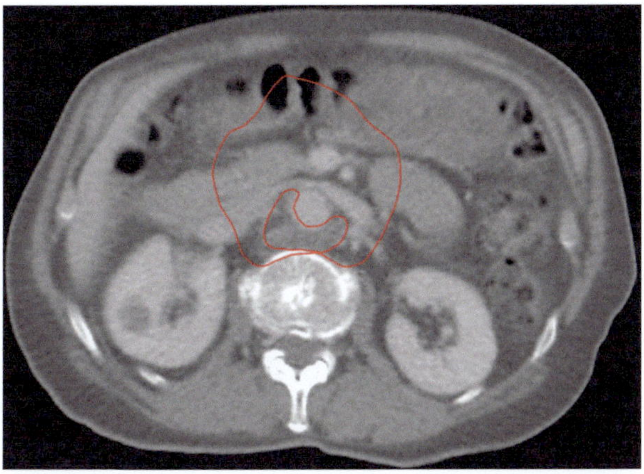

Fig. 4.5 Delineation of post-chemotherapy GTV (inner red structure) shows excellent response to chemotherapy

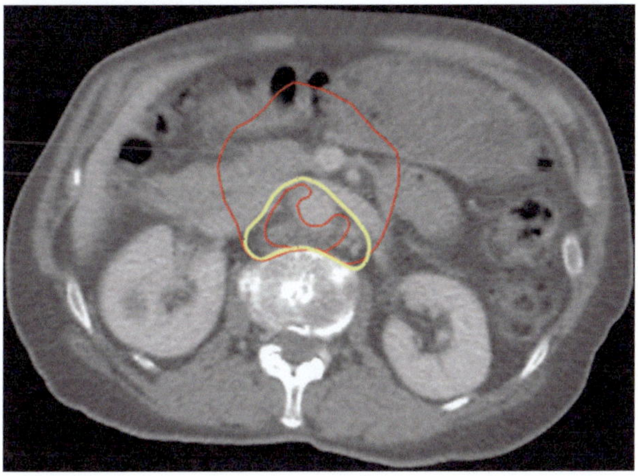

Fig. 4.6 Clinical target volume (CTV, yellow) accounts for possible microscopic spread to surrounding tissue

PET/CT scans) should be performed in the treatment position, using the planned immobilization devices [32], to facilitate the registration with the planning CT scan and to reduce the uncertainties in the contouring process.

- A planning CT scan should be performed in the chosen treatment position, using the planned immobilization devices. Contiguous slices, with a slice thickness of no more than 3–5 mm, should be taken through the regions of interest [32].
- When defining RT targets based on PET-CT scans, the clinician should carefully consider the anatomical information from the CT part of the scan because some small involved nodes with low uptake may be below the PET detection limit. Smaller nodes that are not PET-avid, but visible on CT scan adjacent to (or between) avid nodes, and considered to be involved, should be included in the target volume. For CT masses with partial PET uptake, the entire mass should be included in the target volume [35].
- Volume Definitions for Radiation Therapy Planning are shown in Table 4.2.

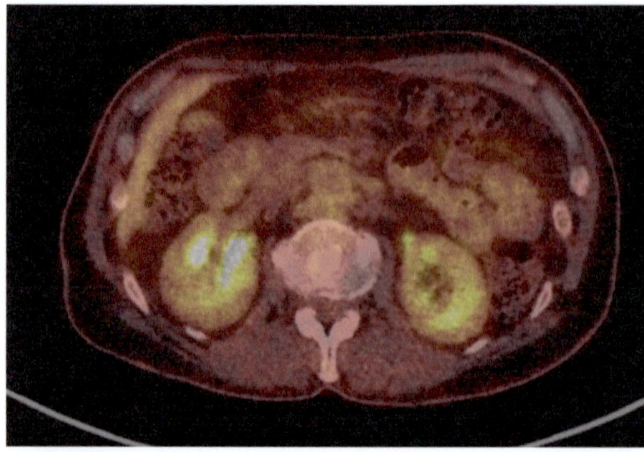

Fig. 4.7 As post-therapy PET/CT scan was negative (5PS of 2), RT was prescribed to 30.6 Gy in 17 fractions of 1.8 Gy

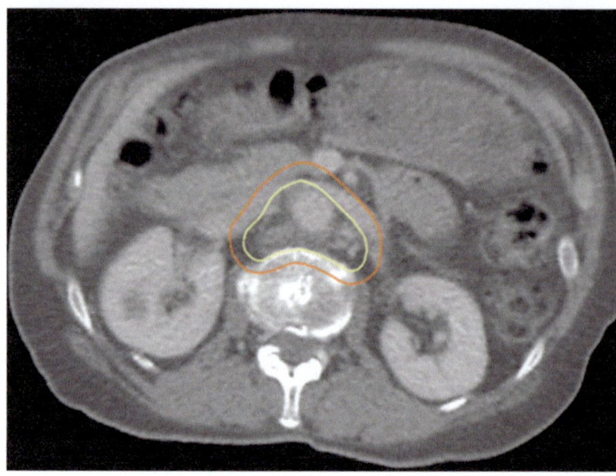

Fig. 4.8 Isometric 5 mm expansion of CTV (yellow) to PTV with the para-aortic region being rather resistant to intra-fractional movements, no ITV was delineated

- Target volumes may be treated with 3D conformal radiation therapy (3D-CRT), static or dynamic IMRT, volumetric modulated arc therapy (VMAT), helical tomotherapy, or proton therapy. In some situations, conventional anteroposterior-posteroanterior techniques may be preferred, because a smaller volume of normal tissue would be irradiated with this technique, albeit to the full-prescribed dose. In other situations, more-conformal techniques, such as IMRT, VMAT, or tomotherapy, may offer significantly better sparing of critical normal structures, usually at the price of a larger total volume of normal tissue irradiated, but with a lower dose [32].
- The selection of the treatment plan should be guided by a clinical judgment of the planning solution estimated to provide the lowest risk of long-term complications on the basis of an individualized approach. Factors such as gender, age, and comorbidities should also be taken into account. A multidisciplinary evaluation must always compare the risk of late RT-induced side effects with the risks of local recurrence if RT is not given. In many situations with aggressive nodal

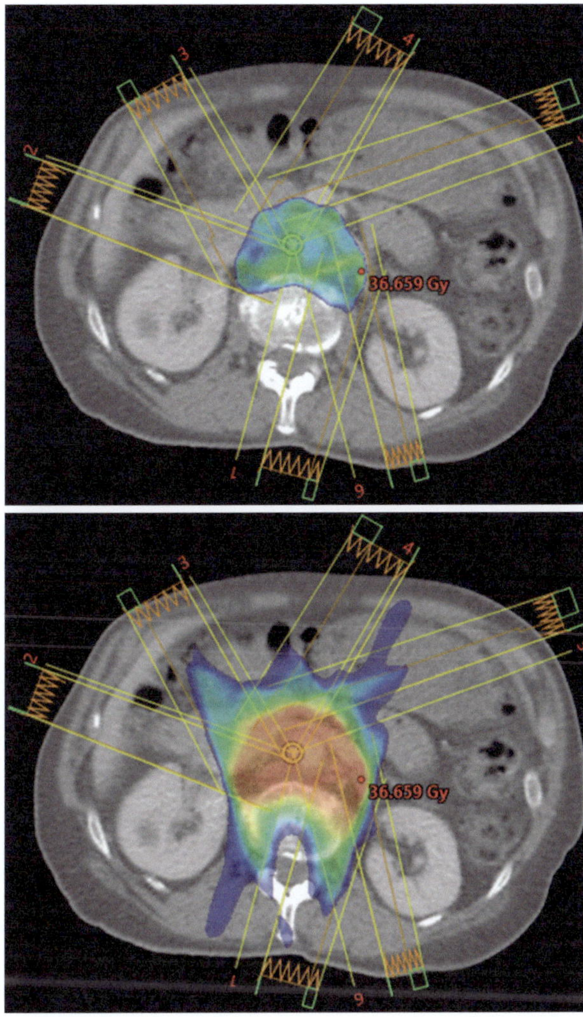

Fig. 4.9 Use of intensity-modulated RT (IMRT) as a 6-field sliding-window technique conferring high-conformity and sparring healthy organs-at-risk. Doses shown as color-wash with a minimum of 95%-isodose (above) and 20 Gy isodose (below). Note the excellent sparing of surrounding spinal cord and kidneys

lymphomas, particularly in older age groups, the risk and morbidity of disease recurrence outweigh the low risk of late effects such as secondary malignancies.

Clinical Case 2: Stage IV DLBCL with Focal Positive Residual PET Uptake after Chemotherapy

A 57-year-old woman presented with a bulky, rapidly evolving, soft tissue mass in right axillary region. An excisional biopsy demonstrated a DLBCL, GCB subtype. The bone marrow biopsy was negative. She was diagnosed with stage IV DLBCL (multiple nodules in the ipsilateral breast gland). She received 6 cycles of R-CHOP chemotherapy and final restaging showed a residual hypermetabolic uptake in the right retropectoral and axillary region (SUV max:6,4; liver uptake:3,2; Deauville

Table 4.2 Planning target definitions of focal residual uptakes after chemotherapy

Volume		Description
Gross tumor volume (GTV)	**Pre-chemotherapy GTV**	Imaging abnormalities suggestive of lymphomatous involvement obtained before any intervention that might have affected tumor volume should be outlined on the simulation study. Pre-chemotherapy images are used for contouring on the CT planning scan
	Post-chemotherapy GTV	The primary imaging of post-chemotherapy macroscopic residual disease should be outlined as GTV on the simulation study and is always part of the CTV
Clinical target volume (CTV)		In principle, the CTV is contoured on the planning CT scan co-registered with post-chemotherapy diagnostic imaging. The CTV encompasses all residual masses containing PET positive areas on the post-chemotherapy scan, with an adequate margin to compensate for all uncertainties (e.g., positioning, microscopic spreading, change in volume since imaging). Healthy structures, such as lungs, kidneys, and muscles, that are clearly uninvolved, should be excluded from the CTV If distinct nodal volumes are involved but are <5 cm apart, they can be encompassed in the same CTV. However, if the involved nodes are >5 cm apart, they are treated with separate fields using the CTV-to-PTV expansion guidelines as described below
Internal target volume (ITV)		The ITV is the CTV plus a margin which takes into account uncertainties in size, shape, and position of the CTV within the patient due to motion [57]
Planning target volume (PTV)		The PTV is the volume that includes the CTV (and ITV when contoured) and accounts for setup uncertainties in patient positioning and alignment of the beams during treatment planning and throughout all treatment sessions. It is often institution dependent and influenced by the type of daily image guidance used for therapy. Generally, it is obtained by adding an isotropic margin of 3–10 mm to the CTV
Organs at risk (OARs)		The OARs relevant to treatment planning and the prescribed dose should be established on the simulation study [32]

Score 4). The case was discussed at the multidisciplinary tumor board and RT was recommended (Figs. 4.10, 4.11, 4.12, 4.13, 4.14, 4.15, 4.16 and 4.17).

Consolidation Radiotherapy of Skeletal Lesions

Management Principles

- *Secondary bone involvement*
  - Skeletal involvement by DLBCL is an extranodal involvement of particular interest for RT.

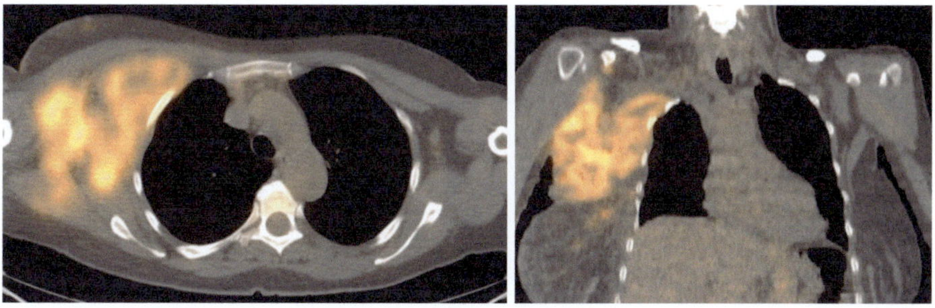

Fig. 4.10 Pre-chemotherapy-staging PET/CT scan showing right bulky axillary mass

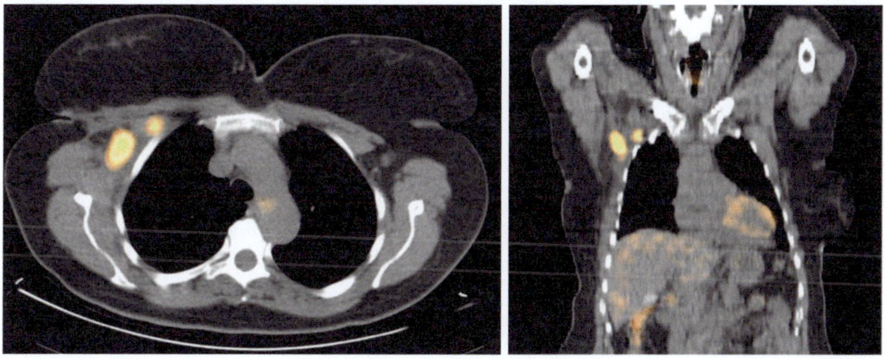

Fig. 4.11 PET/CT after six cycles of R-CHOP showing focal incomplete metabolic response

Fig. 4.12 The pre-chemotherapy GTV was contoured on the baseline diagnostic imaging (CT and PET/CT scan) and then moved to the planning CT scan through a co-registration

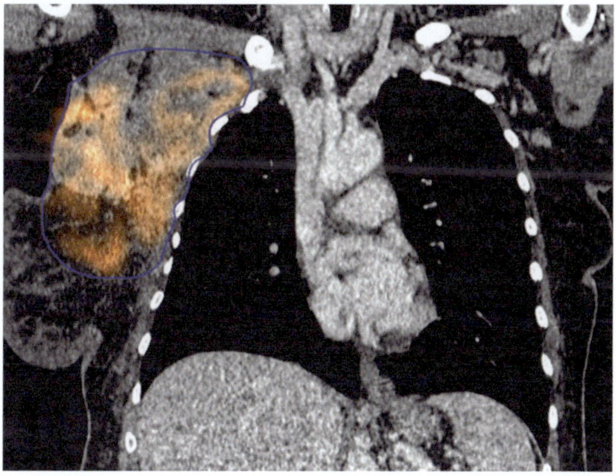

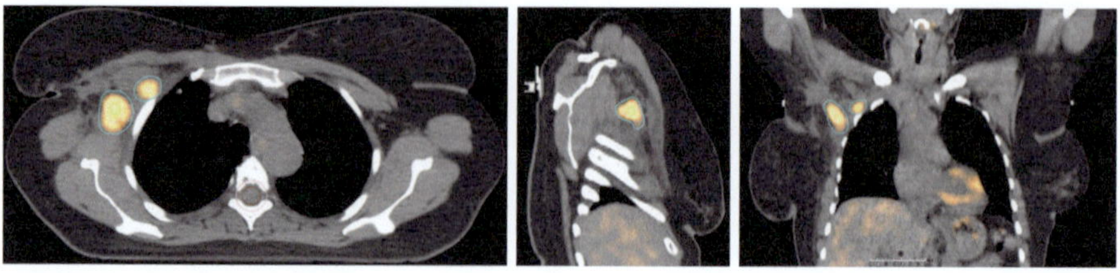

Fig. 4.13 The post chemotherapy GTV was delineated in green on the planning CT scan

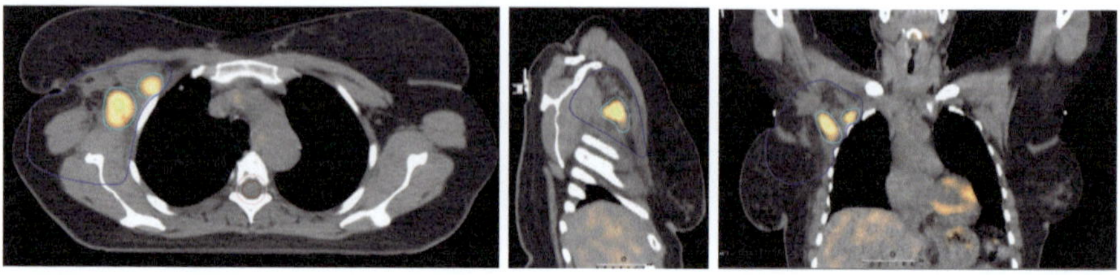

Fig. 4.14 The post-chemotherapy GTV (green) is then transferred to the planning CT scan through a registration with the diagnostic imaging where the target was contoured. Pre-chemotherapy GTV (in blue) is also shown in this figure illustrating the considerable response to chemotherapy

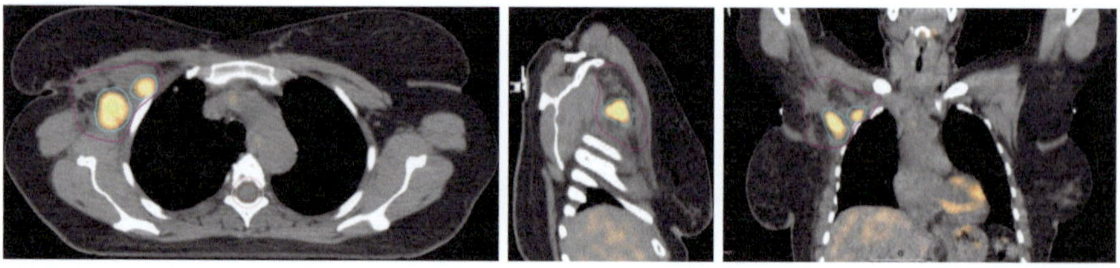

Fig. 4.15 The CTV is shown in pink and includes the post-chemotherapy GTV (green) with an expansion margin to accomplish for all uncertainties

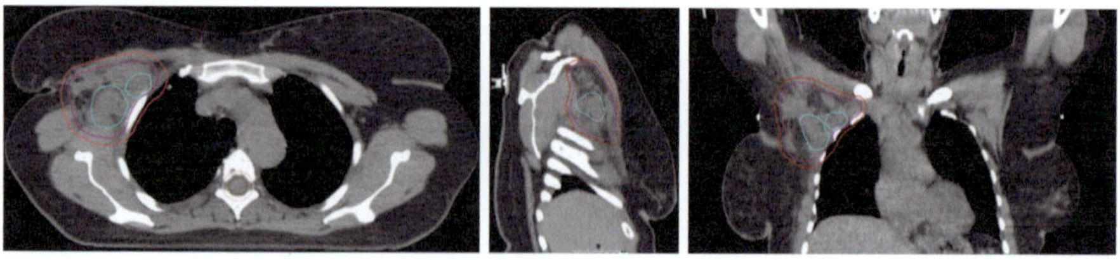

Fig. 4.16 The PTV is shown in red and is obtained by adding an isotropic margin of 5 mm to the CTV

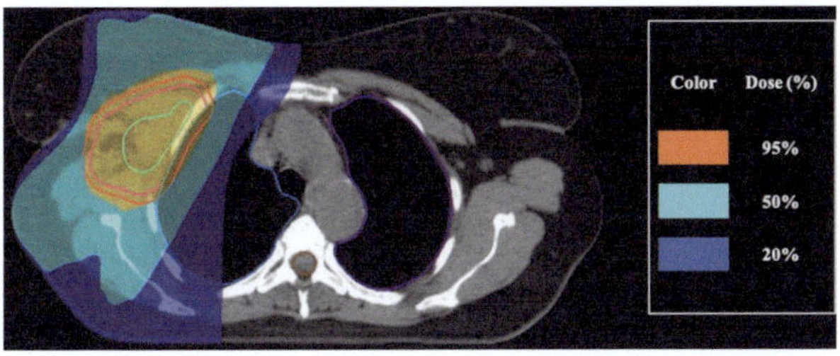

Fig. 4.17 Dose distribution of the helical tomotherapy plan selected in this patient prescribed to 40 Gy in 20 fractions

- A pooled analysis of skeletal involvement in nine consecutive trials of the German High-Grade Non-Hodgkin lymphoma Study Group (DSHNHL) demonstrated a significant benefit for RT, improving 3-year EFS from 36% to 75% [58].
- Interestingly, whereas the introduction of the CD20-antibody rituximab significantly extends EFS and OS in nodal DLBCL, a similar effect could not be observed in DLBCL with skeletal involvement [9, 58]. Consequently, a prognostic "gap" between nodal and bone spread of DLBCL is suspected in times of treatment with R-CHOP chemotherapy, making bone extranodal involvement a risk factor [58].
- In contrast, an analysis of the Surveillance, Epideliology and End Resuts (SEER) database failed to demonstrate a deterioration in OS for osseous involvement which may be attributable to a higher percentage of younger (<60) and limited-stage patients in this category [59].
- It remains unclear whether bone involvement persists as an independent prognostic factor in the era of modern PET-adapted treatment strategies. In the abovementioned study by Freeman et al. [40], **skeletal involvement did not herald a deterioration in PFS in addition to PET-status at the end of immunochemotherapy.**

- *Primary bone lymphoma*
  - A pathological and clinical distinction should be made with the less common primary bone lymphoma which appears either locally or multifocal and bears a favorable prognosis in comparison to advanced-stage DLBCL [60, 61].
  - The prognostic advantage of adding RT to therapy is vividly discussed and postulated for limited [62] or advanced stages [61], respectively and questioned [60, 63].
  - Concerning RT dose, a dose-escalation beyond 36 Gy revealed no amelioration of PFS and OS, which prompted a group from MD Anderson to recommend 30/30.6 Gy for patients that achieve complete remission (5PS of 1–3) after chemotherapy [60, 62].

General Considerations for Radiotherapy and Contouring

- Contouring guidelines are provided by ILROG and require a multi-step CT planning [64].
- MRI acquisition (in addition to PET_CT imaging) prior to systemic therapy is recommended.

- Adequate image fusion with pre-chemotherapy imaging is particularly helpful in cases of osseous involvement. The RT field can be limited to sites of skeletal involvement within a bony structure, irradiation of the whole bone is not necessary (Table 4.3) [60].
- **Dose**: RT dosage vary between 30 and 40 Gy in conventional fractionation.

Clinical Case 4: Consolidation RT of a Skeletal Lesion

A 63-year-old gentleman is diagnosed with DLBCL involving the pelvic bone and several infra-diaphragmatic lymph node areas. He was referred for consolidation RT after completion of 6 cycles of R-CHOP with a 5PS of 3 in the bone, whereas all other involved regions revealed a complete metabolic remission (Figs. 4.18, 4.19, 4.20, 4.21, 4.22, 4.23 and 4.24).

Table 4.3 Planning target definitions for treatment of skeletal lesions

Volume	Description
CTV	Based on pre-chemotherapy GTV (especially MRI) with margins to integrate subclinical disease spread
PTV	CTV+0.5–1 cm based on site, immobilization and daily image guidance

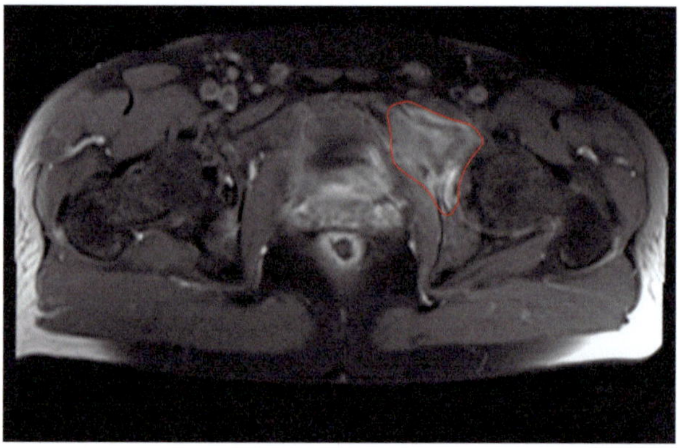

Fig. 4.18 Axial T2-weighted MRI-image of the pelvis showing a hyper-intense mass extending from the left superior pubic ramus into surrounding tissue. Use of different MRI sequences (T1, T2 +/− contrast agent) may be useful to delineate all lymphoma tissue

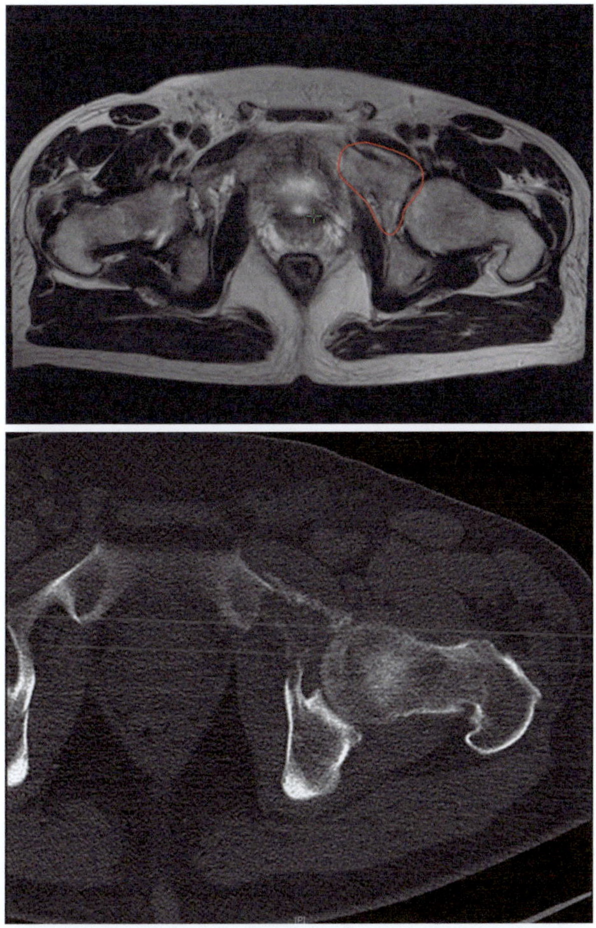

Fig. 4.19 Axial CT scan displaying osteolysis with slight displacement of bony contour

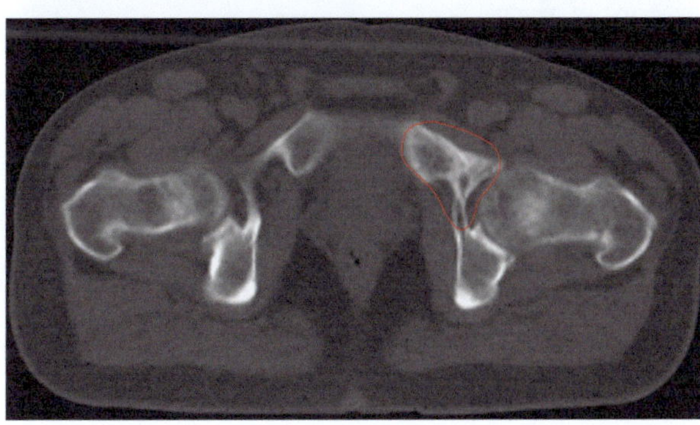

Fig. 4.20 Superimposition of the GTV to the post-chemotherapy planning CT. Note that the bony contour is maintained although microscopic disease in the adjacent tissues cannot be excluded

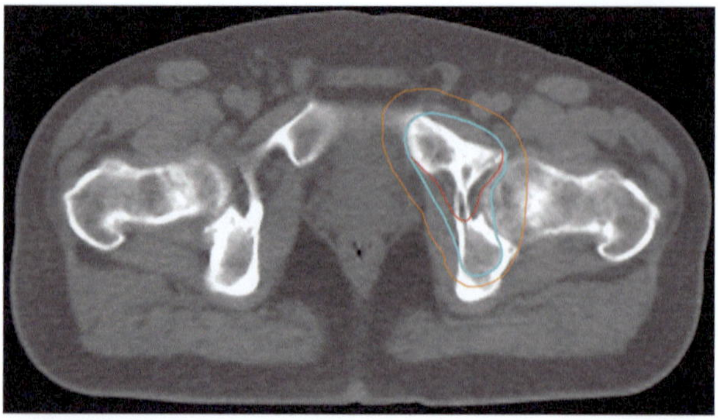

Fig. 4.21 Expansion of the pre-chemotherapy GTV to a CTV (cyan) accounting for subclinical spread. Geometrical isotropic expansion (7 mm) is used to obtain the PTV (orange)

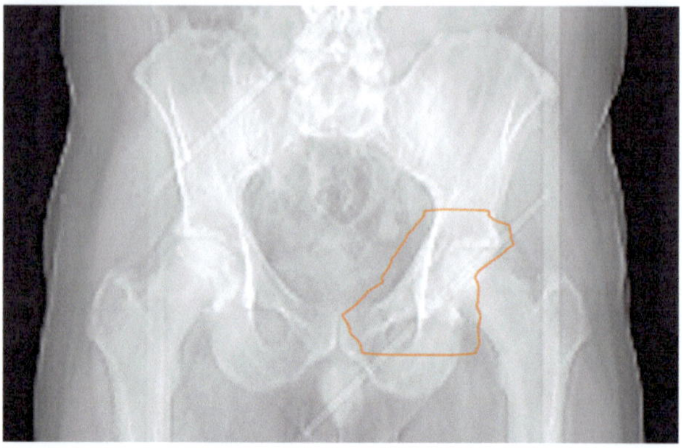

Fig. 4.22 Digitally reconstructed radiograph of the resulting PTV spanning the left superior pubic ramus and the left acetabulum reaching the iliac bone

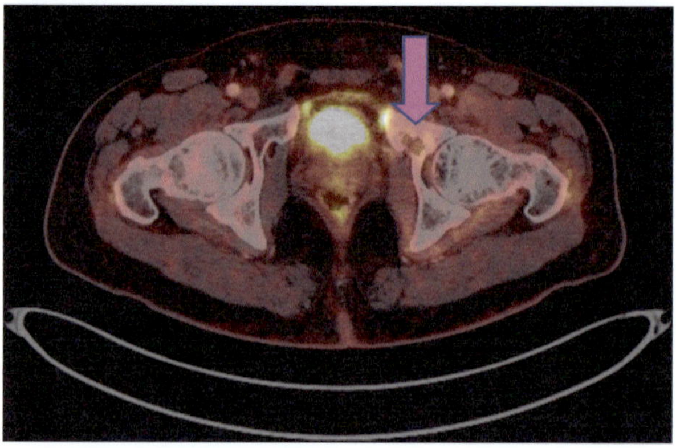

Fig. 4.23 PET-CT imaging 3 months after completion of RT. Residual PET-activity (pink arrow, Deauville 3) is not suggestive of residual disease. Note that surrounding bone is showing signs of (re-) mineralization and sclerosis

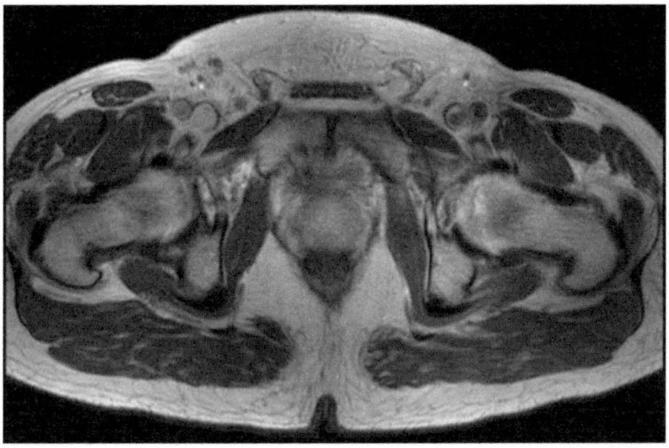

Fig. 4.24 Follow-up MRI (T1-weighted) with only moderate hypo-intensity in the former disease region

References

1. Armitage JO, Weisenburger DD. New approach to classifying non-Hodgkin's lymphomas: clinical features of the major histologic subtypes. Non-Hodgkin's lymphoma classification project. J Clin Oncol. 1998;16(8):2780–95.
2. Siegel RL, Miller KD, Jemal A. Cancer statistics, 2020. CA Cancer J Clin. 2020;70(1):7–30.
3. Sant M, et al. Incidence of hematologic malignancies in Europe by morphologic subtype: results of the HAEMACARE project. Blood. 2010;116(19):3724–34.
4. Tilly H, et al. Diffuse large B-cell lymphoma (DLBCL): ESMO clinical practice guidelines for diagnosis, treatment and follow-up. Ann Oncol. 2015;26(Suppl 5):v116–v25.
5. A clinical evaluation of the international lymphoma study group classification of non-Hodgkin's lymphoma. The non-Hodgkin's lymphoma classification project. Blood. 1997;89(11):3909–18.
6. Wang J, et al. Prognostic value of bone marrow F-18 FDG uptake in patients with advanced-stage diffuse large B-cell lymphoma. Nucl Med Mol Imaging. 2020;54(1):28–34.
7. Ziepert M, et al. Standard international prognostic index remains a valid predictor of outcome for patients with aggressive CD20+ B-cell lymphoma in the rituximab era. J Clin Oncol. 2010;28(14):2373–80.
8. Pfreundschuh M, et al. CHOP-like chemotherapy with or without rituximab in young patients with good-prognosis diffuse large-B-cell lymphoma: 6-year results of an open-label randomised study of the MabThera International Trial (MInT) Group. Lancet Oncol. 2011;12(11):1013–22.
9. Coiffier B, et al. CHOP chemotherapy plus rituximab compared with CHOP alone in elderly patients with diffuse large-B-cell lymphoma. N Engl J Med. 2002;346(4):235–42.
10. Coiffier B, et al. Long-term outcome of patients in the LNH-98.5 trial, the first randomized study comparing rituximab-CHOP to standard CHOP chemotherapy in DLBCL patients: a study by the Groupe d'Etudes des Lymphomes de l'Adulte. Blood. 2010;116(12):2040–5.
11. Habermann TM, et al. Rituximab-CHOP versus CHOP alone or with maintenance rituximab in older patients with diffuse large B-cell lymphoma. J Clin Oncol. 2006;24(19):3121–7.
12. Feugier P, et al. Long-term results of the R-CHOP study in the treatment of elderly patients with diffuse large B-cell lymphoma: a study by the Groupe d'Etude des Lymphomes de l'Adulte. J Clin Oncol. 2005;23(18):4117–26.
13. Pfreundschuh M, et al. Six versus eight cycles of bi-weekly CHOP-14 with or without rituximab in elderly patients with aggressive CD20+ B-cell lymphomas: a randomised controlled trial (RICOVER-60). Lancet Oncol. 2008;9(2):105–16.
14. Rieger M, et al. Primary mediastinal B-cell lymphoma treated with CHOP-like chemotherapy with or without rituximab: results of the Mabthera International Trial Group study. Ann Oncol. 2011;22(3):664–70.

15. Lisenko K, et al. Addition of rituximab to CHOP-like chemotherapy in first line treatment of primary mediastinal B-cell lymphoma. BMC Cancer. 2017;17(1):359.
16. Vassilakopoulos TP, et al. Rituximab, cyclophosphamide, doxorubicin, vincristine, and prednisone with or without radiotherapy in primary mediastinal large B-cell lymphoma: the emerging standard of care. Oncologist. 2012;17(2):239–49.
17. Rosenwald A, et al. The use of molecular profiling to predict survival after chemotherapy for diffuse large-B-cell lymphoma. N Engl J Med. 2002;346(25):1937–47.
18. Vitolo U, et al. Extranodal diffuse large B-cell lymphoma (DLBCL) and primary mediastinal B-cell lymphoma: ESMO Clinical Practice Guidelines for diagnosis, treatment and follow-up. Ann Oncol. 2016;27(suppl 5):v91–v102.
19. Peyrade F, et al. Attenuated immunochemotherapy regimen (R-miniCHOP) in elderly patients older than 80 years with diffuse large B-cell lymphoma: a multicentre, single-arm, phase 2 trial. Lancet Oncol. 2011;12(5):460–8.
20. Swerdlow SH, et al. The 2016 revision of the World Health Organization classification of lymphoid neoplasms. Blood. 2016;127(20):2375–90.
21. Sun H, et al. Outcome of patients with non-Hodgkin lymphomas with concurrent MYC and BCL2 rearrangements treated with CODOX-M/IVAC with rituximab followed by hematopoietic stem cell transplantation. Clin Lymphoma Myeloma Leuk. 2015;15(6):341–8.
22. Puvvada SD, et al. Outcomes of MYC-associated lymphomas after R-CHOP with and without consolidative autologous stem cell transplant: subset analysis of randomized trial intergroup SWOG S9704. Br J Haematol. 2016;174(5):686–91.
23. Dunleavy K, et al. Dose-adjusted EPOCH-R (etoposide, prednisone, vincristine, cyclophosphamide, doxorubicin, and rituximab) in untreated aggressive diffuse large B-cell lymphoma with MYC rearrangement: a prospective, multicentre, single-arm phase 2 study. Lancet Haematol. 2018;5(12):e609–17.
24. Friedberg JW. How I treat double-hit lymphoma. Blood. 2017;130(5):590–6.
25. Dabaja BS, et al. Positron emission tomography/computed tomography findings during therapy predict outcome in patients with diffuse large B-cell lymphoma treated with chemotherapy alone but not in those who receive consolidation radiation. Int J Radiat Oncol Biol Phys. 2014;89(2):384–91.
26. Pregno P, et al. Interim 18-FDG-PET/CT failed to predict the outcome in diffuse large B-cell lymphoma patients treated at the diagnosis with rituximab-CHOP. Blood. 2012;119(9):2066–73.
27. Mamot C, et al. Final results of a prospective evaluation of the predictive value of interim positron emission tomography in patients with diffuse large B-cell lymphoma treated with R-CHOP-14 (SAKK 38/07). J Clin Oncol. 2015;33(23):2523–9.
28. Duhrsen U, et al. Positron emission tomography-guided therapy of aggressive non-Hodgkin lymphomas (PETAL): a multicenter, randomized phase III trial. J Clin Oncol. 2018;36(20):2024–34.
29. Barrington SF, et al. Role of imaging in the staging and response assessment of lymphoma: consensus of the international conference on malignant lymphomas imaging working group. J Clin Oncol. 2014;32(27):3048–58.
30. Zelenetz AD, et al. NCCN guidelines insights: B-cell lymphomas, version 3.2019. J Natl Compr Cancer Netw. 2019;17(6):650–61.
31. Oertel M, et al. The new German evidence-based guideline on diffuse large B-cell lymphoma-key aspects for radiation oncologists. Strahlenther Onkol. 2023;199(2):115–20.
32. Illidge T, et al. Modern radiation therapy for nodal non-Hodgkin lymphoma-target definition and dose guidelines from the International Lymphoma Radiation Oncology Group. Int J Radiat Oncol Biol Phys. 2014;89(1):49–58.
33. Cheson BD. Role of functional imaging in the management of lymphoma. J Clin Oncol. 2011;29(14):1844–54.
34. Spaepen K, et al. Prognostic value of positron emission tomography (PET) with fluorine-18 fluorodeoxyglucose ([18F]FDG) after first-line chemotherapy in non-Hodgkin's lymphoma: is [18F]FDG-PET a valid alternative to conventional diagnostic methods? J Clin Oncol. 2001;19(2):414–9.

35. Mikhaeel NG, et al. The optimal use of imaging in radiation therapy for lymphoma: guidelines from the International Lymphoma Radiation Oncology Group (ILROG). Int J Radiat Oncol Biol Phys. 2019;104(3):501–12.
36. Mikhaeel NG, et al. 18-FDG-PET as a prognostic indicator in the treatment of aggressive non-Hodgkin's lymphoma-comparison with CT. Leuk Lymphoma. 2000;39(5–6):543–53.
37. Cheson BD, et al. Recommendations for initial evaluation, staging, and response assessment of Hodgkin and non-Hodgkin lymphoma: the Lugano classification. J Clin Oncol. 2014;32(27):3059–68.
38. Campbell BA, et al. Balancing the therapeutic ratio in DLBCL requires appropriate, individualized patient selection rather than broad elimination of radiation therapy. Int J Radiat Oncol Biol Phys. 2022;113(3):479–88.
39. Specht L. Does radiation have a role in advanced stage Hodgkin's or non-Hodgkin lymphoma? Curr Treat Options in Oncol. 2016;17(1):4.
40. Freeman CL, et al. Long-term results of PET-guided radiation in patients with advanced-stage diffuse large B-cell lymphoma treated with R-CHOP. Blood. 2021;137(7):929–38.
41. Miller TP, et al. Chemotherapy alone compared with chemotherapy plus radiotherapy for localized intermediate- and high-grade non-Hodgkin's lymphoma. N Engl J Med. 1998;339(1):21–6.
42. Wirth A, et al. Involved site radiation therapy in adult lymphomas: an overview of international lymphoma radiation oncology group guidelines. Int J Radiat Oncol Biol Phys. 2020;107:909.
43. Halasz LM, et al. Combined modality treatment for PET-positive non-Hodgkin lymphoma: favorable outcomes of combined modality treatment for patients with non-Hodgkin lymphoma and positive interim or postchemotherapy FDG-PET. Int J Radiat Oncol Biol Phys. 2012;83(5):e647–54.
44. Pepper NB, et al. Modern PET-guided radiotherapy planning and treatment for malignant lymphoma. Semin Nucl Med. 2023;53(3):389–99.
45. Ferreri AJ, et al. Consolidation radiotherapy to bulky or semibulky lesions in the management of stage III-IV diffuse large B cell lymphomas. Oncology. 2000;58(3):219–26.
46. Aviles A, et al. Residual disease after chemotherapy in aggressive malignant lymphoma: the role of radiotherapy. Med Oncol. 2005;22(4):383–7.
47. Phan J, et al. Benefit of consolidative radiation therapy in patients with diffuse large B-cell lymphoma treated with R-CHOP chemotherapy. J Clin Oncol. 2010;28(27):4170–6.
48. Shi Z, et al. Patterns of failure in advanced stage diffuse large B-cell lymphoma patients after complete response to R-CHOP immunochemotherapy and the emerging role of consolidative radiation therapy. Int J Radiat Oncol Biol Phys. 2013;86(3):569–77.
49. Dorth JA, et al. Impact of consolidation radiation therapy in stage III-IV diffuse large B-cell lymphoma with negative post-chemotherapy radiologic imaging. Int J Radiat Oncol Biol Phys. 2012;84(3):762–7.
50. Pfreundschuh M, et al. Radiotherapy (RT) to bulky (B) and extralymphatic (E) disease in combination with 6 x R-CHOP-14 or R-CHOP-21 in young good-prognosis DLBCL patients: results of the 2 x 2 randomized UNFOLDER trial of the DSHNHL/GLA. J Clin Oncol. 2018;36:7575.
51. Held G, et al. Role of radiotherapy to bulky disease in elderly patients with aggressive B-cell lymphoma. J Clin Oncol. 2014;32(11):1112–8.
52. Pfreundschuh M, et al. Radiotherapy to bulky disease PET-negative after immunochemotherapy in elderly DLBCL patients: results of a planned interim analysis of the first 187 patients with bulky disease treated in the OPTIMAL>60 study of the DSHNHL. J Clin Oncol. 2017;35:7506.
53. Dorth JA, et al. The impact of radiation therapy in patients with diffuse large B-cell lymphoma with positive post-chemotherapy FDG-PET or gallium-67 scans. Ann Oncol. 2011;22(2):405–10.
54. Aviles A, et al. Adjuvant radiotherapy in stage IV diffuse large cell lymphoma improves outcome. Leuk Lymphoma. 2004;45(7):1385–9.
55. Juweid ME, et al. Response assessment of aggressive non-Hodgkin's lymphoma by integrated International Workshop Criteria and fluorine-18-fluorodeoxyglucose positron emission tomography. J Clin Oncol. 2005;23(21):4652–61.

56. Kahn ST, et al. Value of PET restaging after chemotherapy for non-Hodgkin's lymphoma: implications for consolidation radiotherapy. Int J Radiat Oncol Biol Phys. 2006;66(4):961–5.
57. Yu JI, et al. Involved-lesion radiation therapy after chemotherapy in limited-stage head-and-neck diffuse large B cell lymphoma. Int J Radiat Oncol Biol Phys. 2010;78(2):507–12.
58. Held G, et al. Impact of rituximab and radiotherapy on outcome of patients with aggressive B-cell lymphoma and skeletal involvement. J Clin Oncol. 2013;31(32):4115–22.
59. Castillo JJ, Winer ES, Olszewski AJ. Sites of extranodal involvement are prognostic in patients with diffuse large B-cell lymphoma in the rituximab era: an analysis of the surveillance, epidemiology and end results database. Am J Hematol. 2014;89(3):310–4.
60. Bruno Ventre M, et al. Clinical features, management, and prognosis of an international series of 161 patients with limited-stage diffuse large B-cell lymphoma of the bone (the IELSG-14 study). Oncologist. 2014;19(3):291–8.
61. Messina C, et al. Clinical features, management and prognosis of multifocal primary bone lymphoma: a retrospective study of the international extranodal lymphoma study group (the IELSG 14 study). Br J Haematol. 2014;164(6):834–40.
62. Tao R, et al. Benefit of consolidative radiation therapy for primary bone diffuse large B-cell lymphoma. Int J Radiat Oncol Biol Phys. 2015;92(1):122–9.
63. Ramadan KM, et al. A clinicopathological retrospective study of 131 patients with primary bone lymphoma: a population-based study of successively treated cohorts from the British Columbia Cancer Agency. Ann Oncol. 2007;18(1):129–35.
64. Yahalom J, et al. Modern radiation therapy for extranodal lymphomas: field and dose guidelines from the International Lymphoma Radiation Oncology Group. Int J Radiat Oncol Biol Phys. 2015;92(1):11–31.

Further Reading

Barrington SF, Mikhaeel NG, Kostakoglu L, Meignan M, Hutchings M, Mueller SP, et al. Role of imaging in the staging and response assessment of lymphoma: consensus of the International Conference on Malignant Lymphomas Imaging Working Group. J Clin Oncol. 2014;32(27):3048–58.

Campbell BA, Bakst RL, Milgrom SA, Seymour JF. Balancing the therapeutic ratio in DLBCL requires appropriate, individualized patient selection rather than broad elimination of radiation therapy. Int J Radiat Oncol Biol Phys. 2022;113(3):479–88.

Cheson BD, Fisher RI, Barrington SF, Cavalli F, Schwartz LH, Zucca E, et al. Recommendations for initial evaluation, staging, and response assessment of Hodgkin and non-Hodgkin lymphoma: the Lugano classification. J Clin Oncol. 2014;32(27):3059–68.

Illidge T, Specht L, Yahalom J, Aleman B, Berthelsen AK, Constine L, et al. Modern radiation therapy for nodal non-Hodgkin lymphoma-target definition and dose guidelines from the International Lymphoma Radiation Oncology Group. Int J Radiat Oncol Biol Phys. 2014;89(1):49–58.

Mikhaeel NG, Milgrom SA, Terezakis S, Berthelsen AK, Hodgson D, Eich HT, et al. The optimal use of imaging in radiation therapy for lymphoma: guidelines from the International Lymphoma Radiation Oncology Group (ILROG). Int J Radiat Oncol Biol Phys. 2019;104(3):501–12.

Vitolo U, Seymour JF, Martelli M, Illerhaus G, Illidge T, Zucca E, et al. Extranodal diffuse large B-cell lymphoma (DLBCL) and primary mediastinal B-cell lymphoma: ESMO Clinical Practice Guidelines for diagnosis, treatment and follow-up. Ann Oncol. 2016;27(suppl 5):v91–v102.

Wirth A, Mikhaeel NG, Aleman BMP, Pinnix CC, Constine LS, Wilmot JP, et al. Involved site radiation therapy in adult lymphomas: an overview of International Lymphoma Radiation Oncology Group Guidelines. Int J Radiat Oncol Biol Phys. 2020;107(5):909–33

Yahalom J, Illidge T, Specht L, Hoppe RT, Li YX, Tsang R, et al. Modern radiation therapy for extranodal lymphomas: field and dose guidelines from the International Lymphoma Radiation Oncology Group. Int J Radiat Oncol Biol Phys. 2015;92(1):11–31.

Follicular Lymphoma

5

Belinda A. Campbell and N. George Mikhaeel

Contents

B. A. Campbell (✉)
Department of Radiation Oncology, Peter MacCallum Cancer Centre, Melbourne, VIC, Australia

Sir Peter MacCallum Department of Oncology, The University of Melbourne, Parkville, VIC, Australia

Department of Clinical Pathology, The University of Melbourne, Parkville, VIC, Australia
e-mail: belinda.campbell@petermac.org

N. George Mikhaeel
Guy's Cancer Centre, Guy's and St Thomas' Hospital, Great Maze Pond, London, UK

School of Cancer & Pharmaceutical Sciences, Faculty of Life Sciences and Medicine, King's College London, London, UK
e-mail: george.mikhaeel@gstt.nhs.uk

C. Pinnix et al. (eds.), *Target Volume Delineation in Hematologic Malignancies*, Practical Guides in Radiation Oncology,
https://doi.org/10.1007/978-3-031-67722-9_5

Part 1: Background and Epidemiology

- Follicular lymphoma (FL) is the second most common non-Hodgkin lymphoma (NHL), after diffuse large B-cell lymphoma, and constitutes 70% of indolent NHL diagnoses. In the USA, 2.7 new cases of FL are diagnosed per 100,000 people per year, age-adjusted [1, 2].
- FL is most commonly diagnosed in adults aged 55–74 years (median, 63 years) and is rare in children [1, 2]. The incidence is roughly similar in men and women [2]. The aetiology of FL is unclear. Unlike other NHL, there are no definitively known associations with precursor medical conditions [3]. Epidemiological data suggest associations with family history of FL, Sjogren's syndrome, chemical exposures (including agricultural pesticides and herbicides), viral infections, smoking, diet, and lifestyle factors [3–6]. High-grade transformation can occur at an annual risk of 2–3% that continues without a plateau beyond 15 years [7, 8].
- FL is classified by World Health Organisation (WHO) as an indolent non-Hodgkin lymphoma.
  - Microscopically, FL has a predominantly follicular pattern, with closely packed follicles effacing nodal architecture [9]. Centrocytes and centroblasts appear randomly distributed [9].
  - FL expresses the B-cell associated antigens CD19, CD20, CD22, and CD79a. BCL2, BCL6, and CD10 are often positive in FL; CD5 and CD43 are typically absent [9].
  - FL is genetically characterized by t(14;18)(q32;q21) translocation and BCL-2 gene rearrangements, but other variants and genetic alterations are reported [9, 10].
  - As per the fifth edition of the WHO Classification of Haematolymphoid Tumours (WHO-HAEM5), FL is divided into three subtypes: classic FL (cFL), follicular large B-cell lymphoma (FLBL), and FL with uncommon features (uFL) [11].
  - cFL constitutes 85% of FL. cFL comprises a follicular growth pattern, and is composed of centrocytes and centroblasts, and harbours the t(14;18)(q32;q21) translocation associated with *IGH*::*BCL2* fusion [11].
  - The FLBL subtype in the WHO-HAEM5 classification is less common, and largely equates to grade 3B in the WHO-HAEM4R classification [11].
  - The newly introduced uFL subtype displays variant immunophenotypic and genotypic features from cFL. uFL includes two subsets: one with "blastoid" or "large centrocyte" variant cytological features, and the other with a predominantly diffuse growth pattern [11].
  - Recognizing the challenges of reproducibility and consensus, grading is now optional in the updated WHO-HAEM5 classification [11]. However, grading is retained in other classifications (International Consensus Classification) [12].
  - Determination of grade has utility in prognostication and management decisions. Grading of lymph node biopsies reflects the number of centroblasts per high-power field. Grades 1 and 2 (0–5 centroblasts and 6–15 centroblasts per high-power field, respectively) represent a continuum and constitute 80–90% of diagnoses of FL [9]. Grade 3 (>15 centroblasts per high-power field) requires

further classification into Grade 3A and Grade 3B according to the presence or absence of centrocytes, respectively [9]. Grade 3B FL has a more aggressive clinical course and is managed akin to DLBCL; for this reason, distinguishing between Grade 3A and 3B FL by an expert haematopathologist is recommended [13].
  - Variants include paediatric-type and duodenal-type FL, with distinct clinical and biological features. Both variants frequently present as early-stage and have excellent prognoses [9]. Paediatric-type FL occurs more commonly in children and is BCL2 negative. Despite its high-grade morphology, prognosis is excellent with conservative management [9]. Duodenal-type FL often presents as an incidental finding in duodenal polyps and is clinically and microscopically distinct from cFL involving the intestine. The distal small intestine may be involved in 80–85% of cases [9].
- Nodal FLs are more common than extranodal FL. Patients most typically present with slow growing lymphadenopathy and commonly present with advanced stage disease. B symptoms are uncommon.
- Excisional biopsy is preferred for diagnosis of FL; fine needle aspirate is insufficient [13]. Staging of FL is by the Ann Arbor Classification. At a minimum, staging should include a diagnostic computed tomography (CT) scan of the neck, chest, abdomen and pelvis, and bone marrow biopsy/aspirate [13]. The addition of positron emission tomography (PET) is strongly recommended to improve the accuracy of staging and to guide radiotherapeutic management of early-stage disease [13, 14]. Baseline blood tests should include a complete blood count, routine blood chemistry including lactate dehydrogenase (LDH), β2 microglobulin, and uric acid [13]. Consideration should be given to screen for human immunodeficiency virus (HIV), hepatitis B virus (HBV), and hepatitis C [13].
- Standard of care remains contentious in both limited and advanced stages of FL. (Table 5.1).
  - In limited stage disease, definitive involved site radiation therapy (ISRT) remains the backbone of curative-intent treatment [14–18]. In patients with expected longevity, the addition of adjuvant immunochemotherapy or adjuvant immunotherapy may be associated with improved progression-free survival (PFS); however, at the cost of increased risks of toxicities and no proven improvement in OS [19, 20].
  - Advanced stage FL is not curable with current systemic therapies. Asymptomatic patients with no indications for treatment may be managed with observation. For those with indications for systemic therapy (e.g. cytopenia, bulky disease, threatened end-organ function), rituximab-based immunochemotherapy is preferred for fit patients [13].
  - Low-dose ISRT (4Gy in two fractions) has an important role in palliation of symptomatic disease and is extremely well-tolerated [14, 15, 21].
  - In highly-selected, fit patients with stage IIIA FL on PET-staging and low disease burden, total nodal irradiation (TNI) may offer curative potential [22].
  - Cases of extranodal FL are uncommon but are generally managed similar to nodal FL [23].
  - Management of duodenal-type and paediatric-type variants of FL are discussed below in Part 4.

Table 5.1 Management paradigms

Grade	Stage	Management paradigms
1-3A	I, II (contiguous[a])	Curative-intent: 1. Definitive ISRT (24–30Gy) alone 2. Combined modality treatment: ISRT + rituximab-based immunochemotherapy/ immunotherapy
1-3A	II (non-contiguous) III, IV	Palliative-intent: 1. Rituximab-based immunochemotherapy 2. Immunotherapy alone, for patients unlikely to tolerate chemotherapy 3. Radio-immunotherapy 4. Localized, low-dose ISRT (4Gy), to sites of symptomatic disease 5. Watchful waiting Curative-intent: 1. Combined modality treatment (ISRT + rituximab-based immunochemotherapy/ immunotherapy) may be considered for highly selected patients with non-contiguous Stage II FL 2. TNI (24Gy) may be considered for highly selected patients with Stage IIIA FL and low volume of disease
1-3A	Relapsed	Palliative-intent: 1. Watchful waiting 2. Localized, low-dose ISRT (4Gy), to sites of symptomatic disease 3. Rituximab-based immunochemotherapy (non-cross resistant agents) 4. Immunotherapy alone 5. Radio-immunotherapy
3B or follicular large B-cell lymphoma or large cell transformation		As per aggressive lymphoma treatment protocols

ISRT involved site radiation therapy, *TNI* total nodal irradiation

[a]Contiguous stage II is defined as adjacent ipsilateral Ann Arbor nodal regions. For example, involvement of left iliac and left inguinal nodal groups would be contiguous. Examples of non-contiguous involvement include (1) involvement of left para-aortic and left inguinal nodal groups, which are separated by the uninvolved left iliac nodal group; and (2) left and right side nodal involvement in the neck

Pre-Radiotherapy (RT) Imaging and Evaluation

- Pre-treatment imaging is essential for accurate disease mapping and target volume delineation in radiation therapy (RT) planning [14, 24].
- Structural imaging should include CT with intravenous contrast. Functional imaging with 18F-fluorodeoxyglucose (FDG)-PET/CT is recommended, and where possible should be done in the treatment position for ISRT [14].
- For extranodal FL, additional evaluation may be required:
  - Endoscopic evaluation may be required in the cases of FL of the gastro-intestinal tract (consider esophagogastroduodenoscopy, colonoscopy, capsule endoscopy, and endoscopic ultrasonography).

– Magnetic resonance imaging (MRI) is advisable for cases of FL of the head and neck, bone, breast, or abdominal viscera.

Part 2: Management and Treatment of Follicular Lymphoma

Early-Stage Localized FL

Principles of Management

- Patients with clinically localized FL should be fully staged with FDG-PET/CT and bone marrow aspirate and trephine biopsy (BMAT) before treatment.
- The goal of treatment in early-stage FL (stage 1 and contiguous stage 2) is to achieve long-term remission and potential cure. The expected 5-year progression-free survival (PFS) of patients staged with PET/CT and BMAT is approximately 75% for stage 1 and 50% for stage 2 [16].
- Whether definitive, local RT is curative or induces long term remission with eventual relapse has been the subject of debate. However, long-term follow up studies have shown the curative potential of ISRT alone, with approximately 50% of patients remaining relapse-free at 15 years. Relapse beyond 15 years is rare [17, 18].
- Therefore, definitive RT is considered the standard of care for early-stage fit patients as it is associated with low morbidity and is the only potential curative modality [14].
- The role of adjuvant immunochemotherapy continues to be debated. One randomized-controlled trial demonstrated that 10-year PFS was improved from the addition of adjuvant immunochemotherapy after 30Gy of RT. However, this was associated with significantly greater toxicities and no significant improvement over the 10-year overall survival of patients treated with RT alone [19]. Careful patient selection is recommended for this treatment approach [25].

General Considerations for Radiotherapy

- When treating early-stage disease with RT alone, the principles of ISRT as described by the International Lymphoma Radiation Oncology Group (ILROG) [14, 26] are followed with special consideration to the use of adequate margins to account for possible subclinical disease in the absence of chemotherapy. Therefore, ISRT is delivered to all sites of gross disease and adjacent areas at the highest risk of harbouring subclinical disease, but with careful consideration to long-term toxicity.
- Patients should be simulated in supine position with appropriate immobilization. A thermoplastic mask should be used for head and neck areas.
- In sites affected significantly by respiratory movement, the use of deep inspiration breath hold (DIBH) is strongly recommended (e.g. stomach and lung). If DIBH is not available, either 4-dimensional (4D) CT or fluoroscopy should be done to assess organ motion and inform an appropriate patient-specific internal target volume (ITV) margin.

- Axial CT images with intra-venous (IV) contrast should be acquired with ≤2.5 mm slice thickness and should cover the anticipated target volume and the whole extent of the organs at risk (OAR).
- Diagnostic FDG-PET/CT should be fused with planning CT to help define the FDG-avid areas to be included in the target volumes. In some situations, for example, skeletal and head and neck areas, MRI imaging can be fused with planning CT to aid in accurately defining the target volumes.
- Generally, three target volumes are defined for RT planning: gross tumour volume (GTV), clinical target volume (CTV), and planning target volume (PTV). These volumes are further described in Table 5.2.
  - Extra-nodal presentations of FL have a greater variety of location and pattern of spread than their nodal FL. They may be multifocal within the affected organ and may spread along organ walls, cavities, and tissue planes. There may also be a greater uncertainty in determining optimal CTV for extra-nodal presentations. In general, the whole organ or cavity is included whenever feasible and safe, for example, stomach, thyroid, parotid, breast, and orbit. Partial organ irradiation may be considered in other situations, for example, lung, skin, and bone. A detailed discussion of individual extra-nodal sites is provided in the ILROG guidelines for the management of extra-nodal lymphoma [27].
- RT planning may involve 3-dimensional (3D) conformal or inverse planning techniques, including intensity modulated radiotherapy (IMRT) or volumetric modulated arc therapy (VMAT). Beam arrangements and treatment technique should be chosen to minimize dose to organs at risk and are individualized for the specific patient.
- The standard dose for definitive RT in early-stage FL is 24–30 Gy in 2 Gy per fraction [14]. Prospective randomized trials have demonstrated that 24 Gy is as effective as higher doses (40–45 Gy) and provides more durable local control than 4 Gy in two fractions [15, 21, 28].

Advanced Stage FL

Principles of Management

- Advanced stage FL is generally not curable. The goal of treatment is improving quality of life and prolonging survival.
- The mainstay of treatment for advanced stage FL is systemic treatment. An initial "watchful waiting" policy may be appropriate in selected patients with no symptoms and low burden disease and is not associated with survival disadvantage.
- There are many options including single agent immunotherapy (anti-CD20 antibodies), chemo-immunotherapy and more recently novel drugs. The use of maintenance anti-CD20, typically for 2 years, after induction therapy has been shown to prolong the duration of remission.

Table 5.2 Planning target definitions for treatment of FL

Volume	Description	
Gross tumour volume	**GTV**	• **Nodal FL**: The GTV should include: – All FDG-avid nodes. – Any non-FDG-avid but enlarged or equivocal nodes visible on CT. • **Extra-nodal FL**: If the GTV can be identified on imaging (e.g. soft tissue in orbit, bone lesion), this should be outlined as GTV.
Clinical target volume	**CTV**	• **Nodal FL**: The CTV includes the GTV, with consideration to include adjacent visible nodes (even if not enlarged) that are considered to have the highest risk of containing subclinical disease. The CTV may extend to the boundaries of the involved nodal compartment in the axial plane. In the cranio-caudal plane, the CTV also covers potential subclinical disease along the line of the lymphatic pathways, with particular consideration given to avoid significant toxicity, e.g. extensive salivary gland exposure, ovarian/testicular exposure or breast exposure in younger patients. Standardly, this craniocaudal extension is 1–3 cm depending on certainty and accuracy of imaging techniques. • **Extra-nodal FL**: The CTV includes the GTV and: – Whole organ or cavity (e.g. whole stomach, thyroid, parotid gland, breast, and orbit) – Partial organ irradiation may be considered in other settings where whole organ irradiation is not feasible or potentially toxic (e.g. lung, skin) on an individual case basis – Uninvolved local nodes are not routinely included in CTV
Internal target volume	**ITV**	• For sites affected by respiratory motion: a margin is added to CTV to create the ITV as determined by 4D-CT or fluoroscopy. If DIBH is used, this margin is not usually required • For extranodal lymphomas: Consideration should be given for physiological organ filling and changes in shape from day-to-day.
Planning target volume	**PTV**	• Contains CTV (or ITV) plus a margin to account for set-up uncertainties associated with patient position and beam alignment. • Stabilization methods (e.g. thermoplastic mask for head and neck FL) allow for a reduction in the set-up margin. • CTV-to-PTV expansions are patient- and institution-specific. In FL, it is typically 0.5–1 cm.
Organs at risk	**OAR**	• Nearby OAR should be outlined for RT planning optimization to reduce their dose exposure. • Examples of organs to be outlined: Eye, lens, optic nerve, brain stem, cochlea, salivary glands, thyroid, lungs, heart, female breasts, liver, spleen, kidneys, bowel bag, ovaries/testes, urinary bladder, rectum, and spinal cord/canal.

- Low-dose RT is extremely effective in the palliation of advanced stage FL. Objective response rates of >80% (approximately 50% CR rate) are usually obtained with doses as low as 4 Gy in two fractions [15, 21]. This offers a convenient and short treatment option, provides palliation of local symptoms with very little, if any, side effects, and can be used as a means to delay systemic treatment in patients with localized areas of progression. Retreatment with low dose is also possible.

- Higher dose palliation could be considered in selected patients where prevention of local relapse is desirable. A randomized controlled study of 24 Gy in 12 fractions versus 4 Gy in 2 fractions demonstrated high rates of overall response (>80%) but greater local PFS was achieved from 24 Gy (89.9% versus 70.4% at 5 years, respectively) [15, 21]. However, this needs to be weighed against the higher incidence of low-grade toxicities.

General Considerations for Radiotherapy

- The goal of palliative RT is to cover the site of local progression and/or symptoms without an attempt to cover all known disease within the region.
- RT planning should consider prior RT exposure as well as the potential for future RT, in particular to minimise the dose to OAR in patients receiving re-irradiation and/or higher dose palliative RT.
- Pre-treatment simulation, positioning, immobilization, scanning, and use of diagnostic imaging follow the same principles described above.

Part 3: Cases

Case 1

A 67-year-old man presented with a large, left-sided groin mass, first observed approximately 2–3 months earlier. Biopsy of the left groin mass revealed WHO Grade 1–2 FL. Staging PET scan revealed FDG avidity within the 9 cm left inguinal mass and a 3.6 cm left external iliac node. Bone marrow aspirate and biopsy were clear for FL. The patient was staged as Stage IIA FL, with contiguous nodal involvement. Following case discussion and imaging review in a multidisciplinary meeting, definitive treatment with RT alone was recommended. The patient proceeded to definitive ISRT, prescribed to a total dose of 24Gy in 12 fractions, with curative-intent (Fig. 5.1).

Fig. 5.1 (**a**–**f**) ISRT planning for FL of the left inguinal and external iliac nodes. A fused PET/CT simulation study was obtained, with the patient in the treatment position (ideally with the scrotum held by a sling to the contralateral side). The primary advantage of PET/CT simulation includes improved accuracy of delineation of the target volumes: demonstrating both FDG-avid and non-FDG avid structural abnormalities. Due to the increased certainty that comes from PET/CT planning, it is also possible to use relatively tighter margins from GTV to CTV. (**a**) The GTV (orange) is marked on the CT images, derived from the planning PET/CT scan. The FDG-avid nodes are marked in yellow. The GTV includes both the metabolic (yellow) and structural abnormalities seen on PET and CT images, respectively. (**b**) The CTV (red) encompasses the GTV (orange) and is further expanded to cover the entire nodal regions on each axial plane, including non-FDG avid lymph nodes. The CTV is clipped at anatomical boundaries. On this axial plane, the CTV is cropped at the scrotum, musculature, and skin. (**c**) Note the physiological difference in bladder filling which occurred in the time between the CT and PET components of this fused PET/CT scan. (**d**) Beyond the GTV, the CTV (red) is extended distally for 2 cm, following the line of the lymphatic drainage and covering a cluster of subcentimeter, non-FDG-avid nodes. (**e**) Beyond the GTV, the CTV (red) is extended 2 cm proximally along the line of the lymphatics traveling along the vascular bundle. Due to the nonlinear plane of the lymphatics, the CTV is contoured manually on each slice rather than a direct expansion. (**f**) The PTV (blue) is a 1 cm expansion beyond the CTV (red) in all directions

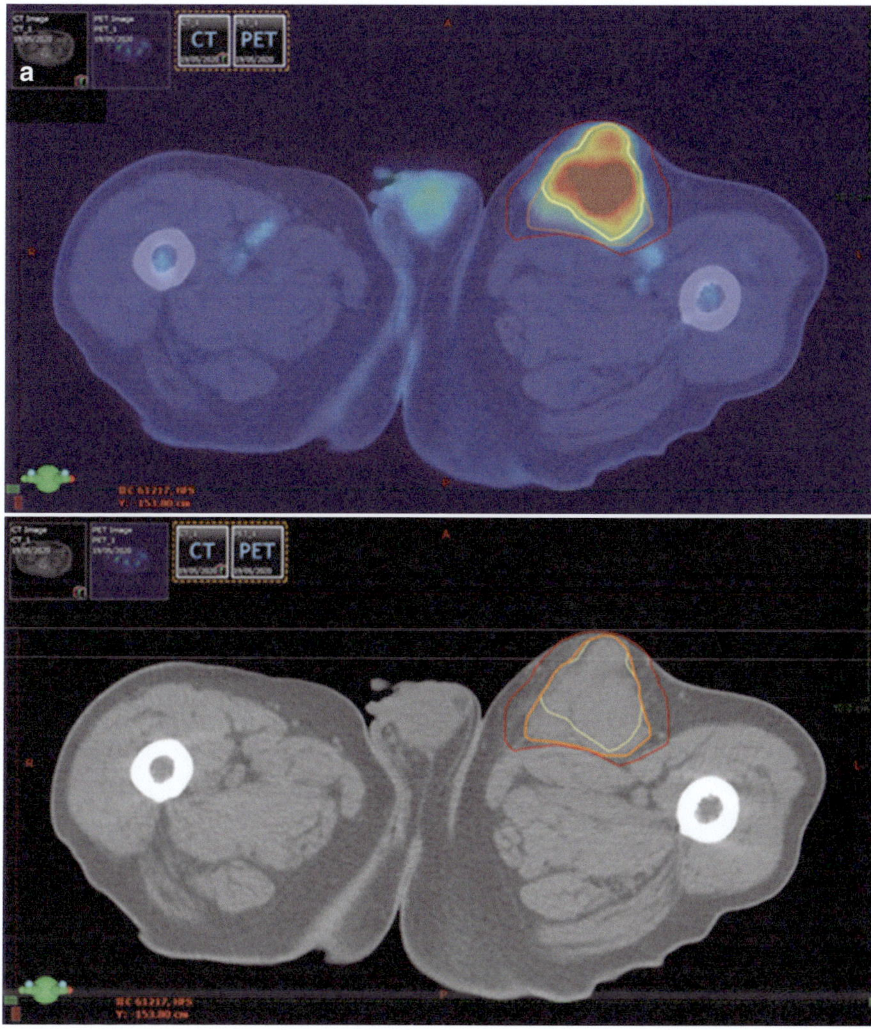
a
CT
PET
CT
PET

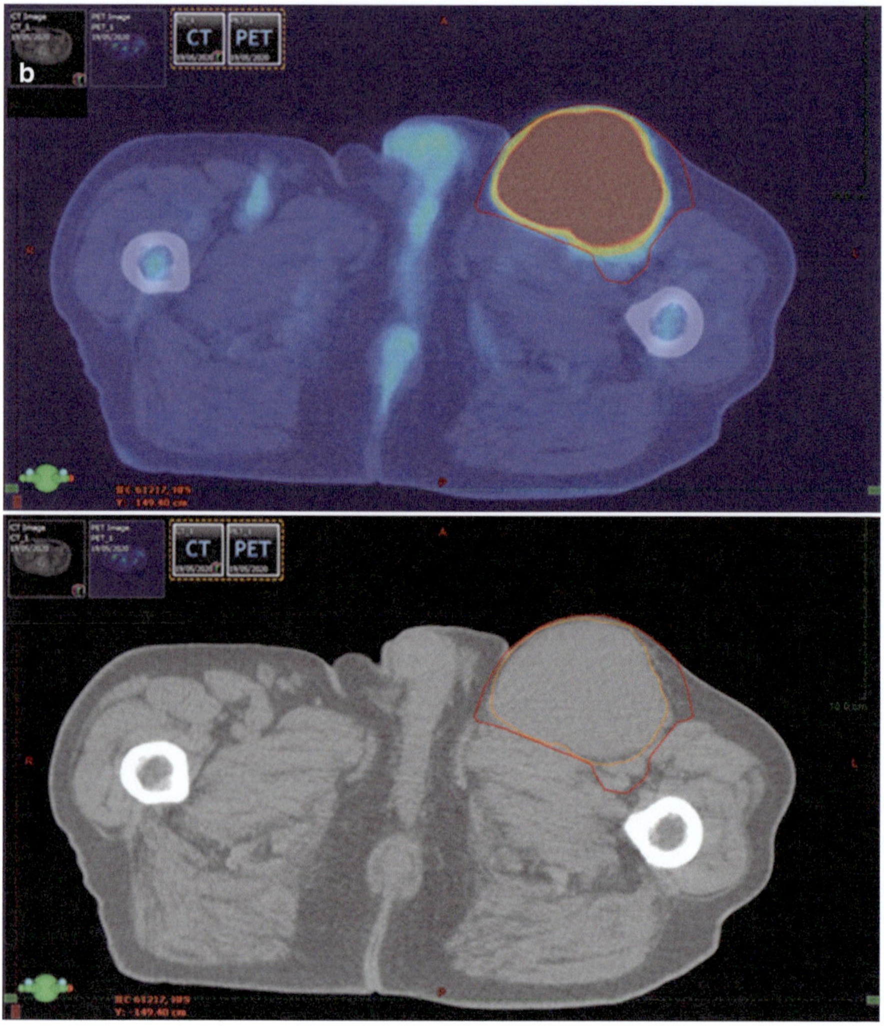

Fig. 5.1 (continued)

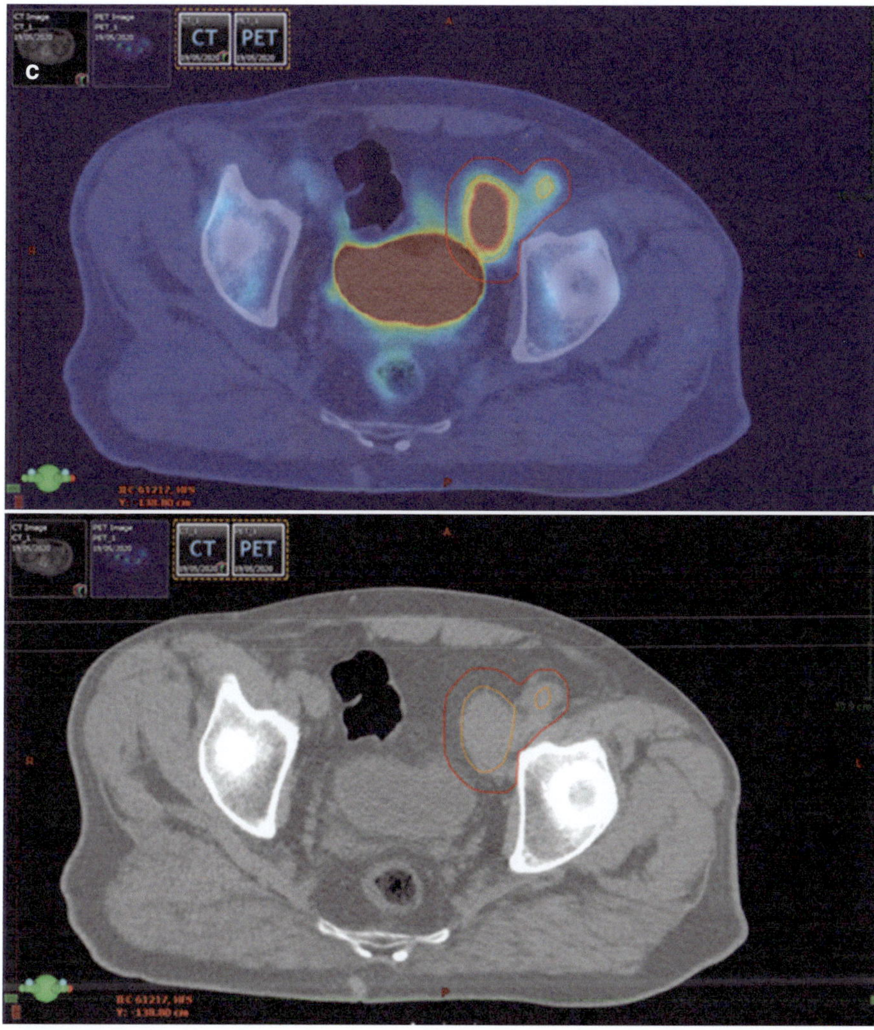

Fig. 5.1 (continued)

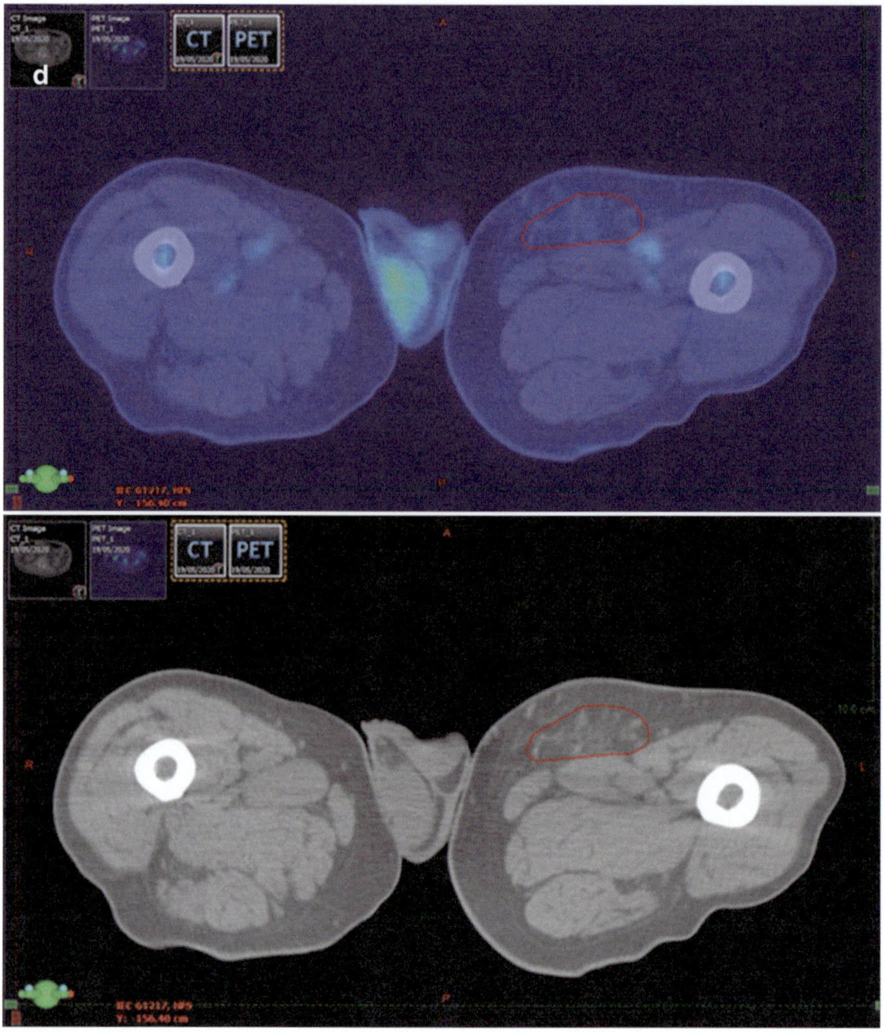

Fig. 5.1 (continued)

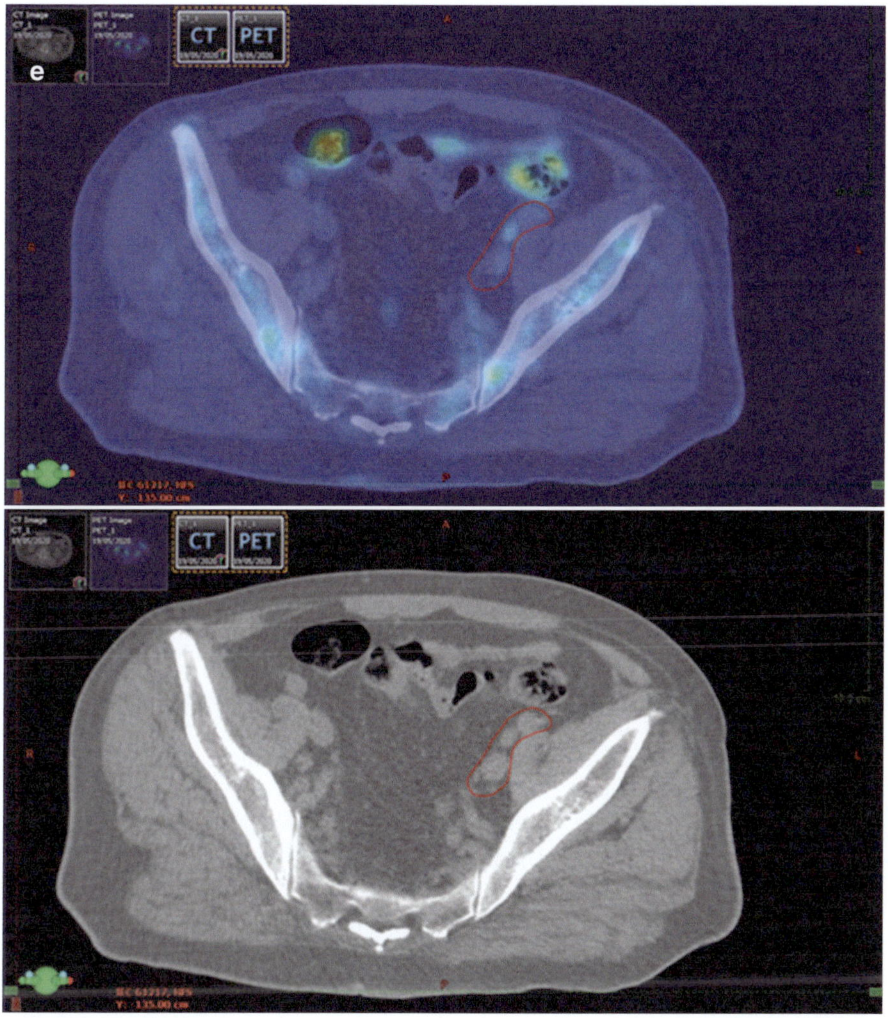

Fig. 5.1 (continued)

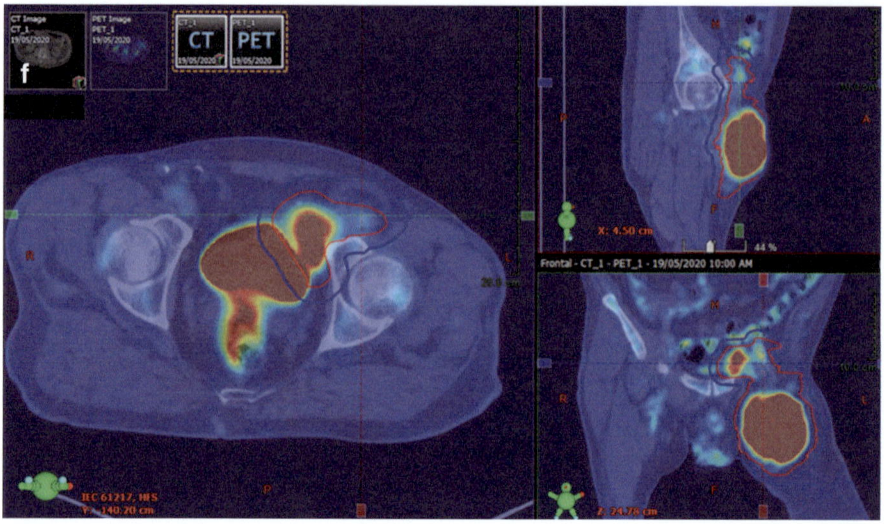

Fig. 5.1 (continued)

Case 2

A 72-year-old man presented with a 6-month history of cough and repeated chest infections. His performance status was WHO-1. He had no B symptoms. His past medical history included smoking, chronic obstructive pulmonary disease, ischaemic heart disease, previous angioplasty, Barrett's oesophagus, and psoriasis. A chest xray showed a mass in lower part of right lung. CT-guided biopsy from the lung mass confirmed follicular lymphoma grade 1–2. Staging FDG-PET/CT scan showed a right lower lung mass measuring 43 mm in maximum dimension with a solid and ground-glass components and partial FDG-avidity (SUVmax 4.5) and an 8 mm right hilar lymph node with low-grade uptake (SUVmax 3.1). Endo-bronchial ultrasound (EBUS)-guided biopsy of station 10R showed reactive changes only, with no evidence of lymphoma. BMAT did not show any evidence of FL. The disease was staged as Stage IAE. The patient was prescribed definitive ISRT, 24Gy in 12 fractions over 2.5 weeks (Fig. 5.2). Following ISRT, repeat PET/CT scan demonstrated complete metabolic and structural response.

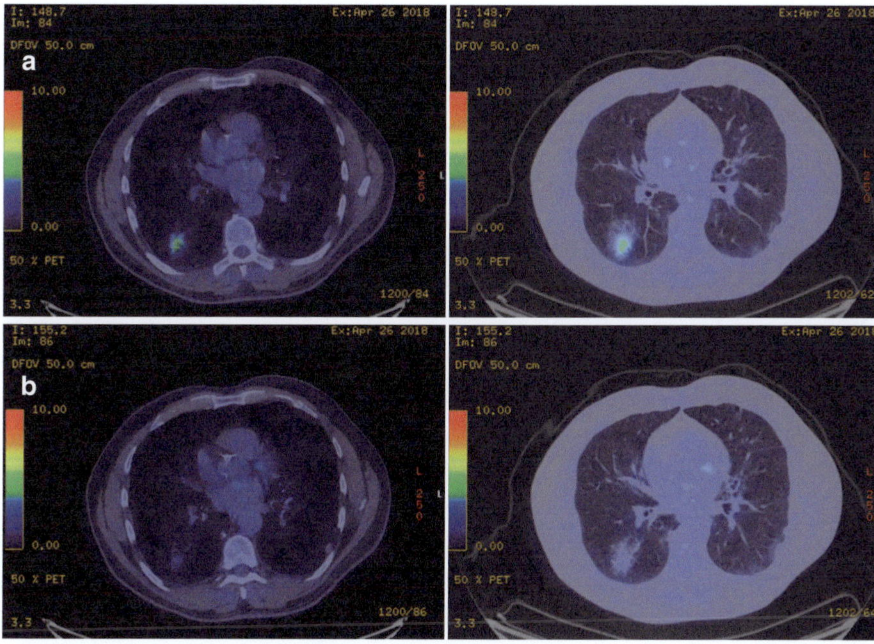

Fig. 5.2 (**a**, **b**) Staging PET/CT scans showing the extent of disease before treatment. The left panels demonstrate normal mediastinal windowing and the right panels show the lung window views. Note that the lesion is partly solid and partly ground-glass, and is only partially FDG-avid. The lung windows show more extensive abnormality than mediastinal windows, which otherwise underestimate the tumour volume. (**c**–**g**) At simulation, the patient is positioned with arms above head. A planning-CT scan was obtained using DIBH and IV contrast. (**c**) The CTV (red) is outlined on lung windows. Both solid and ground-glass components are included as well as FDG-avid and non-avid areas. The right hilum is not included as EBUS-guided biopsy showed only a reactive 8 mm node. Furthermore, it is desirable to reduce the volume of lung irradiated given the patient's COPD. (**d**) The CTV contour (red) is displayed on the corresponding mediastinal window view, to demonstrate that this view underestimates the extent of abnormality. On the mediastinal windows, the heart (purple) and spinal canal (yellow) were outlined as OARs; the lungs were also automatically segmented (not shown). Cardiac substructures were not outlined in this case as the target was reasonably distant from the heart, and the mean heart dose was expected to be low. (**e**) Upper slice of CTV displayed on lung window (left panel) and mediastinal window (right panel). (**f**) Lower slice of CTV displayed on lung window (left panel) and mediastinal window (right panel). (**g**) The PTV (blue) was created directly from CTV by adding 1 cm isotropic margin. As the patient was scanned in DIBH with consistent breath hold, no ITV was required. If DIBH is not available or is poorly tolerated by the patient, 4D-CT can be used to create an ITV accounting for the respiratory motion effect, with the resultant PTV expected to be larger

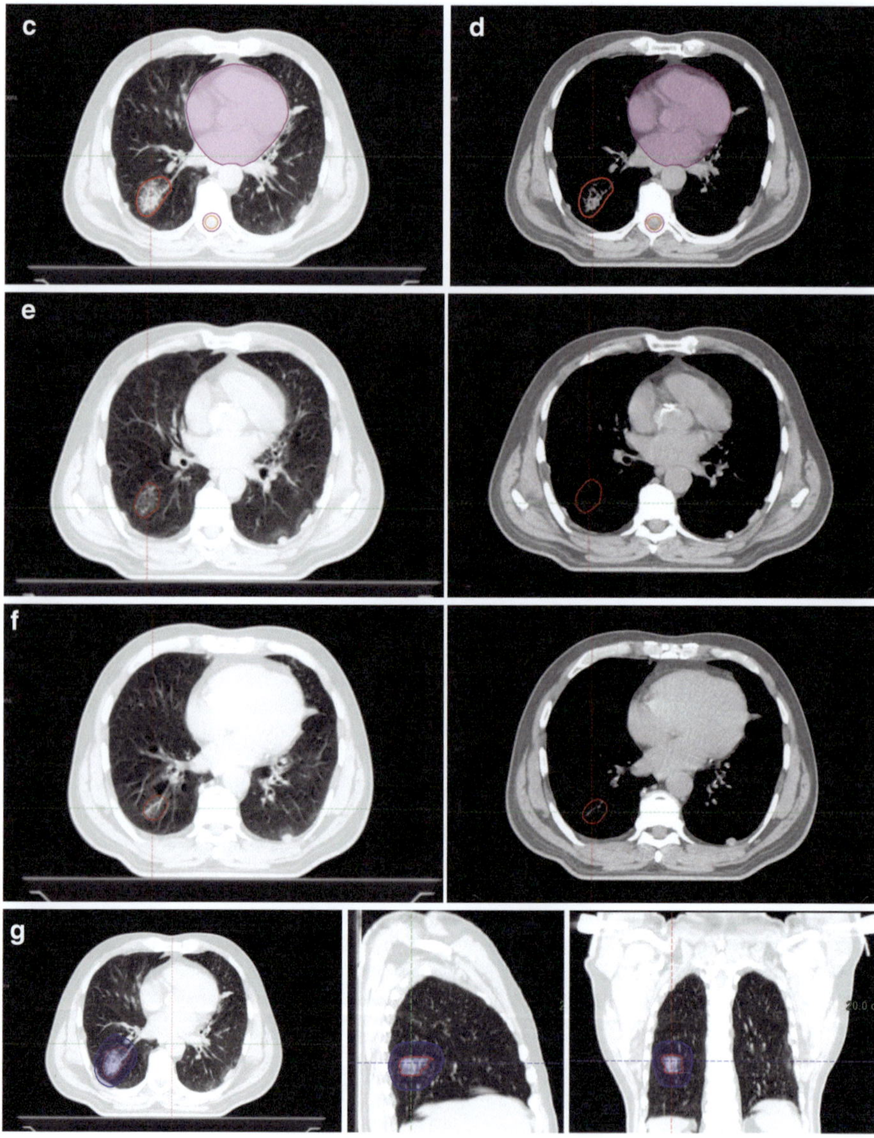

Fig. 5.2 (continued)

Case 3

An 83-year-old woman presented with 3 months of abdominal discomfort and altered bowel habit. A colonoscopy was normal. CT scan of chest, abdomen, and pelvis showed a 7 × 5 cm retroperitoneal mass in the upper abdomen encasing the IVC. A percutaneous CT-guided biopsy revealed Grade 1–2 FL. Staging PET/CT confirmed FDG-avidity within the retroperitoneal mass, with no abnormal uptake elsewhere (Fig. 5.3a). Staging bone marrow aspirate and trephine biopsy was negative. The disease was designated to be stage 1A.

Definitive RT was prescribed to a dose of 24 Gy in 12 fractions over 2.5 weeks (Fig. 5.3 b-d). Intravenous contrast was withheld for the planning CT scan due to renal impairment (chronically raised creatinine and lowered estimated glomerular filtration rate (eGFR)). Treatment was delivered with VMAT plan. Mean kidney dose was kept below 5Gy. Complete metabolic response was achieved on the post-treatment PET/CT scan.

Case 4

A 59-year-old woman, with a 11-year history of Stage IVA FL, was referred for consideration of local radiotherapy for a symptomatic right parotid mass. On clinical examination, the patient had a palpable right parotid mass measuring 5 cm in maximum diameter, with subcutaneous extension over the right temple; the overlying skin was taut and red. Investigations included staging PET/CT, revealing a solitary site of FDG-avidity in the right parotid mass with SUVmax of 15.4, and an ultrasound-guided biopsy confirmed low-grade FL with no evidence of high-grade transformation. Low dose RT was prescribed for symptom control: 4 Gy in two fractions. A planning PET/CT was performed with the head and neck stabilized in a thermoplastic mask (Fig. 5.4). Following RT, complete clinical, radiological, and metabolic responses were achieved at this site.

Case 5

An 89-year-old woman was diagnosed 20 years ago with stage 1A disease and treated with definitive RT to the right groin. Three years ago, she experienced disease relapse and was treated with dose-reduced chemo-immunotherapy, achieving a complete response. The patient now presented with a symptomatic mass in the left axilla. Re-staging PET/CT demonstrated relapse above and below the diaphragm (Stage 3) with prominent nodal relapse in the left axilla. Biopsy of the left axilla mass confirmed Grade 1–2 FL, with no evidence of high-grade transformation. Palliative RT, 4 Gy in two fractions, was prescribed to the site of symptomatic progression in the left axilla, thereby avoiding systemic therapy (Fig. 5.5).

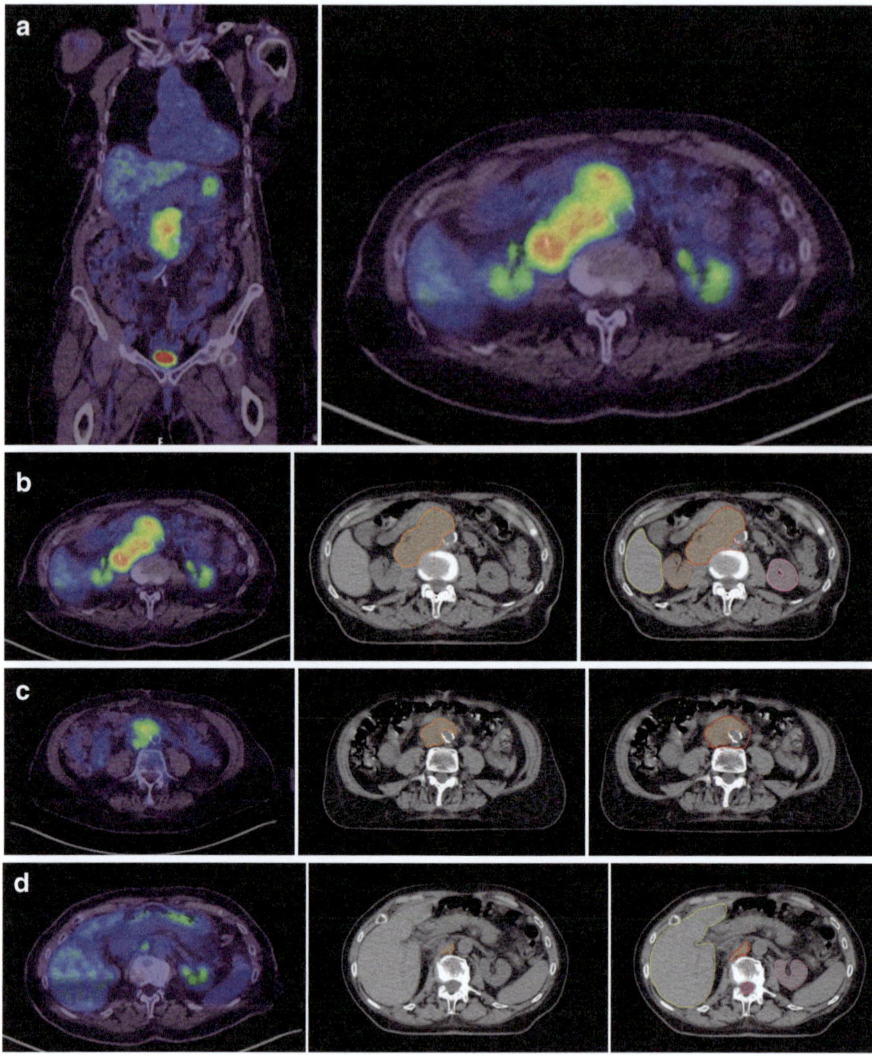

Fig. 5.3 (**a**) Staging FDG-PET/CT. **Left panel:** coronal view. **Right panel:** axial view. (**b–d**) Corresponding axial slices through the target volume on the diagnostic PET/CT and planning CT. **Left panel:** Axial slices on the diagnostic PET/CT. Note the artifact/image degradation in the posterior portion of the image due to placement of the arms by the sides. **Middle panel:** Planning CT with GTV contoured (orange). Note that the kidneys and large vessels are not opacified and the main mass is not enhanced (no IV contrast). **Right panel:** Planning CT with CTV and OAR outlined: CTV (red), liver (yellow), R kidney (orange), L kidney (pink), bowel bag (not shown). (**b**) Axial slice at the level of the maximum width of the mass. Note that CTV (red) is very similar to GTV (orange) with minor extension behind the aorta (calcified); this was deemed appropriate in this case due to confident localization of the well-defined mass and adjacent anatomical boundaries and also to avoid increasing the dose to the kidneys. (**c**) Lower slice of CTV (red). (**d**) Upper slice of CTV (red). PTV was derived using a grown with 10 mm isotropic margin around CTV (not shown)

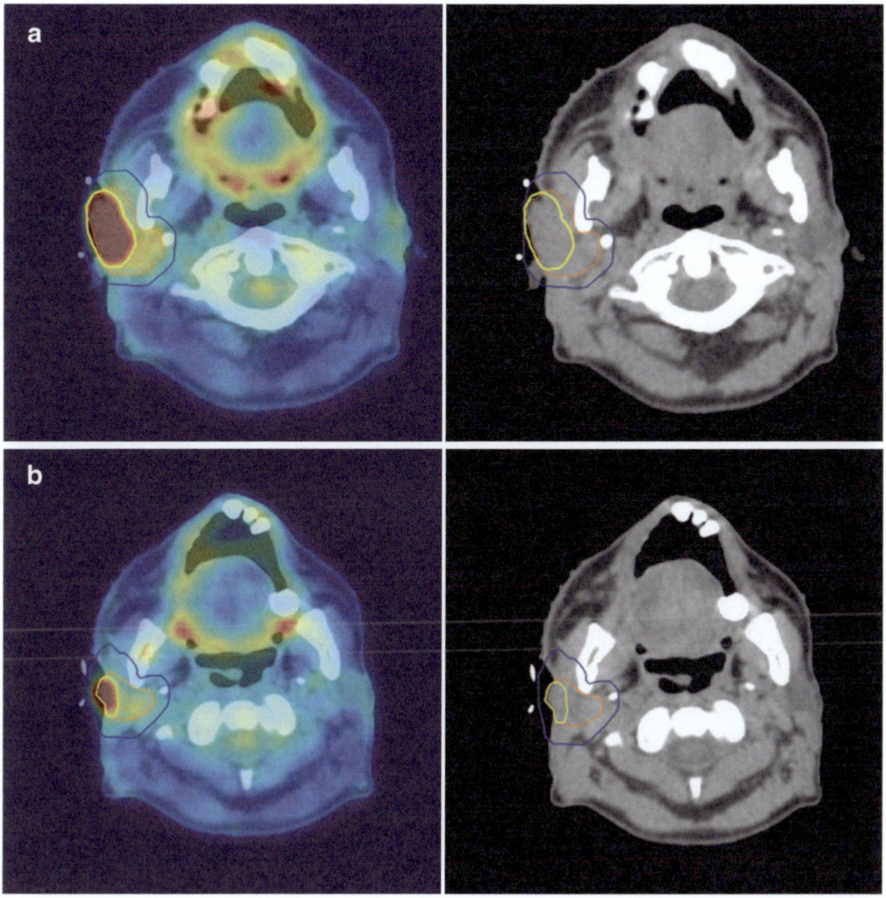

Fig. 5.4 (**a**, **b**) Planning PET/CT images: left panel demonstrates the fused PET and CT axial images, right panel demonstrates CT axial images. The FDG-avid intra-parotid mass is contoured in yellow. The CTV (orange) comprises the whole organ, thus encompassing the less FDG-avid, subclinical disease. The PTV (blue) is a 0.5 cm expansion from the CTV, which is customary for patients with thermoplastic mask stabilization. (**c**, **d**) Clinically and radiologically, the patient had subcutaneous thickening beyond the parotid gland antero-superiorly. The area of intense FDG-avidity is contoured in yellow. The CTV (orange) includes the FDG-avid disease and is extended to cover this subcutaneous thickening on CT. The PTV (blue) is a 0.5 cm expansion of the CTV. (**c**) Axial image. (**d**) Sagittal image

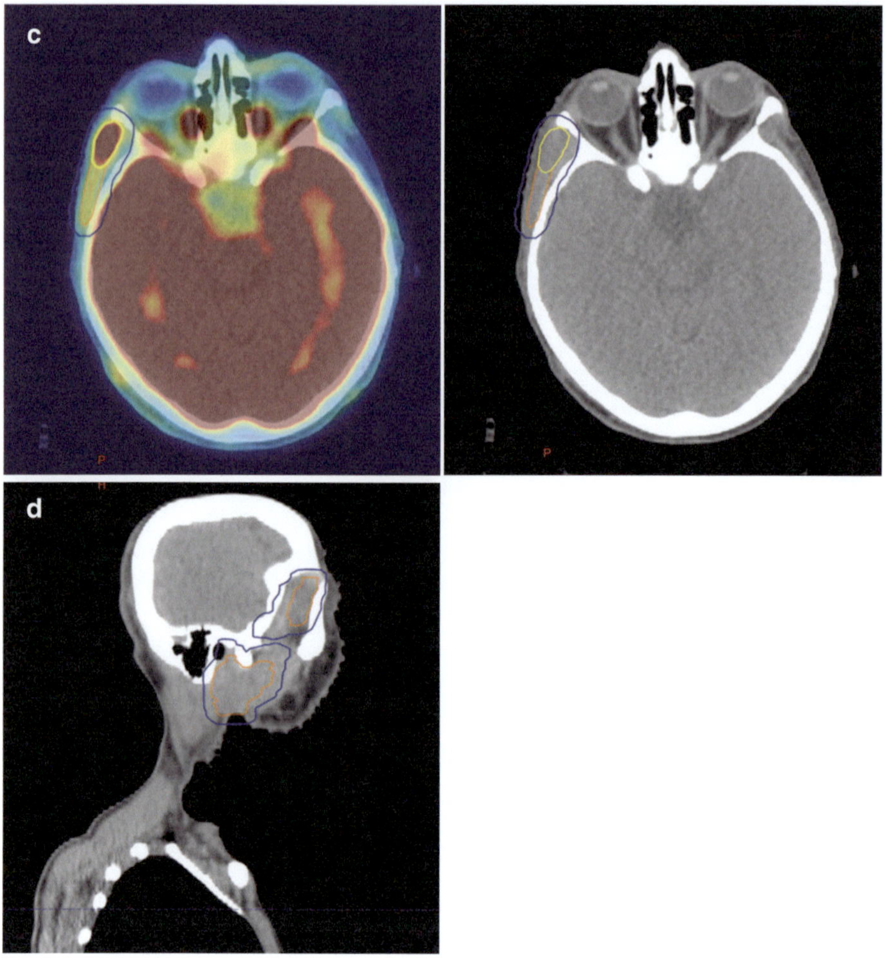

Fig. 5.4 (continued)

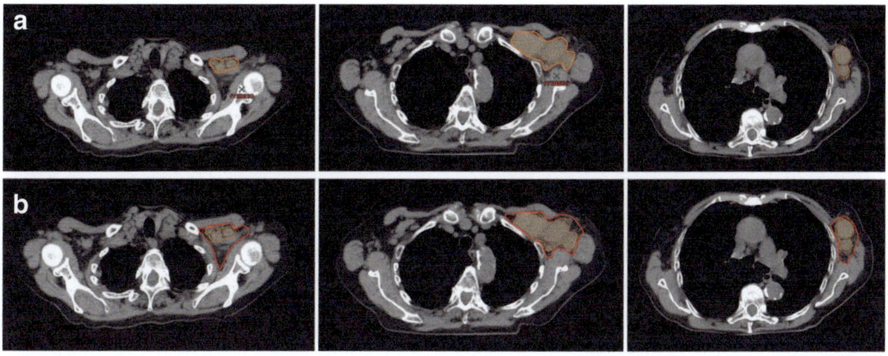

Fig. 5.5 (**a**) Planning CT scan with GTV (orange) and CTV (red) in the left axilla. Note the presence of small volume nodes in right axilla. (**a**) GTV (orange) includes all visible nodes in the left axilla. **Left panel:** upper part of GTV. **Middle panel:** middle of GTV. **Right panel:** lower part of CTV. (**b**) CTV (red) includes the GTV (orange) and extends to the boundaries of the nodal compartment (axilla). **Left panel:** upper part of CTV. **Middle panel:** middle of CTV. **Right panel:** lower part of CTV

Part 4: Special Considerations

- Completely excised stage IA: In cases when all macroscopic disease is completely removed as part of an excisional biopsy, the standard of care is not well defined. However, in fit patients with expected longevity, treatment with ISRT may be considered to eradicate any subclinical disease in the local nodes, with curative intent.
- Variants of FL:
  - Duodenal-type FL: Firstline treatment options include watchful waiting, ISRT, or rituximab. If FL is confined to the duodenum on staging endoscopy/enteroscopy, ISRT may be considered in which the CTV comprises the entire length of the duodenum [27].
  - Paediatric-type FL: This variant is generally associated with limited stage. Patients with completely excised disease may be managed with watchful waiting. Given that paediatric-type FL is commonly diagnosed in young patients and that excellent outcomes are expected from conservative approaches, RT is typically deferred to avoid the risks of secondary radiation-induced malignancies [29].

References

1. Howlader N, Noone AM, Krapcho M, Miller D, Brest A, Yu M, et al. (2020) SEER Cancer Statistics Review, 1975–2017, National Cancer Institute. 12 May 2020 [cited 2020 12 May 2020]. Available from: https://seer.cancer.gov/csr/1975_2017/.
2. Surveillance, epidemiology and end results program, Cancer Stat Facts: NHL—follicular lymphoma Bethesda, MD: National Cancer Institute; 2020 [Available from: https://seer.cancer.gov/statfacts/html/follicular.html.

3. Ambinder AJ, Shenoy PJ, Malik N, Maggioncalda A, Nastoupil LJ, Flowers CR. Exploring risk factors for follicular lymphoma. Adv Hematol. 2012;2012:626035.
4. Chihara D, Nastoupil LJ, Williams JN, Lee P, Koff JL, Flowers CR. New insights into the epidemiology of non-Hodgkin lymphoma and implications for therapy. Expert Rev Anticancer Ther. 2015;15(5):531–44.
5. Ekström Smedby K, Vajdic CM, Falster M, Engels EA, Martínez-Maza O, Turner J, et al. Autoimmune disorders and risk of non-Hodgkin lymphoma subtypes: a pooled analysis within the InterLymph consortium. Blood. 2008;111(8):4029–38.
6. Morton LM, Hartge P, Holford TR, Holly EA, Chiu BC, Vineis P, et al. Cigarette smoking and risk of non-Hodgkin lymphoma: a pooled analysis from the international lymphoma epidemiology consortium (interlymph). Cancer Epidemiol Biomarkers Prev. 2005;14(4):925–33.
7. Bains P, Al Tourah A, Campbell BA, Pickles T, Gascoyne RD, Connors JM, et al. Incidence of transformation to aggressive lymphoma in limited-stage follicular lymphoma treated with radiotherapy. Ann Oncol. 2013;24(2):428–32.
8. Al-Tourah AJ, Gill KK, Chhanabhai M, Hoskins PJ, Klasa RJ, Savage KJ, et al. Population-based analysis of incidence and outcome of transformed non-Hodgkin's lymphoma. J Clin Oncol Off J Am Soc Clin Oncol. 2008;26(32):5165–9.
9. Follicular Lymphoma. In: Swerdlow SH CE, Harris NL, Jaffe ES, Pileri SA, Stein H, Thiele J, editor. WHO Classification of Tumours of Haematopoietic and Lymphoid Tissues Revised Fourth Edition. WHO Classification of Tumours. 2017. p. 266–79.
10. Dada R. Diagnosis and management of follicular lymphoma: a comprehensive review. Eur J Haematol. 2019;103(3):152–63.
11. Alaggio R, Amador C, Anagnostopoulos I, Attygalle AD, Barreto de Oliveira Araujo I, Berti E, et al. The 5th edition of the World Health Organization classification of haematolymphoid tumours: lymphoid neoplasms. Leukemia. 2022;36(7):1720–48.
12. Campo E, Jaffe ES, Cook JR, Quintanilla-Martinez L, Swerdlow SH, Anderson KC, et al. The international consensus classification of mature lymphoid neoplasms: a report from the Clinical Advisory Committee. Blood. 2022;140(11):1229–53.
13. Dreyling M, Ghielmini M, Rule S, Salles G, Vitolo U, Ladetto M. Newly diagnosed and relapsed follicular lymphoma: ESMO clinical practice guidelines for diagnosis, treatment and follow-up. Ann Oncol. 2016;27(suppl 5):v83–90.
14. Illidge T, Specht L, Yahalom J, Aleman B, Berthelsen AK, Constine L, et al. Modern radiation therapy for nodal non-Hodgkin lymphoma-target definition and dose guidelines from the International Lymphoma Radiation Oncology Group. Int J Radiat Oncol Biol Phys. 2014;89(1):49–58.
15. Hoskin PJ, Kirkwood AA, Popova B, Smith P, Robinson M, Gallop-Evans E, et al. 4 Gy versus 24 Gy radiotherapy for patients with indolent lymphoma (FORT): a randomised phase 3 non-inferiority trial. Lancet Oncol. 2014;15(4):457–63.
16. Brady JL, Binkley MS, Hajj C, Chelius M, Chau K, Balogh A, et al. Definitive radiotherapy for localized follicular lymphoma staged by (18)F-FDG PET-CT: a collaborative study by ILROG. Blood. 2019;133(3):237–45.
17. Lo A, Campbell BA, Pickles T, Aquino-Parsons C, Sehn LH, Connors J, et al. Long-term outcomes for patients with limited-stage follicular lymphoma: update of a population-based study. Blood. 2020;136:1006.
18. Campbell BA, Voss N, Woods R, Gascoyne RD, Morris J, Pickles T, et al. Long-term outcomes for patients with limited stage follicular lymphoma: involved regional radiotherapy versus involved node radiotherapy. Cancer. 2010;116(16):3797–806.
19. MacManus M, Fisher R, Roos D, O'Brien P, Macann A, Davis S, et al. Randomized trial of systemic therapy after involved-field radiotherapy in patients with early-stage follicular lymphoma: TROG 9903. J Clin Oncol Off J Am Soc Clin Oncol. 2018;36(29):2918–25.
20. Herfarth K, Borchmann P, Schnaidt S, Hohloch K, Budach V, Engelhard M, et al. Rituximab with involved field irradiation for early-stage nodal follicular lymphoma: results of the MIR study. HemaSphere. 2018;2(6):e160.

21. Hoskin P, Popova B, Schofield O, Brammer C, Robinson M, Brunt AM, et al. 4 Gy versus 24 Gy radiotherapy for follicular and marginal zone lymphoma (FoRT): long-term follow-up of a multi-Centre, randomised, phase 3, non-inferiority trial. Lancet Oncol. 2021;22(3):332–40.
22. MacManus MP, Hicks RJ, Bressel M, Campbell BA, Wirth A, Ryan G, et al. Durable complete remission and long-term survival in FDG-PET staged patients with stage III follicular lymphoma, treated with wide-field radiation therapy. Cancers. 2020;12:4.
23. Andraos T, Ayoub Z, Nastoupil L, Pinnix C, Milgrom S, Gunther J, et al. Early stage extranodal follicular lymphoma: characteristics, management, and outcomes. Clin Lymphoma Myeloma Leuk. 2019;19(6):381–9.
24. Mikhaeel NG, Milgrom SA, Terezakis S, Berthelsen AK, Hodgson D, Eich HT, et al. The optimal use of imaging in radiation therapy for lymphoma: guidelines from the international lymphoma radiation oncology group (ILROG). Int J Radiat Oncol Biol Phys. 2019;104(3):501–12.
25. Campbell BA, Plastaras JP, Savage KJ. Keeping our finger on the pulse: reaffirming the role of radiation therapy in the curative management of early stage follicular lymphoma. Int J Radiat Oncol Biol Phys. 2019;105(3):459–65.
26. Wirth A, Mikhaeel NG, Pauline Aleman BM, Pinnix CC, Constine LS, Wilmot JP, et al. Involved site radiation therapy in adult lymphomas: an overview of international lymphoma radiation oncology group guidelines. Int J Radiat Oncol Biol Phys. 2020;107:909.
27. Yahalom J, Illidge T, Specht L, Hoppe RT, Li YX, Tsang R, et al. Modern radiation therapy for extranodal lymphomas: field and dose guidelines from the International Lymphoma Radiation Oncology Group. Int J Radiat Oncol Biol Phys. 2015;92(1):11–31.
28. Lowry L, Smith P, Qian W, Falk S, Benstead K, Illidge T, et al. Reduced dose radiotherapy for local control in non-Hodgkin lymphoma: a randomised phase III trial. Radiother Oncol. 2011;100(1):86–92.
29. Sandlund JT, Martin MG. Non-Hodgkin lymphoma across the paediatric and adolescent and young adult age spectrum. Hematology Am Soc Hematol Educ Program. 2016;2016(1):589–97.

Further Reading

ILROG Guidelines

Illidge T, Specht L, Yahalom J, Aleman B, Berthelsen AK, Constine L, et al. Modern radiation therapy for nodal non-Hodgkin lymphoma-target definition and dose guidelines from the International Lymphoma Radiation Oncology Group. Int J Radiat Oncol Biol Phys. 2014;89(1):49–58.

Mikhaeel NG, Milgrom SA, Terezakis S, Berthelsen AK, Hodgson D, Eich HT, et al. The optimal use of imaging in radiation therapy for lymphoma: guidelines from the International Lymphoma Radiation Oncology Group (ILROG). Int J Radiat Oncol Biol Phys. 2019;104(3):501–12.

Wirth A, Mikhaeel NG, Pauline Aleman BM, Pinnix CC, Constine LS, Wilmot JP, et al. Involved site radiation therapy in adult lymphomas: an overview of international lymphoma radiation oncology group guidelines. Int J Radiat Oncol Biol Phys. 2020;107:909.

Yahalom J, Illidge T, Specht L, Hoppe RT, Li YX, Tsang R, et al. Modern radiation therapy for extranodal lymphomas: field and dose guidelines from the International Lymphoma Radiation Oncology Group. Int J Radiat Oncol Biol Phys. 2015;92(1):11–31.

6 Extranodal MALT Lymphoma

Yolanda D. Tseng and Richard Tsang

Contents

Y. D. Tseng (✉)
Department of Radiation Oncology, University of Washington, Seattle, WA, USA

Clinical Research Division, Fred Hutchinson Cancer Center, Seattle, WA, USA
e-mail: Ydt2@uw.edu

R. Tsang
Department of Radiation Oncology, Princess Margaret Cancer Centre, Toronto, ON, USA
e-mail: richard.tsang@rmp.uhn.ca

C. Pinnix et al. (eds.), *Target Volume Delineation in Hematologic Malignancies*, Practical Guides in Radiation Oncology,
https://doi.org/10.1007/978-3-031-67722-9_6

Part 1: Background and Epidemiology

- Marginal zone lymphoma (MZL), an indolent, mature B-cell non-Hodgkin lymphoma (NHL), has three subtypes with different clinical characteristics and prognoses [1]:
  - Extranodal Marginal Zone Lymphoma (EMZL) of mucosa-associated lymphoma tissue (MALT) (5–10% of NHL)
  - Nodal MZL (1% of NHL)
  - Splenic MZL (<1% of NHL)
- Patients with EMZL are typically diagnosed in the seventh decade of life (median, 67 years) with a slight predominance among females compared to males (55% vs. 45%). Patients of non-Hispanic white race comprise over 70% of EMZL cases, while patients of white Hispanic, Asian, and African American race each comprise ~10% of cases [1].
- EMZL most commonly involves the gastrointestinal tract, ocular adnexa, lung, skin, and salivary glands, with the distribution of sites varying across race and gender [1].
- Given the close association between EMZL and autoimmune diseases and infectious etiologies (Table 6.1), the pathogenesis of EMZL is hypothesized to occur secondary to chronic antigenic stimulation of the target organ [2].
- Patients with EMZL have variable clinical presentations given the different extranodal organs that may be involved. Most patients (60–70%) present with stage I/II disease, small tumor burden, and excellent performance status.
  - Primary gastric involvement, which comprises 40–50% of EMZL cases, may be associated with dyspepsia with or without signs of chronic bleeding, and less frequently, abdominal pain and/or weight loss.
  - Involvement of the ocular adnexa, which includes the conjunctiva and lacrimal gland, may cause conjunctival swelling and irritation, whereas intra- or retro-orbital involvement may lead to exophthalmos.
- For patients with localized disease, curative-intent treatment options include radiotherapy or in patients whose tumor harbors evidence of infection (e.g., *H. pylori,* typically in gastric MALT lymphoma), appropriate antibiotic ther-

Table 6.1 Disease associations with extranodal marginal zone lymphoma [2]

EMZL site	Chronic immune reaction
Stomach	*Helicobacter pylori*
Intestinal	*Campylobacter jejuni*
Spleen	Hepatitis C virus (HCV)
Ocular adnexa	*Chlamydia psittaci*
Skin	*Borrelia burgdorferi*
Salivary glands	Sjogren syndrome
Thyroid	Chronic autoimmune thyroiditis (Hashimoto disease)

apy for eradication. Radiotherapy is considered first-line therapy for patients without associated infections and/or whose tumor fails to regress after antibiotic therapy.
  - For gastric EMZL that are *H. pylori* positive, testing for t(11;18)(q21;q21) by PCR or FISH should be considered, given the associated higher rates of relapse or no response to antibiotics in the presence of t(11;18) [3].
- Prognosis varies by extranodal site: thyroid and gastric EMZL have the lowest risk of recurrence with 90–100% freedom from progression [4, 5], whereas ocular adnexal and salivary gland EMZL is associated with a 60–70% freedom from progression [4].

Preradiotherapy Imaging and Evaluation

- Multiplanar magnetic resonance imaging (MRI) of the face/orbit with and without gadolinium should be considered for EMZL of orbital structures. Tumors may be T1 and T2 isointense to muscle and generally are homogeneously enhancing. MALT lymphoma of the conjunctiva however may not demonstrate imaging abnormalities on MRI or PET-CT, and therefore clinical examination and documentation with medical photographs are essential.
- Adequate staging procedures are required as up to 25% of patients with gastric MALT and 50% of patients with nongastric MALT have multiorgan involvement [6]. Staging includes contrast-enhanced CT scan of the chest, abdomen, and pelvis and bone marrow biopsy. PET-CT can be considered although only 50% of EMZL are FDG-avid [7], which is influenced by the site and growth pattern. For some sites such as skin and stomach, growth and spread occurs as a thin layer and will often be FDG negative.
  - For patients with gastric EMZL, endoscopy with an adequate number of random biopsies is required to map out the extent of the disease and establish a pathological diagnosis, including the presence of concurrent *H. pylori* infection. Imaging of the ocular adnexa, examination of the ear, nose, and throat, and/or colonoscopy may be considered for patients with clinical symptoms/suspicion of involvement.
  - For patients with nongastric EMZL, endoscopy with multiple biopsies and/or colonoscopy may be considered for patients with clinical symptoms/suspicion of involvement.
- Basic laboratory studies include complete blood count with differential, chemistries with liver and renal function, electrolytes, lactate dehydrogenase, and serum protein electrophoresis.

Part 2: Management and Treatment of Extranodal Marginal Zone Lymphoma

Gastric EMZL: Principles of Management

- In patients whose tumor has evidence of *H. pylori* infection and absence of t(11;18), frontline treatment is antibiotic eradication of *H. pylori*; 80% of these patients will have complete regression of their gastric EMZL on subsequent endoscopies, though the time to complete response may be slow (15% with CR >12 months) [3].
- Radiotherapy is indicated for gastric EMZL without evidence of *H. pylori* infection, or recurrent/persistent disease after antibiotic treatment.
- Given that tumors with t(11;18) predict for suboptimal response to *H. pylori* eradication, radiation may be considered the initial treatment for these tumors. Alternatively, given the low-toxicity profile, antibiotic therapy and close follow-up may be considered with a chance of long-term control in a minority of patients.
- Single-agent rituximab is reserved for patients with recurrent disease after radiotherapy, though this is not considered curative [8].

Gastric EMZL: General Considerations for Radiotherapy

- Radiotherapy for gastric EMZL is delivered to the entire stomach with involved site radiation therapy (ISRT), which utilizes 3D-treatment planning and incorporation of techniques to minimize dose to adjacent normal tissues such as the heart, kidneys, and liver.
  - Given that disease in the stomach can be multifocal, the entire organ is treated in its entirety. Peri-gastric lymph nodes are not routinely included within the CTV/ITV unless they are involved.
- Patients should be simulated supine and immobilized arms up with an armed shuttle or Vaclock cradle.
- To ensure reproducibility in the size of the stomach for daily treatment, patients should be simulated and treated in the fasting state (e.g., at least 4–6 h without anything by mouth).
- Small volume oral contrast (e.g., barium, ~50 cc) may be used to better visualize the stomach; IV contrast may be considered for improved visualization of adjacent lymph nodes.
- As the stomach moves with respiration, motion management should be incorporated as part of treatment planning. These may include:
  - Use of a 4D CT scan and planning on the average intensity projection (AVE-IP).
  - Use of deep inspiration breath hold (DIBH). DIBH has been shown to reduce radiation dose to surrounding normal tissues including the heart, right kidney, lungs, and liver, especially coupled with contemporary planning techniques such as IMRT [9, 10]. End exhalation breath holds may be more challenging

for patients to perform, resulting in shorter breath-hold durations than end inhalation [11]. Whereas breath hold at inspiration may be associated with a lower dose to the heart [9, 10], end exhalation breath holds may increase the distance between upper abdominal organs at risk (OAR) [12]. Generally, at least 2–3 scans are obtained to confirm reproducibility of breath hold.

  - In the absence of patient-specific respiratory motion information through a 4D CT scan or DIBH, one may consider repeat 3D imaging to measure tumor motion between two extreme states of the breathing cycle (e.g., normal inhale and exhale), or an empiric expansion of CTV target volume. This is the least preferred option given the potential of treating a larger target volume and/or missing the target volume if empiric margins do not adequately capture all motion.

- Axial CT images should be acquired in 2.5–3 mm or smaller slices. To ensure adequate dose/volume histograms for OAR, CT simulation scans should include the entire heart, liver, and kidneys. Inclusion of the entire lung may also be considered if feasible (e.g., patient breath hold).
- Generally, three target volumes are useful to construct for radiation planning: gross tumor volume (GTV) if visible on CT scan, clinical target volume (CTV) or internal target volume (ITV), and planning target volume (PTV). These volumes are further described in Table 6.2.

Table 6.2 Planning target definitions for treatment of gastric EMZL lymphoma

Volume	Description
Gross tumor volume (GTV)	• Contains gross tumor volume as identified on diagnostic imaging, if visible
Clinical target volume (CTV)	• Entire stomach from esophageal sphincter to pyloric sphincter
Internal target volume (ITV)	• Contains the CTV plus an internal margin that accounts for variation in CTV shape, size, and position • When a 4D CT scan is available, stomach motion and shape should be assessed over the average intensity projection (AVE-IP), maximum intensity project (MIP), and cine scans • In patients treated with deep inspiration breath hold, the location, size, and shape of the stomach can be evaluated across the serial scans obtained at simulation and incorporated into an ITV
Planning target volume (PTV)	• Contains CTV or ITV plus a margin to account for setup uncertainties associated with patient position and beam alignment • CTV-to-PTV expansions are patient- and institution-specific; any recommendations in this chapter or elsewhere must be adjusted to reflect factors unique to the patient and institution but generally include margins of 7–10 mm
Organs at risk (OAR)	• Includes uninvolved normal structures at risk of RT-related toxicity for which RT planning or dose may be altered. During treatment of the stomach, these generally include both kidneys, liver, heart, lungs, spinal cord, spleen, and bowel

- Acceptable radiation techniques include 3D conformal, intensity-modulated radiotherapy (IMRT), or volumetric-modulated arc therapy (VMAT). DIBH should be used when possible to reduce the dose to the normal tissues, especially the heart [9, 10].
  - 3D conformal techniques typically use four beams from the anterior, posterior, right, and left lateral directions (see Case 1).
  - IMRT/VMAT should be used when possible to further lower the dose to surrounding normal tissues [13].
- Given potential changes in gastric filling, daily volumetric image-guided radiation should be considered (e.g., cone beam CT [CBCT]) to ensure adequate treatment of the stomach, especially when more conformal techniques such as IMRT or VMAT are used.
- Doses between 24 and 30 Gy given in 1.5–2 Gy per fraction are associated with excellent local control and rates of response [14–16]. Recent data suggests that doses of ~24 Gy are adequate [15–17].

Nongastric EMZL: Principles of Management

- Radiotherapy alone, 24–30 Gy in conventional fractionation [17], is considered the definitive treatment for localized EMZL.
  - Curative-intent radiation is appropriate even for the involvement of both orbits, which is considered stage I.
- In patients for whom a generous biopsy or complete resection was performed (e.g., resection of conjunctival or lacrimal gland lesions), adjuvant radiation may be considered for local control, especially in the setting of a positive surgical margin. However, close observation may be considered in older adults and/or asymptomatic patients; risk of clinical recurrence may be 40–50% [18].

Nongastric EMZL: General Considerations for Radiotherapy by Site

- *Thyroid, breast, and salivary glands*: The CTV is the entire extranodal organ using ISRT (Table 6.3).
  - Elective coverage of draining lymph nodes (e.g., upper neck for a parotid lesion) is not required unless there is a radiographic suggestion of involvement or if a portion of the lymph nodes are covered given close proximity to the CTV.
- *Lung and skin*: The CTV is the GTV or iGTV with a margin for potential microscopic disease.
  - For localized, cutaneous lesions, a margin of 1.5–2 cm from GTV to field edge may typically be used. The margin to ensure treatment of microscopic disease beneath the lesion may be modified by the underlying soft tissue thickness and whether there is intact bone and/or fascia that may serve as an

Table 6.3 Planning target definitions for treatment of nongastric EMZL lymphoma

Volume	Description
Gross tumor volume (GTV)	• Contains gross tumor volume as identified on diagnostic imaging and/or physical examination, if visible
Clinical target volume (CTV)	• *Thyroid, breast, and salivary glands*: Resection bed (if applicable) and entire residual extranodal organ • *Lung*: GTV with margin to account for potential microscopic disease, which may vary based on lesion size and ability to safely irradiate a larger volume • *Ocular adnexa* – Conjunctiva and eyelid: Entire upper and lower conjunctiva including reflection to the fornices – Nonconjunctival lesions: Entire bony orbit extending to the orbital apex. Partial orbital radiation may be considered in cases of well-defined disease (i.e., lacrimal gland) [20]
Internal target volume (ITV) [lung]	• Contains the CTV plus an internal margin that accounts for variation in CTV shape, size, and position • When a 4D CT scan is available, the motion of the lesion should be assessed over the average intensity projection (AVE-IP), maximum intensity project (MIP), and cine scans • In patients treated with deep inspiration breath hold, the location, size, and shape of the CTV can be evaluated across the serial scans obtained at simulation and incorporated into the ITV
Planning target volume (PTV)	• Contains CTV or ITV plus a margin to account for setup uncertainties associated with patient position and beam alignment • CTV-to-PTV expansions are patient- and institution-specific; any recommendations in this chapter or elsewhere must be adjusted to reflect factors unique to the patient and institution
Organs at risk (OAR)	• Includes uninvolved normal structures at risk of RT-related toxicity for which RT planning or dose may be altered. The OARs will vary based on extranodal site irradiated and may include: Adjacent salivary glands (parotid, submandibular gland, minor salivary glands of the oral cavity), lacrimal gland, lung, and heart

anatomic barrier. If needed, patients should be scanned to confirm the thickness of the lesion to ensure the proper electron energy is selected.
  - Motion management strategies (4D CT, DIBH) should be incorporated to delineate the ITV or CTV for lung MZL lesions.
- *Ocular adnexa*: Depending on the ocular adnexal structure involved, radiation may be directed to the partial or whole bony orbit.
  - Conjunctival and eyelid lesions may be treated with electrons, sparing the posterior orbit.
  - For retrobulbar lesions, cases of poorly defined orbital EZML involvement, and/or deep conjunctival lesions, the whole bony orbit is generally irradiated. Partial orbital radiation may be associated with a local recurrence outside the irradiated field, which has been seen with older [19] but not in more recent series [20].

Part 3: Cases

Case 1: Gastric EMZL

An 88-year-old man presented with weakness and melena and was found to have a single ulcer of the distal body of the stomach. Biopsy showed chronic inflammation without evidence of *H. pylori* infection. On repeat endoscopy, the ulcer was noted to be healing, but there were residual micronodularities, which on biopsy demonstrated extranodal marginal zone lymphoma, *H. pylori* negative. There was no evidence of distant disease nor abnormal perigastric lymph nodes on staging. The duodenum appeared normal on endoscopy (Fig. 6.1).

Case 2: Cutaneous EMZL

A 49-year-old woman incidentally noted a lump over the right lateral back and was diagnosed with primary cutaneous marginal zone lymphoma. CT scan of the chest, abdomen, and pelvis showed no evidence of distant involvement. In the setting of persistent disease despite intralesional Kenalog for 1 year, she underwent definitive radiotherapy with electrons (Fig. 6.2).

Case 3: Ocular EMZL

A 30-year-old female presented with right eye soreness and swelling for 1 week and was incidentally noted to have a salmon-colored lesion of the right lower lateral conjunctiva. On staging, she was found to have stage IAE right conjunctival MALT (Fig. 6.3).

Case 4: Salivary Gland EMZL

A 64-year-old woman with history of rheumatoid arthritis noted a slowly growing left cheek mass. CT scan demonstrated an enhancing nodularity superficial to the left parotid and masseter muscle. This was observed for 2 years and noted to progress in size and extent. A left superficial parotidectomy with facial nerve dissection demonstrated MZL. CT scan of the chest, abdomen, and pelvis and bone marrow biopsy confirmed no evidence of distant disease (Fig. 6.4).

Case 5: Thyroid EMZL

A 48-year-old man presented with a 2 cm right thyroid nodule. On ultrasound, he had bilateral hypoechoic thyroid nodules, the largest 2 cm on the right and 1 cm on the left. FNA and core needle biopsies of the right-sided nodule yielded small

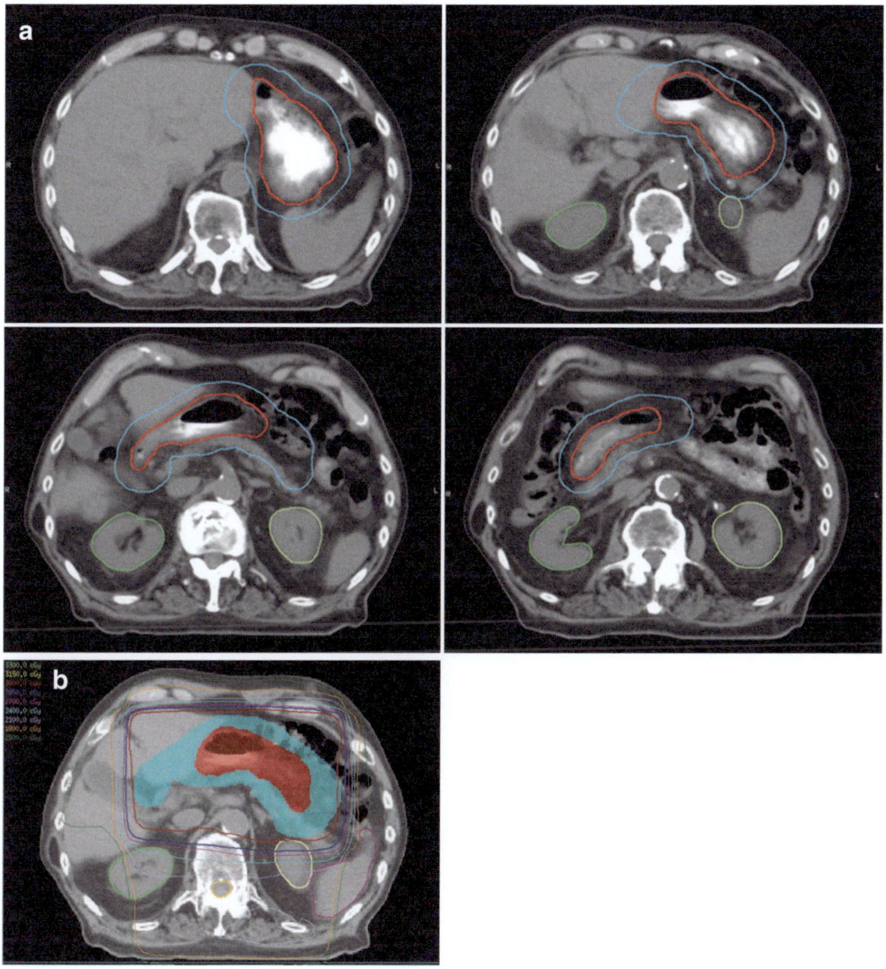

Fig. 6.1 (**a**) Axial AVE-IP images reconstructed from 4D CT scan used for radiation treatment planning. The patient, who fasted for 3 h before the scan, was given 40 cc barium by mouth with a 10 min delay. ITV contours are in red, and PTV contours are in blue. In addition to the AVE-IP, the maximum intensity projection (MIP) and cine are helpful in capturing the entire extent of stomach motion with respiration. (**b**) The patient was treated to 30 Gy in 20 fractions, 1.5 Gy per fraction, with daily CBCT. A 3D conformal technique using a four-field box with 18 MV photons was used. Based on the patient's 4D CT, the stomach target was noted to have a 1.2 cm superior/inferior, 0.5 cm anterior/posterior, and minimal, if any, left/right motion. Because respiratory motion was accounted for in the ITV, a 1 cm PTV margin was used. Note that normal tissue exposure may be reduced with a DIBH technique [9]. (**c**) Dose/volume histogram of radiation plan. The left kidney volume receiving 20 Gy or higher (V20) was 13%, the right kidney V20 was 15%, and liver V30 was 10%

c

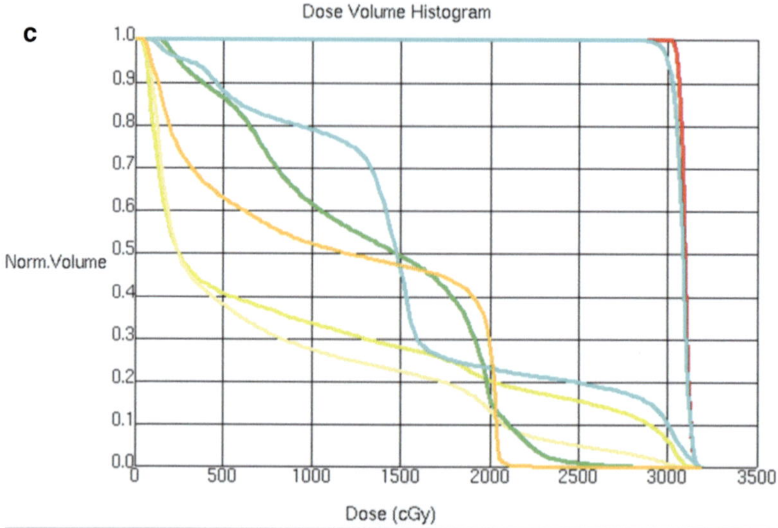

Line Type	ROI	Trial or Record	Min.	Max.	Mean
	ITV_stomach	4 field	2987.2	3167.6	3094.5
	Kidney_L	4 field	52.3	3066.7	731.0
	Kidney_R	4 field	134.5	2803.5	1337.9
	Liver	4 field	75.7	3192.5	1572.5
	PTV_stomach	4 field	2646.7	3189.8	3077.5
	Spinal canal	4 field	48.7	2237.1	1146.1

Fig. 6.1 (continued)

lymphoid cells, kappa restricted, suggestive of lymphoproliferative disorder but not diagnostic of lymphoma. A right hemithyroidectomy, CT scan of the chest, abdomen, and pelvis, and bone marrow biopsy were negative for the disease. PET scan showed abnormal uptake in the remaining left thyroid lobe with SUV_{max} of 9.1. No other significant abnormality was noted, including cervical or mediastinal lymphadenopathy (Fig. 6.5).

Case 6: Lung EMZL

A 61-year-old woman with no smoking history presented with nonspecific shortness of breath. A CT scan showed a spiculated lesion in the left upper lobe, 2.2 cm in maximum dimension, with a high likelihood of malignancy. She had a lung

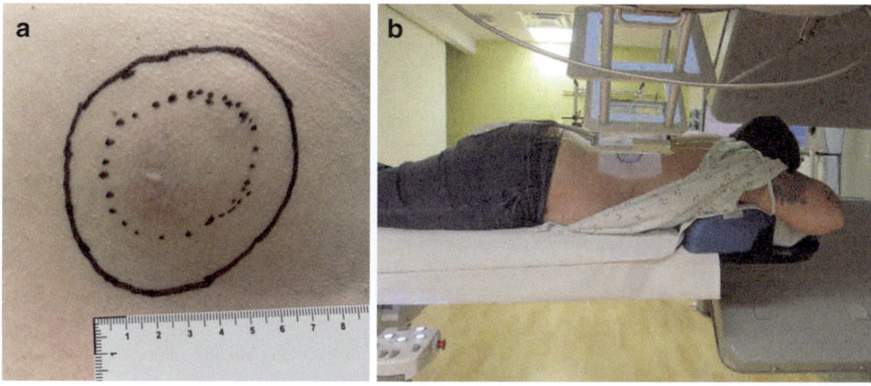

Fig. 6.2 (**a**) GTV in dotted line and block edge (1.5 cm margin from GTV) outlined in solid black. Besides the discoloration of the skin, the GTV was identified by palpation. (**b**) Based on the lesion's maximal thickness of 5 mm, the lesion was treated to 24 Gy in 12 fractions with 6 MeV electrons to the 90% isodose line using daily 5 mm bolus. The gantry angle was selected to be en face with the lesion

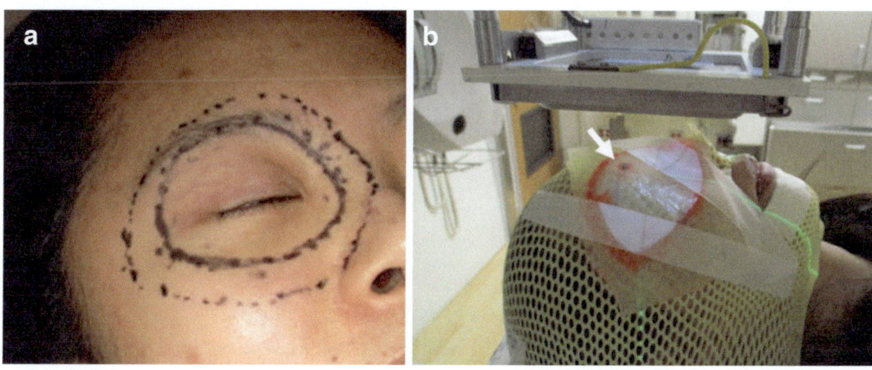

Fig. 6.3 (**a**) The bony orbit was palpated and the CTV delineated with the solid line. A 1 cm margin was given from the CTV to the block edge (dotted line). (**b**) The patient was treated to 25.5 Gy in 17 fractions. 6 MeV electrons with 8 mm bolus were used to spare the posterior orbit and ensure adequate dose buildup, respectively. To spare dose to the lens, a 3 mm lead block (white arrow) was placed over the bolus in the location of her lens. Given that it can be challenging to fixate gaze on an object immediately adjacent to the eye (i.e., lead block), the location of the lens was reproduced by fixating her gaze using her left eye to a mark made on the electron cone

cancer workup, and an FNA biopsy showed monoclonal B cells with an immunophenotype typical for MALT lymphoma. MALT1 gene rearrangement was noted by FISH. Because of the high cellularity of the FNA and the definitive ancillary studies, a further tissue biopsy was not pursued. Bone marrow biopsy was normal. CT and PET scans showed disease localized to the left upper lobe of the lung, with the lesion showing low FDG avidity. Pulmonary function tests were normal. She was treated with definitive radiation therapy (Fig. 6.6).

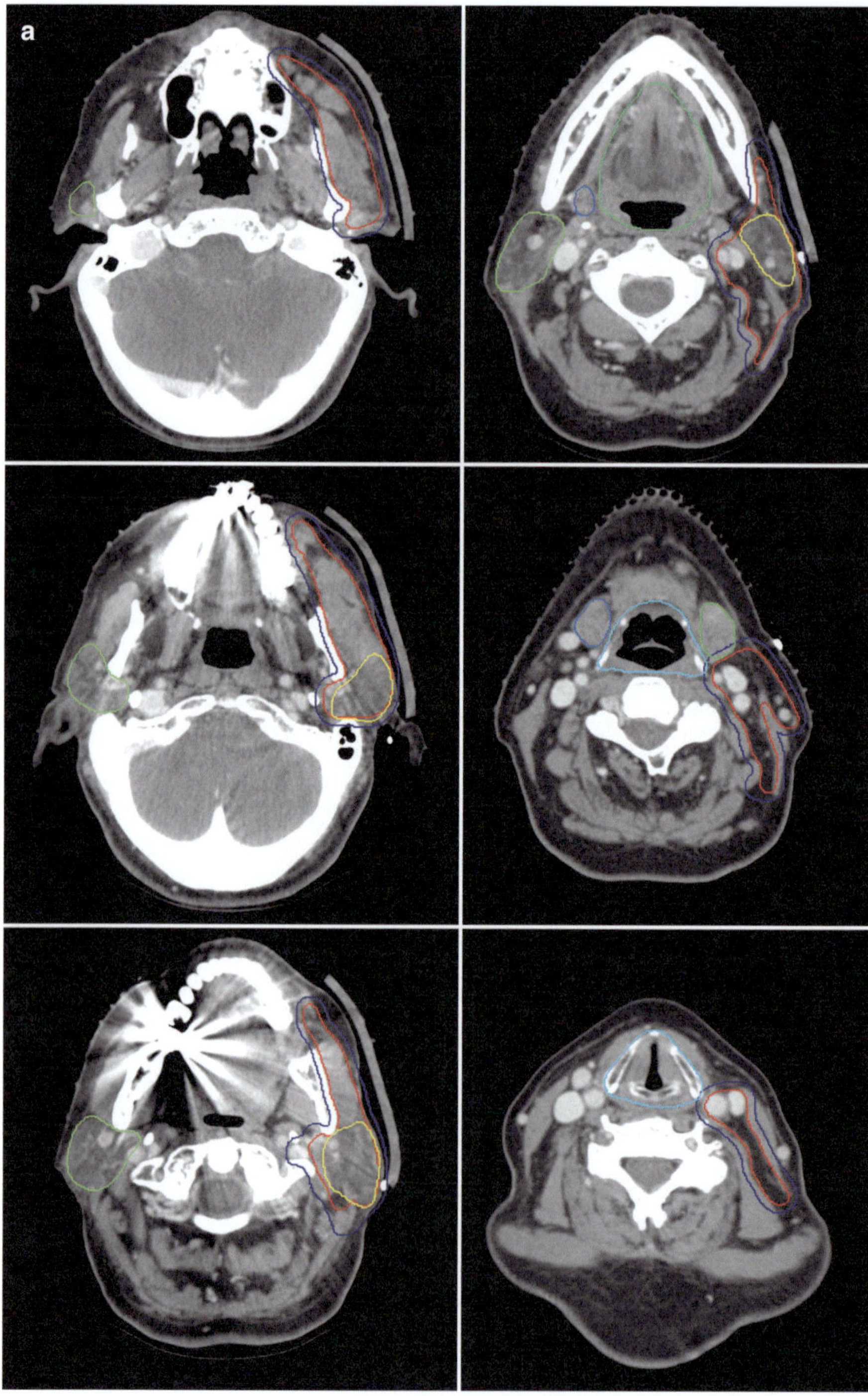
a

Fig. 6.4 (**a**) The patient was immobilized with a thermoplastic mask with a neutral neck. A 5 mm bolus was applied over the left cheek region corresponding to her superficial involvement of the masseter muscle and parotid. Thin cut (1.25 mm) CT scan slices with IV contrast were obtained. CTV contours are in red, and PTV contours (5 mm margin) are in blue, in addition to pertinent OARs including the contralateral parotid, submandibular glands, and larynx. Given that her level of left IA and IV neck nodes appeared slightly larger compared to initial diagnosis, the left neck was included in the CTV given uncertainty of involvement. (**b**) The patient was treated to 24 Gy in 12 fractions using a 3D conformal technique with three fields: slight right anterior oblique, posterior left oblique, and anterior left oblique (left panel). Dose distribution with prescription dose in red and 95% isodose line in blue. (**c**) Dose/volume histogram of the plan. Given the relatively low-prescription dose, the desired target coverage includes CTV V99 $\geq$ 99%, and PTV V99 $\geq$ 95%. The left submandibular gland is unable to be fully spared given that the adjacent level I lymph node level is treated

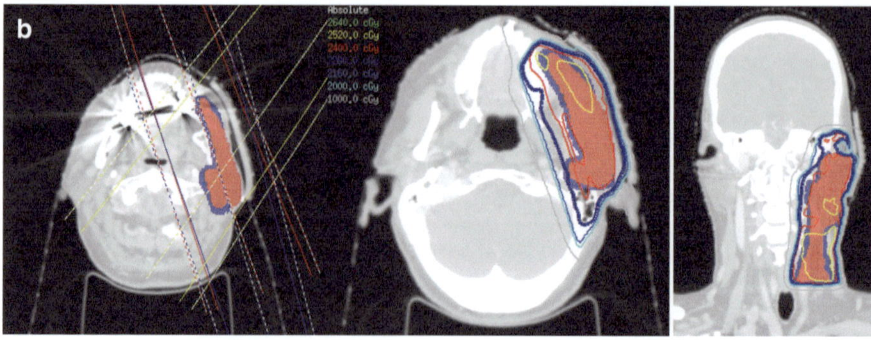

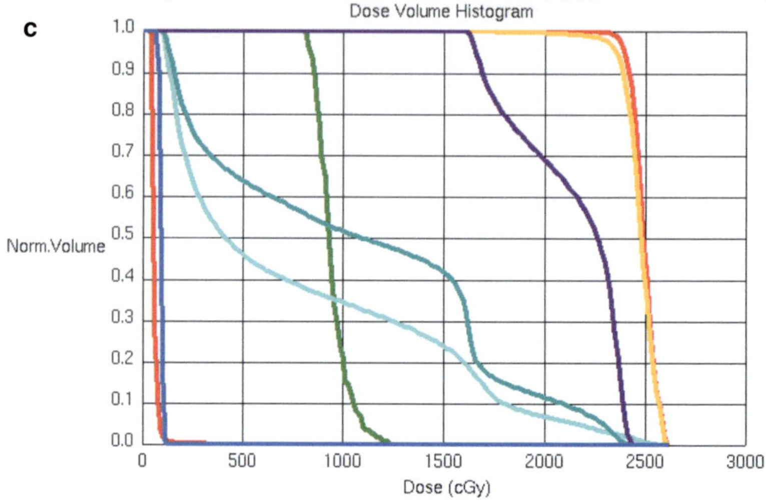

ROI Statistics

Line Type	ROI	Trial or Record	Min.	Max.	Mean	Std. Dev.
(red)	CTV_L parotid neck	Trial_1	1773.7	2611.7	2486.6	59.2
(green)	Cochlea_L	Trial_1	806.3	1234.8	943.3	80.6
(light blue)	Larynx	Trial_1	93.9	2555.1	780.5	706.7
(teal)	Oral cavity	Trial_1	97.7	2448.8	1055.5	739.6
(yellow)	PTV_L parotid neck	Trial_1	--	2615.4	2466.8	108.6
(red)	Parotid_R	Trial_1	36.1	320.3	59.9	17.2
(purple)	SMG_L	Trial_1	1607.9	2440.0	2127.6	266.5
(blue)	SMG_R	Trial_1	70.6	123.7	93.3	10.8

Fig. 6.4 (continued)

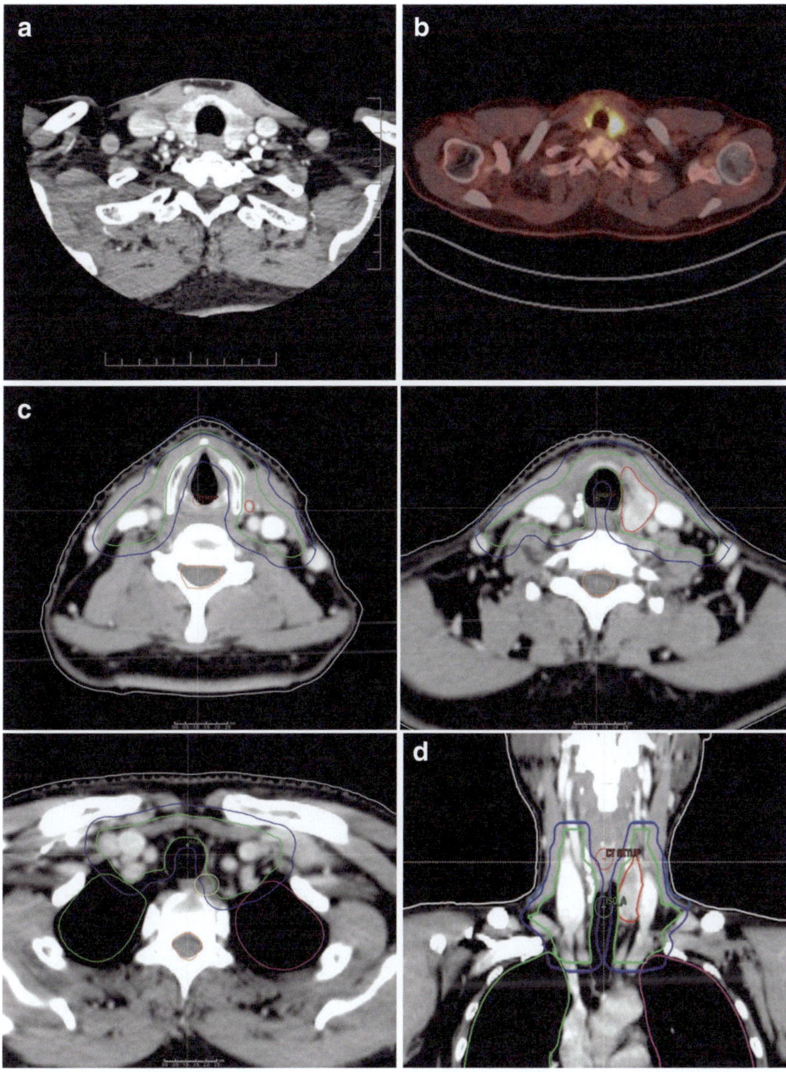

Fig. 6.5 (**a**) CT scan demonstrating thyroid gland nodularity bilaterally with nodules that are less contrast-enhancing than the thyroid gland. The larger nodule is located in the right thyroid lobe. (**b**) FDG PET scan done following a right hemithyroidectomy, showing FDG avidity of the left lobe (SUV_{max} 9.1). Minor uptake in the midline and the right side was interpreted to be normal due to postsurgical healing tissue. (**c**) The patient was treated with definitive RT for stage IE thyroid MALT lymphoma. The patient received IV contrast for a CT simulation scan and immobilization with a thermoplastic mask. GTV (red), CTV (green), and PTV (blue, 5 mm margin) are illustrated in the superior, mid, and inferior aspects of the volume. The CTV covers the residual thyroid left lobe and the entire thyroid surgical bed (postright hemithyroidectomy). (**d**) The coronal perspective is also shown. (**e**) IMRT treatment plan with four beams (beam angles 30°, 70°, 300°, and 345°), delivering 30 Gy in 15 daily fractions. PTV D95 (28.5 Gy) coverage >99%. OAR dose histograms are displayed for the lungs, esophagus, and spinal canal. The patient achieved a complete response and is disease-free 1.5 years posttreatment. Please note that a total prescribed dose of 24 Gy would also be appropriate for this case

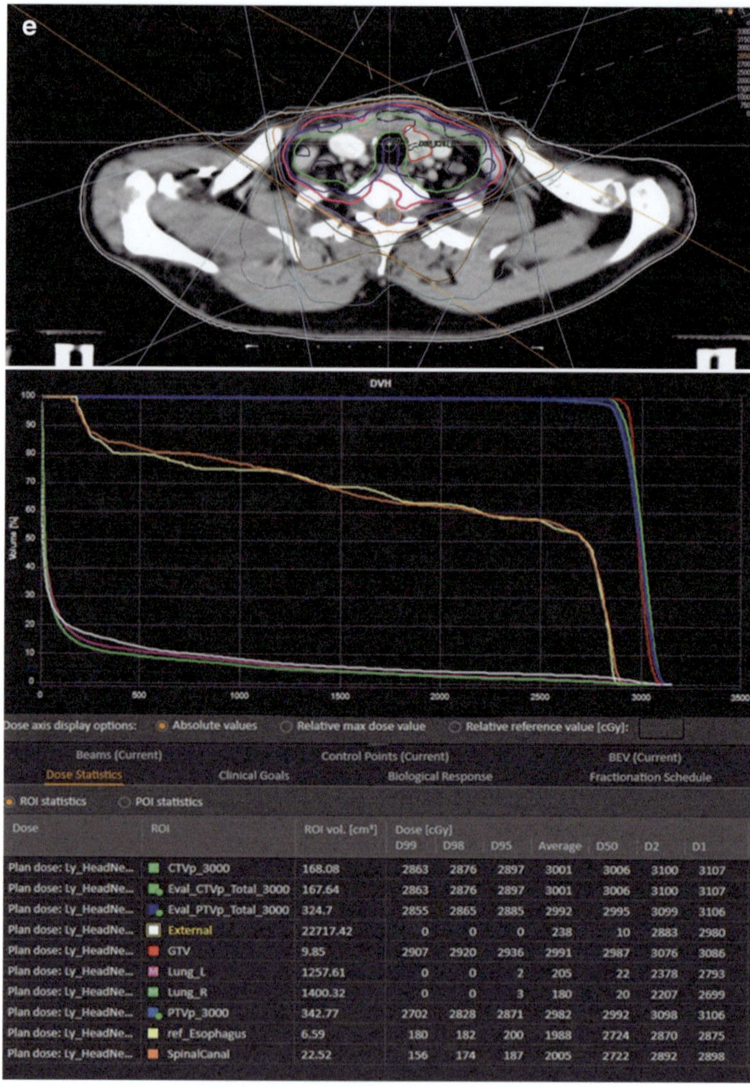

Fig. 6.5 (continued)

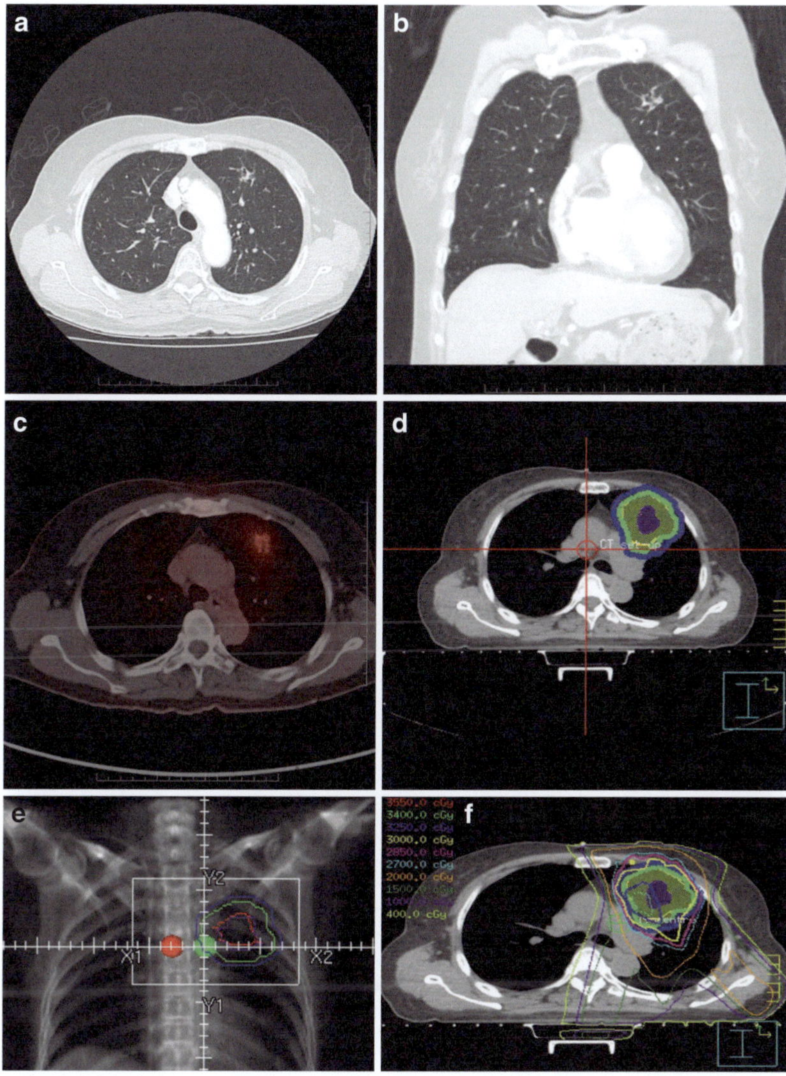

Fig. 6.6 (**a** and **b**) CT scan (lung windows) showed a malignant appearing, spiculated lesion in the left upper lobe, 2.2 cm in maximum size (axial and coronal perspectives). FNA biopsy confirmed MALT lymphoma. (**c**) PET scan showed low FDG avidity of the left upper lobe lung MALT lymphoma, SUV_{max} 2.8. There were no other abnormalities in the lung, mediastinum, or elsewhere. (**d** and **e**) Definitive RT was administered for this patient with stage IE MALT lymphoma of the lung in the left upper lobe. She underwent a 4D CT simulation scan, axial (**d**) and coronal (**e**) perspectives. The GTV was contoured in inhale (purple line) and exhale (red line) phases of quiet respiration. Each was expanded 5 mm to generate the inhale and exhale CTV, then combined and named the ITV (green line). The ITV was then expanded by 5 mm to generate the PTV (blue line). (**f** and **g**) IMRT treatment plan with four beams (beam angles 20°, 140°, 190°, and 340°), delivering 30 Gy in 20 daily fractions. Axial (**f**) and coronal (**g**) perspectives. Please note that a total dose of 24 Gy would also be appropriate for this case. (**h**) DVH of OARs displaying lung and spinal cord doses to be acceptable. (**i**) CT scan (lung windows, axial, and coronal) 6 years following definitive RT 30 Gy. Minor fibrotic changes were noted at the site of treatment. These findings have been stable over time. The patient is presently 10 years posttreatment and doing well with no evidence of lymphoma recurrence

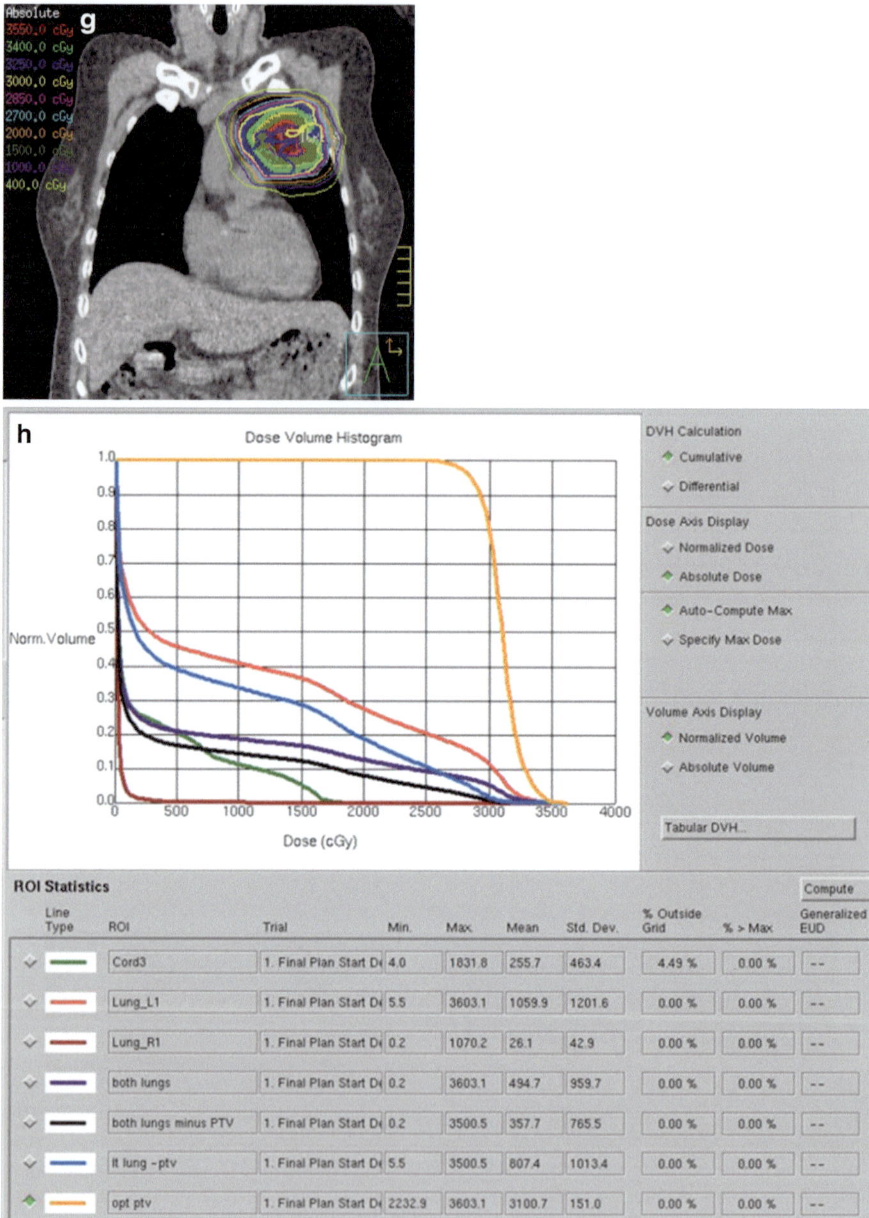

Fig. 6.6 (continued)

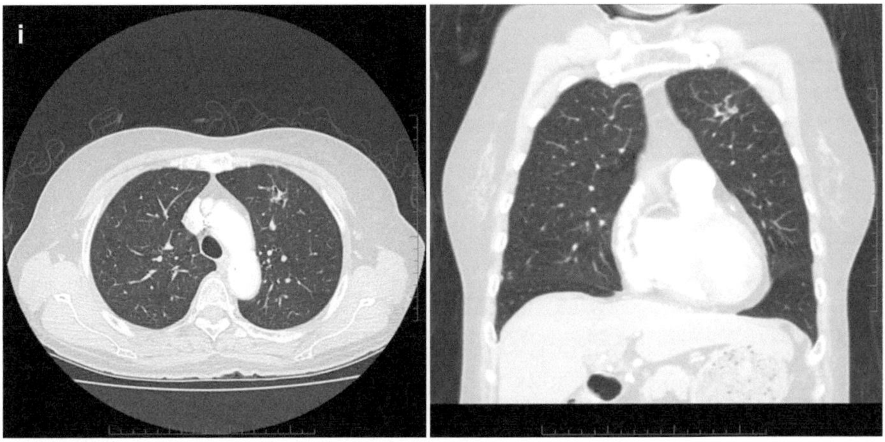

Fig. 6.6 (continued)

Part 4: Special Considerations

- In patients who may not be candidates for definitive treatment or who have advanced disease but with localized, symptomatic disease, low-dose radiotherapy (2 Gy × 2) is associated with 80–90% response rates and minimal, if any toxicity [21, 22]. The multicenter randomized FORT trial compared 24 Gy versus 4 Gy and included patients with EMZL. In this study, 4 Gy was found to be inferior to 24 Gy regarding the duration of local control. More recently response adapted approaches are being explored for patients with EZML with 4 Gy in two fractions as initial therapy, and an additional RT to 20 Gy for incomplete responders (clinicaltrials.gov NCT02494700 and NCT03680586).

References

1. Olszewski AJ, Castillo JJ. Survival of patients with marginal zone lymphoma. Cancer. 2013;119(3):629–38.
2. Raderer M, Kiesewetter B, Ferreri AJ. Clinicopathologic characteristics and treatment of marginal zone lymphoma of mucosa-associated lymphoid tissue (MALT lymphoma). CA Cancer J Clin. 2016;66(2):153–71.
3. Wundisch T, Thiede C, Morgner A, et al. Long-term follow-up of gastric MALT lymphoma after Helicobacter pylori eradication. J Clin Oncol. 2005;23(31):8018–24.
4. Goda JS, Gospodarowicz M, Pintilie M, et al. Long-term outcome in localized extranodal mucosa-associated lymphoid tissue lymphomas treated with radiotherapy. Cancer. 2010;116(16):3815–24.
5. Teckie S, Qi S, Chelius M, et al. Long-term outcome of 487 patients with early-stage extranodal marginal zone lymphoma. Ann Oncol. 2017;28(5):1064–9.
6. Raderer M, Wöhrer S, Streubel B, et al. Assessment of disease dissemination in gastric compared with extragastric mucosa-associated lymphoid tissue lymphoma using extensive staging: a single-center experience. J Clin Oncol. 2006;24(19):3136–41.
7. Weiler-Sagie M, Bushelev O, Epelbaum R, et al. 18F-FDG avidity in lymphoma readdressed: a study of 766 patients. J Nucl Med. 2010;51(1):25–30.

8. Martinelli G, Laszlo D, Ferreri AJM, et al. Clinical activity of rituximab in gastric marginal zone non-Hodgkin's lymphoma resistant to or not eligible for anti-Helicobacter pylori therapy. J Clin Oncol. 2005;23(9):1979–83.
9. Choi SH, Park SH, Lee JJB, Baek JG, Kim JS, Yoon HI. Combining deep-inspiration breath hold and intensity-modulated radiotherapy for gastric mucosa-associated lymphoid tissue lymphoma: dosimetric evaluation using comprehensive plan quality indices. Radiat Oncol. 2019;14(1):59.
10. Christopherson KM, Gunther JR, Fang P, et al. Decreased heart dose with deep inspiration breath hold for the treatment of gastric lymphoma with IMRT. Clin Transl Radiat Oncol. 2020;24:79–82.
11. Wong JW, Sharpe MB, Jaffray DA, et al. The use of active breathing control (ABC) to reduce margin for breathing motion. Int J Radiat Oncol Biol Phys. 1999;44(4):911–9.
12. Taniguchi CM, Murphy JD, Eclov N, et al. Dosimetric analysis of organs at risk during expiratory gating in stereotactic body radiation therapy for pancreatic cancer. Int J Radiat Oncol Biol Phys. 2013;85(4):1090–5.
13. Della Biancia C, Hunt M, Furhang E, Wu E, Yahalom J. Radiation treatment planning techniques for lymphoma of the stomach. Int J Radiat Oncol Biol Phys. 2005;62(3):745–51.
14. Schechter NR, Portlock CS, Yahalom J. Treatment of mucosa-associated lymphoid tissue lymphoma of the stomach with radiation alone. J Clin Oncol. 1998;16(5):1916–21.
15. Schmelz R, Miehlke S, Thiede C, et al. Sequential H. pylori eradication and radiation therapy with reduced dose compared to standard dose for gastric MALT lymphoma stages IE & II1E: a prospective randomized trial. J Gastroenterol. 2019;54(5):388–95.
16. Pinnix CC, Gunther JR, Milgrom SA, et al. Outcomes after reduced-dose intensity-modulated radiation therapy for gastric mucosa-associated lymphoid tissue (MALT) lymphoma. Int J Radiat Oncol Biol Phys. 2019;104(2):447–55.
17. Lowry L, Smith P, Qian W, et al. Reduced dose radiotherapy for local control in non-Hodgkin lymphoma: a randomised phase III trial. Radiother Oncol. 2011;100(1):86–92.
18. Tanimoto K, Kaneko A, Suzuki S, et al. Long-term follow-up results of no initial therapy for ocular adnexal MALT lymphoma. Ann Oncol. 2006;17(1):135–40.
19. Pfeffer MR, Rabin T, Tsvang L, Goffman J, Rosen N, Symon Z. Orbital lymphoma: is it necessary to treat the entire orbit? Int J Radiat Oncol Biol Phys. 2004;60(2):527–30.
20. Binkley MS, Hiniker SM, Donaldson SS, Hoppe RT. Partial orbit irradiation achieves excellent outcomes for primary orbital lymphoma. Pract Radiat Oncol. 2016;6(4):255–61.
21. Hoskin PJ, Kirkwood AA, Popova B, et al. 4 Gy versus 24 Gy radiotherapy for patients with indolent lymphoma (FORT): a randomised phase 3 non-inferiority trial. Lancet Oncol. 2014;15(4):457–63.
22. Hoskin P, Popova B, Schofield O, et al. 4 Gy versus 24 Gy radiotherapy for follicular and marginal zone lymphoma (FoRT): long-term follow-up of a multicentre, randomised, phase 3, non-inferiority trial. Lancet Oncol. 2021;22(3):332–40.

Further Reading

Yahalom J, et al. Modern radiation therapy for extranodal lymphomas: field and dose guidelines from the International Lymphoma Radiation Oncology Group. Int J Radiat Oncol Biol Phys. 2015;92(1):11–31.

Target Volume Delineation for Mycosis Fungoides and Total Skin Electron Beam Treatment

7

Susan Sun, Shunqing Zhang, and Kathryn Dusenbery

Contents

Susan Sun and Shunqing Zhang are co-first authors.

S. Sun (✉)
VA Health Care System, Minneapolis, MN, USA
e-mail: susan.sun@va.gov

S. Zhang
Northwestern Medical Group, Chicago, IL, USA
e-mail: shunqing.zhang@nm.org

K. Dusenbery
University of Minnesota Medical School, Minneapolis, MN, USA
e-mail: dusen001@umn.edu

C. Pinnix et al. (eds.), *Target Volume Delineation in Hematologic Malignancies*, Practical Guides in Radiation Oncology,
https://doi.org/10.1007/978-3-031-67722-9_7

Part 1: Background and Epidemiology

- Cutaneous T-cell lymphomas (CTCLs) constitute approximately 75–80% of primary cutaneous lymphomas, a rare form of lymphomas typically confined to the skin at diagnosis. Mycosis fungoides (MF) is the most common subtype that accounts for 60% of CTCLs [1]. In contrast, Sézary syndrome (SS) is a rare leukemic type of CTCL closely related to MF that has peripheral blood involvement. The age-adjusted incidence rates for MF and SS are approximately 5.5 and 0.1 per million person-years, respectively, in the United States [2].
- MF primarily affects adults and median age at diagnosis is 55–60. The incidence of MF increases with age, and is higher in men and in Blacks [2, 3]. Epidemiological studies have not been able to identify specific causative factors of CTCL. Notably, an association of MF and Human T-Lymphotropic Virus-1/2 infection was reported, but the mechanism remains unclear [4, 5].

Pathology

- *Cells of origin*: The malignant cells in MF/SS originate from mature CD4+ T-helper cells. MF is derived from epidermotropic resident memory cells that remain confined to the skin, while SS involves central memory cells that retain the ability to access the peripheral circulation and lymph nodes [6]. As MF progresses, the malignant cells may undergo large cell transformation and lose epidermotropism. As a result, MF can develop extracutaneous and secondary leukemic involvement [7].
- *Histopathologic findings*: The malignant cells in MF are predominantly small cells with cerebriform nuclei. Patches/plaques involved with MF are typically characterized by a band of papillary lymphoid infiltrates scattered along the base membrane zone of the dermal-epidermal junction, migrating to the epidermis as single cells and sometimes in aggregates [8].
- *Immunophenotypic features*: The clonal T cells in MF/SS are CD4+/CD8−. With large cell transformation, expression of CD20/CD30 may be noted [9, 10].

Typical Presentation

- Classic clinical presentation of early-stage MF includes isolated or limited erythematous patches and/or plaques (<10% body surface area, BSA) in a "bathing suit" distribution that wax and wane over years. In reality, MF patches/plaques vary in size, shape, and color, and their distribution differs in MF variants [1]. Diagnosis at this stage can be challenging, as its presentation shares similarities with common dermatologic etiologies such as dermatitis or psoriasis. It is not uncommon to have a period of months to years between symptom onset and definitive diagnosis.

- In the later stages, ulcerated/exophytic tumors form in a minority of patients. More commonly, the extent of BSA involvement drastically increases until erythroderma is declared with generalized skin erythema involving >80% BSA. Additionally, lymph nodes, viscera, peripheral blood, and bone marrow may become involved. The most commonly involved visceral organs are the lungs, spleen, liver, and gastrointestinal tract [11].
- SS is clinically characterized by erythroderma and significant presence of malignant cells in the peripheral circulation. Other associated symptoms include palmar and plantar hyperkeratosis as well as generalized lymphadenopathy [8, 11].

Staging and Workup

- To diagnose MF, a point-based algorithm by the International Society for Cutaneous Lymphoma (ISCL) incorporates clinical symptoms as well as histopathologic and immunophenotypic findings of the skin biopsy, including an assessment of T cell clonality [10].
- To diagnose SS, one of the following criteria must be met: a significant presence of atypical cerebriform lymphocytes, called Sézary cells, in the peripheral circulation (>1000 cells/μL by cytopathologic assessment or flow cytometry); an expanded CD4+ T-cell population, resulting in a CD4/CD8 ratio ≥10 on flow cytometry; an aberrant expression of pan-T-cell antigens; demonstration of T-cell clonality by Southern blot or PCR-based methods, or cytogenetic demonstration of an abnormal clone [9].
- The clinical staging of MF/SS is based on the characteristics of skin (T), lymph nodes (N), viscera (M), and disease burden in peripheral circulation (B) [12]. Among these characteristics, T staging is highly prognostic and has the greatest influence on overall group staging. (Table 7.1) [12–14].
- Work up includes a thorough dermatologic history. Comprehensive skin exam should include soles, perineum, nails, and auditory canals. Skin photographs are important in tracking the evolution of disease over time and how it responds to treatment. Lymph nodes should be palpated to assess for lymphadenopathy.
- Obtain biopsies from at least two areas of involved skin and from any palpable lymph nodes that are suspicious for involvement. Routine bone marrow examination is generally not necessary unless the patient presents with advanced disease.
- Complete blood count (CBC), complete metabolic panel (CMP), lactate dehydrogenase (LDH), and peripheral blood smear should be obtained. Evaluation for abnormal T-cells using flow cytometry and polymerase chain reaction (PCR)

Table 7.1 Staging of MF and SS

Stage	T	N	M	B	Clinical presentation
IA	1	0	0	0–1	Patch/plaque <10% BSA
IB	2	0	0	0–1	Diffuse patch/plaque ≥10% BSA
IIA	1–2	1–2	0	0–1	Patch/plaque and lymphadenopathy
IIB	3	0–2	0	0–1	Tumor
IIIA	4	0–2	0	0	Erythroderma
IIIB	4	0–2	0	1	Erythroderma and >5% Sezary cells in peripheral blood
IVA1	1–4	0–2	0	2	≥1000 cells/μL in peripheral blood
IVA2	1–4	3	0	0–2	Clinically abnormal, pathologically confirmed lymphadenopathy
IVB	1–4	0–3	1	0–2	Visceral organ involvement

Adapted from Ref. [12]

to detect clonal T-cell receptor gene rearrangement (or other assessment of T cell clonality) should be performed on the specimens from both skin and peripheral blood.

- Imaging with positron emission tomography-computed tomography (PET/CT) or CT scan of the chest, abdomen, and pelvis should be considered if there is high burden of skin involvement, skin tumor, evidence of large cell transformation, or suspicion for lymph node/visceral involvement.

Treatment Approaches

- MF is generally not considered curable. Early-stage MF can be managed with skin-directed therapies including radiation therapy, topical steroids, retinoids, ultraviolet B phototherapy (UVB), and/or photochemotherapy using psoralen plus ultraviolet A (PUVA). These therapies offer similar rates of complete remission.
- Advanced stage MF or SS requires a combination of skin-directed therapy, photopheresis, systemic chemotherapy/immunotherapy, and allogeneic transplantation [15].
- The malignant cells in MF/SS are extremely radiosensitive. Targeted radiation therapy is commonly used for selected skin tumor/lesions that are refractory to other treatments. Radiation therapy may also be used to treat extra-cutaneous sites. If a patient presents with uni-lesional MF (rare), then radiation therapy has potential for disease eradication. When ≥10% of BSA is involved, total skin electron beam therapy (TSEBT) is considered [15, 16].

Pre-radiotherapy Imaging and Evaluation

- Estimate the extent of skin involvement. Wallace Rule of Nines and Palmer Method are the two commonly used methodologies [17, 18].
- Utilize staging imaging studies to supplement the physical exam and better delineate the disease extent.

Part 2: Management and Treatment of Skin Diseases in Mycosis Fungoides and Sézary Syndrome

Principles of Management

Targeted Radiation

- Targeted local radiation is considered when there are isolated sites of skin involvement. Consideration for radiation regimen should include target site, volume, previous radiation history, risk of normal tissue complications, and patient's performance status/comorbidities/preferences.
- Radiation doses ≥8Gy confers a >90% complete response (CR) rate in cutaneous lymphoma [19]. Studies specific to MF/SS have evaluated radiation doses ranging from 6 to 40 Gy, and a dose-response relationship for CR and response durability has been well-documented [20, 21]. Fractionated treatment is favored over single fraction treatment to improve the therapeutic ratio [19], although the convenience of hypofractionation or single fraction regimens are commonly utilized.
- In general, a lower dose regimen of 8–12 Gy in 2–4 fractions is effective, well tolerated, and allows for re-irradiation when indicated.
- A higher radiation dose is considered for patients who present with uni-lesional MF. This is based on two small series, which have found that doses ranging 20–30.6 Gy are successful in achieving durable local control (75–86% at 10 years) as well as relapse-free survival (64–86% at 10 years) [22, 23]. Higher doses should also be considered in patients with advanced T stage and/or large cell transformation for improved durability.
- For patients with poor prognosis and advanced disease refractory to multiple lines of treatments, an ultra-low dose regimen of 2 Gy × 2 fractions may be considered [16].

TSEBT

- TSEBT is considered when disease patches/plaques involve ≥10% BSA.
- Treatment dose can range from 12–36 Gy [14]. It is most commonly delivered in 1–1.5 Gy fractions, four times per week [24], though institutional experiences of hypofractionated regimens have also been reported [25–27].
- 30–36 Gy is the historical standard with high overall response (OR) rates (94.7–100%) and acceptable toxicity profile [28–31]. More durable CR is found among patients treated with ≥25 Gy [32]. Higher T stage and more aggressive MF variant have lower rates of CR and higher risk of disease relapse.
- There is a recent shift towards low dose TSEBT of 12 Gy in recognition that many patients will relapse despite achieving CR and would benefit from re-irradiation. Standard doses of 30–36 Gy precluded physicians from administering more than two lifetime courses of TSEBT due to concern for cumulative toxicity. Low dose TSEBT has shown to have similar OR, progression-free survival (PFS), and overall survival (OS). While CR and durability of response are worse, low dose TSEBT offers shorter treatment course, improved toxicity profile, and may be repeated as indicated [33–35].

- TSEBT is offered only in major radiotherapy centers, primarily because it is a highly specialized radiation technique requiring excellent support from physics and dosimetry.

General Considerations for Radiotherapy

- **Targeted radiation** [36]
  - Electrons are generally preferred, and selection of beam energy depends on thickness of skin lesion and depth of coverage required.
  - Bolus should be added to achieve sufficient skin coverage.
  - Areas of irregular skin surface contours may require use of tissue-equivalent compensator or mega-voltage photon beams using complex field arrangements to ensure homogeneous dose distribution.
  - Margins of 1–2 cm are typically added. More generous margins (≥2 cm) are recommended when treating uni-lesional MF with curative intent.
- **TSEBT**
  - Due to differences in linear accelerator (LINAC) machinery, the specifics of TSEBT procedure are highly variable among institutions. The three principal techniques of TSEBT delivery are: (i) large electron field technique, (ii) rotational technique, and (iii) translational technique [37].

    A common technique is the large electron field technique developed at Stanford. Patients will stand and assume six different positions in relation to the linear accelerator gantry to maximize the exposure of BSA (Fig. 7.1).

    The rotational technique has the patient standing on a rotating platform. Radiation is delivered continuously while the patient rotates at a constant speed about the vertical axis of the body.

    The translational technique is useful in treating patients who cannot tolerate standing or pediatric patients who require general anesthesia. This involves shifting the position of patient, who is lying on a stretcher or a special treatment table that moves along the patient's longitudinal axis. In each position, electron beam of sufficient width to cover the patient's transverse dimensions will be delivered [38, 39].

    Modified large field or rotational techniques have also been used [40, 41].
  - Various techniques involving special filters and beam spoilers are used to create the electron beam used in TSEBT. Commonly, a Lucite plate is placed in front of the patient and serves to scatter the incident electrons and to attenuate photon contamination.
  - A combination of two overlapping treatment fields, known as a dual field, can be used in both large field and rotational TSEBT. Dual field is obtained by rotating the linear accelerator about an axis perpendicular to the patient's skin surface. It allows for treatment with source-to-skin distance (SSD) of 3–5 m, as opposed to the 7 m SSD needed to create a field size which encompasses the entire patient BSA. For instance, with an SSD of 3 m, the dual field is obtained by rotating the gantry to 20° and −20° in relation to the axis perpendicular to the patient's skin surface (Fig. 7.2).

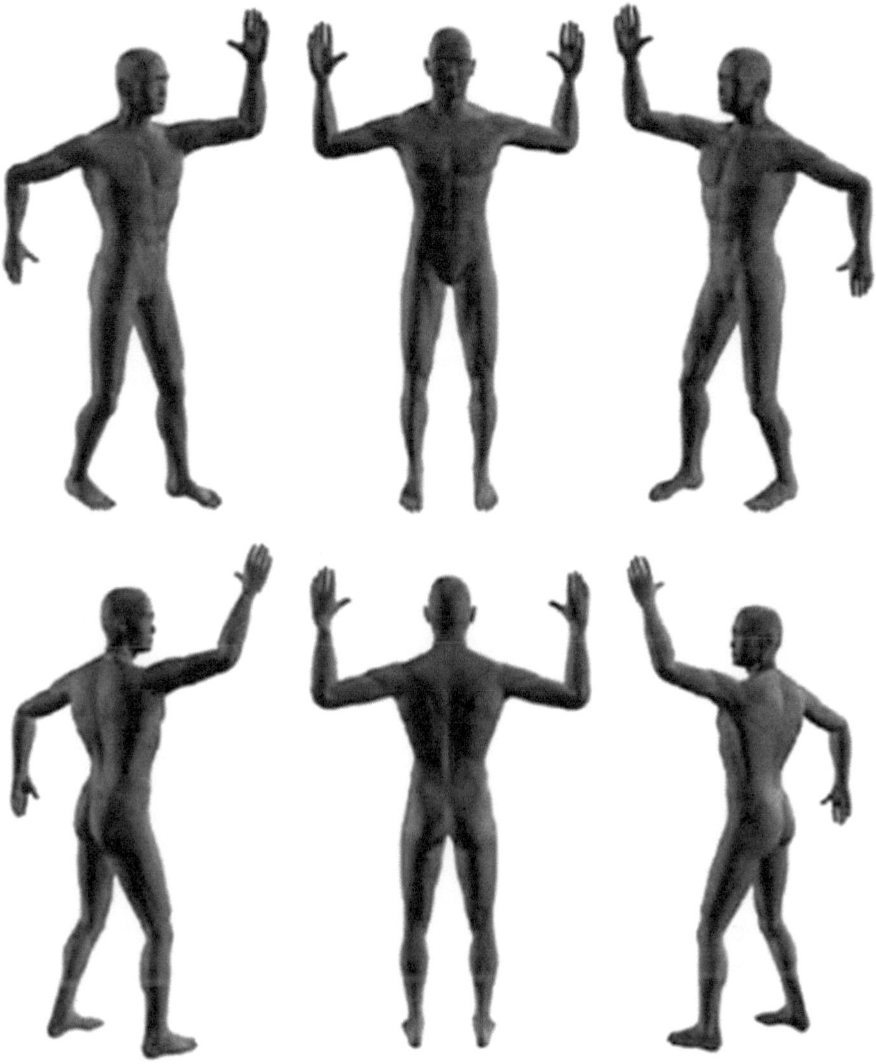

Fig. 7.1 Treatment positions assumed during large electron field TSEBT as per the Stanford technique. (Adapted from Ref. [37])

- To minimize toxicity, the eyes are shielded with external eye shields (if there is no disease near the eyes) or internal contact lens eye shields if skin near the eyelid is involved [42]. Fingernail/toenail shields are considered after 10–15 Gy to avoid nail ridging or loss. Further consideration can be given to shielding of the lips and testes.
- To ensure a homogeneous dose distribution, boosts or shields are often required for top of the scalp, shoulders, axilla, inframammary folds, underneath a panniculus, perineum, groins/medial thighs, and soles. Clinical assessment and in vivo dosimetry are needed to determine appropriate modifications [43].

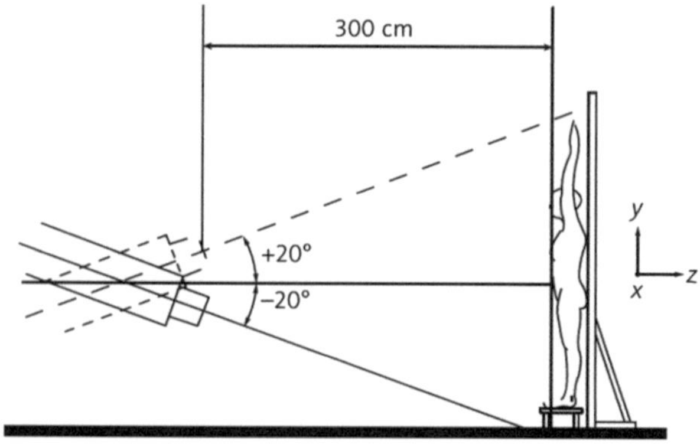

Fig. 7.2 Generation of dual field through rotation of the gantry in relation to the axis perpendicular to the patient's skin surface in large electron field TSEBT. (Adapted from Ref. [37])

Table 7.2 Target volume definitions

	Volume	Description
Targeted radiation, boost radiation to tumors in addition to TSEBT	Gross tumor volume (GTV)	Lesions of interest as determined by clinical assessment
	Clinical target volume (CTV)	(a) 1–2 cm margins from GTV, depend on treatment site and uncertainty in disease extent (b) ≥2 cm margins generally used in treatment of uni-lesional MF
	Planning target volume (PTV)	CTV plus a margin to account for setup uncertainties associated with patient position and beam alignment
	Organs at risk (OAR)	As Low as Reasonably Achievable (ALARA) principle applies, and general constraints for conventional fractionation schemes can be used for extrapolation
TSEBT	Target volume and technical aspects [42]	(a) TSEBT dose is prescribed on the patient's skin surface at the level of the umbilicus (b) The target volume in TSEBT should include epidermis and dermis. ≥4 mm depth from skin surface should be covered by 80% isodose line (c) At the depth of 2 cm, the absorbed dose should not exceed 20% of the prescribed dose (d) The inhomogeneity of dose distribution in the air in the treatment plan should not exceed ± 10% (e) Photon contamination should not exceed 0.7 Gy

- Additional targeted radiation should be planned separately to treat any thickened tumors, involved lymph nodes, and/or diseases in visceral organs.
- Target volume definitions and the specifics of TSEBT plan evaluation are outlined in Table 7.2.

Part 3: Cases

Case 1

An 83-year-old man, otherwise healthy, was diagnosed with a uni-lesional MF, cT1N0M0B0, Stage IA. Physical exam demonstrated a 3 cm skin patch of the medial left buttock (Fig. 7.3a). He received targeted radiation therapy to the left buttock lesion with 30 Gy in 15 fractions (Fig. 7.3a–c).

Case 2

A 33-year-old woman with multiple relapsed/refractory MF presented with rapidly progressive disease and multiple symptomatic cutaneous lesions. She had already progressed through many lines of systemic therapy and her prognosis was very poor. She previously had good relief from targeted radiation therapy to other skin areas and thus underwent another course of palliative radiation therapy with 4 Gy in 2 fractions to the most symptomatic lesions before transition to hospice care (Fig. 7.4).

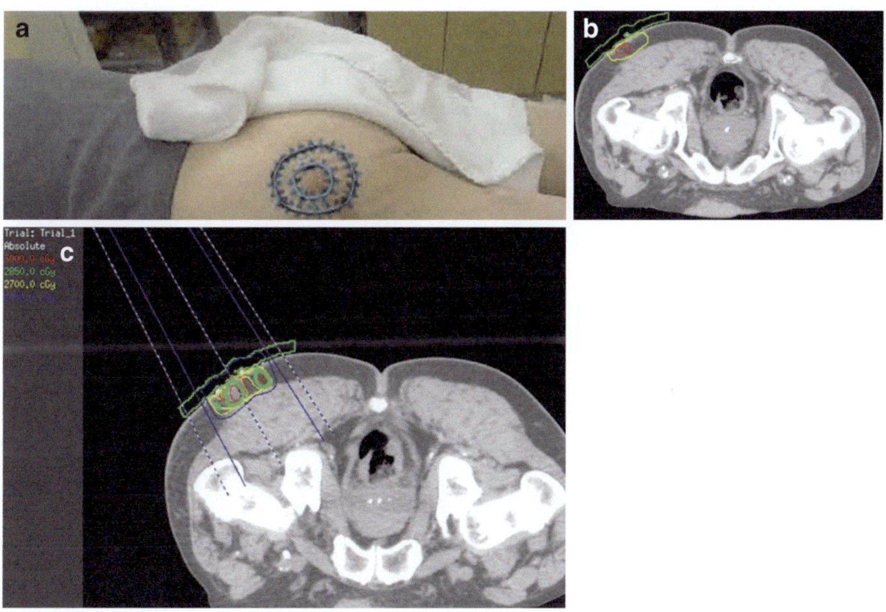

Fig. 7.3 Targeted radiation to a uni-lesional mycosis fungoides: a 2 cm expansion from the gross tumor was marked with wire at the time of simulation (**a**). GTV (red contour) and CTV (yellow contour, 2 cm expansion) were delineated**.** Treatment was delivered with 12 MeV en face electrons with a 1 cm bolus (green contour) (**b**, **c**)

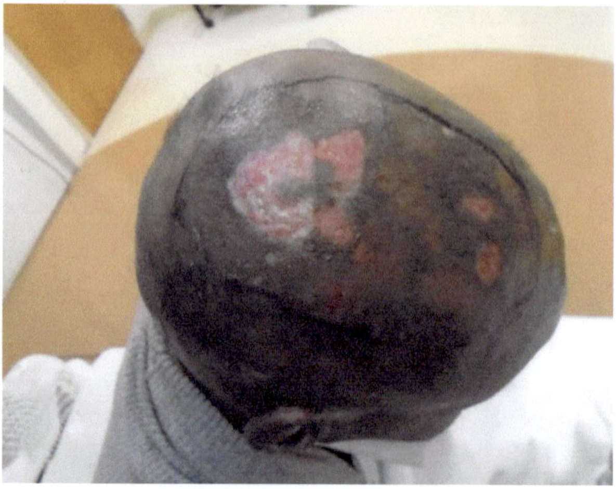

Fig. 7.4 Targeted radiation to the symptomatic scalp patches: Given the patient's poor prognosis, 2 Gy × 2 fractions was chosen. A 1 cm expansion was outlined around the skin involvement. Treatment was delivered using a 6 MeV electron beam and a 5 mm bolus

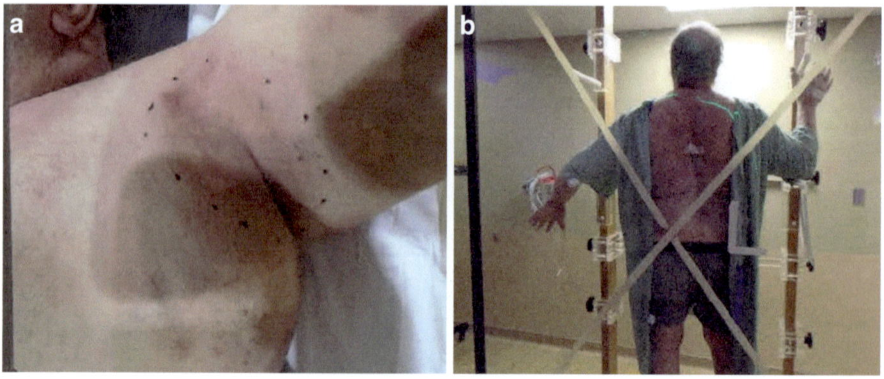

Fig. 7.5 Low dose TSEBT: since the patient had good performance status, treatment was delivered using the Stanford technique: the patient assumed six standing poses as outlined in Fig. 7.1. Dual electron fields were used for treatment at each pose. A polycarbonate beam spoiler was used (**b**). Optically stimulated luminescence dosimeters (OSL) dosimeters were placed on the first day at the axilla, the perineum, under the pannus and at the top of scalp per institutional experience [43] to guide targeted boost to those "shadowed" areas up to a total dose of approximately 12 Gy, the axillary boost is outlined with dotted line (**a**)

Case 3

A 72-year-old male was diagnosed with MF with widespread skin involvement up to 80% BSA, cT2N0M0B0, stage IB. He failed multiple lines of oral and topical agents but previously had good symptomatic relief with targeted radiation therapy (20–24 Gy in 2 Gy/fraction). He then proceeded to TSEBT to 12 Gy in 12 fractions (1 Gy per fraction) over 3 weeks (Fig. 7.5a, b).

Case 4

A 71-year-old male was diagnosed with MF with large cell transformation, cT3N0M0B0, stage IIB. He had painful, ulcerative lesions involving >80% of BSA, including the soles of both feet. His disease was refractory to both topical and systemic therapy. The initial plan involved TSEBT 12 Gy in 8 fractions, four times weekly over 2 weeks. Given concern for poor treatment tolerance, the decision was made to procced with a hypofractionated course with 12 Gy in 3 once-weekly fractions [27]. A reclined TSEBT technique was used per institutional experience (Fig. 7.6a–d) [42, 44]. He was inpatient throughout duration of treatment.

Case 5

A 59-year-old woman, otherwise healthy, was initially diagnosed with MF, cT3N0M0B0, Stage IIB. While her skin disease remained stable on systemic and skin-directed topical therapies, she developed new lymphadenopathy the bilateral groins associated with pain (Fig. 7.7a, **red arrow**). She underwent targeted radiation therapy, 25 Gy in 10 fractions, for symptom palliation (Fig. 7.7b).

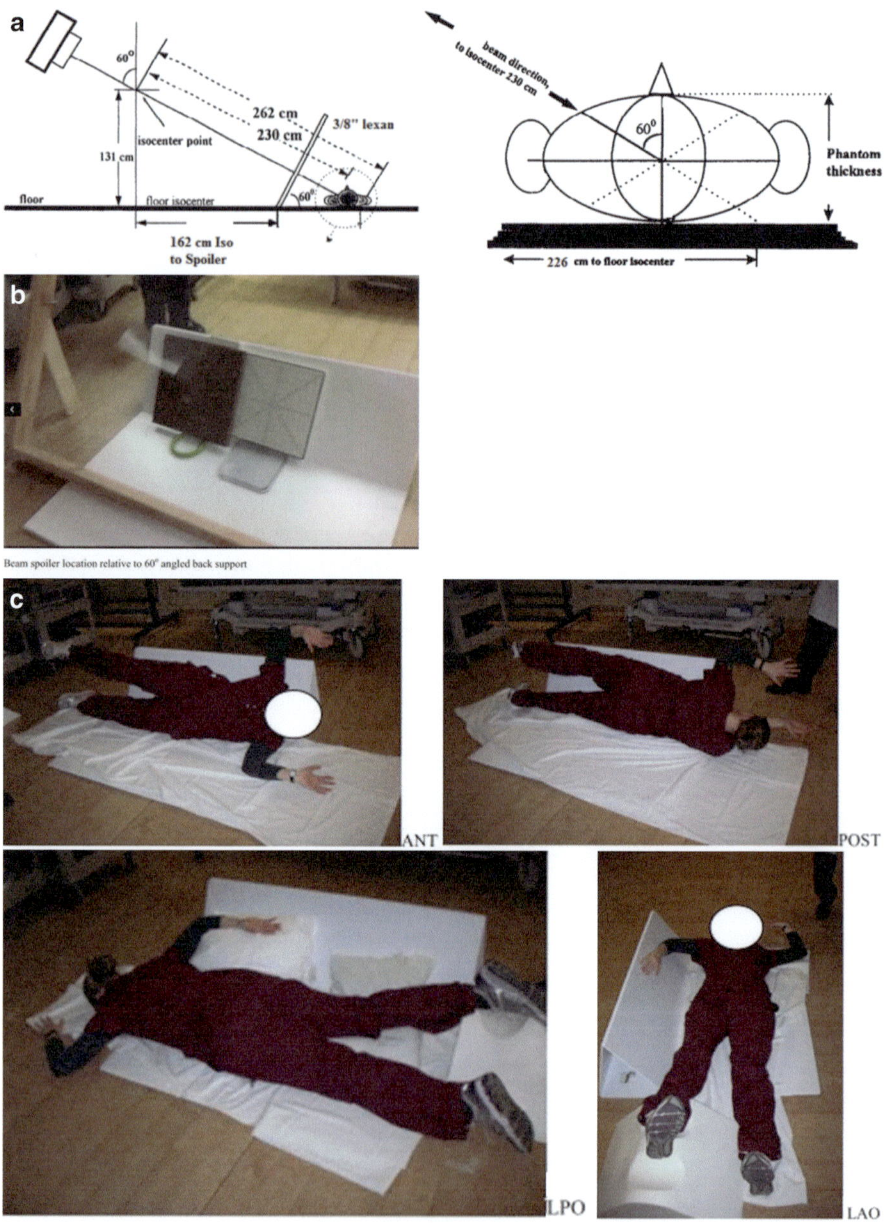

Fig. 7.6 TSEBT in reclined position: The patient was treated with the gantry angled 60° from vertically down, while he was located at a treatment distance of 330 cm SSD along the central axis of the beam. Photos below are of a model posing in the representative positions (**a**). A thin polycarbonate beam spoiler was placed 25 cm from the most proximal surface of the patient for all patient treatment positions (**b**). Adopting with modification the six positions per the Stanford technique, the patient was treated while assuming a reclined position (representative images shown in (**c**)). To produce a flat, uniform field, the patient was moved longitudinally by an experimentally determined distance (**d**)

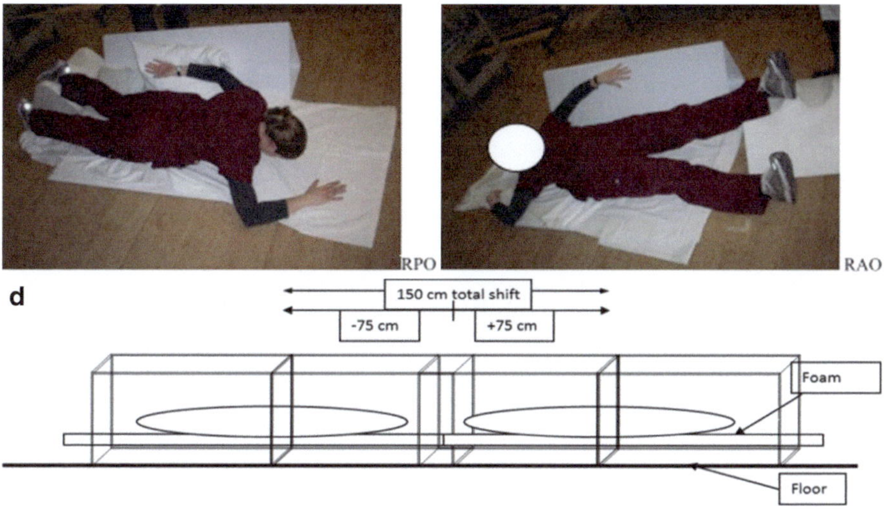

Fig. 7.6 (continued)

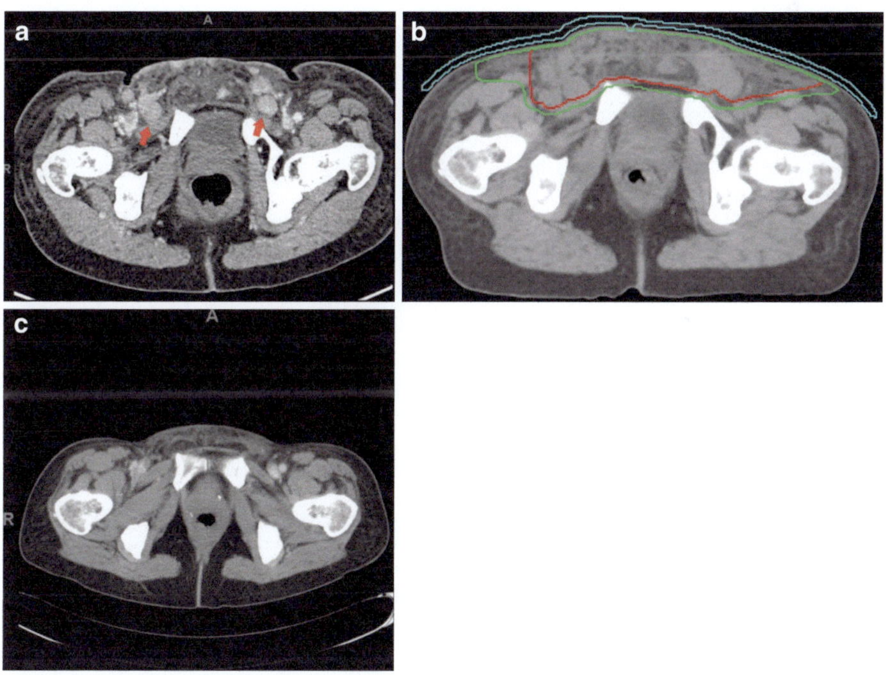

Fig. 7.7 Targeted radiation to symptomatic groin lymphadenopathy: Diagnostic CT was fused with planning CT for target delineation (**a**). CTV is in red, encompassing the gross lymphadenopathy with a 0.5 cm expansion. The PTV is in green (**b**). The 3 month post-treatment CT showed no evidence of residual disease (**c**)

Part 4: Special Consideration

- **General patient management during TSEBT**
  - Common acute side effects can include skin erythema/desquamation, blistering, irritation/pain, hair loss, and nail ridging/loss. These side effects are typically mild and resolve quickly.
  - There is a 5–6% risk of severe skin infection requiring hospitalization [45, 46]. A weekly complete blood count can be used to monitor the patient during TSEBT.
- **Managing patients with erythroderma during TSEBT**
  - Patients with erythrodermic MF are at risk of developing severe and potentially fatal complications, such as septicemia, hyperthermia/hypothermia, and fluid/electrolyte abnormalities.
  - Consider admitting these patients to the hospital for close monitoring during TSEBT.

References

1. Willemze R, Cerroni L, Kempf W, et al. The 2018 update of the WHO-EORTC classification for primary cutaneous lymphomas [published correction appears in Blood. 2019 Sep 26;134(13):1112]. Blood. 2019;133(16):1703–14. https://doi.org/10.1182/blood-2018-11-881268.
2. Imam MH, Shenoy PJ, Flowers CR, Phillips A, Lechowicz MJ. Incidence and survival patterns of cutaneous T-cell lymphomas in the United States. Leuk Lymphoma. 2013;54(4):752–9. https://doi.org/10.3109/10428194.2012.729831.
3. Criscione VD, Weinstock MA. Incidence of cutaneous T-cell lymphoma in the United States, 1973–2002. Arch Dermatol. 2007;143(7):854–9. https://doi.org/10.1001/archderm.143.7.854.
4. Whittemore AS, Holly EA, Lee IM, et al. Mycosis fungoides in relation to environmental exposures and immune response: a case-control study. J Natl Cancer Inst. 1989;81(20):1560–7. https://doi.org/10.1093/jnci/81.20.1560.
5. Pancake BA, Zucker-Franklin D, Coutavas EE. The cutaneous T cell lymphoma, mycosis fungoides, is a human T cell lymphotropic virus-associated disease. A study of 50 patients. J Clin Invest. 1995;95(2):547–54. https://doi.org/10.1172/JCI117697.
6. Campbell JJ, Clark RA, Watanabe R, Kupper TS. Sezary syndrome and mycosis fungoides arise from distinct T-cell subsets: a biologic rationale for their distinct clinical behaviors. Blood. 2010;116(5):767–71. https://doi.org/10.1182/blood-2009-11-251926.
7. Watanabe R, Gehad A, Yang C, et al. Human skin is protected by four functionally and phenotypically discrete populations of resident and recirculating memory T cells. Sci Transl Med. 2015;7(279):279ra39. https://doi.org/10.1126/scitranslmed.3010302.
8. Hsu MY, Murphy GF. Chapter 31. Cutaneous lymphomas and leukemias. In: Elder DE, Elenitsas RE, Johnson Jr BL, et al., editors. Lever's histopathology of the skin. 10th ed. Lippincott Williams & Wilkins; 2009.
9. Vonderheid EC, Bernengo MG, Burg G, et al. Update on erythrodermic cutaneous T-cell lymphoma: report of the International Society for Cutaneous Lymphomas. J Am Acad Dermatol. 2002;46(1):95–106. https://doi.org/10.1067/mjd.2002.118538.
10. Kirsch IR, Watanabe R, O'Malley JT, et al. TCR sequencing facilitates diagnosis and identifies mature T cells as the cell of origin in CTCL. Sci Transl Med. 2015;7(308):308ra158. https://doi.org/10.1126/scitranslmed.aaa9122.
11. Lessin SR. Alibert lymphoma: renaming mycosis fungoides. Arch Dermatol. 2009;145(2):209–10. https://doi.org/10.1001/archdermatol.2008.567.

12. Olsen E, Vonderheid E, Pimpinelli N, et al. Revisions to the staging and classification of mycosis fungoides and Sezary syndrome: a proposal of the International Society for Cutaneous Lymphomas (ISCL) and the cutaneous lymphoma task force of the European Organization of Research and Treatment of Cancer (EORTC) [published correction appears in Blood. 2008 May 1;111(9):4830]. Blood. 2007;110(6):1713–22. https://doi.org/10.1182/blood-2007-03-055749.
13. Agar NS, Wedgeworth E, Crichton S, et al. Survival outcomes and prognostic factors in mycosis fungoides/Sézary syndrome: validation of the revised International Society for Cutaneous Lymphomas/European Organisation for Research and Treatment of Cancer staging proposal. J Clin Oncol. 2010;28(31):4730–9. https://doi.org/10.1200/JCO.2009.27.7665.
14. Mehta-Shah N, Horwitz SM, Ansell S, et al. NCCN guidelines insights: primary cutaneous lymphomas, version 2.2020. J Natl Compr Cancer Netw. 2020;18(5):522–36. https://doi.org/10.6004/jnccn.2020.0022.
15. Hoppe RT. Mycosis fungoides: radiation therapy. Dermatol Ther. 2003;16(4):347–54. https://doi.org/10.1111/j.1396-0296.2003.01647.x.
16. Neelis KJ, Schimmel EC, Vermeer MH, Senff NJ, Willemze R, Noordijk EM. Low-dose palliative radiotherapy for cutaneous B- and T-cell lymphomas. Int J Radiat Oncol Biol Phys. 2009;74(1):154–8. https://doi.org/10.1016/j.ijrobp.2008.06.1918.
17. Wallace AB. The exposure treatment of burns. Lancet. 1951;1(6653):501–4. https://doi.org/10.1016/s0140-6736(51)91975-7.
18. Louden BA, Pearce DJ, Lang W, Feldman SR. A Simplified Psoriasis Area Severity Index (SPASI) for rating psoriasis severity in clinic patients. Dermatol Online J. 2004;10(2):7. Published 2004 Oct 15.
19. Kim JH, Nisce LZ, D'Anglo GJ. Dose-time fractionation study in patients with mycosis fungoides and lymphoma cutis. Radiology. 1976;119(2):439–42. https://doi.org/10.1148/119.2.439.
20. Cotter GW, Baglan RJ, Wasserman TH, Mill W. Palliative radiation treatment of cutaneous mycosis fungoides—a dose response. Int J Radiat Oncol Biol Phys. 1983;9(10):1477–80. https://doi.org/10.1016/0360-3016(83)90321-8.
21. Russo AL, Chen YH, Martin NE, et al. Low-dose involved-field radiation in the treatment of non-Hodgkin lymphoma: predictors of response and treatment failure. Int J Radiat Oncol Biol Phys. 2013;86:121–7. https://doi.org/10.1016/j.ijrobp.2012.12.024.
22. Wilson LD, Kacinski BM, Jones GW. Local superficial radiotherapy in the management of minimal stage IA cutaneous T-cell lymphoma (mycosis fungoides). Int J Radiat Oncol Biol Phys. 1998;40(1):109–15. https://doi.org/10.1016/s0360-3016(97)00553-1.
23. Micaily B, Miyamoto C, Kantor G, et al. Radiotherapy for unilesional mycosis fungoides. Int J Radiat Oncol Biol Phys. 1998;42(2):361–4. https://doi.org/10.1016/s0360-3016(98)00218-1.
24. Moraes FY, Carvalho Hde A, Hanna SA, Silva JL, Marta GN. Literature review of clinical results of total skin electron irradiation (TSEBT) of mycosis fungoides in adults. Rep Pract Oncol Radiother. 2013;19(2):92–8. https://doi.org/10.1016/j.rpor.2013.08.003. Published 2013 Sep 27.
25. Le Bourgeois JP, Haddad E, Marinello G, Marin L, Mazeron JJ, Ganem G. The indications for total cutaneous electron beam radiation therapy of mycosis fungoides. Int J Radiat Oncol Biol Phys. 1987;13(2):189–93. https://doi.org/10.1016/0360-3016(87)90126-x.
26. Nisce LZ, Chu FC, Lee HS, Filippa D, Kempin S, Coleman M. Total skin electron beam therapy for cutaneous lymphomas and leukemias. Int J Radiat Oncol Biol Phys. 1982;8(9):1587–92. https://doi.org/10.1016/0360-3016(82)90621-6.
27. Jeans EB, Hu YH, Stish BJ, et al. Low-dose hypofractionated total skin electron beam therapy for adult cutaneous T-cell lymphoma. Pract Radiat Oncol. 2020;10(6):e529–37. https://doi.org/10.1016/j.prro.2020.08.001.
28. Quirós PA, Jones GW, Kacinski BM, et al. Total skin electron beam therapy followed by adjuvant psoralen/ultraviolet-a light in the management of patients with T1 and T2 cutaneous T-cell lymphoma (mycosis fungoides). Int J Radiat Oncol Biol Phys. 1997;38(5):1027–35. https://doi.org/10.1016/s0360-3016(97)00127-2.

29. Ysebaert L, Truc G, Dalac S, et al. Ultimate results of radiation therapy for T1-T2 mycosis fungoides (including reirradiation). Int J Radiat Oncol Biol Phys. 2004;58(4):1128–34. https://doi.org/10.1016/j.ijrobp.2003.08.007.
30. Navi D, Riaz N, Levin YS, Sullivan NC, Kim YH, Hoppe RT. The Stanford University experience with conventional-dose, total skin electron-beam therapy in the treatment of generalized patch or plaque (T2) and tumor (T3) mycosis fungoides. Arch Dermatol. 2011;147(5):561–7. https://doi.org/10.1001/archdermatol.2011.98.
31. Heumann TR, Esiashvili N, Parker S, et al. Total skin electron therapy for cutaneous T-cell lymphoma using a modern dual-field rotational technique [published correction appears in Int J Radiat Oncol Biol Phys. 2015 Nov 1;93(3):729–30]. Int J Radiat Oncol Biol Phys. 2015;92(1):183–91. https://doi.org/10.1016/j.ijrobp.2014.11.033.
32. Hoppe RT, Fuks Z, Bagshaw MA. The rationale for curative radiotherapy in mycosis fungoides. Int J Radiat Oncol Biol Phys. 1977;2(9–10):843–51. https://doi.org/10.1016/0360-3016(77)90182-1.
33. Hoppe RT, Harrison C, Tavallaee M, et al. Low-dose total skin electron beam therapy as an effective modality to reduce disease burden in patients with mycosis fungoides: results of a pooled analysis from 3 phase-II clinical trials. J Am Acad Dermatol. 2015;72(2):286–92. https://doi.org/10.1016/j.jaad.2014.10.014.
34. Elsayad K, Kriz J, Moustakis C, et al. Total skin electron beam for primary cutaneous T-cell lymphoma. Int J Radiat Oncol Biol Phys. 2015;93(5):1077–86. https://doi.org/10.1016/j.ijrobp.2015.08.041.
35. Morris S, Scarisbrick J, Frew J, et al. The results of low-dose total skin electron beam radiation therapy (TSEB) in patients with mycosis fungoides from the UK Cutaneous Lymphoma Group. Int J Radiat Oncol Biol Phys. 2017;99(3):627–33. https://doi.org/10.1016/j.ijrobp.2017.05.052.
36. Specht L, Dabaja B, Illidge T, Wilson LD, Hoppe RT, International Lymphoma Radiation Oncology Group. Modern radiation therapy for primary cutaneous lymphomas: field and dose guidelines from the International Lymphoma Radiation Oncology Group. Int J Radiat Oncol Biol Phys. 2015;92(1):32–9. https://doi.org/10.1016/j.ijrobp.2015.01.008.
37. Piotrowski T, Milecki P, Skórska M, Fundowicz D. Total skin electron irradiation techniques: a review. Postepy Dermatol Alergol. 2013;30(1):50–5. https://doi.org/10.5114/pdia.2013.33379.
38. Williams PC, Hunter RD, Jackson SM. Whole body electron therapy in mycosis fungoides—a successful translational technique achieved by modification of an established linear accelerator. Br J Radiol. 1979;52(616):302–7. https://doi.org/10.1259/0007-1285-52-616-302.
39. Kron T, Donahoo G, Lonski P, Wheeler G. A technique for total skin electron therapy (TSET) of an anesthetized pediatric patient. J Appl Clin Med Phys. 2018;19(6):109–16. https://doi.org/10.1002/acm2.12457.
40. Gerbi BJ, Khan FM, Deibel FC, Kim TH. Total skin electron arc irradiation using a reclined patient position. Int J Radiat Oncol Biol Phys. 1989;17(2):397–404. https://doi.org/10.1016/0360-3016(89)90457-4.
41. Skórska M. Total skin electron beam (TSEB) therapy in pediatric patients: a review of the literature. Rep Pract Oncol Radiother. 2013;19(2):109–13. https://doi.org/10.1016/j.rpor.2013.06.003. Published 2013 Jul 19.
42. Jones GW, Kacinski BM, Wilson LD, et al. Total skin electron radiation in the management of mycosis fungoides: consensus of the European Organization for Research and Treatment of Cancer (EORTC) Cutaneous Lymphoma Project Group. J Am Acad Dermatol. 2002;47(3):364–70. https://doi.org/10.1067/mjd.2002.123482.
43. Weaver RD, Gerbi BJ, Dusenbery KE. Evaluation of dose variation during total skin electron irradiation using thermoluminescent dosimeters. Int J Radiat Oncol Biol Phys. 1995;33(2):475–8. https://doi.org/10.1016/0360-3016(95)00161-Q.
44. Mathew D, Gerbi B. SU-G-TeP1-13: reclined total skin electron treatment technique. Med Phys. 2016;43(6Part26):3654–5.
45. Desai KR, Pezner RD, Lipsett JA, et al. Total skin electron irradiation for mycosis fungoides: relationship between acute toxicities and measured dose at different anatomic sites [published

correction appears in Int J Radiat Oncol Biol Phys 1989 Jan;16(1):A1]. Int J Radiat Oncol Biol Phys. 1988;15(3):641–5. https://doi.org/10.1016/0360-3016(88)90306-9.
46. Meyler TS, Blumberg AL, Purser P. Total skin electron beam therapy in mycosis fungoides. Cancer. 1978;42(3):1171–6. https://doi.org/10.1002/1097-0142(197809)42:3<1171::aid-cncr2820420321>3.0.co;2-8.

Cutaneous Lymphoma

8

Jillian R. Gunther and Bouthaina S. Dabaja

Contents

Cutaneous B Cell Malignancies

Part 1: Background and Epidemiology

- Epidemiology
  - Most common subtypes of cutaneous B cell lymphoma:
    Primary cutaneous marginal zone B-cell lymphoma (PCMZL).
    Primary cutaneous follicle center lymphoma (PCFCL).

J. R. Gunther (✉) · B. S. Dabaja
Division of Radiation Oncology, Department of Radiation Oncology, The University of Texas MD Anderson Cancer Center, Houston, TX, USA
e-mail: jgunther@mdanderson.org; bdabaja@mdanderson.org

C. Pinnix et al. (eds.), *Target Volume Delineation in Hematologic Malignancies*, Practical Guides in Radiation Oncology,
https://doi.org/10.1007/978-3-031-67722-9_8

Primary cutaneous diffuse large B-cell lymphoma, leg-type (PCLBCL, LT) (will not be discussed further in this chapter).

- Patients commonly affected, age of diagnosis, gender predilection, and risk factors.
  - No strong age or gender predilection.
  - Reported links with *B. burgdorferi* infection, tattoos, acrodermatitis chronica atrophicans, and vaccination sites [1, 2].
- Pathology details
  - Small to medium lymphocytes in nodular to diffuse infiltrates of the skin with epidermal sparing.
  - Marginal zone: B-cells express CD20, CD79, and Bcl-2, most often negative for CD5, CD10, and Bcl-6.
  - Primary cutaneous follicle center (PCFCL): monotonous large follicle center cells in nodular or diffuse infiltrates of the skin with epidermal sparing. Cells are CD20+, CD79a+, and Bcl-6+, with surrounding CD21+ or CD35+ follicular dendritic cells. Rarely expressing t(14;18) or Bcl-2 [3].
- Typical presentation
  - Red to violaceous papules, plaques, or nodules. Non-ulcerative and typically asymptomatic (non-painful, non-itchy).
  - PCMZL is more common on trunk and extremities. PCFCL is more common on scalp and forehead.
  - Slow rate of growth.
- Staging and workup
  - A full dermatologic examination should be performed to identify all sites of possible disease with biopsies as appropriate.
  - Diagnostic imaging to rule out systemic disease involvement with contrasted CTs or positron emission tomography (PET)-CT should be performed.
  - History of autoimmune diseases, and immunosuppressive therapy.
  - Labs including complete blood count (CBC), comprehensive metabolic panel (CMP), lactate dehydrogenase (LDH).
  - Additional workup including hepatitis B/C testing, peripheral blood flow cytometry, Serum protein electrophoresis (SPEP)/immunoglobulins, Borrelia burgdorferi testing, *H. pylori* testing, and/or bone marrow biopsy considered for select cases.
- Overview of standard of care treatment approaches
  - Therapy can include antibiotics, surgical excision (although discouraged), intralesional steroid, or radiation therapy. If multifocal or larger disease burden, systemic therapy such as rituximab can be employed [3, 4].
  - Published series report excellent responses to radiation therapy, even with doses as low as 4–12 Gy [5, 6].
  - Full response to treatment can take up to 4–8 weeks.
  - Disease-specific survival approaches 100%. Cutaneous relapses are common, but can be salvaged successfully.

Pre-radiotherapy Imaging and Evaluation

- A full dermatologic examination should be performed to identify all sites of possible disease and delineate the extent of the skin lesion if there is any question for RT field design. Diagnostic imaging can be utilized/reviewed to determine lesion depth.

Part 2: Management and Treatment of Cutaneous B Cell Lymphomas

Principles of Management

- PCMZL and PCFCL are indolent lymphomas which rarely affect the overall lifespan of the patient. Therefore, consideration of any toxicity associated with treatment is of utmost importance.
- RT is incredibly effective and can be given at initial presentation or if other treatments (topical steroid, intra-lesional kenalog) have failed, radiation is also considered as an ideal alternative to any surgical excision for optimized cosmetic outcomes. Treatment with doses as low as 4 Gy are effective. Dose escalation can be performed in the setting of insufficient response or relapse.
- Patients are encouraged to commit to regular and long-term follow-up with dermatology, as out-of-field cutaneous relapses are common.

General Considerations for Radiotherapy

- Radiation therapy is typically used to treat the identified skin lesion with margin. Elective, uninvolved nodes are not treated. The disease-specific survival rates for patients with cutaneous B cell lymphoma are excellent, approaching 100%. Therefore, it is imperative that treatment does not impart unacceptable toxicity. The lowest effective dose should be used.
- As lesions are cutaneous/superficial, clinical simulation can often be performed in lieu of CT-based simulation.
  - For thick, nodular lesions with unavailable diagnostic imaging, CT simulation can be performed to inform the appropriate electron energy.
  - CT simulation is also helpful in cases where the lesion abuts critical structures such as the eye, salivary glands, etc., so that dose to normal structures can be monitored/recorded.
- Some centers have access to orthovoltage technology, which can be helpful for superficial, small lesions.
- Planning of Target Volumes (Table 8.1):

  For clinical skin treatments using electrons (without CT simulation), a 1.5–3 cm margin is typically drawn around the border of the visible skin lesion which accounts for CTV margin (microscopic disease), PTV, and adequate dose buildup. In critical locations like the face, skin collimation is indicated to allow smaller margins around the lesion of 0.5 cm. The total margin is chosen based on

Table 8.1 Planning target definitions for treatment of cutaneous lymphoma

Volume	Description	
Gross tumor volume (GTV)	GTV	• Contains gross tumor volume as identified by direct visualization of skin (wired at time of CT simulation) and by skin changes identified on diagnostic and simulation imaging (if applicable)
	Post-excision GTV	• If the lesion has been surgically excised, a virtual GTV should be estimated using pre-excision photographs and/or diagnostic imaging
Clinical target volume (CTV)	CTV	• 1–2 cm margin on the GTV, depending upon the clarity/demarcation of the lesion border
Internal target volume (ITV)	• n/a	
Planning target volume (PTV)	• PTV margin of 0.5–1cm can be added based on physician oversight of setup and site. For clinical electron therapy treatments, additional margin (0.5–1 cm) to block edge must be added to allow for adequate dose buildup depending upon treatment technique • For planned external beam treatments, CTV-to-PTV expansions should be individualized based on the treatment site, expected patient setup reproducibility, Image-guided radiation therapy (IGRT) utilized, etc.	
Organs at risk (OAR)	• Skin directed radiation is typically delivered using superficial electron treatment. However, it is possible that Organs at Risk (OARs) including but not limited to the eye, salivary glands, thyroid, brain, oral mucosa, and even spinal cord (depending on the size of the patient and the electron energy) could receive dose, which should be considered during treatment planning. This is particularly important during clinical treatment performed without CT simulation as contouring and documentation of OAR doses is not part of the workflow	

the clarity of lesion borders and the dosimetry of the planned radiation technique to ensure adequate dose buildup. The size of the treatment field is recorded and used for dosimetric calculations and future treatment delivery.

- When CT simulation is performed for use in treatment planning, the lesion and/or intended treatment field is often wired at the time of simulation. A 1–2 cm CTV (depending upon certainty of lesion demarcation and treatment site) should be used. A site-specific PTV of 0.5–1 cm can be added based on physician oversight of setup, immobilization, and image-guidance.
  - When treatment of the lesion abuts critical structures, these margins can be narrowed slightly. Critical structures can also be better protected through the use of additional shielding in the way of skin collimation, eye shields, testicular clam shell, etc.
- The vast majority of cutaneous lymphomas require treatment of only the superficial skin, which is effectively accomplished using electron therapy. The lesion depth should be measured and an appropriate electron energy chosen to ensure adequate coverage. Bolus should be used for lower energy electron treatments to achieve full skin dose. Bolus using soaking wet towels can be used in areas with irregular surface to achieve better bolus conformality, with attention to the thickness of the towel. Custom aquaplast or 3D printed bolus is also an acceptable option.
- Complete response rates as high as 99–100% have been reported [5, 7].

Part 3: Cases

Case 1: Primary Cutaneous Marginal Zone Lymphoma

A 40-year-old woman presented with a lesion that grew over 2 months. It was biopsied and consistent with low grade B-cell lymphoma consistent with extranodal marginal zone lymphoma. Histologic sections showed a nodular dermal infiltrate composed of predominantly small lymphocytes. Immunohistochemical studies demonstrated the infiltrate comprised CD20 positive B cells positive for Bcl-2 and CD23. The patient underwent staging contrasted CTs of the neck, chest, abdomen, and pelvis, which were negative for any evidence of active lymphoma. She was recommended treatment with local radiation therapy alone (Fig. 8.1).

Case 2: Primary Cutaneous Follicle Center Lymphoma

A 45-year-old male patient noticed a raised lesion on his left frontal scalp for about a year. Biopsy was performed and consistent with low grade B cell lymphoma involving the skin. The lymphocytes were CD10+ and Bcl-6+ with large cells suggestive of cutaneous follicle center cell lymphoma. Contrasted CTs were performed and negative for evidence of systemic lymphoma. Labs were performed and unremarkable. He was recommended treatment with RT to a total dose of 4 Gy (Figs. 8.2, 8.3, and 8.4).

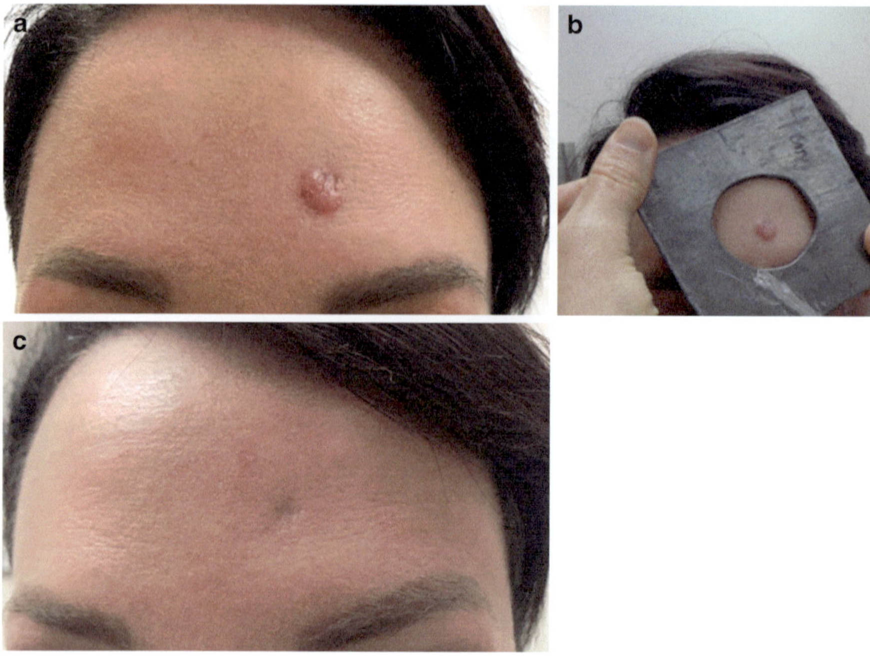

Fig. 8.1 Pre-treatment patient evaluation and clinical simulation. (**a**) Pre-treatment photograph showing the 1.2 cm nodular lesion on the patient's forehead. (**b**) Approximately 1.5 cm margin around the lesion was chosen. A 4 cm circle skin collimation was used to provide full radiation dose distribution at the edge of the field, as the electron penumbra falls outside the target and on the collimation. The collimation was positioned to completely block the eyebrow, orbit, and the hair line. The patient was treated using 9 MeV electrons with 1 cm bolus. (**c**) Five weeks after RT completion, the patient achieved a complete response. A small scar remained in the location of the prior nodule

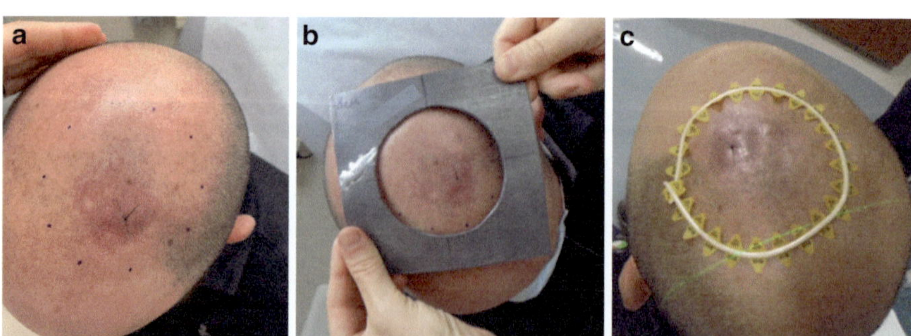

Fig. 8.2 Pretreatment patient evaluation, clinical simulation, and CT simulation. The target was delineated during the initial consultation in clinic, which included the lesion with approximately 1.5 cm margin. A pre-cut skin collimation which approximated the drawn treatment field was used. At time of CT simulation, the opening of the skin collimation was wired to facilitate identification of the lesion on the CT simulation images. An aquaplast mask was made and cut out around the wire. (**a**) Vertex scalp of patient with marked dots outlining the intended treatment field. (**b**) Skin collimation (8 cm circle) centered on skin lesion. (**c**) Wire at the time of simulation outlining the opening of the skin collimation

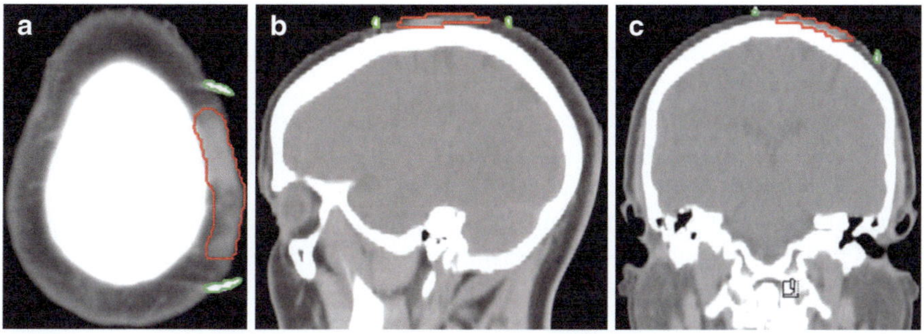

Fig. 8.3 CT simulation images showing the wire (green) marking the inside opening of the skin collimation and the contoured GTV (red) in the (**a**) axial, (**b**) sagittal, and (**c**) coronal planes

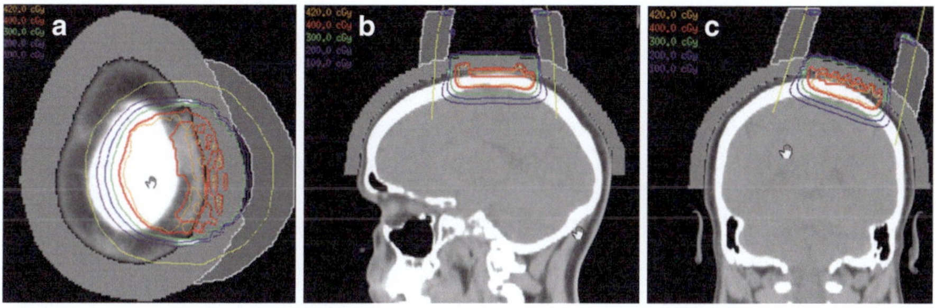

Fig. 8.4 Radiation was delivered using 9 MeV electrons with 1 cm bolus. Virtual skin collimation (grey with outline) and 1 cm virtual bolus (grey) were modeled during the planning process. Representative images of the final treatment plan in the (**a**) axial, (**b**) sagittal, and (**c**) coronal planes

Cutaneous T Cell Lymphoma: Mycosis Fungoides

Part 1: Background and Epidemiology

- Epidemiology/background
  - Most common cutaneous T cell lymphoma (CTCL), about 2/3 of all CTCL cases.
  - Patients are often treated for various other skin disorders (e.g., psoriasis) before a diagnostic biopsy is obtained.
  - Generally displays indolent behavior and is considered incurable unless aggressive treatment with stem cell transplant is considered.
- Patients commonly affected, age of diagnosis, gender predilection, and risk factors.
  - More common in males and older patients (>50).
  - External triggers for disease include hydrochlorothiazide diuretics, immuno-suppression, chemical exposure, and putative bacterial and viral agents [8].

- Pathology details
  - Pathology characterized by clonal T-cells grouped at the epidermal basement membrane
  - Typical immunophenotype: CD2+, CD3+, CD5+, CD4+, CD8+, CCR4+, TCR-beta+, and CD45RO+ without typical T cell markers including CD7 and CD26 [9].
  - Confirmation of clonal T-cell receptor (TCR) gene rearrangement can support the diagnosis and rule out other inflammatory conditions
- Typical presentation
  - Early-stage disease presents with patches, which are often scaly and erythematous. Often patients had skin lesions for years if not decades where multiple biopsies failed to diagnose it. Disease can progress to plaques or tumors and can include generalized erythroderma.
  - Patient frequently have co-existing skin infections that can worsen disease.
- Staging and workup
  - Full dermatologic exam and skin photography to document the involved body surface area (BSA), and the Modified Severity-Weighted Assessment Tool (mSWAT). Location and extent of patch, plaque, and tumor disease should be noted for initial staging and subsequent response assessment. Clinical nodal exam should be performed.
  - General labs including CBC, CMP, LDH, and flow cytometry to assess blood involvement.
  - Imaging and bone marrow biopsy are sometimes considered based on the extent of disease involvement. Consider biopsy of enlarged/suspicious nodes for staging.
  - If skin-limited disease, T1 and T2 disease includes patches and/or plaques involving less than or greater than 10% of the skin, respectively. Any tumor is T3 and ≥80% of confluent skin erythema is T4. Nodal staging requires histologic confirmation. Blood involvement is determined by number/percentage of abnormal cells on flow cytometry.
- Overview of standard of care treatment approaches
  - Skin directed therapies include topical agents, phototherapy, and radiation therapy [10].
  - Systemic therapies include retinoids, interferon, methotrexate, histone deacetylase inhibitors, targeted therapy, cytotoxic chemotherapy, and clinical trial agents.
  - Focal radiation therapy can be used to palliate limited skin lesions
  - Total skin electron beam therapy (TSEBT) is used to treat the entire skin surface for patients with greater disease burden [11, 12].

Pre-radiotherapy Imaging and Evaluation

- Contrasted CTs or PET-CT can be used during initial staging to rule out systemic disease involvement.
- Patients should be evaluated by a dermatologist for a full skin exam and BSA documentation, ideally at a high volume CTCL center. Medical oncology consultation is recommended unless disease burden is minimal.

- Radiation therapy for CTCL is effective at low to moderate doses and is typically well tolerated. Topical therapies can be continued on non-irradiated lesions during focal treatment. Systemic therapies such as bexarotene, interferon, extracorporeal photophoresis, and brentuximab vedotin can typically be continued during focal treatment and considered even for patients undergoing TSEBT. Methotrexate/pralatrexate should be discontinued during RT [13].

Part 2: Management and Treatment of Mycosis Fungoides

Principles of Management

- Skin directed therapies include topical agents (steroids, chemotherapy, bexarotene gel, imiquimod), phototherapy (Psoralen plus ultraviolet A (PUVA), ultraviolet B (UVB)), and radiation therapy (focal treatment, total skin electron beam therapy (TSEBT).
- Systemic therapies include retinoids/bexarotene, interferon, methotrexate/pralatrexate, histone deacetylase inhibitors, targeted therapy, cytotoxic chemotherapy, and clinical trial agents.
- Focal radiation therapy can be used for palliation of a limited number of symptomatic and/or progressing sites of disease.
  - Doses as low as 4–12 Gy are typically effective, with higher doses of 8–12 Gy typically given for thicker, ulcerative disease [6].
- TSEBT, which treats the entire skin surface, is reserved for higher percentage BSA involvement.
  - Often given twice weekly with 2 Gy per fraction treatments. Supplemental boost fields include the axillae, shoulders, inframammary and other skin folds, groins, perineum, perianal area, and soles.
  - 10–12 Gy overall response rates of >80% with mild toxicity [12].
  - 28–36 Gy for pre-transplant conditioning [14].
  - Full response may require up to 8–12 weeks.

General Considerations for Radiotherapy

- Patients with mycosis fungoides are not generally considered curable; therefore, all treatments are palliative in nature [3].
  - Treatment should be directed at symptomatic (itching, painful) and or problematic (infection risk, encroaching critical structure such as the eye) lesions
  - The lowest possible dose should be given to minimize toxicity and allow for future treatment (re-treatment).
- As lesions are cutaneous/superficial, clinical simulation can often be performed in lieu of CT-based simulation.
  - For plaque and tumor lesions with unavailable diagnostic imaging, CT simulation can be performed to assess depth and inform the appropriate electron energy.
  - CT simulation is also helpful in cases where the lesion abuts critical structures such as the eye, salivary glands, etc., so that dose to OARs can be monitored/recorded.

- Some centers have access to orthovoltage technology, which can be helpful for superficial, small lesions.
- Centers with a high volume of CTCL patients are often equipped for TSEBT, which requires special workflows and training of the dosimetry/physics/therapy/ and physician treatment teams.
- Planning of target volumes (Table 8.2):
- For clinical skin treatments using electrons (without CT simulation), a 1.5–3 cm margin is typically drawn around the border of the visible skin lesion which accounts for CTV margin (microscopic disease), PTV, and adequate dose buildup. In critical locations like the face, skin collimation is indicated to allow

Table 8.2 Planning target definitions for treatment of cutaneous lymphoma

Volume	Description	
Gross tumor volume (GTV)	GTV	• Contains gross tumor volume as identified by direct visualization of skin (wired at the time of CT simulation) and by skin changes identified on diagnostic and simulation imaging (if applicable)
	Post-excision GTV	• If the lesion has been surgically excised, a virtual GTV should be estimated using pre-excision photographs and/or diagnostic imaging
Clinical target volume (CTV)	CTV	• 1–2 cm margin on the GTV, depending upon the clarity/demarcation of the lesion border
Internal target volume (ITV)	• n/a	
Planning target volume (PTV)	• PTV margin of 0.5–1 cm can be added based on physician oversight of setup and site. For clinical treatments, additional margin (0.5–1 cm) to block edge must be added to allow for adequate dose buildup depending upon treatment technique • For planned external beam treatments, CTV-to-PTV expansions should be individualized based on the treatment site, expected patient setup reproducibility, IGRT utilized, etc.	
Organs at risk (OAR)	• Skin directed radiation is typically delivered using superficial electron treatment. However, it is possible that Organs at Risk (OARs) including but not limited to the eye, salivary glands, thyroid, brain, oral mucosa, and even spinal cord (depending on the size of the patient and the electron energy) could receive dose should be considered during treatment planning. This is particularly important during clinical treatment performed without CT simulation as contouring and documentation of OAR doses is not part of the workflow (avoiding organs at risk takes priority over comprehensively including lesions)	

using smaller margins around the lesion of 0.5 cm. The total margin is chosen based on the clarity of lesion borders and the dosimetry of the planned radiation technique to ensure adequate dose buildup. The size of the treatment field is recorded and used for dosimetric calculations and future treatment delivery.

- When CT simulation is performed for use in treatment planning, the lesion is often wired at time of simulation. A 1–2 cm CTV (depending upon certainty of lesion demarcation and treatment site) should be used. A site-specific PTV of 0.5–1 cm can be added based on physician oversight of setup, immobilization, and image-guidance.
  - When treatment of the lesion abuts critical structures, these margins can be narrowed slightly. Critical structures can also be better protected using additional shielding in the way of skin collimation, eye shields, testicular clam shell, etc. For instance, when treating next to the face, additional bolus can be placed on top of the parotid to avoid unnecessary radiation to underlying salivary glands.
  - When treating the surface of curved structures, for instance extremities or the scalp, avoid using high energy abutting electrons to avoid double dose at depth.
- The vast majority of cutaneous lymphomas require treatment of only the superficial skin, which is effectively accomplished using electron therapy. The lesion depth should be measured, and an appropriate electron energy chosen to ensure adequate coverage. Covering the dermis and appendages is advised to get to the location of the disease formation. Bolus should be used for lower energy electron treatments to achieve full skin dose. For superficial patch disease on the trunk or extremities, 9 MeV electrons with 1 cm of bolus often provide adequate coverage. Bolus using soaking wet towels (measured carefully) can be used in areas with irregular surface to achieve better bolus conformality. Custom aquaplast or 3D printed bolus is also an acceptable option.
- Response assessment in cutaneous lymphoma is challenging given the irregular tumor borders, difficulty in visualization of early-stage lesions on diagnostic imaging such as CT or PET-CT, and inflammatory changes that persist after treatment. Given the incurable nature of the disease, regular interval follow-up is less common than for solid tumors or systemic lymphomas. As such, data are limited on the dose-response relationship of cutaneous T cell lymphomas. Complete response rates of 92% have been reported for doses as low as 8 Gy in 2 fractions [6].

Part 3: Cases

Case 1: CD30+ Cutaneous T Cell Lymphoma, Clinically Consistent with Cutaneous Anaplastic Large Cell Lymphoma

A 70-year-old female with long history of cutaneous T cell lymphoma. She had been treated with numerous prior topical and systemic therapies. She had also received numerous prior radiation therapy courses with good response. She presented with a new lesion on the nose that progressed rapidly over 20 days as shown below (Fig. 8.5). She was recommended focal radiation therapy. She received 7.5 Gy in 3 fractions (Fig. 8.6).

Cutaneous T cell lymphomas can present with coexisting features of both mycosis fungoides and other T cell histologies such as primary cutaneous anaplastic large cell lymphoma (pcALCL). Clinical presentation as well as pathologic analysis are critical in the proper characterization of each disease process. Primary cutaneous ALCL is the second most common CTCL. Patients commonly present with rapidly growing ulcerative lesions with black eschar. Prior studies support excellent response to local radiation therapy with doses less than 20 Gy having equal efficacy to higher dose treatments [15, 16].

Case 2: Mycosis Fungoides with Large Cell Transformation

A 36-year-old patient had a 10-year history of skin rashes, biopsied 6 years prior as mycosis fungoides. He had only been treated with topical steroids. He then presented with rapid worsening of his skin lesions and tumor development. Biopsy confirmed large cell transformation of MF. Dermatologic exam confirmed 2% patch, 44.5% plaque, and 1.5% tumor on BSA assessment. PET-CT revealed avid cutaneous/subcutaneous disease as well as sub-centimeter occipital and cervical lymph nodes, likely reactive and draining from the lesion. He was initiated on oral Targretin and referred for radiation therapy. Given his diffuse skin involvement and uncontrolled itching, he was recommended total skin electron beam therapy with a boost to the tumor involving the occipital scalp. TSEBT was delivered at 2 Gy per fraction twice weekly. The scalp tumor was treated with an additional 9.6 Gy given as 1.2 Gy per day treated 4 days per week including standing TSEBT days (Figs. 8.7, 8.8, 8.9, and 8.10).

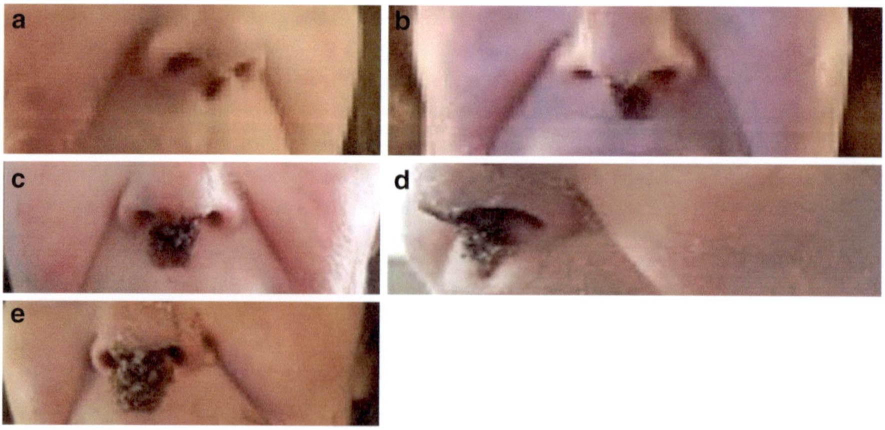

Fig. 8.5 Progressive worsening of the lesion over a period of 20 days

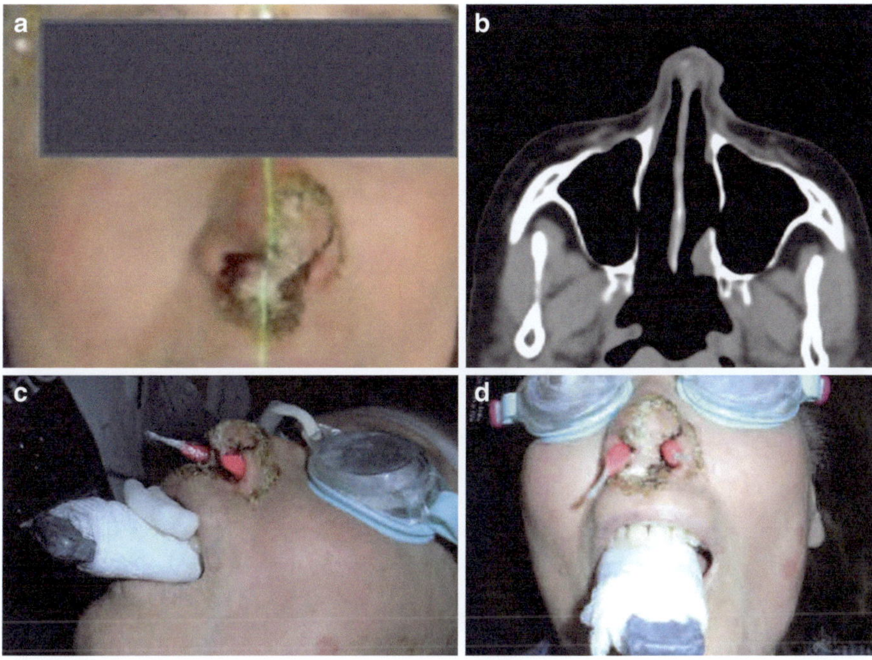

Fig. 8.6 (**a**–**d**) CT simulation and patient setup for treatment delivery. (**a**) Photograph of patient setup during CT simulation. Simulation was performed to confirm the depth of the tumor as no diagnostic imaging was available. (**b**) Axial CT image demonstrating involvement of the nasal skin with no deeper involvement of the nasal cavity. (**c**) Lateral, and (**d**) frontal photographs of patient setup at time of treatment delivery. Tissue compensator material (pink material) was placed in both nostrils. Swimming goggles filled with Cerrobend were used to block and protect the orbital structures. Cotton roll was used to elevate the lip and decrease dose to oral cavity structures as well to decrease the back scatter to the inner upper lip mucosa when the electrons strike the bone of the maxilla. To decrease the dose to the tongue and lower jaw the mouth was kept open with cerrobend block half way in the patient's mouth. The field size was calculated as 6.5 cm × 6.5 cm to encompass the visible skin disease with margin. She was treated with 12 MeV electrons. 1 cm bolus was used for treatment

Case 3: Mycosis Fungoides with Focal Patch Disease

A 58-year-old male with a longstanding history of mycosis fungoides (more than 16 years). He had previously used multiple topical treatments including steroid, bexarotene gel, and light therapy with narrowband UVB. He presented with painful, refractory disease in several focal locations (Fig. 8.11). He was treated with radiation therapy to a total dose of 4 Gy in 2 fractions (Figs. 8.12 and 8.13).

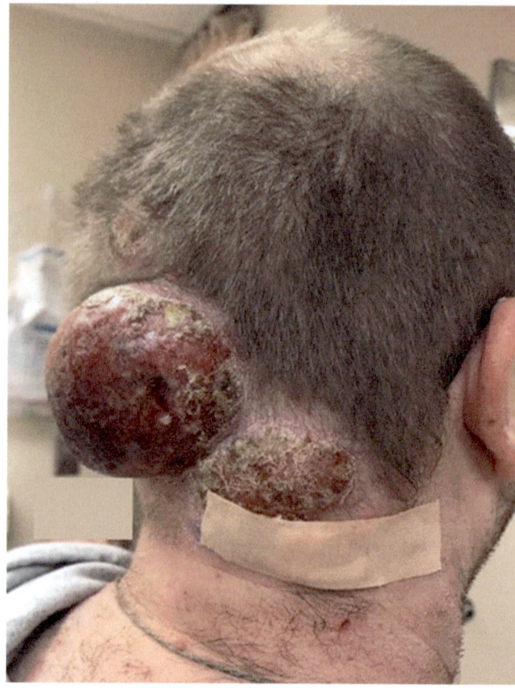

Fig. 8.7 Patient presentation. The patient presented with an MSWAT of 97% including diffuse plaque involvement of the trunk and extremities. He also had tumor disease occupying the occipital scalp

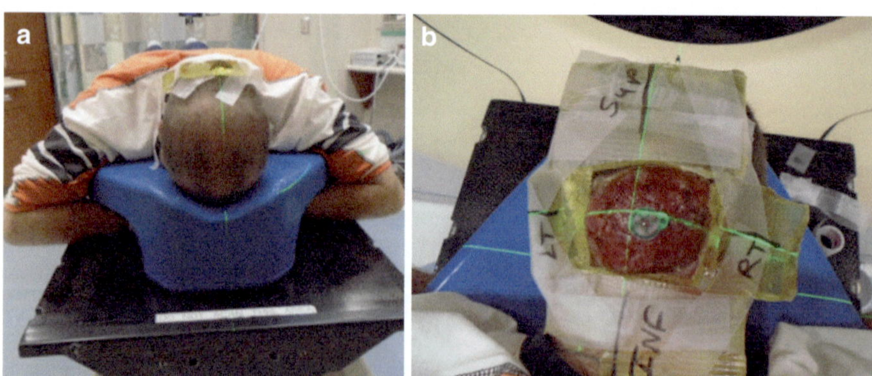

Fig. 8.8 CT simulation. (**a**) The patient was simulated prone. (**b**) Bolus (2 cm thickness) was used to surround the tumor

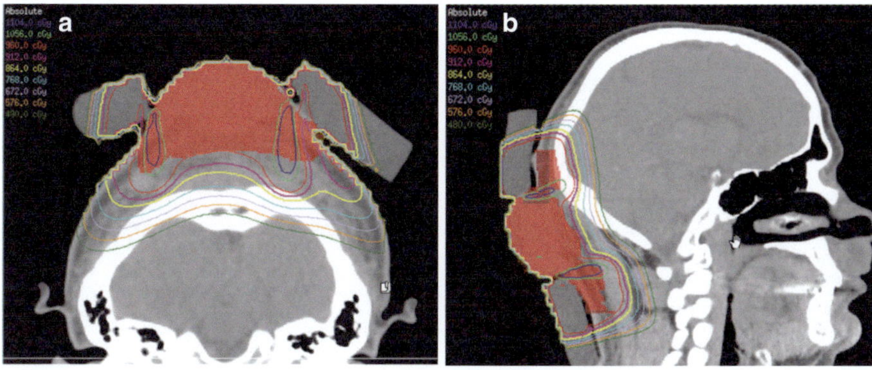

Fig. 8.9 Target delineation and treatment planning. CT simulation images in the (**a**) axial and (**b**) sagittal planes. Coverage of GTV (red) expanded by 1 cm with the prescription isodose line. 16 MeV electrons were used, which covered the superficial skin with near full dose, obviating the need for bolus over the lesion. Bolus was placed on the sides of the tumor to decrease the dose to adjacent brain and other normal tissues. The patient received concurrent TSEBT, which provided additional superficial skin coverage

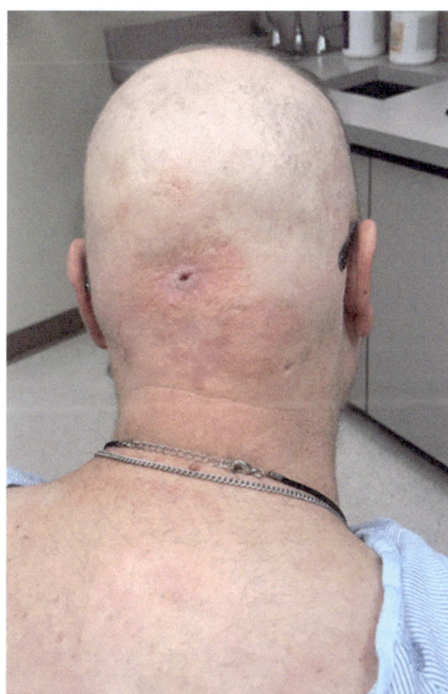

Fig. 8.10 Response assessment of the scalp. The patient had a complete response at follow-up evaluation at 10 weeks after RT completion

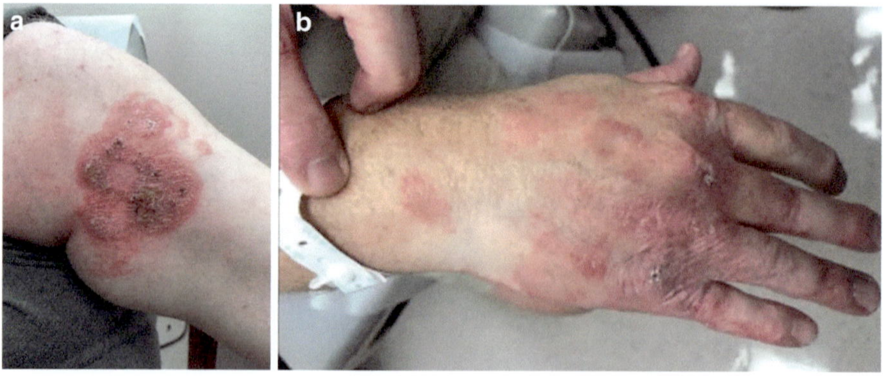

Fig. 8.11 Patient presentation. He had erythematous patch disease with superficial scaling and erosions involving the (**a**) left upper arm and (**b**) right dorsal hand

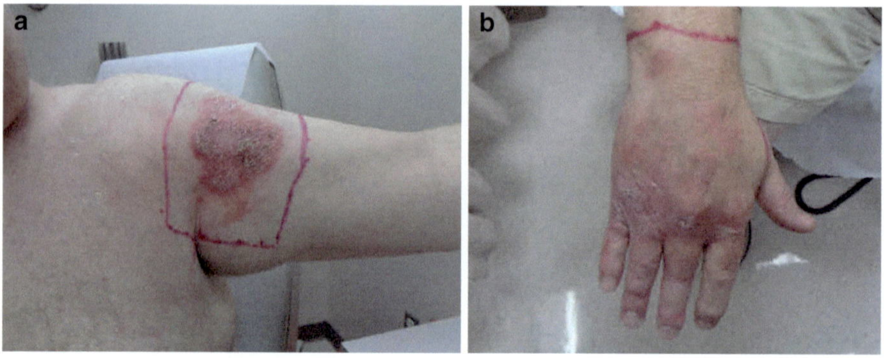

Fig. 8.12 Treatment planning. Treatment fields were drawn on the patient's skin encompassing the disease in the (**a**) left upper arm and (**b**) right dorsal hand with 1–2 cm margin. Note that when treating the hand even with superficial electrons, the radiation dose can penetrate through the full thickness of hand and fingers. Therefore, in cases where a lesion exists on the opposite side, both sides can be covered with a single field

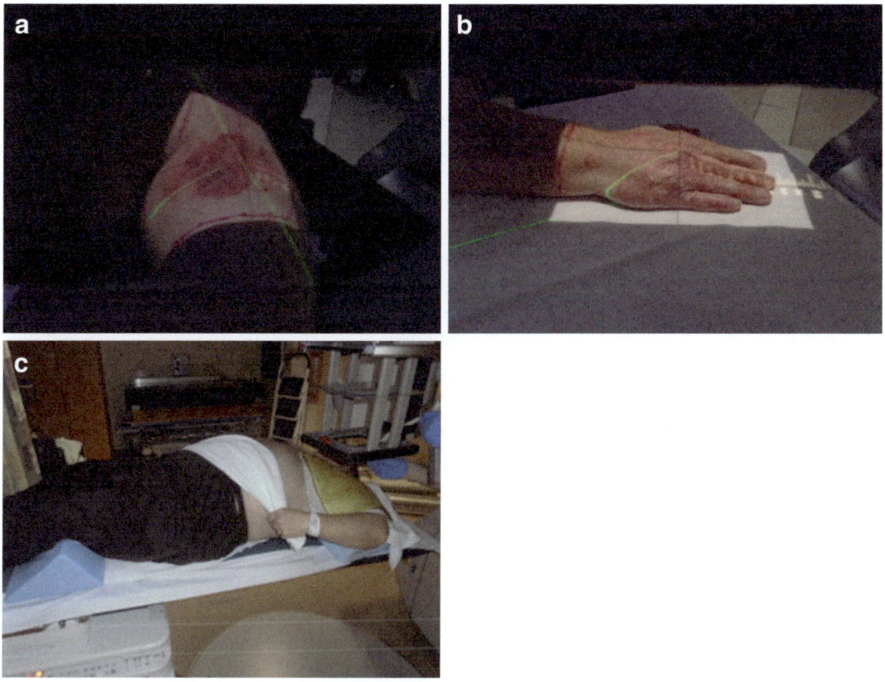

Fig. 8.13 Treatment delivery. For treatment delivery, the fields were redrawn on the patient's skin. Hand blocking was used to approximate the desired field borders for the (**a**) left upper arm and (**b**) right dorsal hand fields. (**c**) Bolus (1 cm) was applied over the entire treatment field prior to dose delivery. Each field was treated using 9 MeV electrons

References

1. Garbe C, et al. Borrelia burgdorferi-associated cutaneous B cell lymphoma: clinical and immunohistologic characterization of four cases. J Am Acad Dermatol. 1991;24(4):584–90.
2. May SA, et al. Cutaneous lymphoid hyperplasia and marginal zone B-cell lymphoma following vaccination. J Am Acad Dermatol. 2005;53(3):512–6.
3. Dabaja B. Renaissance of low-dose radiotherapy concepts for cutaneous lymphomas. Oncol Res Treat. 2017;40(5):255–60. https://doi.org/10.1159/000470845. Epub 2017 Apr 6.PMID: 28380490.
4. Specht L, et al. Modern radiation therapy for primary cutaneous lymphomas: field and dose guidelines from the International Lymphoma Radiation Oncology Group. Int J Radiat Oncol Biol Phys. 2015;92(1):32–9.
5. Akhtari M, et al. Primary cutaneous B-cell lymphoma (non-leg type) has excellent outcomes even after very low dose radiation as single-modality therapy. Leuk Lymphoma. 2016;57(1):34–8.
6. Neelis KJ, et al. Low-dose palliative radiotherapy for cutaneous B- and T-cell lymphomas. Int J Radiat Oncol Biol Phys. 2009;74(1):154–8.
7. Senff NJ, et al. Results of radiotherapy in 153 primary cutaneous B-cell lymphomas classified according to the WHO-EORTC classification. Arch Dermatol. 2007;143(12):1520–6.
8. Ghazawi FM, et al. Environmental and other extrinsic risk factors contributing to the pathogenesis of cutaneous T cell lymphoma (CTCL). Front Oncol. 2019;9:300.

9. NCCN guidelines version 2.2020. 2020 [cited 2020].
10. Whittaker S, Hoppe R, Prince HM. How I treat mycosis fungoides and Sézary syndrome. Blood. 2016;127(25):3142–53.
11. Hoppe RT, et al. Low-dose total skin electron beam therapy as an effective modality to reduce disease burden in patients with mycosis fungoides: results of a pooled analysis from 3 phase-II clinical trials. J Am Acad Dermatol. 2015;72(2):286–92.
12. Morris S, et al. The results of low-dose total skin electron beam radiation therapy (TSEB) in patients with mycosis fungoides from the UK Cutaneous Lymphoma Group. Int J Radiat Oncol Biol Phys. 2017;99(3):627–33.
13. Wilson LD, et al. Experience with total skin electron beam therapy in combination with extracorporeal photopheresis in the management of patients with erythrodermic (T4) mycosis fungoides. J Am Acad Dermatol. 2000;43(1 Pt 1):54–60.
14. Hosing C, et al. Allogeneic stem-cell transplantation in patients with cutaneous lymphoma: updated results from a single institution. Ann Oncol. 2015;26(12):2490–5.
15. Million L, et al. Radiation therapy for primary cutaneous anaplastic large cell lymphoma: an International Lymphoma Radiation Oncology Group multi-institutional experience. Int J Radiat Oncol Biol Phys. 2016;95(5):1454–9.
16. Smith GL, et al. Effectiveness of low-dose radiation for primary cutaneous anaplastic large cell lymphoma. Adv Radiat Oncol. 2017;2(3):363–9.

Further Reading

Feature important publications, book chapters here. For instance, relevant ILROG guidelines.

Specht L, Dabaja B, Illidge T, Wilson LD, Hoppe RT, International Lymphoma Radiation Oncology Group, Modern radiation therapy for primary cutaneous lymphomas: field and dose guidelines from the International Lymphoma Radiation Oncology Group. Int J Radiat Oncol Biol Phys. 2015;92(1):32–9. https://doi.org/10.1016/j.ijrobp.2015.01.008.

Extranodal Natural Killer (NK)/T-Cell Lymphoma, Nasal Type

9

Shu-Nan Qi and Ye-Xiong Li

Contents

Part 1: Background and Epidemiology

Extranodal natural killer (NK)/T-cell lymphoma, nasal-type (ENKTCL) is a distinct clinicopathologic entity with aggressive, heterogeneous clinical behavior.

- ENKTCL is rare globally, but more prevalent in East Asia and South America [1, 2]. In China, ENKTCL is the most common subtype of T- and NK-cell neoplasms, accounting for approximately 50% of all newly diagnosed cases [3].

S.-N. Qi (✉) · Y.-X. Li
Department of Radiation Oncology, National Cancer Center/Cancer Hospital, Chinese Academy of Medical Sciences (CAMS) and Peking Union Medical College (PUMC), Beijing, China

C. Pinnix et al. (eds.), *Target Volume Delineation in Hematologic Malignancies*, Practical Guides in Radiation Oncology,
https://doi.org/10.1007/978-3-031-67722-9_9

- The World Health Organization (WHO) classification unifies ENKTCLs from all extranodal origins as the nasal type. The histological features of ENKTCL are similar irrespective of the site of involvement. ENKTCL rarely occurs in the lymph node.
- ENKTCL diagnosis peaks between 40–55 years of age, and are more common in males than female (ratio, 2.0–2.5:1) [3, 4].
- The clinical features of ENKTCL vary according to primary location within the nasal cavity, extranasal upper aerodigestive tract (UADT) and extra-UADT sites [5].
  - There is no standard definition for primary location in the WHO classification. The definition of "nasal type" is part of the name of the histopathological entity, both for cases originating in the nasal cavity and elsewhere. To avoid this confusing terms, the disease could anatomically be classified into nasal, extranasal-UADT and extra-UADT, although cases arising outside of the UADT are often called "extranasal type" in the literature.
  - The majority localizes to the UADT, including the nasal cavity and extranasal UADT (the Waldeyer's ring, paranasal sinuses, larynx and oral cavity). Extranasal-UADT ENKTCLs have more regional lymph node involvement, advanced-stage disease and poorer performance status [5].
  - ENKTCL can have extra-UADT presentation, with skin and soft tissues, gastrointestinal tract, testes and lung being the most common sites. Most patients with extra-UADT ENKTCL have advanced-stage disease and poor prognosis.
- 70–90% patients with ENKTCL present with localized disease, among whom 10–30% will develop distant progression after treatment [6, 7]. The primary tumor tends to extend through the mucosa into neighboring structures or tissues (PTI), indicating a decreased prognosis. PTI is defined as growth of the primary tumor beyond the original single site to a neighboring structure or tissue, or continuous multisite involvement, regardless of stage [8]. 10–30% of ENKTCLs present as disseminated disease at diagnosis. ENKTCLs tend to disseminate to extranodal organs.
- Progressed ENKTCL patients frequently develop hemophagocytic syndrome (HPS) that almost inevitably leads to death [9, 10].

Part 2: Pre-treatment Evaluation and Imaging

Assessment of tumor extension before treatment is essential for ENKTCL. The disease is characteristic of mucosa invasion which demand multi-modality assessment methods.

- Physical examination, blood chemistry, computed tomography of the head and neck, abdomen and pelvis, and bone marrow examination are standard evaluation at initial diagnosis.

- Physical examination and fiberoptic endoscopy of the UADT prior to treatment are essential for staging and radiation planning in that they can identify superficial mucosa lesions beyond the resolution of imaging.
- MRI of the head and neck is the recommended imaging modality for staging. MRI has high soft tissue resolution that could differentiate tumor from concomitant inflammation.
- PET/CT is recommended, particularly for locally advanced disease or advanced-stage disease. PET/CT can detect latent distant extranodal lesions.
- Quantitative measurement of circulating EBV-DNA viral load is recommended because of its usefulness in the initial diagnosis, monitoring and predicting prognosis of the disease [11, 12].

Part 3: Stage, Risk Stratification and Definition

Stage, risk stratification and primary site provide essential information and aid in estimating the prognosis and determining treatment plan.

- The Ann Arbor staging system is recommended for all patients. Accordingly, stage IE disease is defined as primary extranodal lesion with or without invasion of adjacent structure or organs (PTI), whereas stage IIE disease is defined as primary extranodal lesion with drainage lymph nodes involvement on the same side of the diaphragm.
- Patients can be classified into low-, intermediate-low, intermediate-high-, high- or very high-risk groups using nomogram-revised risk index (NRI, Table 9.1) [13]. Patients with advanced-stage disease can be stratified into the intermediate- to very high-risk group.
- Early-stage patients can be classified into low-, intermediate-low-, intermediate-high- or high-risk groups using early-stage adjusted NRI (EA-NRI, Table 9.1) [13].
- Primary tumor invasion (PTI) is an important, independent prognostic factor, and should be clarified for all patients, particularly for early-stage disease.
- PTI is defined as extensive growth of the primary tumor beyond the original site to a neighboring structure or tissue, or simultaneous involvement of continuous multiple sites (especially in the UADT site), regardless of stage.
- Detailed definition of PTI is explained in Figs. 9.1 and 9.2 according to origin [8].

Part 4: Management of ENKTCL

Principles of Management

Early-stage or localized ENKTCL should be managed differently from advanced-stage or disseminated disease. There is no evidence supporting that extra-UADT ENKTCL should be managed differently from UADT ENKTCL.

Table 9.1 NRI-defined risk groups for all patients and early-stage adjusted NRI for early-stage patients

Risk factors[a]	Risk groups	5-year OS
NRI		
Age >60 years (vs. ≤60 years)	0 = Low risk	85
Ann Arbor stage (vs. I)	1 = Intermediate low risk	79
II (*1 point*)	2 = Intermediate high risk	68
III–IV (*2 point*)	3 = High risk	53
ECOG score ≥2 (vs. 0–1)	≥4 = Very high risk	33
Elevated LDH (vs. normal)		
PTI present (vs. absent)		
EA-NRI		
Age >60 years (vs. ≤60 years)	0 = Low risk	85
Ann Arbor stage II (vs. I)	1 = Intermediate low risk	79
ECOG score ≥2 (vs. 0–1)	2 = Intermediate high risk	70
Elevated LDH (vs. normal)	≥3 = High risk	56
PTI present (vs. absent)		

[a] Each binary risk factor was defined as 1 point, except for stage III/IV as 2 points. *NRI* Nomogram-revised risk index, *EA-NRI* early-stage adjusted NRI, *OS* overall survival, *ECOG* Eastern Cooperative Oncology Group, *LDH* lactate dehydrogenase, *PTI* primary tumor invasion

- In early-stage disease, radiotherapy is the backbone of curative treatment.
  - Radiotherapy significantly improves locoregional control and long-term survival [4, 14].
  - Radiotherapy is essential even after complete response to asparaginase-based chemotherapy in early-stage patients [15].
  - Radiotherapy techniques, including target definition, dose, and delivery modality, are crucial for the chance of curing patients with early-stage ENKTCL [16–18].
  - Adding chemotherapy into radiotherapy significantly improved survival in intermediate- to high-risk early-stage patients [19].
- Risk-adapted therapy is recommended for early-stage patients [19] (Table 9.2).
  - Radiotherapy alone is a viable option for low-risk patients (without PTI, LDH elevation or stage II disease) and for fragile or elder patients who could not tolerate chemotherapy [19, 20].
  - Combined modality treatment (radiotherapy and chemotherapy) is recommended for intermediate- to high-risk patients with any risk factors (with PTI, LDH elevation or stage II disease) except age [8, 19].
- Upfront radiotherapy and non-anthracycline (ANT)-based chemotherapy have improved ENKTCL treatment outcomes in the past decade. Based on published literature, choices of combined modality treatment for intermediate- to high-risk early-stage patients include [21]:
  - Radiotherapy followed by non-ANT-based chemotherapy [19, 22].
  - Short-course chemotherapy followed by radiotherapy [23].

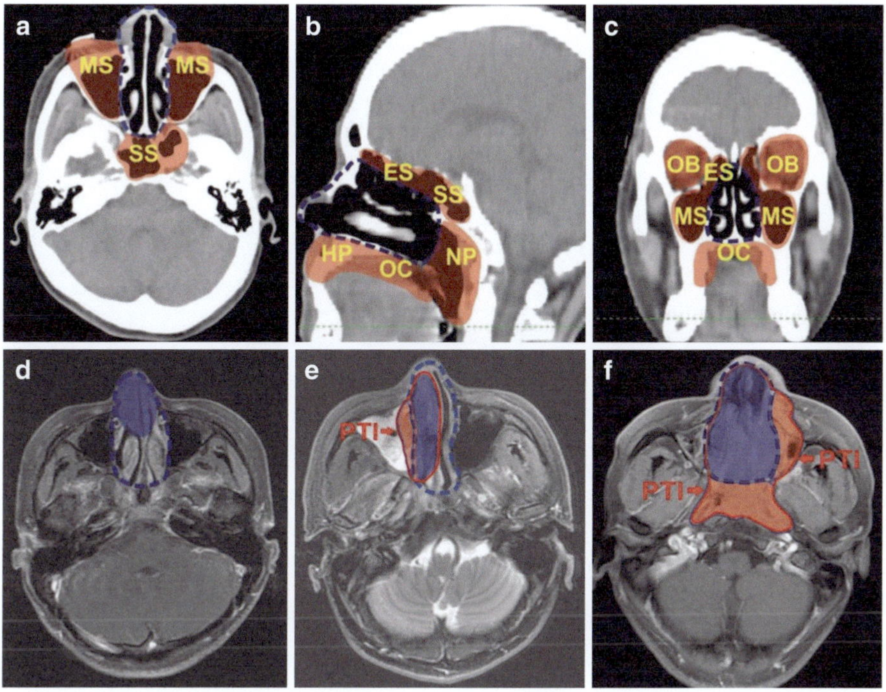

Fig. 9.1 (**a**–**f**) Definitions of primary tumor invasion (PTI) for nasal-ENKTCL. (**a**) Commonly involved adjacent structures for ENKTCL of the nasal cavity in transverse plane, (**b**) in sagittal plane and (**c**) in coronal plane. *MS* maxillary sinus, *SS* sphenoid sinus, *ES* ethmoid sinus, *NP* nasopharynx, *HP* hard palate, *OC* oral cavity, *OB* orbit. If the nasal tumor was confined to the bilateral nasal cavity (dashed blue line), it is PTI negative. If the tumor invaded any of the above structures (red areas), it is PTI positive. (**d**) Negative PTI example of ENKTCL of the nasal cavity; (**e**) and (**f**) positive PTI with ENKTCL of the nasal cavity extended into maxillary sinus and nasopharynx (red area with an arrow)

  - Sandwich chemoradiation [24, 25].
  - Concurrent chemoradiation [26–28].
- Non-ANT-based chemotherapy with or without radiotherapy is the primary treatment for advanced-stage patients.

General Considerations for Radiotherapy

High dosage and adequate coverage of the primary tumor and potential subclinical extent of involvement constitute the principles of radiotherapy in ENKTCL.

- Unlike diffuse large B cell lymphoma and other aggressive lymphomas, ENKTCL is relatively resistant to chemotherapy, while sensitive to radiotherapy.

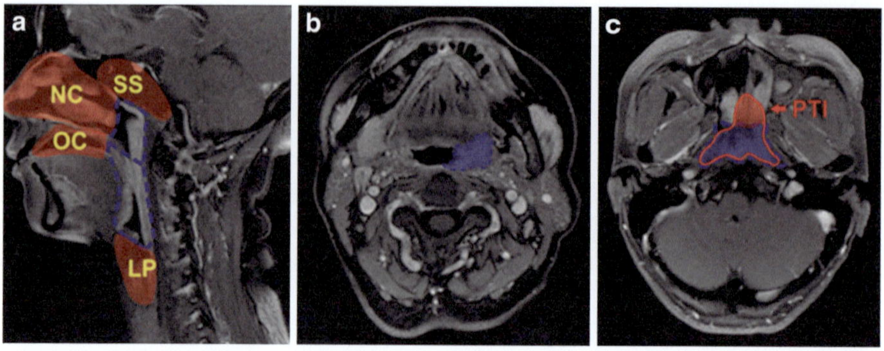

Fig. 9.2 (**a**–**c**) Definitions of primary tumor invasion (PTI) for Waldeyer's Ring (WR)-ENKTCL. (**a**) Commonly involved structures for ENKTCL in the sagittal plane. *NC* nasal cavity, *LP* laryngopharynx; (**b**) negative PTI example of ENKTCL of the extra-nasal upper aerodigestive tract; (**c**) positive PTI example of ENKTCL of the extra-nasal upper aerodigestive tract extended to the nasal cavity (red area with an arrow)

Table 9.2 Risk-adapted treatments for ENKTCL according to stage and NRI-defined risk group

Stage	Risk factor	Risk group	Treatment
IE	No	Low-risk	• Radiotherapy alone (preferred) • Combined modality treatment
IE	Presence	Intermediate- to high-risk	• Radiotherapy followed by non-ANT-chemotherapy • Short-course (≤3 cycles) non-ANT-chemotherapy followed by radiotherapy • Concurrent chemoradiation
IIE	Any	Intermediate- to high-risk	• Radiotherapy followed by non-ANT-chemotherapy • Short-course (≤3 cycles) non-ANT-chemotherapy followed by radiotherapy • Concurrent chemoradiation
III/IV	Any	Intermediate/high- to very high-risk	• Clinical trial • Non-ANT-based chemotherapy with or without radiotherapy

Risk factors: PTI, stage II or III/IV, elevated LDH, ECOG score ≥2

Appropriate radiotherapy (target definition, dose and delivery modality) is crucial in curing early-stage patients.

- In contrast to involved site radiotherapy (ISRT) in chemo-sensitive lymphomas, the extended involved-site radiotherapy (E-ISRT) principles are advocated in ENKTCLs. Smaller treatment volume is associated with higher locoregional failure.

- Radiotherapy is the most effective treatment with curative-intent for early-stage disease; increasing dose is associated with improved tumor control and long-term survival.
- High dose (≥50 Gy) is recommended for ENKTCL based on the dose-survival curve in the CLCG study [14] and multivariate analysis result with NCDB database [4].
  - However, in small prospective series, 45 Gy among cases with complete response to short-course modified-SMILE chemotherapy [23] and 45 Gy concurrent chemoradiation was also used [27].

Part 5: Treatment Volume for Localized ENKTCL

RT planning incorporates the current concepts of volume determination as outlined in the International Commission on Radiation Units and Measurements (ICRU) report 83.

- Patients should be simulated supine and in a thermoplastic mask for immobilization.
- Axial CT images should be acquired in 3 mm or smaller increments. Some centers may use an MR simulator. MR images are useful for radiation planning [29].
- Generally, 3 target volumes are useful to construct for radiation planning: Gross tumor volume (GTV), Clinical target volume (CTV) and planning target volume (PTV). These volumes are further described in Table 9.3 and displayed in Figs. 9.3 and 9.4.
- Target volumes should be treated with intensity-modulated radiotherapy (IMRT). Beam arrangements should be chosen to minimize dose to organs at risk (OARs), including the parotid gland, brainstem, spinal cord, temporal lobes, lens and cornea.
- Radiation dose is a predictor of response and survival, with better outcomes observed in patients who receive at least 50 Gy.
- Suggested OARs and constraints are listed in Table 9.4.

Table 9.3 Treatment volume definitions for radiotherapy of ENKTCL

Volume	Description
GTV	• Contains gross tumor volume as identified on diagnostic imaging, physical examination and endoscope • In cases receiving chemotherapy first, combining information before and after chemotherapy to identify the maximum tumor extension

(continued)

Table 9.3 (continued)

Volume	Description	
CTV	• The current CTV is based on the study of involved frequency with each anatomic site [30] • The CTV should include the entire primarily involved site and adjacent structures of potential contiguous spread • Includes consideration of the following: – Image accuracy and quality – Adjacent organ dose constraints	
	Nasal cavity origin	• Whole nasal cavity, ipsilateral maxillary and anterior ethmoid sinuses are at high risk of involvement and should be routinely covered • Facial skin, oropharynx, hard palate, orbit, floor of the nasopharynx and other local sites are at intermediate- or low-risk, should be covered if disease is close to them • Prophylactic cervical lymph node irradiation is not recommended based on the low lymph node failure rate in the absence of irradiation (<6%) • The retropharyngeal node and level II cervical lymph nodes represent the most commonly involved regional LNs; if involved, the whole ipsilateral neck or at least upper neck irradiation is recommended
	Extranasal-UADT site	• Extranasal-UADT ENKTCLs tend to have multisite involvement or PTI (59%) and a high frequency of regional lymph node involvement (60–80%) • The whole WR (nasopharynx, tonsillar regions, base of the tongue and oropharynx), posterior nasal aperture, and adjacent organs or structures are recommended to be covered • Prophylactic upper neck irradiation is recommended • If cervical lymph node is involved, the whole neck needs to be encompassed
	Extra-UADT site	• Refer to the general principles for extranodal lymphoma irradiation • Consider a 2 cm margin around GTV for ENKTCL arising in skin, soft tissues, intestine, and lung et al • Consider the entire stomach and peri-gastric LNs for gastric ENKTCL
PTV	• Contains CTV plus a margin to account for setup uncertainties associated with patient position and beam alignment • CTV-to-PTV expansions are patient- and institution-specific; any recommendations in this chapter or elsewhere must be adjusted to reflect factors unique to the patient and institution	
OAR	• Includes uninvolved normal structures at risk of RT-related toxicity for which RT planning or dose may be altered • OARs in UADT irradiation include: Parotid gland, brainstem, spinal cord, temporal lobes, lens and cornea	

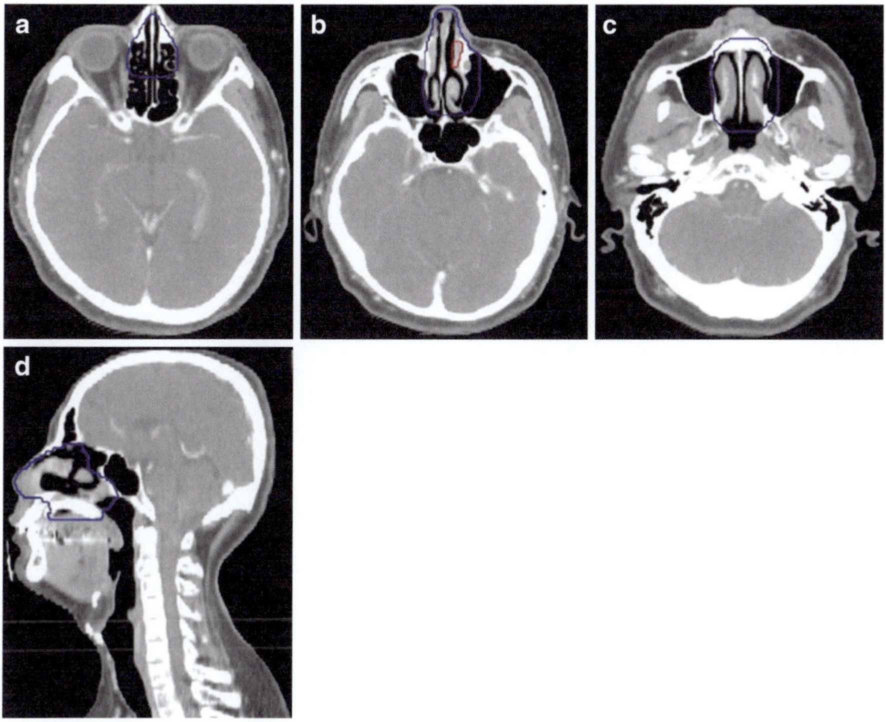

Fig. 9.3 Radiotherapy planning for localized NKTCL origined from nasal cavity. The total prescription dose is 50 Gy. (**a-d**) Representative imaging planes for an ENKTCL case with disease confined to the left nasal cavity. The GTV is delineated in red on the planning CT scan. The CTV is shown in blue as a 1 cm expansion from the GTV (red) along the mucosa and is modified to include the adjacent anatomic structures, but is cropped back from bone: whole nasal cavity, ipsilateral maxillary (at least medial half), anterior ethmoid sinuses and hard palate

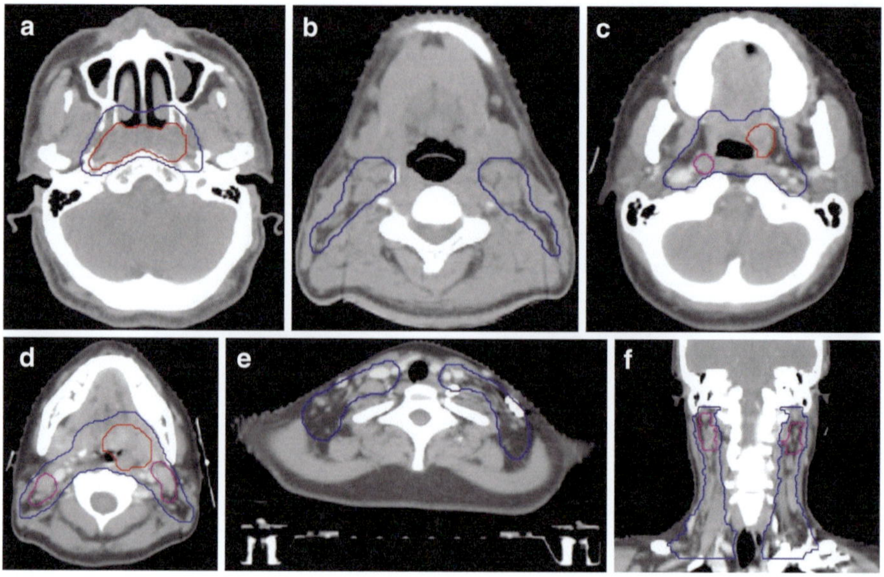

Fig. 9.4 Radiotherapy planning for localized NKTCL origined from nasal pharynx (Waldeyer's Ring). The total prescription dose is 50 Gy, alternatively coming down to the primary tumor with a boost of 6–10 Gy. (**a**–**f**) Representative imaging planes for an ENKTCL case with naso pharynx and oro pharynx disease and cervical LNs involvement. The GTV is delineated in red and GTV-LN in purple on the planning CT scan. The CTV is shown in blue as a 1 cm expansion from the GTV (red) along the mucosa and is modified to include the adjacent anatomic structures, but is cropped back from bone: whole mucosa of WR, posterior nasal aperture and bilateral cervical LNs

Table 9.4 Recommended constraints for OARs in UADT irradiation

OAR	Constraints
Brainstem	The maximum dose <50 Gy
Spinal cord	The maximum dose ≤40 Gy
Optic nerve and chiasm	The maximum dose ≤50 Gy
Lens	The maximum dose ≤10 Gy
Parotid glands	• The mean dose ≤26 Gy for WR ENKTCL • The mean dose ≤18 Gy for nasal ENKTCL • As there is a linear relationship between the mean dose to the parotid glands and ≥Grade II xerostomia, the dose constraint should be kept as low as possible

Part 6: Special Considerations

Radiotherapy for Advanced-Stage ENKTCL

- Retrospective data suggests that consolidation radiotherapy associated with better prognosis in advanced-stage ENKTCL [31].
- Similar principles of treatment volume and dose borrowed from the localized disease are applied for these cases.

Re-irradiation for Localized-Recurrent UADT ENKTCL

- Patients with localized recurrence had a better prognosis than those with systemic recurrence. Salvage radiotherapy or re-irradiation resulted in a favorable prognosis for patients with localized recurrent disease [32].
- Careful evaluation of the treatment benefit versus potential damage associating with re-irradiation should be made basing on clinical judgement.
- We recommend at least 1–2 cm margin adding to GTV as the treatment volume to avoid significant toxicity. However, a wide margin is recommended when OARs are safe after dose evaluation.
- We recommend a higher dose (40–50 Gy) whenever possible.

Surveillance After Treatment

- Studies on failure patterns show majority treatment failures occur within 24 months. Patients who achieve progression-free survival within 24 months after initial treatment had favorable long-term outcomes that are comparable to the general population.
- The hazards of failure decreased in a risk-dependent manner among patients with early NKTCL after radiotherapy: intermediate- and high-risk patients had an initially higher but progressively declining risk of failure and death over time, whereas low-risk patients had a consistently lower risk [33].
- A risk-dependent time-varying surveillance plan is recommended: intense follow-up among intermediate- and high-risk patients for the first 2 years after treatment; low-risk cases and cases that achieve progression-free survival at 2 years have low relapse risks and could be considered for a less intense follow-up plan.

References

1. Vose J, Armitage J, Weisenburger D, International TCLP. International peripheral T-cell and natural killer/T-cell lymphoma study: pathology findings and clinical outcomes. J Clin Oncol. 2008;26(25):4124–30.

2. Au WY, Weisenburger DD, Intragumtornchai T, Nakamura S, Kim WS, Sng I, et al. Clinical differences between nasal and extranasal natural killer/T-cell lymphoma: a study of 136 cases from the International Peripheral T-Cell Lymphoma Project. Blood. 2009;113(17):3931–7.
3. Sun J, Yang Q, Lu Z, He M, Gao L, Zhu M, et al. Distribution of lymphoid neoplasms in China: analysis of 4638 cases according to the World Health Organization classification. Am J Clin Pathol. 2012;138(3):429–34.
4. Vargo JA, Patel A, Glaser SM, Balasubramani GK, Farah RJ, Marks SM, et al. The impact of the omission or inadequate dosing of radiotherapy in extranodal natural killer T-cell lymphoma, nasal type, in the United States. Cancer. 2017;123(16):3176–85.
5. Li YX, Liu QF, Fang H, Qi SN, Wang H, Wang WH, et al. Variable clinical presentations of nasal and Waldeyer ring natural killer/T-cell lymphoma. Clin Cancer Res. 2009;15(8):2905–12.
6. Yang Y, Zhang YJ, Zhu Y, Cao JZ, Yuan ZY, Xu LM, et al. Prognostic nomogram for overall survival in previously untreated patients with extranodal NK/T-cell lymphoma, nasal-type: a multicenter study. Leukemia. 2015;29(7):1571–7.
7. Yamaguchi M, Suzuki R, Oguchi M, Asano N, Amaki J, Akiba T, et al. Treatments and outcomes of patients with extranodal natural killer/T-cell lymphoma diagnosed between 2000 and 2013: a cooperative study in Japan. J Clin Oncol. 2017;35(1):32–9.
8. Qi SN, Xu LM, Yuan ZY, Wu T, Zhu SY, Shi M, et al. Effect of primary tumor invasion on treatment and survival in extranodal nasal-type NK/T-cell lymphoma in the modern chemotherapy era: a multicenter study from the China Lymphoma Collaborative Group (CLCG). Leuk Lymphoma. 2019;60(11):2669–78.
9. Han L, Li L, Wu J, Li X, Zhang L, Wang X, et al. Clinical features and treatment of natural killer/T cell lymphoma associated with hemophagocytic syndrome: comparison with other T cell lymphoma associated with hemophagocytic syndrome. Leuk Lymphoma. 2014;55(9):2048–55.
10. Wen H, Ma H, Cai Q, Lin S, Lei X, He B, et al. Recurrent ECSIT mutation encoding V140A triggers hyperinflammation and promotes hemophagocytic syndrome in extranodal NK/T cell lymphoma. Nat Med. 2018;24(2):154–64.
11. Wang ZY, Liu QF, Wang H, Jin J, Wang WH, Wang SL, Song YW, Liu YP, Fang H, Ren H, Wu RY, Chen B, Zhang XM, Lu NN, Zhou LQ, Li YX. Clinical implications of plasma Epstein-Barr virus DNA in early-stage extra nodal nasal-type NK/T-cell lymphoma patients receiving primary radiotherapy. Blood. 2012;120(10):2003–10.
12. Kwong YL, Pang AWK, Leung AYH, et al. Quantification of circulating Epstein-Barr virus DNA in NK/T-cell lymphoma treated with the SMILE protocol: diagnostic and prognostic significance. Leukemia. 2014;28:265–870.
13. Chen SY, Yang Y, Qi SN, Wang Y, Hu C, He X, et al. Validation of nomogram-revised risk index and comparison with other models for extranodal nasal-type NK/T-cell lymphoma in the modern chemotherapy era: indication for prognostication and clinical decision-making. Leukemia. 2020;35(1):130–42. https://doi.org/10.1038/s41375-020-0791-3.
14. Li YX, Yao B, Jin J, Wang WH, Liu YP, Song YW, et al. Radiotherapy as primary treatment for stage IE and IIE nasal natural killer/T-cell lymphoma. J Clin Oncol. 2006;24(1):181–9.
15. Deng XW, Wu JX, Wu T, Zhu SY, Shi M, Su H, et al. Radiotherapy is essential after complete response to asparaginase-containing chemotherapy in early-stage extranodal nasal-type NK/T--cell lymphoma: a multicenter study from the China Lymphoma Collaborative Group (CLCG). Radiother Oncol. 2018;129(1):3–9.
16. Isobe K, Uno T, Tamaru J, Kawakami H, Ueno N, Wakita H, et al. Extranodal natural killer/T-cell lymphoma, nasal type: the significance of radiotherapeutic parameters. Cancer. 2006;106(3):609–15.
17. Yang Y, Cao JZ, Lan SM, Wu JX, Wu T, Zhu SY, et al. Association of improved locoregional control with prolonged survival in early-stage extranodal nasal-type natural killer/T-cell lymphoma. JAMA Oncol. 2017;3(1):83–91.
18. Wu T, Yang Y, Zhu SY, Shi M, Su H, Wang Y, et al. Risk-adapted survival benefit of IMRT in early-stage NKTCL: a multicenter study from the China Lymphoma Collaborative Group. Blood Adv. 2018;2(18):2369–77.

19. Yang Y, Zhu Y, Cao JZ, Zhang YJ, Xu LM, Yuan ZY, et al. Risk-adapted therapy for early-stage extranodal nasal-type NK/T-cell lymphoma: analysis from a multicenter study. Blood. 2015;126(12):1424–32.
20. Li YX, Wang H, Jin J, Wang WH, Liu QF, Song YW, et al. Radiotherapy alone with curative intent in patients with stage I extranodal nasal-type NK/T-cell lymphoma. Int J Radiat Oncol Biol Phys. 2012;82(5):1809–15.
21. Qi SN, Yang Y, Zhang YJ, et al. Risk-based, response-adapted therapy for early-stage extranodal nasal-type NK/T-cell lymphoma in the modern chemotherapy era: a China Lymphoma Collaborative Group (CLCG) study. Am J Hematol. 2020;95(9):1047–56. https://doi.org/10.1002/ajh.25878.
22. Qi F, Wang WH, He XH, Chen B, Gui L, Fang H, et al. Phase 2 study of first-line intensity modulated radiation therapy followed by gemcitabine, dexamethasone, and cisplatin for high-risk, early stage extranodal nasal-type NK/T-cell lymphoma: the GREEN Study. Int J Radiat Oncol Biol Phys. 2018;102(1):61–70.
23. Qi SN, Yahalom J, Hsu M, Chelius M, Lunning M, Moskowitz A, et al. Encouraging experience in the treatment of nasal type extra-nodal NK/T-cell lymphoma in a non-Asian population. Leuk Lymphoma. 2016;57(11):2575–83.
24. Xu PP, Xiong J, Cheng S, Zhao X, Wang CF, Cai G, et al. A phase II study of methotrexate, etoposide, dexamethasone and pegaspargase sandwiched with radiotherapy in the treatment of newly diagnosed, stage IE to IIE extranodal natural-killer/T-cell lymphoma, nasal-type. EBioMedicine. 2017;25:41–9.
25. Jiang M, Zhang H, Jiang Y, Yang Q, Xie L, Liu W, et al. Phase 2 trial of "sandwich" L-asparaginase, vincristine, and prednisone chemotherapy with radiotherapy in newly diagnosed, stage IE to IIE, nasal type, extranodal natural killer/T-cell lymphoma. Cancer. 2012;118(13):3294–301.
26. Yamaguchi M, Tobinai K, Oguchi M, Ishizuka N, Kobayashi Y, Isobe Y, et al. Phase I/II study of concurrent chemoradiotherapy for localized nasal natural killer/T-cell lymphoma: Japan Clinical Oncology Group Study JCOG0211. J Clin Oncol. 2009;27(33):5594–600.
27. Kim SJ, Kim K, Kim BS, Kim CY, Suh C, Huh J, et al. Phase II trial of concurrent radiation and weekly cisplatin followed by VIPD chemotherapy in newly diagnosed, stage IE to IIE, nasal, extranodal NK/T-Cell Lymphoma: Consortium for Improving Survival of Lymphoma study. J Clin Oncol. 2009;27(35):6027–32.
28. Kwong YL, Kim SJ, Tse E, Oh SY, Kwak JY, Eom HS, et al. Sequential chemotherapy/radiotherapy was comparable with concurrent chemoradiotherapy for stage I/II NK/T-cell lymphoma. Ann Oncol. 2018;29:256–63.
29. Mikhaeel NG, Milgrom SA, Terezakis S, Berthelsen AK, Hodgson D, Eich HT, et al. The optimal use of imaging in radiation therapy for lymphoma—guidelines from the International Lymphoma Radiation Oncology Group (ILROG). Int J Radiat Oncol Biol Phys. 2019;104(3):501–12.
30. Wu RY, Liu K, Wang WH, Jin J, Song YW, Wang SL, et al. Patterns of primary tumor invasion and regional lymph node spread based on magnetic resonance imaging in early-stage nasal NK/T-cell lymphoma: implications for clinical target volume definition and prognostic significance. Int J Radiat Oncol Biol Phys. 2017;97(1):50–9.
31. Bi XW, Jiang WQ, Zhang WW, Huang JJ, Xia Y, Wang Y, et al. Treatment outcome of patients with advanced stage natural killer/T-cell lymphoma: elucidating the effects of asparaginase and postchemotherapeutic radiotherapy. Ann Hematol. 2015;94(7):1175–84.
32. Zhao T, Li YX, Wang SL, Jin J, Wang WH, Song YW, Liu YP, Liu XF, Fang H, Ren H, Chen B, Qi SN, Liu QF, Lu NN, Yu ZH. Survival benefit with salvage radiotherapy for patients with locoregionally recurrent extranodal nasal-type NK/T-cell lymphoma. Ann Hematol. 2013;92:325–32.
33. Liu X, Wu T, Zhu SY, Shi M, Su H, Wang Y, et al. Risk-dependent conditional survival and failure hazard after radiotherapy for early-stage extranodal natural killer/T-cell lymphoma. JAMA Netw Open. 2019;2(3):e190194.

Further Reading

Consensus on extranodal lymphomas irradiation: field and dose: Yahalom J, Illidge T, Specht L, Hoppe RT, Li YX, Tsang R, et al. Modern radiation therapy for extranodal lymphomas: field and dose guidelines from the International Lymphoma Radiation Oncology Group. Int J Radiat Oncol Biol Phys. 2015;92(1):11–31.

Prognosis for individual patient: Yang Y, Zhang YJ, Zhu Y, Cao JZ, Yuan ZY, Xu LM, et al. Prognostic nomogram for overall survival in previously untreated patients with extranodal NK/T-cell lymphoma, nasal-type: a multicenter study. Leukemia. 2015;29(7):1571–7.

Risk stratification for early-stage disease: Chen SY, Yang Y, Qi SN, Wang Y, Hu C, He X, et al. Validation of nomogram-revised risk index and comparison with other models for extranodal nasal-type NK/T-cell lymphoma in the modern chemotherapy era: indication for prognostication and clinical decision-making. Leukemia. 2020. https://doi.org/10.1038/s41375-020-0791-3.

Risk-adapted therapy for early-stage disease: Yang Y, Zhu Y, Cao JZ, Zhang YJ, Xu LM, Yuan ZY, et al. Risk-adapted therapy for early-stage extranodal nasal-type NK/T-cell lymphoma: analysis from a multicenter study. Blood. 2015;126(12):1424–32.

Risk-based, response-adapted therapy for early-stage disease: Qi SN, Yang Y, Zhang YJ, et al. Risk-based, response-adapted therapy for early-stage extranodal nasal-type NK/T-cell lymphoma in the modern chemotherapy era: a China Lymphoma Collaborative Group (CLCG) study. Am J Hematol. 2020. https://doi.org/10.1002/ajh.25878.

Pediatric Hodgkin Lymphoma

10

James E. Bates, Bradford S. Hoppe,
and Raymond B. Mailhot-Vega

Contents

Part 1: Background and Epidemiology

- Hodgkin lymphoma (HL) is a rare malignancy with a bimodal distribution of incidence throughout the age spectrum with one peak in adolescence and young adulthood and another in those over 60 years old [1].
- HL is very rare in children under the age of 14 years, representing only 3% of all malignancies in that population, but more common in children aged 14–19 years,

J. E. Bates (✉)
Department of Radiation Oncology, Emory University, Atlanta, GA, USA
e-mail: James.edward.bates@emory.edu

B. S. Hoppe
Department of Radiation Oncology, Mayo Clinic, Jacksonville, FL, USA
e-mail: hoppe.bradford@mayo.edu

R. B. Mailhot-Vega
Department of Radiation Oncology, University of Florida College of Medicine, Jacksonville, FL, USA

C. Pinnix et al. (eds.), *Target Volume Delineation in Hematologic Malignancies*, Practical Guides in Radiation Oncology,
https://doi.org/10.1007/978-3-031-67722-9_10

representing 13% of malignancies in adolescents. It is among the most common malignancies in adolescents [2].
- Histologically, there are several subtypes of Hodgkin lymphoma, which can be split into two primary categories that drive treatment decisions [3].
  - *Classic Hodgkin Lymphoma* (cHL): A CD20-negative histology characterized by "Reed-Sternberg cells" including nodular sclerosing, lymphocyte-rich, lymphocyte-deplete, and mixed cellularity HL.
  - *Nodular Lymphocyte-Predominate Hodgkin Lymphoma* (NLPHL): A CD20-positive histology resembling a non-HL.
- Pediatric HL is an extremely curable disease with 5-year overall survival rates exceeding 90% [4].
- Late effects of cancer therapies, such as second malignancies (especially of the thyroid, lung, and breasts of female survivors) and cardiac disease, are a significant concern in this population of often very long-term survivors.
- Consequently, contemporary clinical trials have focused on reducing the intensity of therapies, often through the elimination of radiotherapy, to reduce the late effect burden.

Pre-radiotherapy Imaging and Evaluation

- Diagnostic imaging and laboratory results obtained before initiating chemotherapy can significantly influence radiotherapy decisions in pediatric HL.
- After a diagnosis of HL is established, preferably by excisional biopsy, a positron emission tomography (PET)/computed tomography (CT) scan should be performed.
  - If the diagnosis indicates that radiotherapy is likely needed, this PET/CT scan should be performed with the patient in the approximate treatment planning position.
  - A dedicated CT scan with contrast of the involved areas taken before the initiation of chemotherapy may also be helpful in radiotherapy planning.
- Pre-chemotherapy laboratory results including a comprehensive metabolic panel, complete blood counts, serum albumin, and a sedimentation rate are helpful in prognostication and may be used in the selection of patients for radiotherapy.
- Nearly every child with HL will receive chemotherapy prior to the initiation of radiotherapy. The radiation oncologist must obtain and evaluate all imaging taken during and after chemotherapy.

Part 2: Management and Treatment of Pediatric Hodgkin Lymphoma

Principles of Management

- Children with HL can be categorized into three risk groups based on recent Children's Oncology Group prospective trials.
  - *Low Risk*—Patients with stage IA/IIA disease without B symptoms or bulky disease, generally with 3 or fewer sites of involvement.

- *Intermediate Risk*—Patients with stage I/II disease with any risk factor including bulky disease, B symptoms, or extranodal disease. Some studies include patients with stage IIIA/IVA disease without the aforementioned risk factors.
- *High Risk*—Patients with stage IIIB/IVB disease; in some studies patients with stage IIB bulky disease.

- The management of pediatric HL is driven by chemotherapy and PET-adapted therapy. General guidelines for target delineation are described in Table 10.1 and Fig. 10.1. Tables 10.2 and 10.3 describe treatment paradigms, complete response, and rapid early response as defined in recent Children's Oncology Group and

Table 10.1 Planning target definitions for treatment of pediatric Hodgkin lymphoma [17]

Volume	Description	
Gross tumor volume (GTV)	Pre-chemotherapy GTV	• Contains the GTV as identified on diagnostic imaging prior to chemotherapy. This should be contoured on prechemotherapy PET/CT that is fused to simulation scan
	Post-chemotherapy GTV	• Contains any residual tumor after chemotherapy
Clinical target volume (CTV)	CTV	• There is no traditional distance-based expansion for the GTV-to-CTV volume in Hodgkin lymphoma treatment • The CTV should be drawn based on clinical judgement to include all areas of prechemotherapy disease, edited off uninvolved normal structures • Separate nodal volumes that are greater than 5 cm apart should be contoured as separate volumes; those closer should be combined into one CTV
	Boost CTV	• In some situations, with residual PET-avid disease, a boost field may be considered. This should be contoured as a relatively tight field around residual disease
Internal target volume (ITV)	• Contains the CTV plus an internal margin that accounts for variation in CTV shape, size, and position with internal motion. The ITV is most relevant for tumors that move with the respiratory cycle (those of the thorax or upper abdomen) • Efforts should be taken either to minimize internal motion with breath-hold techniques and/or abdominal compression if the patient can tolerate or to account for internal motion with a 4DCT scan	

(continued)

Table 10.1 (continued)

Volume	Description
Planning target volume (PTV)	• Contains CTV or ITV plus a margin to account for setup uncertainties associated with patient position and beam alignment • CTV-to-PTV expansions are anatomic location-, patient-, and institution-specific. We recommend using your institutional standard expansions • In the absence of other guidance, we recommend a 0.3-cm expansion for tumors in the head and neck region, a 0.5-cm expansion for those in the thoracic region (if using 4DCT), and a 0.7-cm expansion for abdominal tumors
Organs at risk (OAR)	• Includes uninvolved normal structures at risk of radiotherapy-related toxicity for which radiotherapy planning or dose may be altered. The OARs that should be contoured are dependent on the location of the primary tumor. We recommend placing high focus on the heart, lungs, thyroid, and breasts for tumors that are near those structures. Additionally, when planning with IMRT or proton therapy, plans can be optimized to reduce the dose to the cardiac substructures, such as the coronary vessels and ventricles

CT computed tomography, *IMRT* intensity-modulated radiotherapy, *PET* positron emission tomography, *4D* four-dimensional

EuroNet-Pediatric Hodgkin Lymphoma Group studies. Therapy is primarily driven by the protocol chosen by the referring pediatric oncologist; radiation oncologists should refer to the protocol for exact radiotherapy guidelines (Fig. 10.2).

General Considerations for Radiotherapy

- *Treatment Technique*—Given the high likelihood of survival and consequent risk of late effects, children with HL should be treated using advanced radiation treatment modalities such as intensity-modulated radiotherapy (IMRT), volumetric modulated arc therapy (VMAT), or proton therapy.
  - *Proton Therapy*—If available and feasible for the patient and family, children with HL should be considered for treatment with proton therapy, especially those with mediastinal disease who have an increased risk of late radiation-induced cardiac toxicity and second cancers.

    Proton therapy is most beneficial to patients with lower mediastinal disease (below the level of the T7 vertebral body) and females with axillary disease [5].

    Proton therapy is equivalently efficacious to photon therapy in pediatric HL [6, 7].

    Proton therapy is capable of reducing RT doses to nearly all organs at risk when compared to VMAT-based plans [8].

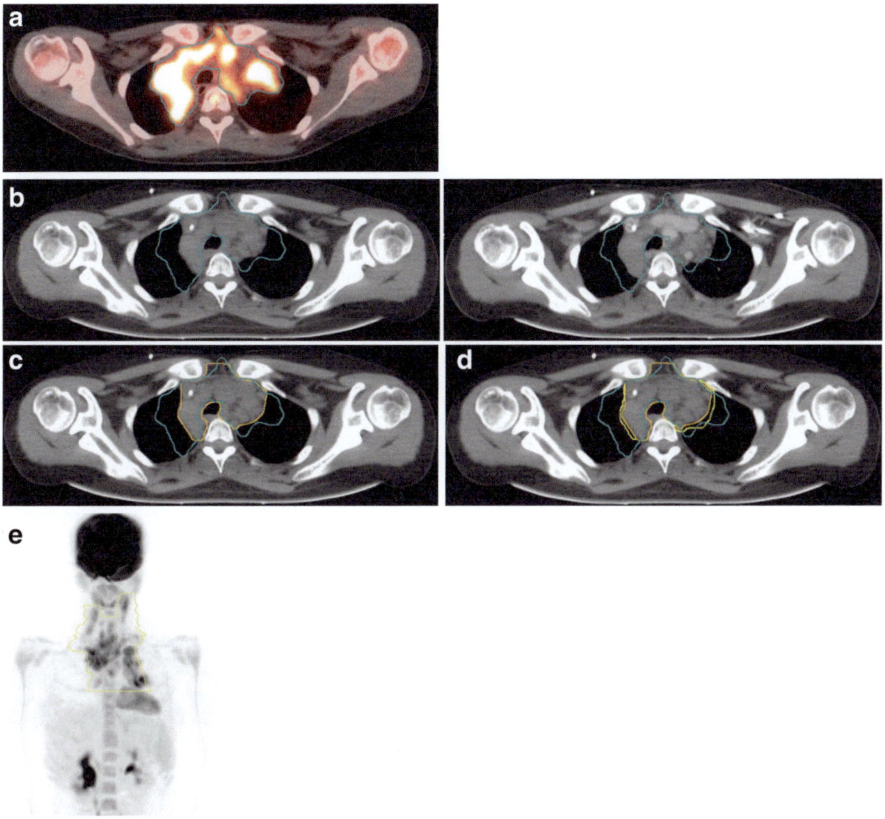

Fig. 10.1 Consolidative radiotherapy planning for intermediate-risk classical Hodgkin lymphoma treated as per AHOD0031. (**a**) The prechemotherapy gross tumor volume (GTV) is delineated on the prechemotherapy positron emission tomography (PET)-computed tomography (CT) image (blue). The volume is constructed from the gross disease as defined by CT and PET from the prechemotherapy PET-CT images. (**b**) The prechemotherapy PET-CT is fused with the CT-simulation images. For thoracic tumors requiring motion management, a 4-dimensional (4D) scan and a separate CT with contrast may be obtained to allow better visualization of vasculature. After fusion, the prechemotherapy GTV is visible on the 4D planning scan (left) and simulation (right). (**c**) With the prechemotherapy GTV fused to the simulation images, a CTV is created (gold). The CTV captures prechemotherapy disease, edited off uninvolved structures. The reduction in disease from the prechemotherapy GTV (blue) to CTV can be appreciated. (**d**) Utilizing the 4D CT to account for motion management, an ITV is created (yellow). (**e**) As a final check at our institution, we evaluate a deformed registration of the prechemotherapy PET-CT to our simulation scan to evaluate internal target volume (ITV) delineation (yellow)

Table 10.2 Children's Oncology Group studies for pediatric Hodgkin lymphoma

Study	Risk group	Chemotherapy schema	Response criteria	Radiotherapy
AHOD 0431 [18]	*Low risk*: Stage IA or IIA without bulky disease	Three cycles of AV-PC	**CR:** ≥80% reduction in PPD *and* negative PET *and* no mass >2 cm outside of the mediastinum on PET *after first cycle of chemotherapy*	If CR, no RT If no CR, 21 Gy at 1.5 Gy/fraction to all sites of initial disease and recurrent disease (if any)
AHOD 0031 [19, 20]	*Intermediate risk:* Stage I–II if patients have B symptoms, bulky disease, or extranodal disease Stage IIIA–IVA regardless of bulk	Two cycles of ABVE-PC → PET scan → two further cycles of ABVE-PC	**RER**: ≥60% reduction in PPD of all lesions on CT, regardless of PET response (after 2 cycles) **CR**: ≥80% reduction in PPD of all lesions *and* no mass >2 cm outside of the mediastinum *and* negative PET	If RER *and* CR, no RT If RER *without* CR *or* no RER, 21 Gy at 1.5 Gy/fraction to all initially involved sites of disease
AHOD 0831 [21]	*High risk:* Stage IIIB or IVB disease	Two cycles of ABVE-PC → PET scan → two further cycles of ABVE-PC (with two cycles of ifosfamide and vinorelbine if no RER)	**RER**: PET-negative, regardless of size of mass	RT only given to sites of bulky disease, splenic macronodular involvement, and regions of SER (21 Gy at 1.5 Gy/fraction)

AV-PC doxorubicin, vincristine, prednisone, and cyclophosphamide, *ABVE-PC* doxorubicin, bleomycin, vincristine, etoposide, prednisone, and cyclophosphamide, *CR* complete response, *PET* positron emission tomography, *PPD* product of perpendicular dimension, *RER* rapid early response, *RT* radiotherapy

- *IMRT/VMAT-Based Photon Therapy*—In cases where photon therapy is used, advanced treatment planning techniques should be incorporated.

  One potential treatment planning option is the IMRT-based "butterfly technique" which uses 5–7 total beams, all of which are anterior obliques (300–30°) or posterior obliques (160–210°) [9].

  A similar technique can be done with multiple VMAT arcs; this method may help reduce late toxicity risk when compared to fixed-field IMRT [10].

Table 10.3 EuroNet Pediatric Hodgkin Lymphoma Group C1 study schema [22]

Risk group	Chemotherapy schema	Response criteria	Radiotherapy
Low risk: Stage IA/B without extranodal disease Stage IIA without extranodal disease	Two cycles of OEPA	**CR**: All symptoms disappeared, no new disease, all initial sites of disease ≤5% of initial volume *or* ≤ 2 cm^3 **CRu**: Any individual site of disease ≤25% of initial volume of disease **PR**: Any individual site of disease ≤50% of initial volume of disease **AR1**: All patients in CR, regardless of PET results **AR2**: All patients in CRu or PR with a negative PET	If in AR1 or AR2, no RT All other patients receive 19.8 Gy at 1.8 Gy/fraction to all initially involved sites of disease If poor response and/or bulky residual disease, add 10 Gy at 2 Gy/fraction boost to residual disease
Intermediate risk: Stage IA/B with extranodal disease Stage IIA with extranodal disease Stage IIB without extranodal disease Stage IIIA without extranodal disease	Two cycles of OEPA followed by either two cycles of COPP or COPDAC		
High risk: Stage IIB with extranodal disease Stage IIIA with extranodal disease Stage IIIB Stage IV	Two cycles of OEPA followed by four cycles of COPP or COPDAC		

AR1 adequate response group 1, *AR2* adequate response group 2, *COPDAC* cyclophosphamide, vincristine sulfate, prednisone, and dacarbazine, *COPP* cyclophosphamide, vincristine, procarbazine and prednisone, *CR* complete response, *CRu* complete response unconfirmed, *OEPA* vincristine, etoposide, and doxorubicin, *PR* partial response, *RT* radiotherapy

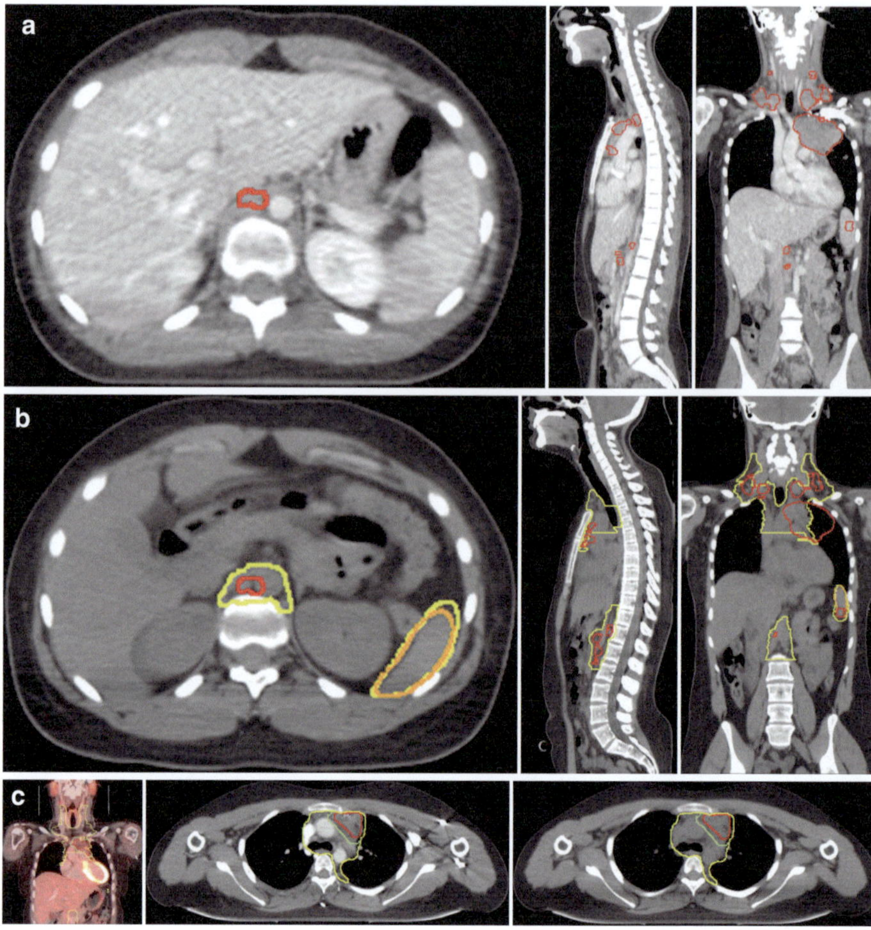

Fig. 10.2 Consolidative radiotherapy planning for a high-risk Hodgkin lymphoma patient with splenic involvement and persistent positron emission tomography (PET)-positivity at end of systemic treatment treated as per EURONET C2. (**a**) The prechemotherapy gross tumor volume (GTV; red) can be appreciated on the representative axial (left), sagittal (middle), and coronal slices (right) of the computed tomography (CT) portion of the prechemotherapy imaging. (**b**) The methodology of prechemotherapy GTV to clinical target volume (CTV) to internal target volume (ITV) creation is as above. For this case, one can appreciate on the prechemotherapy PET the presence of disease above and below the diaphragm. For splenic treatment, the patient must fast before treatment to reduce gastric-related displacement of the spleen. A 4D scan was obtained for both respiratory motion of the mediastinal volume as well as respiratory motion of the spleen. The ITV is depicted in yellow with the 3D depiction of spleen in gold. Slices from 4D simulation planning show the axial (left), sagittal (middle), and coronal (right) planes. (**c**) A coronal slice of the residual PET active disease is shown (left). The end of systemic therapy PET-CT was registered to the simulation scan. A GTV of the boost volume (including anatomic and metabolic residual disease) is delineated (red) and shown on axial slices of the planning contrast and 4D scan (middle and right, respectively). An ITV accounting for respiratory motion is also shown (light green). The ITV from the standard risk volume is shown as reference (yellow)

- *Organs at Risk*—The normal tissues that are at risk for late complications from radiotherapy depend on the anatomic distribution of disease; clinical judgement must be used to determine which of the following organs to consider. Suggested dose constraints are presented below.
  - *Heart* [11]—Radiotherapy increases the risk of various cardiac diseases in a dose-dependent manner. This effect is exacerbated by the presence of anthracycline-based chemotherapies in all HL regimens. **Mean heart doses in excess of 5–10 Gy increase the risk of late cardiac disease.** For situations where consolidative RT after a complete response to chemotherapy in the frontline setting would result in a mean heart dose of 15 Gy or higher, omission of RT should be contemplated.

    We also recommend contouring the left anterior descending artery and bilateral ventricles, and manually reviewing plans to avoid hot spots in those regions and minimize the amount of those structures receiving 15 Gy [12, 13].
  - *Breast*—The risk of breast cancer increases linearly both with increasing radiation dose and with increasing anthracycline dose [14]. No clear guidance exists to suggest a breast dose which does not increase this risk. **The volume of breast tissue receiving 4 Gy should be minimal**.
  - *Lung* [15]– Pediatric-specific data regarding the relationship between radiation dose and risk of radiation pneumonitis is sparse [16]. We extrapolate from adult lymphoma data that **the V20 must be kept <30% and the mean lung dose <13.5 Gy** (PMID 29730281).

Part 3: Special Considerations

- *Nodular Lymphocyte-Predominate Hodgkin Lymphoma* [23] (NLPHL)—NLPHL is a distinct clinical entity from classical HL. It typically presents as early-stage (stage I/II) disease.
  - *One Positive Lymph Node*—Patients with a single lymph node with NLPHL can be treated with surgery alone if a gross total resection is achieved. Patients have an approximately 20% risk of relapse within 5 years after surgery alone, so close clinical monitoring is important. Chemotherapy can be used to salvage any treatment failures.

Other Stage IA/IIA Disease—**Patients with multiple involved lymph nodes can be treated as low-risk pediatric HL patients.**

Funding None.

Disclosures BSH is a Scientific Consultant for Merck & Co., Inc. and Bristol-Myers Squibb. RBM is a recipient of an educational grant from Ion Beam Applications (IBA).

References

1. Cartwright RA, Watkins G. Epidemiology of Hodgkin's disease: a review. Hematol Oncol. 2004;22:11–26.
2. Special section: cancer in adolescents and young adults. 2020. https://www.cancer.org/content/dam/cancer-org/research/cancer-facts-and-statistics/annual-cancer-facts-and-figures/2020/special-section-cancer-in-adolescents-and-young-adults-2020.pdf. Accessed 14 Apr 2020.
3. Eberle FC, Mani H, Jaffe ES. Histopathology of Hodgkin's lymphoma. Cancer J. 2009;15:129–37.
4. Mauz-Körholz C, Metzger ML, Kelly KM, et al. Pediatric Hodgkin lymphoma. J Clin Oncol. 2015;33:2975–85.
5. Ntentas G, Dedeckova K, Andrlik M, et al. Clinical intensity modulated proton therapy for Hodgkin lymphoma: which patients benefit the most? Pract Radiat Oncol. 2019;9:179–87.
6. Wray J, Flampouri S, Slayton W, et al. Proton therapy for pediatric Hodgkin lymphoma. Pediatr Blood Cancer. 2016;63:1522–6.
7. Hoppe BS, Hill-Kayser CE, Tseng YD, et al. Consolidative proton therapy after chemotherapy for patients with Hodgkin lymphoma. Ann Oncol. 2017;28:2179–84. https://www.ncbi.nlm.nih.gov/pubmed/28911093
8. Guan C, Wu B, Yu T, et al. Spatial auxin signaling controls leaf flattening in Arabidopsis. Curr Biol. 2017;27:2940–50.e2944.
9. Voong KR, McSpadden K, Pinnix CC, et al. Dosimetric advantages of a "butterfly" technique for intensity-modulated radiation therapy for young female patients with mediastinal Hodgkin's lymphoma. Radiat Oncol. 2014;9:94. https://www.ncbi.nlm.nih.gov/pubmed/24735767
10. Levis M, Filippi AR, Fiandra C, et al. Inclusion of heart substructures in the optimization process of volumetric modulated arc therapy techniques may reduce the risk of heart disease in Hodgkin's lymphoma patients. Radiother Oncol. 2019;138:52–8.
11. Bates JE, Howell RM, Liu Q, et al. Therapy-related cardiac risk in childhood cancer survivors: an analysis of the childhood cancer survivor study. J Clin Oncol. 2019;37:1090–101.
12. Feng M, Moran JM, Koelling T, et al. Development and validation of a heart atlas to study cardiac exposure to radiation following treatment for breast cancer. Int J Radiat Oncol Biol Phys. 2011;79:10–8.
13. Duane F, Aznar MC, Bartlett F, et al. A cardiac contouring atlas for radiotherapy. Radiother Oncol. 2017;122:416–22.
14. Moskowitz CS, Chou JF, Wolden SL, et al. Breast cancer after chest radiation therapy for childhood cancer. J Clin Oncol. 2014;32:2217–23.
15. Pinnix CC, Smith GL, Milgrom S, et al. Predictors of radiation pneumonitis in patients receiving intensity modulated radiation therapy for Hodgkin and non-Hodgkin lymphoma. Int J Radiat Oncol Biol Phys. 2015;92:175–82.
16. Nanda R, Flampouri S, Mendenhall NP, et al. Pulmonary toxicity following proton therapy for thoracic lymphoma. Int J Radiat Oncol Biol Phys. 2017;99:494–7.
17. Specht L, Yahalom J, Illidge T, et al. Modern radiation therapy for Hodgkin lymphoma: field and dose guidelines from the international lymphoma radiation oncology group (ILROG). Int J Radiat Oncol Biol Phys. 2014;89:854–62.
18. Keller FG, Castellino SM, Chen L, et al. Results of the AHOD0431 trial of response adapted therapy and a salvage strategy for limited stage, classical Hodgkin lymphoma: a report from the Children's Oncology Group. Cancer. 2018;124:3210–9.
19. Friedman DL, Chen L, Wolden S, et al. Dose-intensive response-based chemotherapy and radiation therapy for children and adolescents with newly diagnosed intermediate-risk Hodgkin lymphoma: a report from the Children's Oncology Group Study AHOD0031. J Clin Oncol. 2014;32:3651–8.
20. Charpentier AM, Friedman DL, Wolden S, et al. Predictive factor analysis of response-adapted radiation therapy for chemotherapy-sensitive pediatric Hodgkin lymphoma: analysis of the Children's Oncology Group AHOD 0031 trial. Int J Radiat Oncol Biol Phys. 2016;96:943–50.

21. Kelly KM, Cole PD, Pei Q, et al. Response-adapted therapy for the treatment of children with newly diagnosed high risk Hodgkin lymphoma (AHOD0831): a report from the Children's Oncology Group. Br J Haematol. 2019;187:39–48.
22. Interim results of EURONET-PHL-C1. 2016. https://www.hodgkinsymposium.org/archive/2016/recording/57. Accessed 25 May 2020.
23. Appel BE, Chen L, Buxton AB, et al. Minimal treatment of low-risk, pediatric lymphocyte-predominant Hodgkin lymphoma: a report from the Children's Oncology Group. J Clin Oncol. 2016;34:2372–9.

Target Volume Delineation and Radiation Planning Considerations for Total Body Irradiation

11

Jeffrey Y. C. Wong, Mario Levis, An Liu, and Umberto Ricardi

Contents

J. Y. C. Wong (✉) · A. Liu
Department of Radiation Oncology, City of Hope, Duarte, CA, USA
e-mail: jwong@coh.org; aliu@coh.org

M. Levis (✉) · U. Ricardi
Department of Oncology, University of Torino, Torino, Italy
e-mail: mario.levis@unito.it; umberto.ricardi@unito.it

C. Pinnix et al. (eds.), *Target Volume Delineation in Hematologic Malignancies*, Practical Guides in Radiation Oncology,
https://doi.org/10.1007/978-3-031-67722-9_11

Part 1: Introduction

Background and Epidemiology

- Total body irradiation (TBI) is an important part of the conditioning regimen for patients receiving allogeneic stem cell transplantation (SCT) [1, 2], in particular those with acute lymphoid leukemia (ALL) and acute myeloid leukemia (AML). Rarely, it has been used as part of conditioning for patients receiving autologous stem cell transplantation with the goal to eradicate residual disease.
- TBI was developed with a myeloablative intent. The most common myeloablative TBI schedule is twice-daily 2-Gy fractions given over 3 days (total dose 12 Gy) [3, 4]. Patients that cannot tolerate myeloablative conditioning regimens are offered reduced-intensity regimens consisting of either chemotherapy-only or reduced-dose TBI, most often 2–4 Gy given in one or two fractions [5].
- The effects of TBI depend on dose. Goals of myeloablative TBI include eradication of residual disease, eradication of existing stem cells, and immunosuppression to prevent rejection of donor hematopoietic cells. In contrast, the goal of non-myeloablative TBI is to induce immunosuppression and facilitate engraftment of donor hematopoietic cells.
- ALL affects mainly pediatric patients, with a peak incidence between 1 and 4 years. The incidence is estimated at 1–2 per 100,000 in the USA. Older adults (>40 years) and patients with relapsed or refractory disease have a poorer prognosis [6]. In ALL, indications for SCT include:
  - Philadelphia chromosome-positive disease in first remission, or Philadelphia chromosome-negative disease with poor risk features in first remission;
  - Disease that is refractory, including lack of response to induction chemotherapy;
  - Disease relapse after a remission;
  - Disease that is refractory after relapse.
- Several studies have shown a superiority for TBI-containing myeloablative regimens compared to chemotherapy alone (e.g. cyclophosphamide (CY)/busulfan (BU)), for ALL [7–9]. Therefore, radiotherapy-containing regimens are usually preferred for these patients [10].
- AML is the most common acute leukemia in the adulthood. The incidence ranges 3–5 per 100,000 in the USA. The median age at diagnosis is 69 years old. Despite significant advances in treatment options, prognosis remains poor for elderly patients, who account for the majority of new cases [11]. In AML, indications for SCT include:
  - Disease with intermediate- to poor-risk molecular and cytogenetic features in first remission;

  - Disease that is refractory, including lack of response to induction chemotherapy;
  - Disease relapse after a remission;
  - Disease that is refractory after relapse.
- In AML patients, the combination of myeloablative CY/TBI achieved similar outcomes to CY/BU in many randomized trials [12–15]. Non-myeloablative conditioning regimens are associated with lower toxicity and treatment-related mortality [16], especially among older patients [17]. However, an increased relapse risk in younger patients has been noted in some studies [18, 19].
- Other diseases, such as multiple myeloma (MM), chronic myeloid leukemia, Hodgkin (HL) and non-Hodgkin (NHL) lymphomas, might benefit from TBI in the transplant setting (either autologous or allogeneic), but the indications are still controversial and limited to select cases [20–24].
- The use of conventional TBI is declining due to associated toxicities and availability of alternate non-TBI approaches. More targeted forms of TBI directed to the bone (total marrow irradiation, TMI) or bone and lymphoid regions (total marrow and lymphoid irradiation, TMLI) are needed to address these challenges. TMI is now being performed at multiple centers worldwide. Clinical results have been encouraging and demonstrate:
  - Feasibility, with acceptable toxicities [25];
  - The ability to offer radiation containing conditioning regimens to older patients or those with co-morbidities [26, 27]:
  - The ability to safely dose escalate with encouraging response and survival rates in advanced disease [28, 29];
  - Reduced intermediate and long-term toxicities compared to conventional TBI [30].

Patient Evaluation

- Tumor histology, prior therapies (including radiotherapy), and current disease status based on the last bone marrow and cerebrospinal fluid cytologic tests should be reviewed.
- Preexisting conditions that could affect lung, cardiac, hepatic, or renal function should be evaluated to assess the relative safety of TBI. Patients that are actively smoking prior to radiotherapy should be counseled about smoking cessation.
- Evaluation of the testes by physical exam and, if necessary, testicular ultrasound should be performed to rule out leukemic involvement.
- Fertility preservation should be discussed with patients that are fertile at time of SCT evaluation given the high probability of permanent sterility.

Part 2: Radiation Conditioning Regimens for Hematopoietic Stem Cell Transplantation

Myeloablative TBI

Clinical Aspects

- The main aims of myeloablative TBI in conditioning regimens for allogeneic SCT are:
  - Possible eradication of residual chemo-resistant malignant cells, in which efficacy is independent of metabolism, bio-distribution, or clearance kinetics.
  - Immunosuppression to prevent rejection of the transplanted hematopoietic cells.
  - Sterilization of potential sanctuary sites (e.g. brain and testis).
- TBI-based conditioning regimens are preferred for patients with higher risk factors to enhance disease eradication, immunosuppression, or both.
- Myeloablative TBI (10–16 Gy) is typically combined with single-agent chemotherapy, often cyclophosphamide. The most commonly used schedules include:
  - 12 Gy in 6 fractions (2 Gy fraction) delivered twice-daily (usually with 4–6 h between fractions)
  - 12 Gy in 4 fractions (3 Gy fraction) delivered once daily
  - 12–13.5 Gy in 8–9 fractions (1.5 Gy fraction) delivered twice-daily
  - 12–13.2 Gy in 10–11 fractions (1.2 Gy fraction) three-times-daily

  All these fractionation schedules have been tested with similar results; the 12 Gy in 6 fractions given twice daily schedule remains popular worldwide [3, 4, 31].
- At many centers, an additional 4-Gy single-fraction testicular boost is delivered with electrons to male patients with ALL to reduce the risk of relapse in this sanctuary site [32].
- Single-dose TBI (10 Gy) was popular decades ago. However, hyperfractionated schedules improved the therapeutic ratio by reducing toxic effects [33–35] (e.g. veno-occlusive disease of the liver and pneumonitis).
- Though there are no randomized trials, a myeloablative regimen is preferred over non-myeloablative regimen in patients with ALL. Patients with AML are offered myeloablative TBI whenever possible. However, as these patients are often elderly and/or have co-morbidities, they are more frequently treated with a reduced-intensity regimen [1].
- Myeloablative regimens are associated with high treatment-related mortality (20–30%). Thus, unfit and/or older patients (>60 years) are rarely suitable to this intensive schedule and require a less intensive conditioning regimen.
- Radiation-induced pneumonitis is one of the most relevant TBI-related side effect and may compromise a patient's outcome. Most centers adopt lung shielding to keep the mean lung dose below 8–10 Gy [34, 36].

Technical Issues

- TBI delivery varies across centers and countries in terms of prescribed dose, patient positioning and immobilization, organ shielding, and RT techniques [37]. This makes standardization challenging.
- Most commonly, conventional TBI is delivered with a single beam at an extended source-to-skin distance (SSD) (e.g. ~4 m) with the patient standing, laying in the lateral decubitus position, sitting, or lying down [1, 38, 39]. The large SSD not only permits use of a larger field but also reduces the dose rate to about 10% of that typically used in RT.
- The collimator is often rotated by 45°, which allows use of the diagonal dimension of the field (i.e. longest aspect of field is aligned to the length of the patient). Anterior and posterior fields are most often used. High-energy photon beams between 4 and 18 MV are preferred. A beam spoiler may be used to prevent skin sparing of high-energy photons.
- Variable separation along the patient's length (e.g. chest versus knee) can result in dose heterogeneity. Compensating filters with lead strips are inserted in the beam's path to achieve a uniform dose (at midline) from head to foot. Thinner portions of the body (e.g. ankles, knees) have more lead strips. In vivo dosimetry is used to measure the dose at several points on the patient's body. If needed, compensating filters may be adjusted during treatment to achieve a uniform dose within ±10%.
- Myeloablative TBI incorporates lung shielding. Lung blocks are customized from a chest radiograph or chest CT scan of the patient in the treatment position. The blocks cover the central portion of the lung. A ~1 cm margin of unblocked lung is generally given from the clavicle, chest wall, and diaphragm, whereas a ~2 cm margin of unblocked lung is typically given from the vertebral bodies medially. At some centers, supplemental electron fields are used to boost areas of the chest wall that are otherwise shielded by the lung blocks.
- Many studies have investigated the effect of dose rate on risk of interstitial pneumonitis with conflicting results. Only one prospective study was conducted, showing no differences in survival and in lung toxicity profile between 6 and 15 cGy/min dose rates [40]. With adoption of hyperfractionated regimens, a dose rate below 15–20 cGy/min seems to be safe and well tolerated [33, 41].
- TBI toxicities in the short term include interstitial pneumonitis, parotitis, nausea and vomiting, dry mouth and mucositis, diarrhea, fatigue, decreased appetite, erythema, esophagitis, and alopecia [42–44]. Long-term toxicities include cataract formation, gonadal failure, hypothyroidism, kidney dysfunction, decreased bone mineral density, sinusoidal obstructive syndrome of the liver, and secondary cancers [45–53]. Children are at higher risk of developing multiple endocrine disorders and short stature.
- The most common methods for delivering TBI are illustrated in the following clinical cases.

Case 1: Standing Myeloablative TBI

- The patient stands in a harness anchored to the ceiling to provide support during treatment (Fig. 11.1). Additional support and immobilization are achieved with hand grips and shoulder rests. A plastic tray sits anterior to the patient, which lung transmission blocks are mounted to. For the posterior–anterior treatment, the patient turns away and has the back facing forward.
- Lung blocks are designed from radiographs in the standing position (Fig. 11.2). Typically used margins are 2–2.5 cm from the vertebral edge and 1–1.5 cm from the rib cage, bottom edge of the clavicle, and diaphragm. A portal image is taken for verification of block placement.
- Axial dose distribution (Fig. 11.3) within the thorax demonstrating the effect of 50% transmission lung blocks reducing dose to the lung in a patient undergoing TBI to 12 Gy. Nine mega electron-volt electrons were used to boost the chest wall.

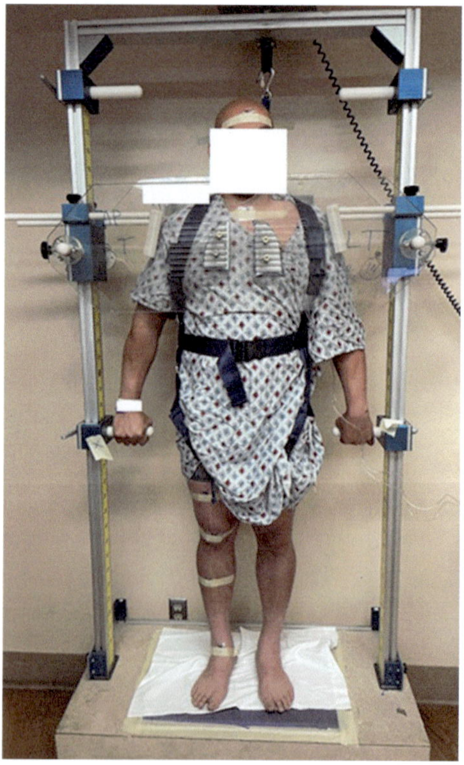

Fig. 11.1 Picture of patient standing in harness for TBI

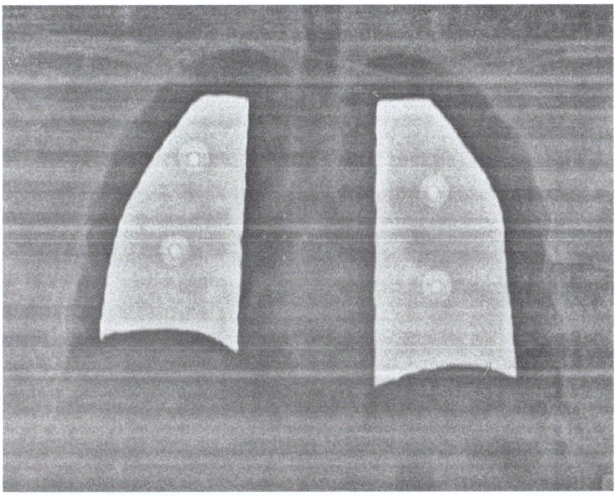

Fig. 11.2 Portal image to verify lung block placement for TBI

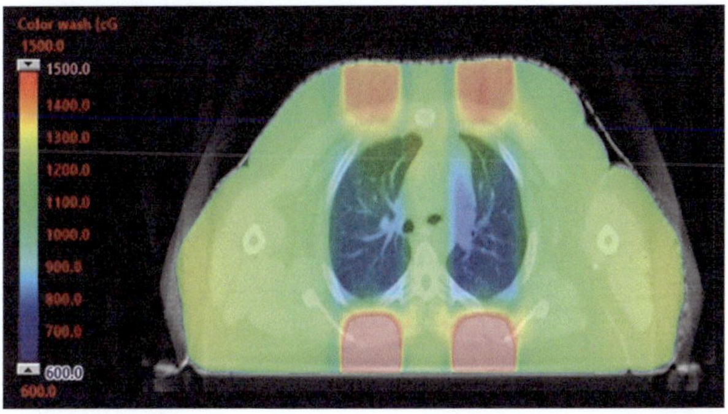

Fig. 11.3 Axial dose distribution with 50% transmission lung blocks

Case 2: Seated Myeloablative TBI

- The patient sits on a stand designed for TBI (Fig. 11.4). Hand grips and abdominal strips provide additional immobilization and support. Lung transmission blocks are mounted on a slotted plastic tray, which is attached to the stand. The patient's position is reversed for posterior–anterior treatment.
- Treatment simulation is done with a planning CT scan. Lung blocks are then designed on the CT scan (Fig. 11.5a), with a 1–2 cm margin from the diaphragm, vertebral edge, rib cage, and bottom edge of the clavicle. Dose calculation may require the addition of a simulated bolus to compensate for displacements of visceral organs and abdominal fat between the planning (supine) and the treating (seated) position, particularly in obese patients. The anteroposterior abdominal diameter in seated position is measured during the planning CT scan to account for the bolus dimension (Fig. 11.5b).
- Dose distribution shown in axial (Fig. 11.6a) and coronal (Fig. 11.6b) slice through the thorax, demonstrating reduction of lung dose achievable with a

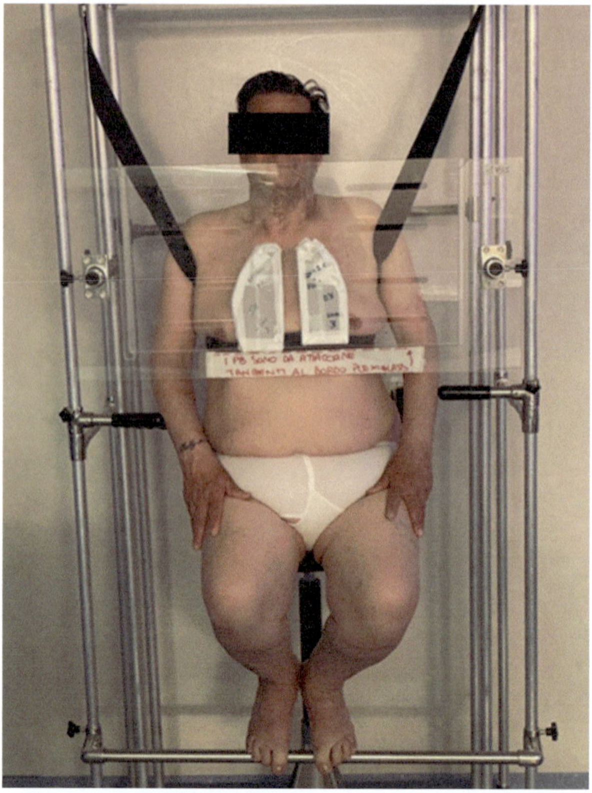

Fig. 11.4 Picture of patient sitting on stand designed for TBI

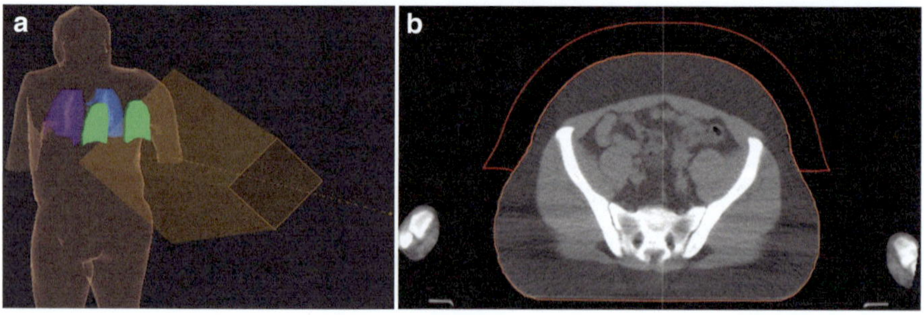

Fig. 11.5 (**a**) Lung block design and (**b**) use of simulated bolus for dose calculation

conventional technique for a patient undergoing TBI to 12 Gy, with transmission blocks over the lungs.

- In room management: A 1–2 cm thick Plexiglass barrier (indicated by the yellow arrow in Fig. 11.7) is placed in front of the patient to produce electrons. These electrons increase the surface dose to at least 90% of the prescribed dose.
- In room management [2]: the source-axis distance can be up to 5 m (4 m in the example case). The gantry is rotated roughly 90° (Fig. 11.8a). The central axis of

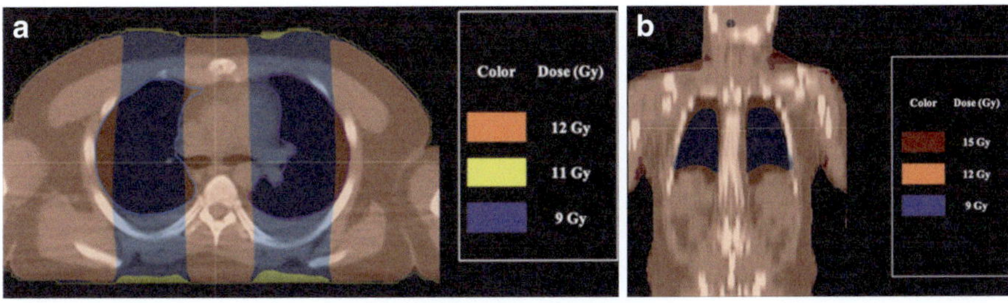

Fig. 11.6 Dose distribution through the lungs on (**a**) axial and (**b**) coronal slices

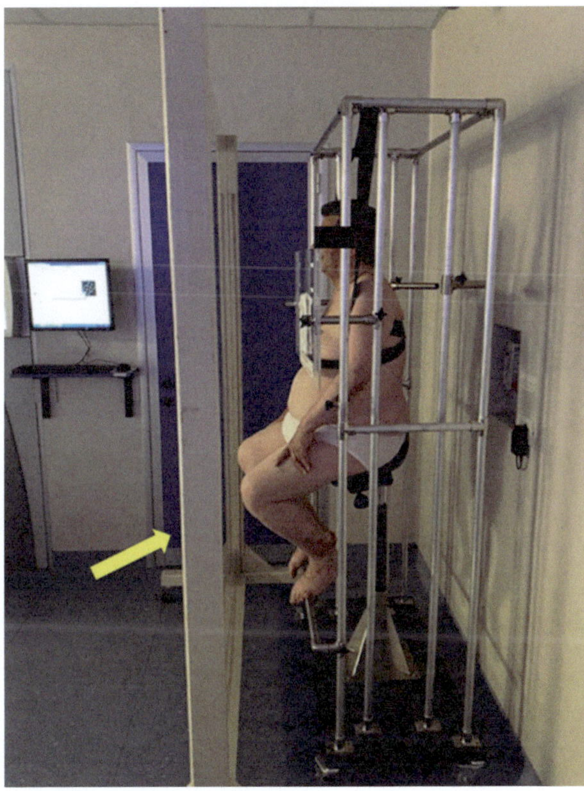

Fig. 11.7 Plexiglass placed in front of patient (yellow arrow) to generate electron scatter

the beam should be incident at the umbilicus; occasionally, this could require a minimal additional gantry angling (±5°). The collimator is usually opened to its maximum size (40 × 40 cm) and is rotated to 45° to use the diagonal dimension and maximize the height of the field (Fig. 11.8b).

- In room management [3]: A visual inspection is mandatory before every fraction, to ascertain that the patient is entirely included in the treating field (Fig. 11.9).

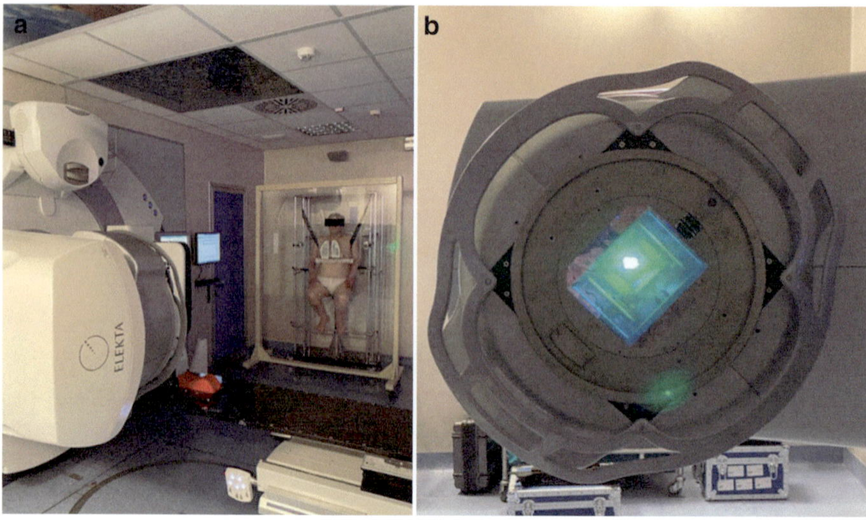

Fig. 11.8 Picture of (**a**) gantry rotated 90 degrees and (**b**) collimator rotated to 45 degrees

Fig. 11.9 Confirmation that patient is within treatment field

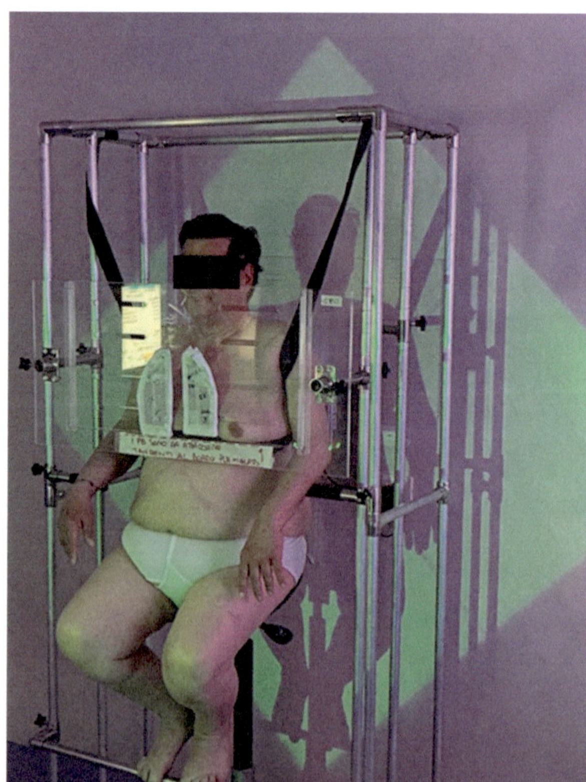

Reduced-Intensity (Non-myeloablative) TBI

Clinical Aspects

- Reduced intensity conditioning regimens utilize reduced chemotherapy and TBI dose. Non-myeloablative regimens result in reversible pancytopenia and sufficient immunosuppression for engraftment. These conditioning regimens are less toxic and were developed to offer allogeneic SCT to unfit patients (older age, comorbidities, previously received myeloablative regimen, or heavily pretreated for relapsed/refractory disease), who cannot tolerate standard myeloablative schedules [5].
- TBI is usually delivered at doses ≤4 Gy in a single fraction, ≤8 Gy fractionated for reduced intensity regimen, and ≤2 Gy for non-myeloablative regimens.
- Reduced-intensity TBI may be integrated in the conditioning regimen to enhance immunosuppression when engraftment of donor cells is expected to be more challenging (e.g. myelofibrosis, myelodysplastic disorders) [5].
- The main aim of these regimens is to provide immunosuppression that favors engraftment of donor cells. Disease control primarily relies on graft-versus-tumor (GVT) effect [54]. As with graft versus host disease (GvHD), GVT is due to the genetic differences between the donor and recipient. Donor-derived T-cells play an important role. Though GVT is strongly associated with GvHD development, it can also occur independent of clinically significant GvHD [55]. GVT can be observed in patients undergoing myeloablative and reduced intensity conditioning regimens. After non-myeloablative SCT, patients may have an initial mixed donor–host chimerism. Achievement of full donor engraftment can take several months. Although mixed chimerism may be sufficient to correct congenital nonmalignant disorders, full donor chimerism is more important to exert GVT effects [56].
- GVT seems more effective for patients with lymphoid malignancies (ALL, chronic lymphocytic leukemia, NHL, MM) in complete remission before transplant. Myeloid malignancies are at higher risk for relapse after non-myeloablative TBI. Thus, the addition of pre-transplant chemotherapy or post-transplant maintenance therapy may be required to achieve valuable disease control in this latter group [57].
- AML is more frequently treated with low-dose TBI compared to ALL given the patient demographics at presentation (older age, comorbidities) [16, 18, 19].
- The combination of low-dose TBI (2 Gy) + fludarabine was associated with improved survival compared to TBI alone, based on a randomized phase III trial including patients diagnosed with both lymphoid (mainly NHL) and myeloid malignancies. Moreover, fludarabine contributed to a better engraftment of donor cells [58].
- Conversely, the superiority of a combined TBI + chemotherapy approach over chemotherapy alone is still debated in the non-myeloablative setting of AML. Two studies have shown no differences in survival or treatment-related mortality between TBI and TBI + chemotherapy when a fludarabine-based regimen is used and an HLA-identical donor is available [59, 60].

- As it is for myeloablative regimens, the decision to include or not TBI in non-myeloablative conditioning is left to the discretion of treating physicians after a personalized analysis of the risk–benefit ratio.
- Table 11.1 summarizes the main differences between myeloablative and non-myeloablative TBI.

Technical Issues

- Technical issues of reduced intensity TBI are similar to myeloablative regimens in terms of planning, patient positioning, and treatment delivery. The only difference is that lung shielding is not required, given the lower doses delivered (most commonly 2–4 Gy).

Total Marrow Irradiation (TMI), Total Marrow and Lymphoid Irradiation (TMLI), and TBI Delivered Using IMRT

- *Background and Rationale:* The utilization of TBI is declining [61] due to additional resources required to perform TBI and concerns for TBI-related acute and late effects, including second malignancies [62]. As a result, there has been increasing use of chemotherapy-only myeloablative conditioning and reduced-intensity conditioning regimens [63]. In addition, the perspective has evolved from viewing allogeneic SCT primarily as a cytotoxic tool to more of an immunologic tool, which relies more on graft versus tumor effects for disease control. In an increasing number of clinical scenarios, TBI is no longer the primary modality but added when increased cytoreduction and/or immunosuppression are needed, and only if it can be added without significant additional toxicity. More targeted forms of TBI are needed to address these challenges and to redefine and expand the role of radiotherapy in SCT.
- Advances in radiotherapy systems now permit the use of helical tomographic [64–66] or volumetric arc-based IMRT [67] devices to deliver IMRT to large regions of the body, allowing for more targeted forms of TBI. The term total marrow irradiation (TMI) has been used if the target structure is bone. The term total marrow and lymphoid irradiation (TMLI) has been used to reflect the addition of the major lymph node chains and spleen as target regions. In some clinical studies, liver and brain have been included as target regions.
- Clinical strategies that are being evaluated using TMI or TMLI include:
  - Escalation of TMI or TMLI doses over standard TBI doses to improve disease control in advanced, refractory patients [25, 28, 29, 68–71].
  - Addition to reduced intensity conditioning regimens to improve disease control with acceptable toxicity in older patients [26, 27, 72, 73].
  - IMRT to deliver TBI as an alternative to conventional TBI to further reduce lung dose and toxicities [74–80].
- *Patient immobilization and CT acquisition*: TMI/TMLI treatment is performed in the supine position. Frequently used immobilization devices include thermoplastic masks and whole-body vacuum bags (Vac-Lok). Wong et al. [64] uses a

Table 11.1 Comparison of clinical factors and prescription doses between myeloablative and non-myeloablative TBI

Regimen	Clinical factors	Main indications	Intent	Common RT doses	Risk–benefit ratio
Myeloablative	***Low-risk profile*** Young age (≤ 55) No comorbidities Remission after systemic therapy HLA-matched donor Low risk of post-transplant relapse	ALL AML	1. Eradication of residual malignant cells 2. Immunosuppression 3. Penetration in sanctuary sites where CT is less effective (brain, testis)	12 Gy/6fr/3d 12 Gy/4fr/4d 13.5 Gy/9fr/4.5d 13.2/11fr/3.5d	**Pros** High cure rates **Cons** Higher toxicity Limited to younger patents
Non-myeloablative (reduced intensity)	***High risk profile*** Older age Comorbidities Refractory/relapsing disease Aggressive prior systemic therapy Complex karyotype	Myelodysplastic disorders Myelofibrosis Aplastic anemia CML MM—HL—NHL ALL[a] and AML[a]	1. Immunosuppression 2. Exploit GVT	2 Gy/1 fr 4 Gy/2 fr	**Pros** Less toxic Allows transplant in unfit patients **Cons** Higher risk of relapse

ALL acute lymphoblastic leukemia, *AML* acute myeloid leukemia, *CML* chronic myeloid leukemia, *MM* multiple myeloma, *HL* Hodgkin's lymphoma, *NHL* non-Hodgkin lymphoma, *GVT* graft-versus-tumor, *fr* fraction, *d* days

[a] If unsuitable to myeloablative regimens

type-S thermoplastics head frame (Civco, Kalona, Iowa, USA) coupled with customized Accuform™ cushion to immobilize the head and shoulder. A whole-body Vac-Lok bag (Civco, Kalona, Iowa, USA) is used to immobilize the entire body (Fig. 11.10). Two CT scans are typically needed to cover the entire patient body. A head-first supine scan is obtained of the upper body, starting 3 cm above the top of the skull to the mid-thigh. A feet-first supine scan covers the lower extremity from the upper thigh to 3 cm past the soles of the feet. It is recommended to scan patient at 5–8 mm thickness to balance the image resolution and contouring workload. While a shallow normal breathing CT scan is used for planning, additional 4D CT or breath-hold CT scans at the end of shallow inspiration and expiration can be acquired to evaluate target and organ motion of ribs, lungs, heart, liver, kidneys, and spleen.

- *Target delineation and normal organ contours*. For TMI, the clinical target volume (CTV) is skeletal bone. For TMLI, major lymph node chains and potentially spleen, testes, liver, brain, and PET avid regions of disease can be added as targets. Table 11.2 lists the possible organs at risk (OAR) and targets for planning. Spinal cord is contoured separately to control the hotspots inside the cord. Ribs/sternum and mandible are contoured separately to aid in dose sparing of the lung and oral cavity, respectively. Figures 11.11, 11.12 and 11.13 show contours of target structures and OARs at representative CT slices.
- Margins added to the OAR and target contours have varied between centers [81–87]. In our opinion, instead of uniform margins applied to each CTV throughout the body, variable margins can be used depending on the setup reproducibility [65]. For bone target structures, the auto threshold tool is used to initially outline bone targets. Bone contours are then modified to connect islands and remove gaps. A 5–10 mm margin is added for CTV targets in regions with more set up uncertainty and that are further from critical normal organs such as shoulders and spinous processes. For the arms and thighs, a 10-mm margin is used. For all other bones including the skull, anterior spine, and pelvic bones where set up is reproducible, no additional margin is added. Ribs, liver, spleen, and kidneys contours are modified to account for respiratory motion using registered inspiration/expiration CT images. Contours for these organs need to be enlarged to compensate the breathing motion. No additional margin is added to the other normal critical organs.
- *Fractionation and total doses*. The most common TMI fractionation schedules use 1.5–2 Gy fractions administered twice a day. These are derived from fractionation schedules used for conventional TBI. Total doses have ranged from 12 to 20 Gy. A few centers have utilized larger daily fractions ranging from 3 to 5 Gy for conventional TBI and have applied similar fractionation schedules to TMI delivery [70, 88].
- *Toxicities associated with TMI/TMLI*: The long-term toxicity data for TMI or TMLI is favorable and potentially reduced compared to historical controls: among 142 patients treated to a median 14 Gy (range 10–19 Gy), rates of hypothyroidism and cataract formation were 6.0% and 7.0%, respectively. No radiation-induced renal toxicity was noted. Rates of radiation pneumonitis (RP)

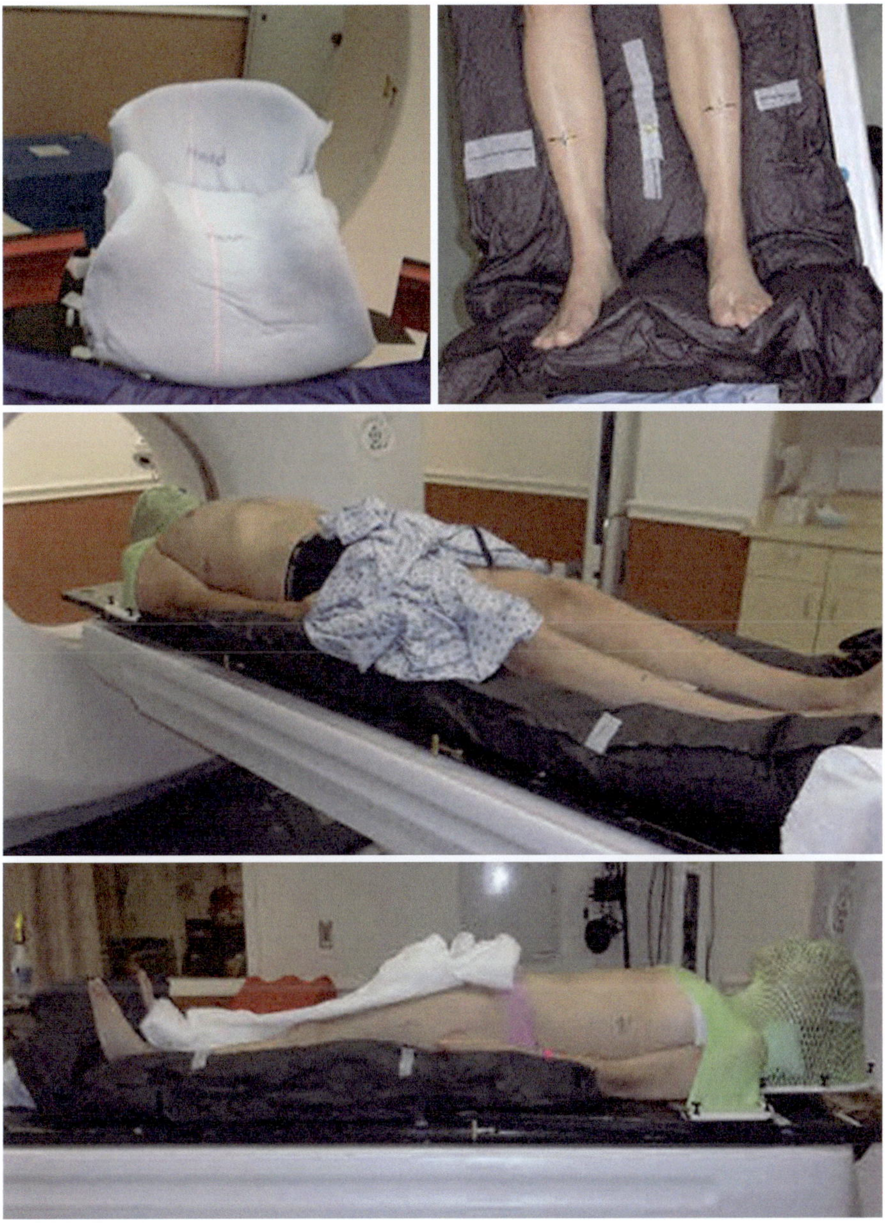

Fig. 11.10 Type S thermoplastic mask, Accuform cushion, and whole body Vac Lok bag are used in patient immobilization

was 0.7% (crude) and that of infection and RP (I/RP) was 22.7% at 2 years and 32.3% at 6 years. Risk of I/RP was associated with mean lung dose (MLD); as such, a MLD ≤8 Gy is recommended to limit the risk of pulmonary I/RP. In addi-

Table 11.2 Potential list of critical organs to spare and target organs. Some organs such as brain (* in the table) can be organ at risk or a target region depending on the clinical scenario

Organs to spare	Targets
Bladder	Bone
Brain*	Brain*
Breast	Liver*
Esophagus	Lymph nodes
Eyes	Mandible
Heart	Ribs/sternum
Kidneys	Skull
Lens	Spinal cord
Liver*	Spleen
Lungs	Testes*
Oral cavity	
Ovaries	
Parotid glands	
Rectum	
Small intestine	
Stomach	
Testes*	
Thyroid	

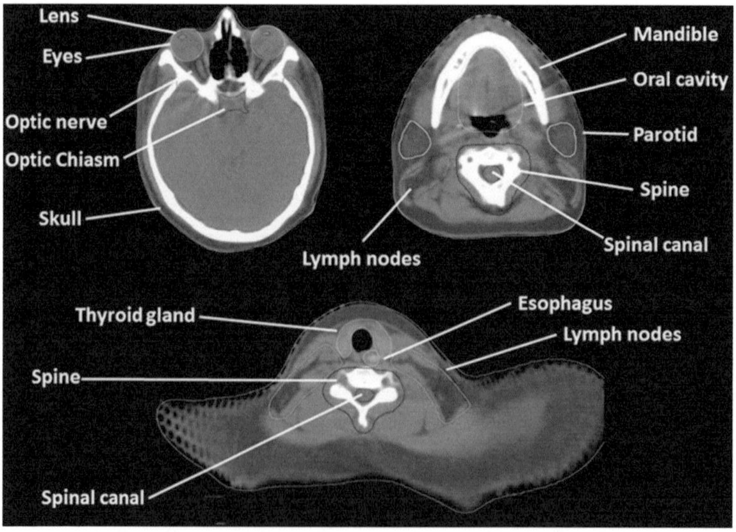

Fig. 11.11 Contours of target structures and organs at risk at level of head and neck

tion, an increase in non-engraftment has not been reported with doses up to 20 Gy. The low incidence of late toxicities also suggests that the higher dose rate with TMI/TMLI at ≥200 cGy/min as compared to conventional TBI of <30 cGy/min did not contribute to organ dysfunction, which is consistent with predictions from previously published studies [30].

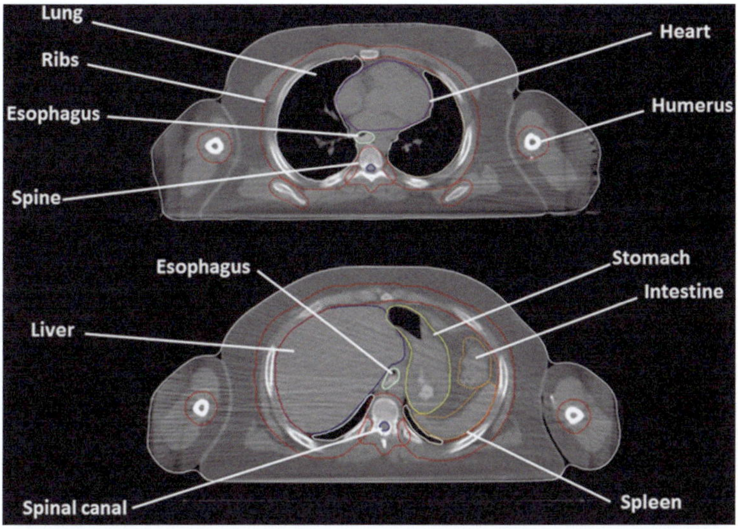

Fig. 11.12 Contours of target structures and organs at risk at level of thorax

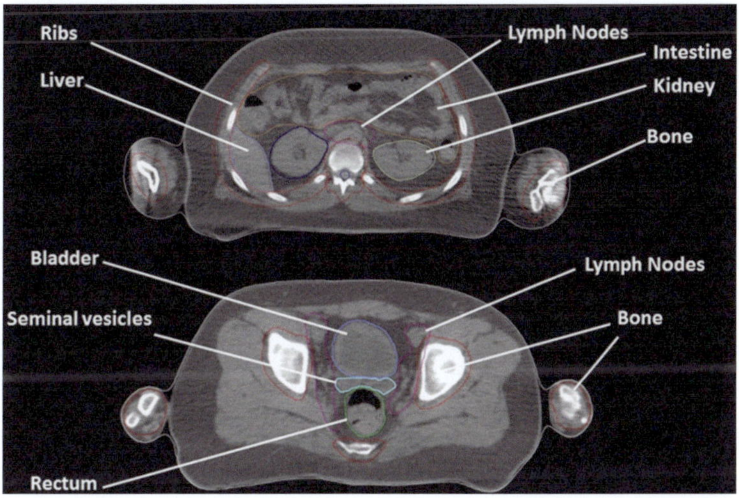

Fig. 11.13 Contours of target structures and organs at risk at level of abdomen and pelvis

- *Organ sparing and recurrence rates*. Organ sparing with TMI and TMLI has raised concerns of sparing of leukemia cells in these regions and increased recurrence rates. Patterns of extramedullary recurrence after TMI or TMLI do not appear dose dependent, nor do they appear different from those historically reported after TBI [89]. Similar concerns have been raised that non-simultaneous dose delivery to all parts of the body could result in reduction of dose to circulating leukemia cells, leading to an increase in relapse rates. Molloy et al. [90] demonstrated that for typical blood circulation times, dose heterogeneity to circulating blood was clinically acceptable if the dose was fractionated and the treatment times for each fraction were 20 min or greater.

Case 3: IMRT-Based TBI (12 Gy) with Lung Blocking

- Clinical rationale: MLD of 8 Gy or less is associated with improved survival among pediatric leukemia patients undergoing TBI [36]. Intensity-modulated radiation therapy (IMRT) may achieve better lung-sparing compared to conventional 2D techniques (35–40% reduction in median lung in one study) [91].
- Figure 11.14 compares 12 Gy TBI using a conventional approach versus TBI delivered using IMRT (using Tomotherapy).

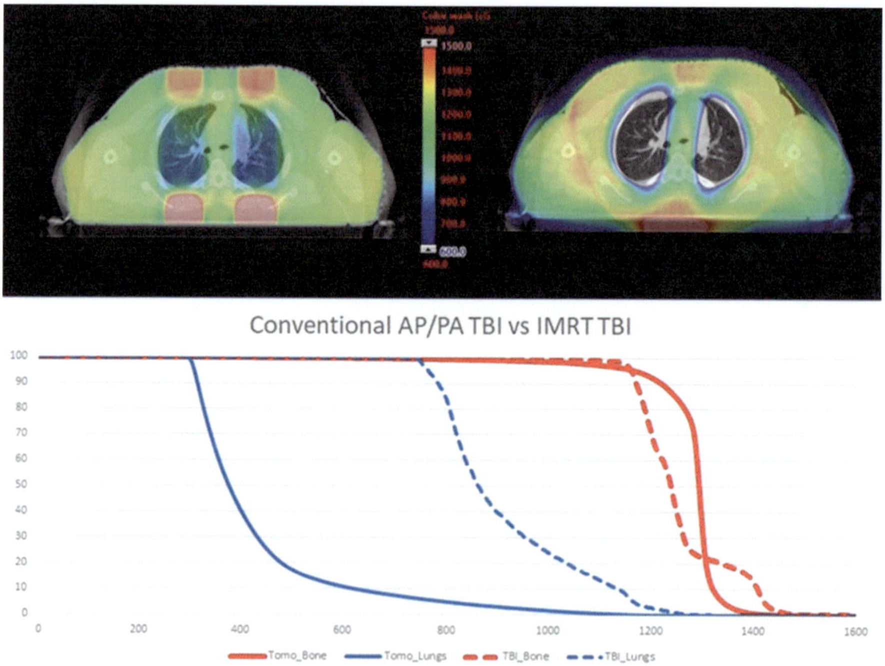

Fig. 11.14 The top panel compares dose color washes of conventional AP/PA (left) versus IMRT (right) demonstrating superior sparing of lung using IMRT. The bottom panel compares DVHs of lung (blue) and bone (red) for conventional (dashed line) and IMRT (solid line). The use of IMRT results in lower lung doses and better dose uniformity in bone

Cases 4, 5, and 6: TMI (12 Gy) vs. TMLI 12 Gy vs. TMLI 20 Gy (12 Gy to Brain and Liver)

- Clinical rationale and summary:
  - TMI, where the target structure is bone, is being evaluated as part of autologous or allogeneic SCT with melphalan for multiple myeloma [71, 92, 93]. It is also being evaluated as part of allogeneic SCT for acute leukemia.
  - TMLI is being evaluated as part of the conditioning regimen in allogenic SCT. In addition to bone, the lymph nodes and spleen are also targeted to augment immunosuppression. TMLI (12 Gy) was first used in patients with acute leukemia older than 55 years old as a means of safely escalating dose in an otherwise reduced-intensity conditioning regimen to further reduce relapse rates [26, 27, 72, 73].
  - Higher doses of TBI have been shown to result in reduced relapse rates in patients with acute and chronic leukemia undergoing SCT but is associated with an unacceptable increase in toxicities [15]. TMLI dose escalation up to 20 Gy is being evaluated in clinical trials [25, 28, 29, 68–71].
- Figure 11.15 compares dose color washes in the axial and coronal planes for TMI 12 Gy (target is bone), TMLI 12 Gy (targets are bone, lymph nodes, and spleen), and TMLI 20 Gy (with 12 Gy to liver and brain) (Table 11.3). All plans were done in the same patient with acute myelogenous leukemia.

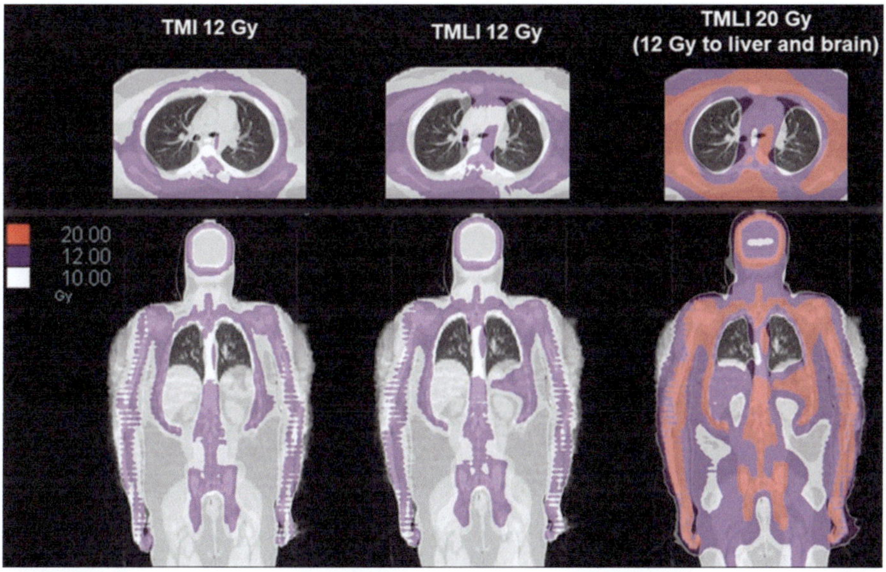

Fig. 11.15 Comparison of dose color washes in axial (upper) and coronal planes (lower) for TMI 12 Gy (target is bone), TMLI 12 Gy (targets are bone, lymph nodes, and spleen) and TMLI 20 Gy (with 12 Gy to liver and brain)

Table 11.3 Compares mean organ doses for each of the three plans. There is a small increase in organ doses with TMLI 12 Gy compared to TMI 12 Gy. With dose escalation to 20 Gy and the inclusion of brain and liver as target organs to 12 Gy, there is an increase in organ doses though mean lung, kidney, heart, esophagus, oral cavity and thyroid remain below 8 Gy

Organs	TMI 12 Gy Mean dose (Gy)	TMLI 12 Gy Mean dose (Gy)	TMLI 20 Gy (liver and brain 12 Gy) Mean dose (Gy)
Bladder	5.51	6.38	9.39
Brain	6.85	7.12	14.64
Esophagus	4.03	4.21	6.42
Eyes	3.4	4.12	4.71
Heart	4.97	5.21	7.6
Kidneys	4.68	5.11	7.53
Lens	1.88	2.34	2.56
Liver	5.15	5.82	12.68
Lungs	5.55	5.63	7.78
Oral cavity	3.29	3.48	7.99
Parotid glands	5.33	6.04	8.74
Rectum	4.35	5.07	8.61
Small intestine	7.58	7.13	11.16
Stomach	5.8	6.27	10.13
Thyroid	3.75	4.37	7.31

References

1. Wong JYC, Filippi AR, Dabaja BS, Yahalom J, Specht L. Total body irradiation: guidelines from the International Lymphoma Radiation Oncology Group (ILROG). Int J Radiat Oncol Biol Phys. 2018;101(3):521–9.
2. Paix A, Antoni D, Waissi W, Ledoux MP, Bilger K, Fornecker L, et al. Total body irradiation in allogeneic bone marrow transplantation conditioning regimens: a review. Crit Rev Oncol Hematol. 2018;123:138–48.
3. Ishibashi N, Soejima T, Kawaguchi H, Akiba T, Hasegawa M, Isobe K, et al. National survey of myeloablative total body irradiation prior to hematopoietic stem cell transplantation in Japan: survey of the Japanese Radiation Oncology Study Group (JROSG). J Radiat Res. 2018;59(4):477–83.
4. Gopal R, Ha CS, Tucker SL, Khouri IF, Giralt SA, Gajewski JL, et al. Comparison of two total body irradiation fractionation regimens with respect to acute and late pulmonary toxicity. Cancer. 2001;92(7):1949–58.
5. Deeg HJ, Sandmaier BM. Who is fit for allogeneic transplantation? Blood. 2010;116(23):4762–70.
6. Malard F, Mohty M. Acute lymphoblastic leukaemia. Lancet. 2020;395(10230):1146–62.
7. Bunin N, Aplenc R, Kamani N, Shaw K, Cnaan A, Simms S. Randomized trial of busulfan vs total body irradiation containing conditioning regimens for children with acute lymphoblastic leukemia: a Pediatric Blood and Marrow Transplant Consortium study. Bone Marrow Transplant. 2003;32(6):543–8.
8. Kato M, Ishida H, Koh K, Inagaki J, Kato K, Goto H, et al. Comparison of chemotherapeutic agents as a myeloablative conditioning with total body irradiation for pediatric acute lymphoblastic leukemia: a study from the pediatric ALL working group of the Japan Society for Hematopoietic Cell Transplantation. Pediatr Blood Cancer. 2015;62(10):1844–50.

9. Davies SM, Ramsay NK, Klein JP, Weisdorf DJ, Bolwell B, Cahn JY, et al. Comparison of preparative regimens in transplants for children with acute lymphoblastic leukemia. J Clin Oncol. 2000;18(2):340–7.
10. Marks DI, Wang T, Perez WS, Antin JH, Copelan E, Gale RP, et al. The outcome of full-intensity and reduced-intensity conditioning matched sibling or unrelated donor transplantation in adults with Philadelphia chromosome-negative acute lymphoblastic leukemia in first and second complete remission. Blood. 2010;116(3):366–74.
11. De Kouchkovsky I, Abdul-Hay M. Acute myeloid leukemia: a comprehensive review and 2016 update. Blood Cancer J. 2016;6(7):e441.
12. Dusenbery KE, Daniels KA, McClure JS, McGlave PB, Ramsay NK, Blazar BR, et al. Randomized comparison of cyclophosphamide-total body irradiation versus busulfan-cyclophosphamide conditioning in autologous bone marrow transplantation for acute myeloid leukemia. Int J Radiat Oncol Biol Phys. 1995;31(1):119–28.
13. Hartman AR, Williams SF, Dillon JJ. Survival, disease-free survival and adverse effects of conditioning for allogeneic bone marrow transplantation with busulfan/cyclophosphamide vs total body irradiation: a meta-analysis. Bone Marrow Transplant. 1998;22(5):439–43.
14. Ringden O, Ruutu T, Remberger M, Nikoskelainen J, Volin L, Vindelov L, et al. A randomized trial comparing busulfan vs total body irradiation in allogeneic marrow transplant recipients with hematological malignancies. Transplant Proc. 1994;26(3):1831–2.
15. Clift RA, Buckner CD, Appelbaum FR, Sullivan KM, Storb R, Thomas ED. Long-term follow-up of a randomized trial of two irradiation regimens for patients receiving allogeneic marrow transplants during first remission of acute myeloid leukemia. Blood. 1998;92(4):1455–6.
16. Bornhauser M, Kienast J, Trenschel R, Burchert A, Hegenbart U, Stadler M, et al. Reduced-intensity conditioning versus standard conditioning before allogeneic haemopoietic cell transplantation in patients with acute myeloid leukaemia in first complete remission: a prospective, open-label randomised phase 3 trial. Lancet Oncol. 2012;13(10):1035–44.
17. Aoudjhane M, Labopin M, Gorin NC, Shimoni A, Ruutu T, Kolb HJ, et al. Comparative outcome of reduced intensity and myeloablative conditioning regimen in HLA identical sibling allogeneic haematopoietic stem cell transplantation for patients older than 50 years of age with acute myeloblastic leukaemia: a retrospective survey from the Acute Leukemia Working Party (ALWP) of the European group for Blood and Marrow Transplantation (EBMT). Leukemia. 2005;19(12):2304–12.
18. Ringden O, Labopin M, Ehninger G, Niederwieser D, Olsson R, Basara N, et al. Reduced intensity conditioning compared with myeloablative conditioning using unrelated donor transplants in patients with acute myeloid leukemia. J Clin Oncol. 2009;27(27):4570–7.
19. Scott BL, Pasquini MC, Logan BR, Wu J, Devine SM, Porter DL, et al. Myeloablative versus reduced-intensity hematopoietic cell transplantation for acute myeloid leukemia and myelodysplastic syndromes. J Clin Oncol. 2017;35(11):1154–61.
20. Gauthier J, Castagna L, Garnier F, Guillaume T, Socie G, Maury S, et al. Reduced-intensity and non-myeloablative allogeneic stem cell transplantation from alternative HLA-mismatched donors for Hodgkin lymphoma: a study by the French Society of Bone Marrow Transplantation and Cellular Therapy. Bone Marrow Transplant. 2017;52(5):689–96.
21. Maeng CH, Ko YH, Lim DH, Kang ES, Choi JY, Kim WS, et al. Comparison of total body irradiation (TBI) conditioning with non-TBI for autologous stem cell transplantation in newly diagnosed or relapsed mature T- and NK-cell non-Hodgkin lymphoma. Cancer Res Treat. 2017;49(1):92–103.
22. Tseng YD, Stevenson PA, Cassaday RD, Cowan A, Till BG, Shadman M, et al. Total body irradiation is safe and similarly effective as chemotherapy-only conditioning in autologous stem cell transplantation for mantle cell lymphoma. Biol Blood Marrow Transplant. 2018;24(2):282–7.
23. Kato H, Taji H, Ogura M, Kagami Y, Oki Y, Tsujimura A, et al. Favorable consolidative effect of high-dose melphalan and total-body irradiation followed by autologous peripheral blood stem

cell transplantation after rituximab-containing induction chemotherapy with in vivo purging in relapsed or refractory follicular lymphoma. Clin Lymphoma Myeloma. 2009;9(6):443–8.
24. Munker R, Baghian A, Koleva Y, Andrews P, Matharoo GS, Wright AE, et al. Long-term follow-up of patients with multiple myeloma treated with total body irradiation-melphalan conditioning. Eur J Haematol. 2017;99(1):56–9.
25. Wong JYC. Total body irradiation: redefining the role of radiotherapy in bone marrow transplantation. In: Wong JYC, Hui SK, editors. Total marrow irradiation. New York: Springer Nature; 2020. p. 1–28.
26. Rosenthal J, Wong J, Stein A, Qian D, Hitt D, Naeem H, et al. Phase 1/2 trial of total marrow and lymph node irradiation to augment reduced-intensity transplantation for advanced hematologic malignancies. Blood. 2011;117(1):309–15.
27. Jensen LG, Stiller T, Wong JYC, Palmer J, Stein A, Rosenthal J. Total marrow lymphoid irradiation/fludarabine/melphalan conditioning for allogeneic hematopoietic cell transplantation. Biol Blood Marrow Transplant. 2018;24(2):301–7.
28. Stein A. Dose escalation of total marrow and lymphoid irradiation in advanced acute leukemia. In: Wong JYC, Hui SK, editors. Total marrow irradiation. New York: Springer Nature; 2020. p. 69–76.
29. Stein A, Palmer J, Tsai NC, Al Malki MM, Aldoss I, Ali H, et al. Phase I trial of total marrow and lymphoid irradiation transplantation conditioning in patients with relapsed/refractory acute leukemia. Biol Blood Marrow Transplant. 2017;23(4):618–24.
30. Shinde A, Yang D, Frankel P, Liu A, Han C, Del Vecchio B, et al. Radiation-related toxicities using organ sparing total marrow irradiation transplant conditioning regimens. Int J Radiat Oncol Biol Phys. 2019;105(5):1025–33.
31. Wingard JR, Piantadosi S, Santos GW, Saral R, Vriesendorp HM, Yeager AM, et al. Allogeneic bone marrow transplantation for patients with high-risk acute lymphoblastic leukemia. J Clin Oncol. 1990;8(5):820–30.
32. Shank B, O'Reilly RJ, Cunningham I, Kernan N, Yaholom J, Brochstein J, et al. Total body irradiation for bone marrow transplantation: the Memorial Sloan-Kettering Cancer Center experience. Radiother Oncol. 1990;18(Suppl 1):68–81.
33. Girinsky T, Benhamou E, Bourhis JH, Dhermain F, Guillot-Valls D, Ganansia V, et al. Prospective randomized comparison of single-dose versus hyperfractionated total-body irradiation in patients with hematologic malignancies. J Clin Oncol. 2000;18(5):981–6.
34. Labar B, Bogdanic V, Nemet D, Mrsic M, Vrtar M, Grgic-Markulin L, et al. Total body irradiation with or without lung shielding for allogeneic bone marrow transplantation. Bone Marrow Transplant. 1992;9(5):343–7.
35. Deeg HJ, Sullivan KM, Buckner CD, Storb R, Appelbaum FR, Clift RA, et al. Marrow transplantation for acute nonlymphoblastic leukemia in first remission: toxicity and long-term follow-up of patients conditioned with single dose or fractionated total body irradiation. Bone Marrow Transplant. 1986;1(2):151–7.
36. Esiashvili N, Lu X, Ulin K, Laurie F, Kessel S, Kalapurakal JA, et al. Higher reported lung dose received during total body irradiation for allogeneic hematopoietic stem cell transplantation in children with acute lymphoblastic leukemia is associated with inferior survival: a report from the Children's Oncology Group. Int J Radiat Oncol Biol Phys. 2019;104(3):513–21.
37. Giebel S, Miszczyk L, Slosarek K, Moukhtari L, Ciceri F, Esteve J, et al. Extreme heterogeneity of myeloablative total body irradiation techniques in clinical practice: a survey of the Acute Leukemia Working Party of the European Group for Blood and Marrow Transplantation. Cancer. 2014;120(17):2760–5.
38. Wong JYC, Schultheiss T. Total body irradiation. In: Appelbaum FR, Forman SJ, Negrin RS, Blume KG, editors. Thomas' hematopoietic cell transplantation. 5th ed. Livingston: Wiley; 2016.
39. Barker CA, Wong JYC, Yahalom J. Total body irradiation. In: Tepper JE, Foote RL, Michalski JM, editors. Clinical radiation oncology. Philadelphia: Elsevier; 2020. p. 388–407.
40. Ozsahin M, Pene F, Touboul E, Gindrey-Vie B, Dominique C, Lefkopoulos D, et al. Total-body irradiation before bone marrow transplantation. Results of two randomized instantaneous dose rates in 157 patients. Cancer. 1992;69(11):2853–65.

41. Oya N, Sasai K, Tachiiri S, Sakamoto T, Nagata Y, Okada T, et al. Influence of radiation dose rate and lung dose on interstitial pneumonitis after fractionated total body irradiation: acute parotitis may predict interstitial pneumonitis. Int J Hematol. 2006;83(1):86–91.
42. Keane TJ, Van Dyk J, Rider WD. Idiopathic interstitial pneumonia following bone marrow transplantation: the relationship with total body irradiation. Int J Radiat Oncol Biol Phys. 1981;7(10):1365–70.
43. Buchali A, Feyer P, Groll J, Massenkeil G, Arnold R, Budach V. Immediate toxicity during fractionated total body irradiation as conditioning for bone marrow transplantation. Radiother Oncol. 2000;54(2):157–62.
44. Valls A, Granena A, Carreras E, Ferrer E, Algara M. Total body irradiation in bone marrow transplantation: fractionated vs single dose. Acute toxicity and preliminary results. Bull Cancer. 1989;76(8):797–804.
45. Benyunes MC, Sullivan KM, Deeg HJ, Mori M, Meyer W, Fisher L, et al. Cataracts after bone marrow transplantation: long-term follow-up of adults treated with fractionated total body irradiation. Int J Radiat Oncol Biol Phys. 1995;32(3):661–70.
46. Tauchmanova L, Selleri C, Rosa GD, Pagano L, Orio F, Lombardi G, et al. High prevalence of endocrine dysfunction in long-term survivors after allogeneic bone marrow transplantation for hematologic diseases. Cancer. 2002;95(5):1076–84.
47. Gerstein J, Meyer A, Sykora KW, Fruhauf J, Karstens JH, Bremer M. Long-term renal toxicity in children following fractionated total-body irradiation (TBI) before allogeneic stem cell transplantation (SCT). Strahlenther Onkol. 2009;185(11):751–5.
48. Abboud I, Porcher R, Robin M, de Latour RP, Glotz D, Socie G, et al. Chronic kidney dysfunction in patients alive without relapse 2 years after allogeneic hematopoietic stem cell transplantation. Biol Blood Marrow Transplant. 2009;15(10):1251–7.
49. Benmiloud S, Steffens M, Beauloye V, de Wandeleer A, Devogelaer JP, Brichard B, et al. Long-term effects on bone mineral density of different therapeutic schemes for acute lymphoblastic leukemia or non-Hodgkin lymphoma during childhood. Horm Res Paediatr. 2010;74(4):241–50.
50. Ishida Y, Sakamoto N, Kamibeppu K, Kakee N, Iwai T, Ozono S, et al. Late effects and quality of life of childhood cancer survivors: part 2. Impact of radiotherapy. Int J Hematol. 2010;92(1):95–104.
51. Ricardi U, Filippi AR, Biasin E, Ciammella P, Botticella A, Franco P, et al. Late toxicity in children undergoing hematopoietic stem cell transplantation with TBI-containing conditioning regimens for hematological malignancies. Strahlenther Onkol. 2009;185(Suppl 2):17–20.
52. Carreras E. Veno-occlusive disease of the liver after hemopoietic cell transplantation. Eur J Haematol. 2000;64(5):281–91.
53. Rizzo JD, Curtis RE, Socie G, Sobocinski KA, Gilbert E, Landgren O, et al. Solid cancers after allogeneic hematopoietic cell transplantation. Blood. 2009;113(5):1175–83.
54. Pingali SR, Champlin RE. Pushing the envelope-nonmyeloablative and reduced intensity preparative regimens for allogeneic hematopoietic transplantation. Bone Marrow Transplant. 2015;50(9):1157–67.
55. Horowitz MM, Gale RP, Sondel PM, Goldman JM, Kersey J, Kolb HJ, et al. Graft-versus-leukemia reactions after bone marrow transplantation. Blood. 1990;75(3):555–62.
56. Gyurkocza B, Sandmaier BM. Conditioning regimens for hematopoietic cell transplantation: one size does not fit all. Blood. 2014;124(3):344–53.
57. Kahl C, Storer BE, Sandmaier BM, Mielcarek M, Maris MB, Blume KG, et al. Relapse risk in patients with malignant diseases given allogeneic hematopoietic cell transplantation after nonmyeloablative conditioning. Blood. 2007;110(7):2744–8.
58. Kornblit B, Maloney DG, Storb R, Storek J, Hari P, Vucinic V, et al. Fludarabine and 2-Gy TBI is superior to 2 Gy TBI as conditioning for HLA-matched related hematopoietic cell transplantation: a phase III randomized trial. Biol Blood Marrow Transplant. 2013;19(9):1340–7.
59. Mohty M, Labopin M, Janssen JJWM, Mufti GJ, Cornelissen JJ, Milpied NJ, et al. Comparison of low dose total body irradiation (TBI)-based reduced intensity conditioning (RIC) vs. chemotherapy-based RIC prior to allogeneic stem cell transplantation (allo-SCT) from an HLA identical sibling donor for acute myeloid leukemia (AML) in first complete remission

(CR1): a retrospective analysis of 1200 patients from the Acute Leukemia Working Party of EBMT. Blood. 2009;114(22):489.
60. Aoki J, Seo S, Kanamori H, Tanaka M, Fukuda T, Onizuka M, et al. Impact of low-dose TBI on outcomes of reduced intensity conditioning allogeneic hematopoietic stem cell transplantation for AML. Bone Marrow Transplant. 2016;51(4):604–6.
61. Hong S, Barker CA, Klein JP, Shaw P, Bredeson C, Angelina A, et al. Trends in utilization of total body irradiation (TBI) prior to hematopoietic cell transplantation (HCT) worldwide. Biol Blood Marrow Transplant. 2012;18:2.
62. Mohty M, Malard F, Savani BN. High-dose total body irradiation and myeloablative conditioning before allogeneic hematopoietic cell transplantation: time to rethink? Biol Blood Marrow Transplant. 2015;21(4):620–4.
63. Sandmaier BM, Mackinnon S, Childs RW. Reduced intensity conditioning for allogeneic hematopoietic cell transplantation: current perspectives. Biol Blood Marrow Transplant. 2007;13(1 Suppl 1):87–97.
64. Wong JY, Liu A, Schultheiss T, Popplewell L, Stein A, Rosenthal J, et al. Targeted total marrow irradiation using three-dimensional image-guided tomographic intensity-modulated radiation therapy: an alternative to standard total body irradiation. Biol Blood Marrow Transplant. 2006;12(3):306–15.
65. Schultheiss TE, Wong J, Liu A, Olivera G, Somlo G. Image-guided total marrow and total lymphatic irradiation using helical tomotherapy. Int J Radiat Oncol Biol Phys. 2007;67(4):1259–67.
66. Hui SK, Kapatoes J, Fowler J, Henderson D, Olivera G, Manon RR, et al. Feasibility study of helical tomotherapy for total body or total marrow irradiation. Med Phys. 2005;32(10):3214–24.
67. Aydogan B, Yeginer M, Kavak GO, Fan J, Radosevich JA, Gwe-Ya K. Total marrow irradiation with RapidArc volumetric arc therapy. Int J Radiat Oncol Biol Phys. 2011;81(2):592–9.
68. Wong JY, Forman S, Somlo G, Rosenthal J, Liu A, Schultheiss T, et al. Dose escalation of total marrow irradiation with concurrent chemotherapy in patients with advanced acute leukemia undergoing allogeneic hematopoietic cell transplantation. Int J Radiat Oncol Biol Phys. 2013;85(1):148–56.
69. Patel P, Aydogan B, Koshy M, Mahmud D, Oh A, Saraf SL, et al. Combination of linear accelerator-based intensity-modulated total marrow irradiation and myeloablative fludarabine/busulfan: a phase I study. Biol Blood Marrow Transplant. 2014;20(12):2034–41.
70. Hui S, Brunstein C, Takahashi Y, DeFor T, Holtan SG, Bachanova V, et al. Dose escalation of total marrow irradiation in high-risk patients undergoing allogeneic hematopoietic stem cell transplantation. Biol Blood Marrow Transplant. 2017;23(7):1110–6.
71. Somlo G, Spielberger R, Frankel P, Karanes C, Krishnan A, Parker P, et al. Total marrow irradiation: a new ablative regimen as part of tandem autologous stem cell transplantation for patients with multiple myeloma. Clin Cancer Res. 2011;17(1):174–82.
72. Arslan S, Al Malki MM. Total marrow and lymphoid irradiation in patient undergoing haplo-identical transplants. In: Wong JYC, Hui SK, editors. Total marrow irradiation. 1st ed. New York: Springer Nature; 2020. p. 123–34.
73. Aristei C, Saldi S, Pierini A, Ruggeri L, Piccine S, Ingrosso G. Total marrow/lymphoid irradiation in the conditioning regimen for haploidentical T-cell depleted hematopoietic stem cell transplantation for acute myeloid leukemia. The Perugia experience. In: Wong JYC, Hui SK, editors. Total marrow irradiation. New York: Springer Nature; 2020. p. 111–22.
74. Penagaricano JA, Chao M, Van Rhee F, Moros EG, Corry PM, Ratanatharathorn V. Clinical feasibility of TBI with helical tomotherapy. Bone Marrow Transplant. 2011;46(7):929–35.
75. Gruen A, Ebell W, Wlodarczyk W, Neumann O, Kuehl JS, Stromberger C, et al. Total body irradiation (TBI) using helical tomotherapy in children and young adults undergoing stem cell transplantation. Radiat Oncol. 2013;8:92.

76. Tas B, Durmus IF, Okumus A, Uzel OE, Gokce M, Goksoy HS, et al. Total-body irradiation using linac-based volumetric modulated arc therapy: its clinical accuracy, feasibility and reliability. Radiother Oncol. 2018;129(3):527–33.
77. Sarradin V, Simon L, Huynh A, Gilhodes J, Filleron T, Izar F. Total body irradiation using Helical Tomotherapy((R)): treatment technique, dosimetric results and initial clinical experience. Cancer Radiother. 2018;22(1):17–24.
78. Sun R, Cuenca X, Itti R, Nguyen Quoc S, Vernant JP, Mazeron JJ, et al. First French experiences of total body irradiations using helical TomoTherapy((R)). Cancer Radiother. 2017;21(5):365–72.
79. Jiang Z, Jia J, Yue C, Pang Y, Liu Z, Ouyang L, et al. Haploidentical hematopoietic SCT using helical tomotherapy for total-body irradiation and targeted dose boost in patients with high-risk/refractory acute lymphoblastic leukemia. Bone Marrow Transplant. 2018;53(4):438–48.
80. Dandapani S, Wong JYC. Modern total body irradiation (TBI): intensity modulated radiation treatment (IMRT). In: Wong JYC, Hui SK, editors. Total marrow irradiation. New York: Springer Nature; 2020. p. 177–86.
81. Wilkie JR, Tiryaki H, Smith BD, Roeske JC, Radosevich JA, Aydogan B. Feasibility study for linac-based intensity modulated total marrow irradiation. Med Phys. 2008;35(12):5609–18.
82. Jiang B, Dai J, Zhang Y, Zhang K. Feasibility study of a novel rotational and translational method for linac-based intensity modulated total marrow irradiation. Technol Cancer Res Treat. 2012;11(3):237–47.
83. Cherpak AJ, Monajemi T, Chytyk-Praznik K, Mulroy L. Energy-dependent OAR sparing and dose conformity for total marrow irradiation of obese patients. J Appl Clin Med Phys. 2018;19(5):532–8.
84. Mancosu P, Navarria P, Castagna L, Reggiori G, Sarina B, Tomatis S, et al. Interplay effects between dose distribution quality and positioning accuracy in total marrow irradiation with volumetric modulated arc therapy. Med Phys. 2013;40(11):111713.
85. Corvo R, Zeverino M, Vagge S, Agostinelli S, Barra S, Taccini G, et al. Helical tomotherapy targeting total bone marrow after total body irradiation for patients with relapsed acute leukemia undergoing an allogeneic stem cell transplant. Radiother Oncol. 2011;98(3):382–6.
86. Lin SC, Hsieh PY, Shueng PW, Tien HJ, Wang LY, Hsieh CH. Total marrow irradiation as part of autologous stem cell transplantation for Asian patients with multiple myeloma. Biomed Res Int. 2013;2013:321762.
87. Shueng PW, Lin SC, Chong NS, Lee HY, Tien HJ, Wu LJ, et al. Total marrow irradiation with helical tomotherapy for bone marrow transplantation of multiple myeloma: first experience in Asia. Technol Cancer Res Treat. 2009;8(1):29–38.
88. Bao Z, Zhao H, Wang D, Gong J, Zhong Y, Xiong Y, et al. Feasibility of a novel dose fractionation strategy in TMI/TMLI. Radiat Oncol. 2018;13(1):248.
89. Kim JH, Stein A, Tsai N, Schultheiss TE, Palmer J, Liu A, et al. Extramedullary relapse following total marrow and lymphoid irradiation in patients undergoing allogeneic hematopoietic cell transplantation. Int J Radiat Oncol Biol Phys. 2014;89(1):75–81.
90. Molloy JA. Statistical analysis of dose heterogeneity in circulating blood: implications for sequential methods of total body irradiation. Med Phys. 2010;37(11):5568–78.
91. Zhuang AH, Liu A, Schultheiss TE, Wong JY. Dosimetric study and verification of total body irradiation using helical tomotherapy and its comparison to extended SSD technique. Med Dosim. 2010;35(4):243–9.
92. Mahe M, Liagostera C, Moreau P, Meyer A, Lioure B, Batard S. Total marrow irradiation in multiple myeloma—the French Myeloma Group Experience. In: Wong JYC, Hui SK, editors. Total marrow irradiation. New York: Springer Nature; 2020. p. 135–44.
93. Sahebi F. Total marrow irradiation in multiple myeloma—the City of Hope experience. In: Wong JYC, Hui SK, editors. Total marrow irradiation. New York: Springer Nature; 2020. p. 145–54.

Further Reading

Barker CA, Wong JYC, Yahalom J. Total body irradiation. In: Tepper JE, Foote RL, Michalski JM, editors. Clinical radiation oncology. Philadelphia: Elsevier; 2020. p. 388–407.

Esiashvili N, Lu X, Ulin K, et al. Higher reported lung dose received during total body irradiation for allogeneic hematopoietic stem cell transplantation in children with acute lymphoblastic leukemia is associated with inferior survival: a report from the Children's Oncology Group. Int J Radiat Oncol Biol Phys. 2019;104(3):513–21.

Gyurkocza B, Sandmaier B. Conditioning regimens for hematopoietic cell transplantation: one size does not fit all. Blood. 2014;124(3):344–53.

Scott BL, Pasquini MC, Logan BR, et al. Myeloablative versus reduced-intensity hematopoietic cell transplantation for acute myeloid leukemia and myelodysplastic syndromes. J Clin Oncol. 2017;35:1154–61.

Wong JYC. Total marrow irradiation: redefining the role of radiotherapy in bone marrow transplantation. In: Wong JYC, Hui SK, editors. Total marrow irradiation. New York: Springer Nature; 2020. p. 1–28.

Wong JYC, Schultheiss T. Radiotherapeutic principles of hematopoietic cell transplantation. In: Forman SJ, Negrin RS, Antin JH, Appelbaum FR, editors. Thomas' hematopoietic cell transplantation. 5th ed. West Sussex: John Wiley & Sons, Ltd; 2016. p. 244–57.

Wong JYC, Filippi AR, Dabaja BS, Yahalom J, Specht L. Total body irradiation: guidelines from the International Lymphoma Radiation Oncology Group (ILROG). Int J Radiat Oncol Biol Phys. 2018;101(3):521–9.

Target Volume Delineation for Plasmacytoma and Multiple Myeloma

12

Leslie K. Ballas, Youlia Kirova, and Michael J. Yunes

Contents

L. K. Ballas (✉)
Department of Radiation Oncology, Cedars-Sinai Medical Center, Los Angeles, CA, USA
e-mail: leslie.ballas@cshs.org

Y. Kirova
Department of Radiation Oncology, Institut Curie, Paris, France
e-mail: youlia.kirova@curie.fr

M. J. Yunes
Division of Radiology/Oncology, Radiation Oncology, Springfield, MA, USA
e-mail: michael.yunes@baystatehealth.org

C. Pinnix et al. (eds.), *Target Volume Delineation in Hematologic Malignancies*, Practical Guides in Radiation Oncology,
https://doi.org/10.1007/978-3-031-67722-9_12

Part 1: Background and Epidemiology

- Plasma cell neoplasms are mature B-cell monoclonal populations of cells and include the diagnoses of monoclonal gammopathy of undetermined significance (MGUS), isolated or solitary plasmacytoma of bone (SBP), extramedullary plasmacytoma (SEP), and multiple myeloma (MM). All of these diagnoses are the result of a malignant transformation of a post-germinal center B-cell.
- Based on the SEER database plasmacytomas and multiple myeloma account for approximately one quarter of all mature B-cell neoplasms and <6% are plasmacytomas [1].
- SBP and SEP arise outside the bone marrow in the absence of signs or symptoms of multiple myeloma.
- SBP and SEP occur in a slightly younger age group (55–65 years) than MM (>65 years) [2].
- The annual incidence of new MM cases is approximately 6.9 per 100,000 men and women with a slight preponderance of males. An estimated 32,270 new cases are expected in 2020 representing approximately 1.8% of all new cancer diagnoses [3].
- MGUS appears to precede a diagnosis of MM in most, if not all patients [4–6].

Diagnosis	Common marrow/M protein features	Clinical presentation	Transformation rate to MM
MGUS [4]	<10% plasma cells in marrow	Asymptomatic	0.5–1% per year (van Nieuwenhuijzen PMID 29703720)
Solitary plasmacytoma of bone (SBP) [7]	Solitary bone lesion, <10% plasma cells in marrow	May be symptomatic or asymptomatic	70% with median time to progression 19 months (de Waal PMID 27605358)
Extramedullary plasmacytoma (SEP) [8]	Solitary soft tissue lesion (most often nasopharynx, tonsils, paranasal sinuses)	May be symptomatic or asymptomatic	14% at 3 years (Paiva PMID 24876564)
Multiple myeloma (MM)	Multiple bone lesions or ≥10% monoclonal plasma cells in marrow or EMP	Symptomatic with a myeloma-defining event	

- Patients with MGUS (up to 3–5% of the population >70 years) and asymptomatic multiple myeloma are often diagnosed incidentally or as part of a routine hematological workup.
- Patients with SBP frequently present with pain (vertebrae most commonly), neurologic changes, or pathologic fractures.
- Patients with SEP frequently present with local compressive symptoms (upper aerodigestive system most commonly).
- Patients with MM may present with any end-organ damage symptoms. Fatigue and bone pain due to anemia are the most common, followed by other end-organ

symptoms such as pathologic fractures, renal impairment, neurologic changes, and infections.

- Evaluation of a patient with MGUS, plasmacytoma and multiple myeloma should include the following tests.
  - H&P.
  - CBC with differential and blood smear.
  - Chemistries including calcium and creatinine looking for end-organ damage.
  - Bone marrow biopsy and biopsy of the mass (clonality, labeling index, immunophenotype, and cytogenetics).
  - Serum B2 microglobulin, albumin, C-reactive protein, LDH.
  - Quantitative M component evaluation.
    - Serum protein electrophoresis and immunofixation.
    - Urine protein electrophoresis (Bence Jones proteinuria).
    - Free light chain measurements.
  - Imaging.
    - Skeletal survey (still considered standard for screening at diagnosis as not all facilities may have advanced imaging capability).
      - Low sensitivity.
      - Cannot detect marrow positivity or extra-osseous disease.
    - CT as indicated for local disease assessment for diagnosis, staging, and guiding treatment.
      - CT-guided biopsy is often the standard approach to obtain initial tissue for diagnosis.
    - MRI preferred for determining the extent of disease in medullary cavity and is essential in head and neck, spine, epidural, soft tissue, and cord compression presentations.
      - Becoming the favored screening method to assess bone marrow involvement due to lack of radiation exposure to the patient.
    - PET/CT for complete assessment of potential occult disease.
      - High sensitivity (approx. 30% of MRI negative patients have additional disease based on PET/CT) [9–11].
      - Limited utility in very small lesions and early marrow involvement.
      - Poor spatial resolution with CT.
    - ILROG recommendations.
      - MRI should be the routine staging procedure for workup of SBP and SEP [9, 12, 13].
      - PET/CT is mandatory for confirming diagnosis of SBP and SEP [9, 14].

Pre-radiotherapy Imaging and Evaluation

- The imaging used in staging and confirmation of a diagnosis of SBP/SEP or MM should also be the preferred imaging for treatment planning. Examples:
  - Head and neck—MRI & PET/CT to determine extent of disease and treatment volume.

- Spine—MRI to assist delineation of bone, marrow and soft tissue involvement.
- Long bones—MRI to localize lesion. Use a preop MRI if fixation or stabilization required prior to RT.

• Fusion of primary imaging should be standard when possible.

Part 2: Management and Treatment of Solitary Plasmacytoma and Multiple Myeloma

Principles of Management

• Preoperative vs. postoperative RT.
  - Preoperatively, it is not necessary to treat the whole bone [9, 15].
  - Postoperatively, if instrumentation or implant disrupts the plasmacytoma, consider radiation to the entire surgical hardware. Radiation is recommended after surgery to reduce the risk of repeat fracture/hardware failure, promote healing and improve pain control [16, 17].
  - For palliation, entire surgical hardware does not have to be included, but treating hardware may decrease local recurrence [18] (see discussion for Case 2, below).
  - Whole bone RT is not necessary but may be required in some cases where additional risk is limited. For example, vertebral body.
  - Limit marrow in treatment fields when feasible. (For example, additional uninvolved vertebral levels do not require treatment.)
  - Generally recommended postoperative timing is 2–4 weeks following surgery to allow adequate wound healing.
• Elective nodal coverage in SEP is not recommended if quality imaging does not identify suspicious nodes.
• Vertebroplasty/Kyphoplasty.
  - Pain from an unstable spine will likely not be relieved with radiation alone [19].
  - Radiation is recommended with vertebroplasty or kyphoplasty [20, 21].
  - Generally used for patients with symptomatic vertebral body fractures or retropulsion of bone in the SBP or MM setting.
• Radiofrequency ablation, cryoablation, and focused ultrasound may have a role for refractory pain after radiation. There is no clear role as initial management of symptoms in hematologic malignancies when compared to radiation.
• Integration with chemotherapy or novel medications.
  - Osteoclast inhibitors may prevent repeat fracture but do not delay disease progression [22].
  - Data suggests that moderate dose RT (20–30 Gy in 2–3 Gy fractions) may be safely delivered with concurrent myeloma systemic therapy (Salgado et al., PMID 30706018); however, care should be taken to limit dose to surrounding normal tissues as much as possible.

Palliative radiotherapy given concurrently with Bortezomib, Carfilzomib, or Daratumumab showed no significant increase in acute toxicity (including CBC lab values) compared to RT without these agents (Salgado PMID 30706018).

- Post-transplant considerations.
  - MM patients who have undergone a transplant can pose a difficult clinical situation. Treatment recommendations vary in the setting of a limited relapse, particularly in a single bony site. With limited guidance in the literature, the options are to treat this area as an SBP or a MM. The clinical decision is often left to the radiation oncologist based on other factors such as performance status, volume of marrow potentially radiated and anatomic location.

General Considerations for Radiotherapy

- Definitive RT for SBP.
  - Local control rates of 94% were reported with a dose of 40 Gy or above compared with 69% for doses lower than 40 Gy [23]. A multi-institutional study of 258 patients showed no dose–response relationship beyond 30–35 Gy [7].
  - There has been no improvement in local control with doses of 50–60 Gy [7, 24, 25]. Princess Margaret reported a lack of dose–response above 35 Gy for tumors <5 cm and suggested that higher doses should be used in patients with tumors >5 cm [26].
  - In single center study, the combination of Lenalidomide-dexamethasone in association with IMRT 40 Gy/20 fractions in the treatment of solitary plasmacytoma was reported as safe and improves MMFS and PFS and the local control was 100% in irradiated volumes [27].
  - The NCCN guidelines recommend a minimum dose of 40 Gy independent of tumor size (NCCN Multiple myeloma guidelines v3.2023 accessed 6.30.2023).
  - ILROG offers the following dosing guidelines (Tsang PMID 29976492):

    SBP <5 cm: 35–40 Gy.

    SBP >5 cm 40–50 Gy.

    SEP: 40–50 Gy, with 40 Gy being acceptable for small, well defined, or post-excision with positive surgical margin.
- Palliative RT for MM.
  - Lower doses are sufficient to alleviate symptoms in MM patients; however, no consensus on dose has been reached.

    Retrospective comparison of 8 Gy in 1 fraction or 20 Gy in 5 fractions compared to 30 Gy in 10 fractions or 37.5 Gy in 15 fractions and even 40 Gy in 20 fractions for cord compression from vertebral body disease showed that the longer course treatments had higher rates of motor function at 6 and 12 months [28].

Randomized trial comparing 30 Gy in 10 fractions to 8 Gy in 1 fraction for symptomatic bone lesions found similar pain relief between fractionation but improved QOL with the fractionated regimen [29].

- Based on the data available, ILROG recommends:

  8–30 Gy hypofractionated treatment (8 Gy × 1, 20 Gy in 5 fractions or 30 Gy in 10 fractions) with a single 8 Gy × 1 if prognosis is poor.

  20–30 Gy conventional fractionation for retreatment or for large treatment volumes.

  30 Gy in 10–15 fractions for epidural disease, spinal cord compression, or a bulky mass when durable local control is desired.

- OAR.
  - Because SBP/SEP/MM can appear anywhere in the body, it is important to keep the dose to OAR "as low as reasonably possible" and respecting known tolerances. This is also important because neighboring locations may require treatment in the future.
  - Total bone marrow reserve is important for MM patients, therefore limiting dose to the bone marrow and using RT sparingly is essential. Novel systemic agents and bisphosphonates may provide better PFS, consequently local therapy may not be used as frequently, particularly in relatively asymptomatic patients.
- Technique.
  - Technique for the treatment of SBP/SEP/MM varies depending on anatomic location, neighboring critical structures, and dosing. Patients can receive 2D, 3D CRT, IMRT, or VMAT based on clinician judgment. When appropriate, comparative treatment planning is encouraged to limit dosing based on technique (Table 12.1).

Table 12.1 Planning target definitions for treatment SBP, SEP, and MM

Volume	Description	
Gross tumor volume (GTV)	GTV	Using the primary imaging of untreated lesions, the GTV should be outlined on the simulation study and is always part of the clinical target volume (CTV). When feasible, fusion of the primary imaging (for example, PET/CT or MRI) with the simulation study can be helpful to define the GTV

(continued)

Table 12.1 (continued)

Volume	Description	
Clinical target volume (CTV)	CTV	By definition, the CTV encompasses the original GTV and suspected microscopic subclinical disease. In the setting of definitive RT for SP, it is reasonable that the CTV includes the GTV plus a margin of 0.5–3 cm expanded in all directions, respecting anatomical boundaries. An axial GTV to CTV expansion of 0.5–1 cm may be appropriate for potential microscopic extension in soft tissues (e.g. in the head and neck area, see Case 1). However, for a long bone site, the proximal and distal expansion should be increased to 2–3 cm depending on the availability of accurate imaging with MRI and PET/CT. Adjacent normal structures that are clearly uninvolved or at low risk of subclinical disease should be excluded from the CTV. In outlining the CTV, the following points should be considered: • Quality and accuracy of imaging (ideally MRI and PET information taken into account) • Concerns of changes in volume since imaging • Local spread of disease (MRI very useful) • Potential subclinical involvement (e.g. potential nodal involvement with head and neck sites) • Adjacent organs and constraints
	Palliative irradiation in the setting of multiple myeloma	In the palliative setting, it is reasonable to omit an additional margin from GTV to CTV as it is not critical to cover adjacent subclinical disease in the context of wider systemic disease. Whole bone coverage is generally not required
Internal target volume (ITV)	In situations where there is expected physiological movement (for example, respiration) affecting the CTV, an additional margin (ITV) should be added to the CTV to account for this movement. The optimal method is to use 4D CT simulation to identify the required ITV margins	
Planning target volume (PTV)	The PTV is the volume that takes into account the CTV (or ITV, when relevant) and is expanded to account for setup uncertainties during radiotherapy planning and treatment sessions. This margin depends on estimated setup variations that are a function of the immobilization device, body site, and patient compliance. In general, margins for uncertainties should be added quadratically to avoid excessive margins based on the most extreme (and least likely) situations	

(continued)

Table 12.1 (continued)

Volume	Description
Organs at risk (OAR)	OARs relevant to treatment planning should be outlined on the CT-based simulation study. The dosimetry/physics team should calculate dose-volume histograms, and the plan should be evaluated in consideration of the expected normal tissue complication probability. The objective is to deposit dose to OAR "as low as reasonably achievable" (ALARA principle), rather than a set dose level to keep within traditional tolerance limits. Consideration should also be given to factors such as gender, age, and co-morbidities of the patient. Some structures, such as spinal cord, lung, heart, and kidneys are more critical than others. Based on comparative treatment planning (comparison dose-volume histogram [DVH]) and a determination of the priority of the OARs to protect, the radiation oncology team should make a clinical judgment as to which treatment technique to use. Bone marrow dose should be tracked in all cases

Part 3: Cases

Case 1: SEP of the Head and Neck

A 44-year-old female with 3 months of difficulty swallowing. A CT of the head and neck showed a 2.5 cm × 2.6 cm region of fullness in the right nasopharynx. An MRI showed a mass in the right tonsillar tissue extending into the upper part of the oropharynx. A biopsy revealed a kappa-restricted plasma cell neoplasm and PET scan showed uptake in the right nasopharynx into the right tonsil with an SUV of 4.5. There were no other PET-avid lesions confirming a solitary extramedullary plasmacytoma (SEP). The plan was designed to treat the nasopharyngeal mass to 4500 cGy in 25 fractions using VMAT with 6MV photons.

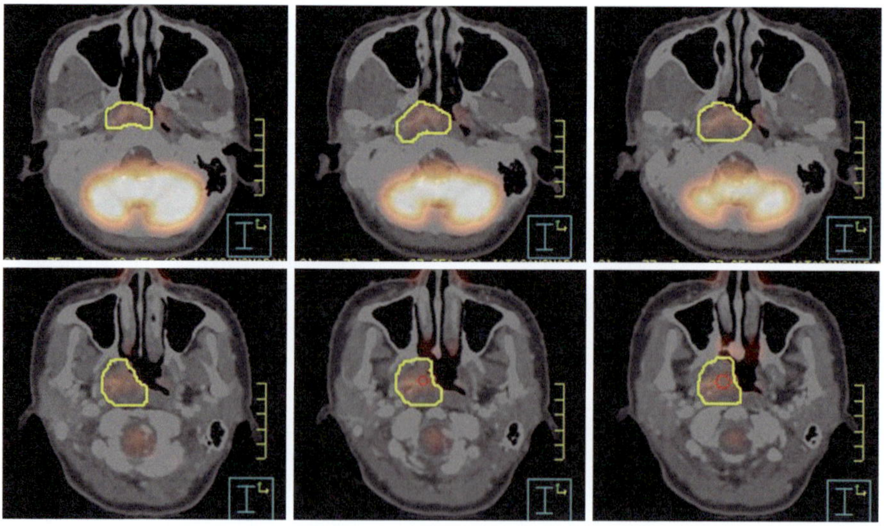

CT simulation fused with staging PET-CT. GTV outlined in yellow.

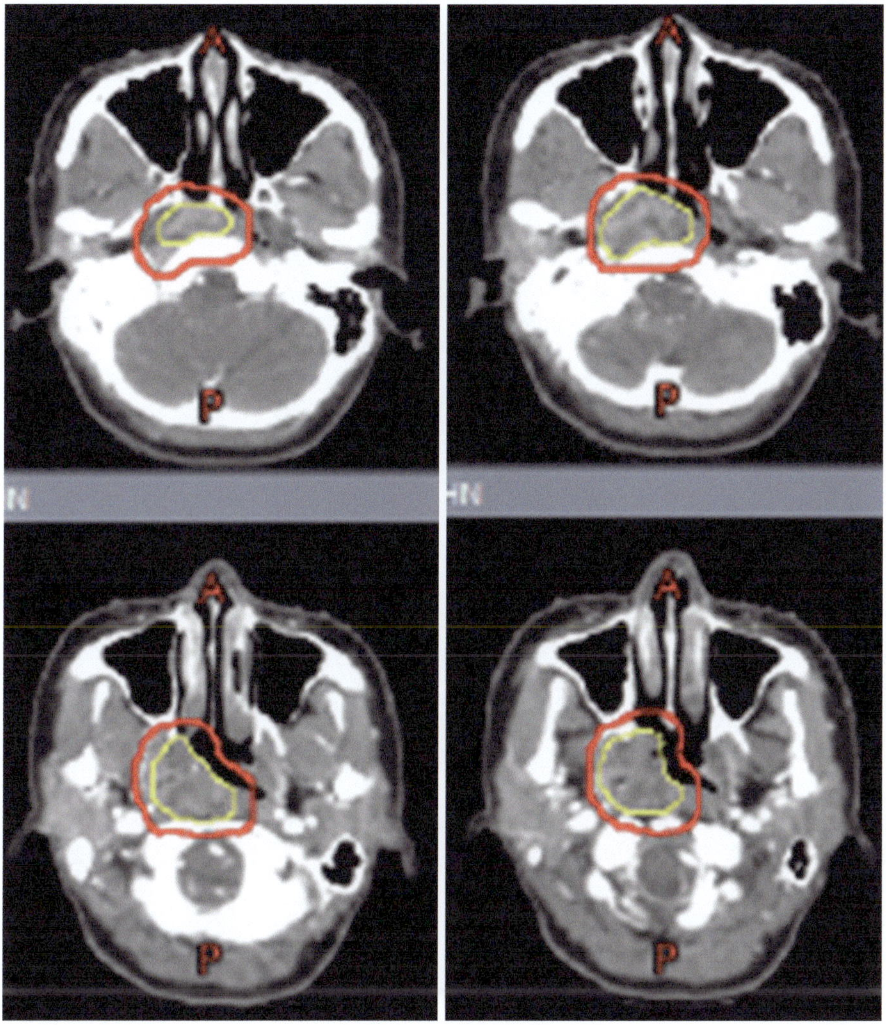

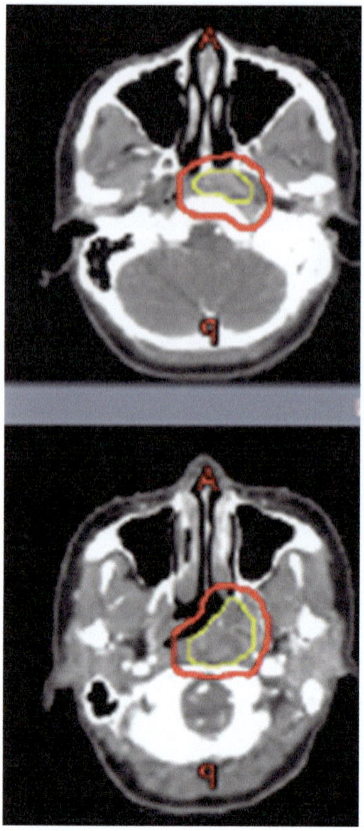

GTV outlined in yellow with 0.5 cm expansion to CTV (red).

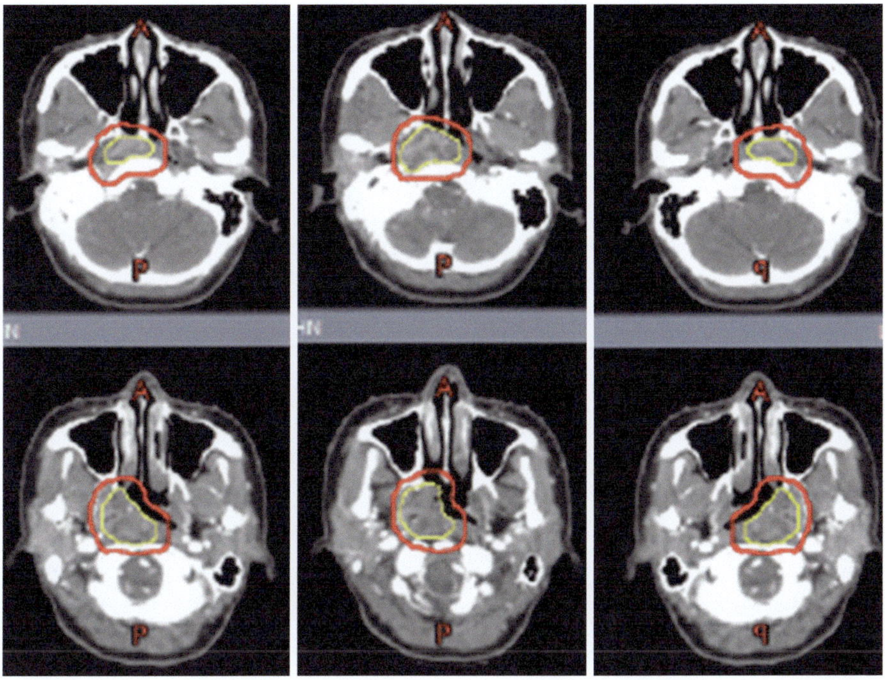

CTV (red) expansion by 0.3 cm to PTV (blue). Patient in aquaplast mask and so expansion to PTV based on immobilization.

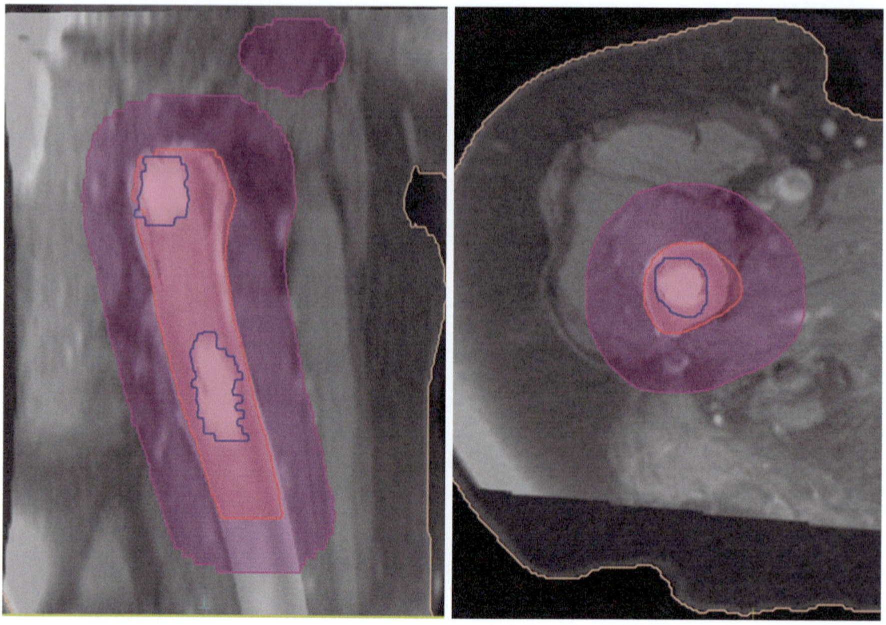

Isodose distribution.

Case 2: Multiple Myeloma Long Bone s/p Surgical Stabilization

A 75-year-old female with known diagnosis of MM who had progressing pain in the left hip and underwent an MRI revealing multiple lesions in the acetabulum and proximal left femur. Due to the cortical narrowing, the risk of fracture was felt to be significant and she underwent prophylactic intramedullary nail stabilization followed by postoperative radiotherapy. Plan was to treat the area of preoperative disease to 2000 cGy in 10 fractions using AP-PA beams with 6 MV photons.

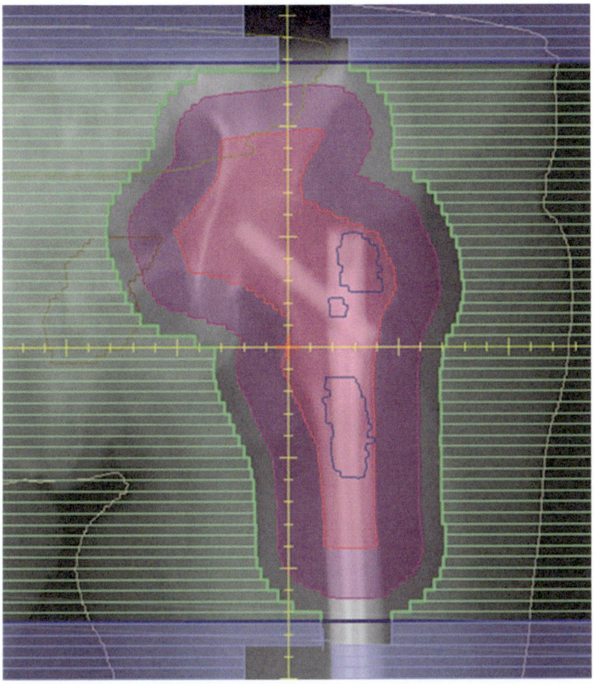

CT simulation fused with pre-op MRI shown in sagittal and axial planes. GTV outlined in blue. CTV (red) = GTV + 3 cm confined to bone outlined in red. Expansion from CTV to PTV (pink) is 1 cm.

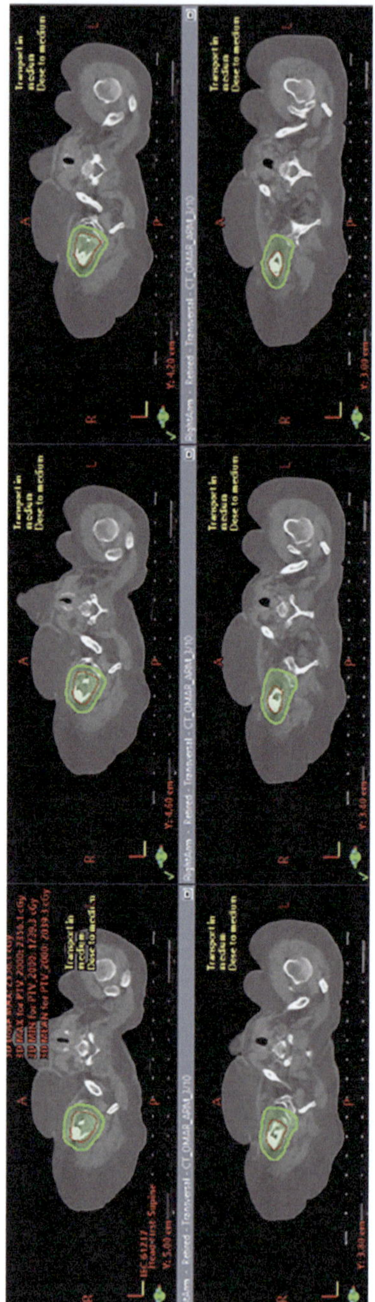

Beams eye view with MLC. GTV (blue), CTV (red), and PTV (pink) all displayed.

There is some controversy regarding treatment of the entire surgical hardware. The ILROG guidelines suggest that for SBP, including the whole bone in the CTV when there is uncertainty regarding extent of disease in the bone and when expansion to include the whole bone will not add additional morbidity. In the setting of MM, whole bone coverage is generally not required. Since the ILROG guidelines were published, a retrospective study evaluating local failure along the surgical hardware has been published. In this study, 3/40 (7.5%) of patients had local failure along the surgical hardware outside of the RT field. The extent of hardware coverage (>80% vs. <80%) predicted disease relapse along the hardware ($p = 0.04$) [18].

Case 3: SBP Long Bone s/p Surgical Stabilization

A 51-year-old female who presented to the ED with a fracture in her right humeral shaft. The patient underwent intramedullary nailing. Pathology revealed a plasma cell neoplasm. Bone marrow biopsy showed 5% plasma cells with no other bone lesions on imaging confirming solitary plasmacytoma of bone. She presented for consideration of postoperative radiotherapy. Plan was for 4500 cGy AP-PA using 6 MV photons.

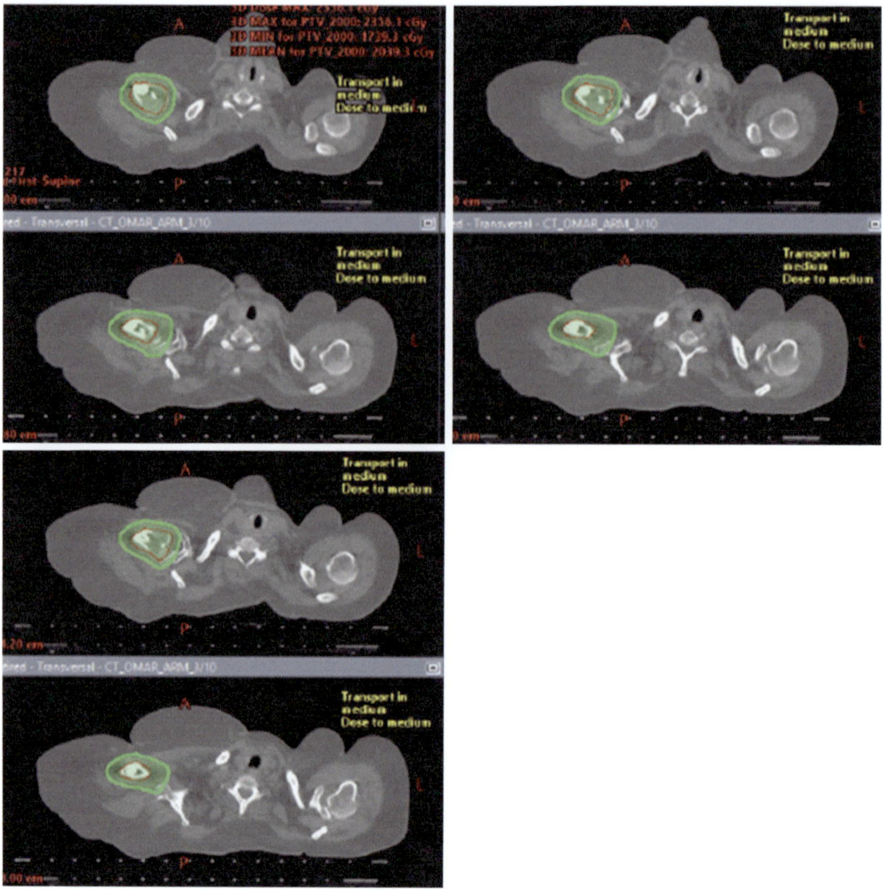

CTV (red) is entire extent of intramedullary rod. PTV (green) is 1 cm expansion from CTV.

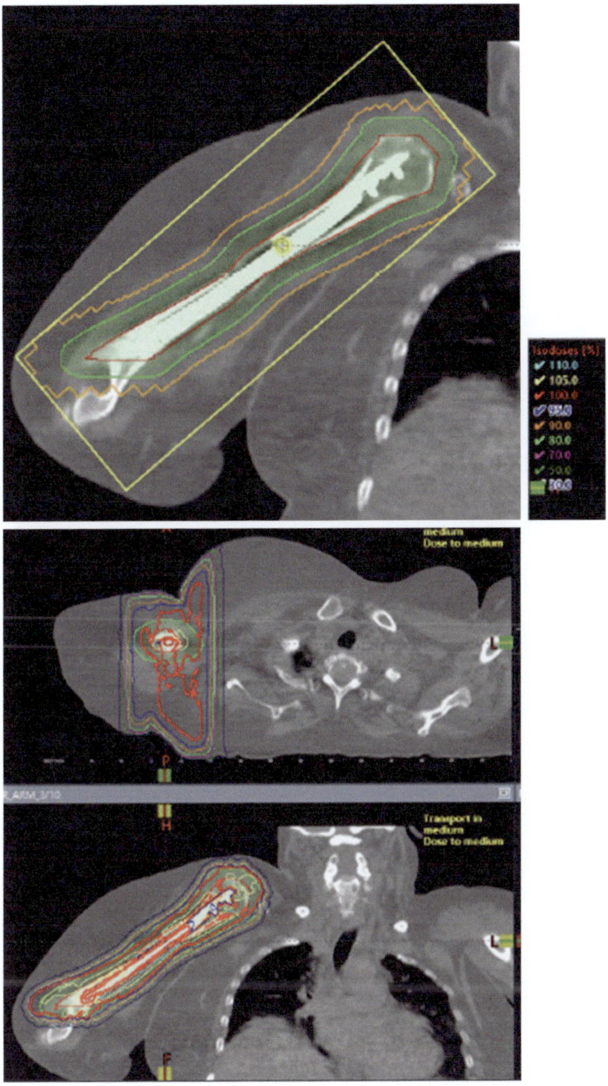

Coronal view of CTV, PTV, and block edge (pink). Isodose distribution with AP-PA beams.

Case 4: SEP

A 61-year-old male presented with abdominal pain. An ultrasound was performed to rule out cholecystitis and identified a mass in the pancreas. MRI revealed a 5.3 × 3.8 cm non-cystic mass in the head of the pancreas. ERCP biopsy revealed a plasma cell neoplasm. Kappa light chain was positive. Bone marrow biopsy found <10% plasma cells. PET/CT scan and skeletal survey was negative confirming SEP. Plan was 4500 cGy using VMAT with 6MV photons.

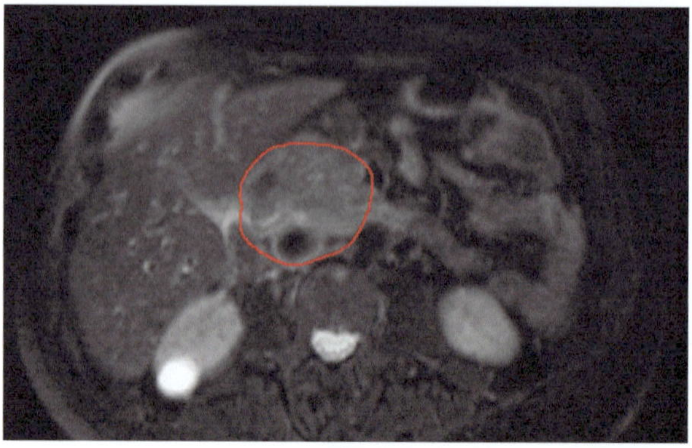

MRI Fusion with GTV contoured in red.

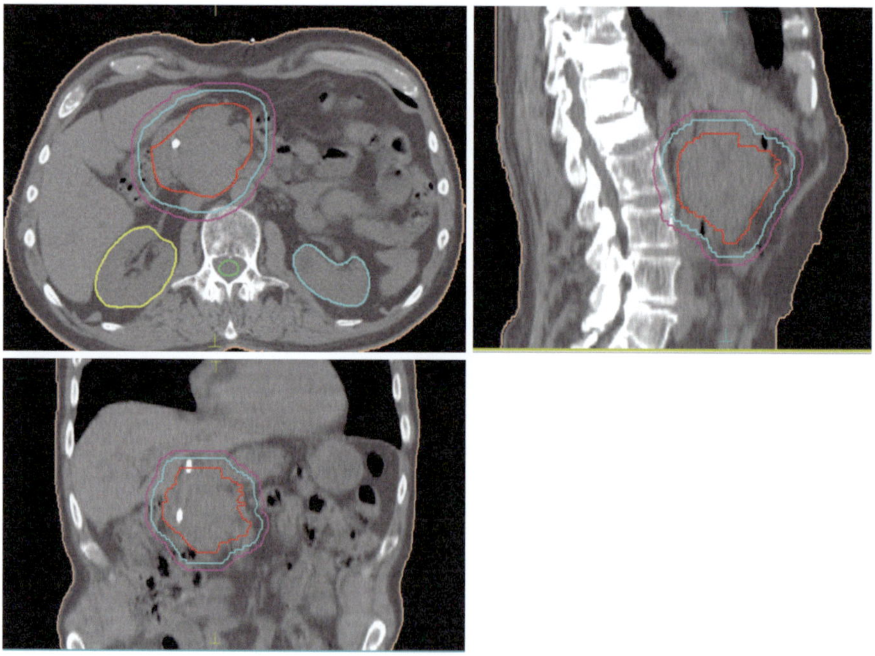

GTV (red) expanded by 1 cm to CTV (blue). CTV sculpted off bone which is seen nicely on the sagittal image. PTV (purple) has 0.5 cm margin on CTV.

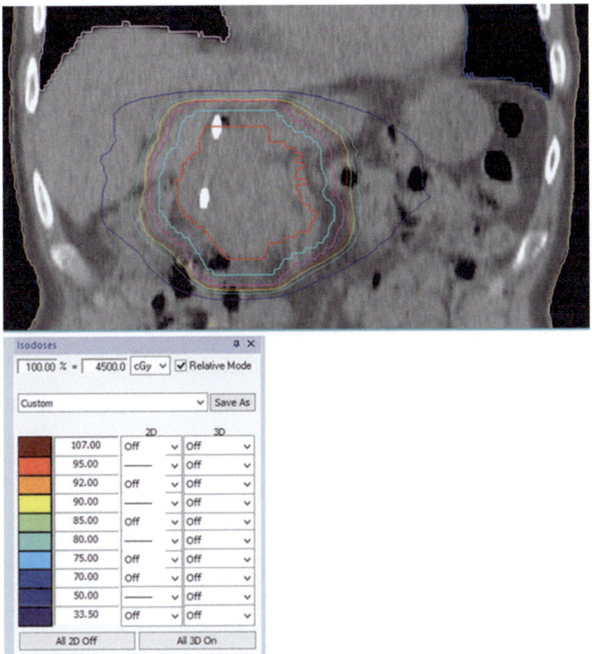

Isodose distribution.

Case 5: MM of Vertebral Body

A 51-year-old man presented with back pain. MRI of spine showed T8 compression fracture with bony retropulsion and moderate cord compression. The workup confirmed a diagnosis of MM. Planed for 2000 cGy in 10 fractions using 3D conformal technique with 15MV photons.

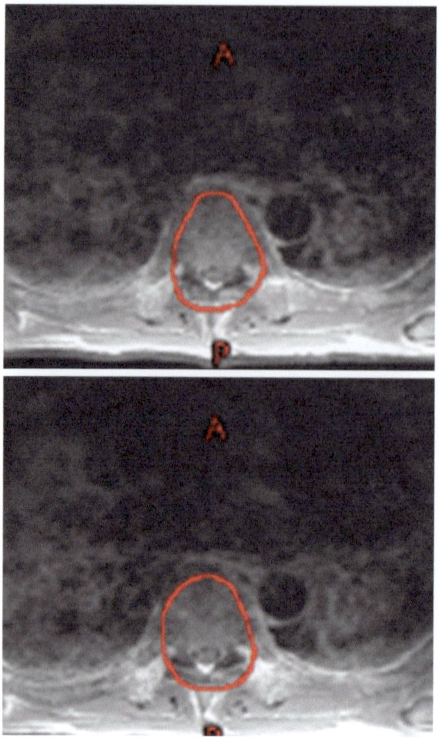

CTV contoured in red on fused MRI.

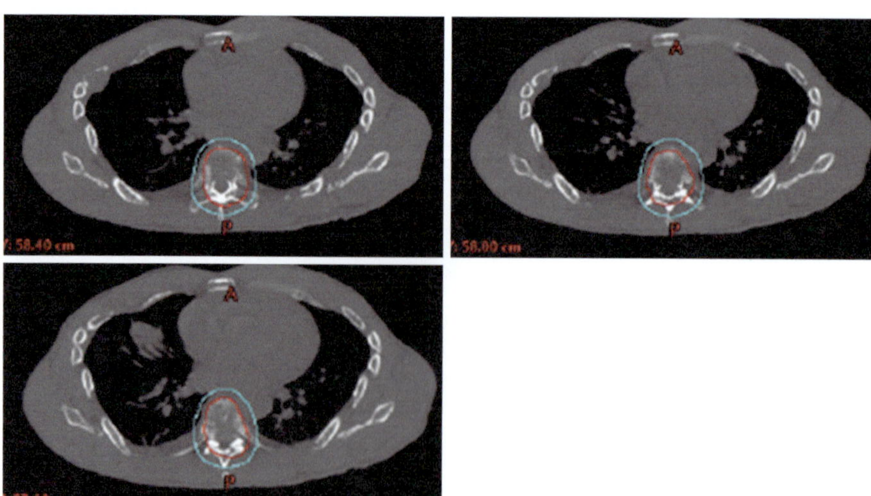

CTV (red) with 1 cm expansion to PTV (blue).

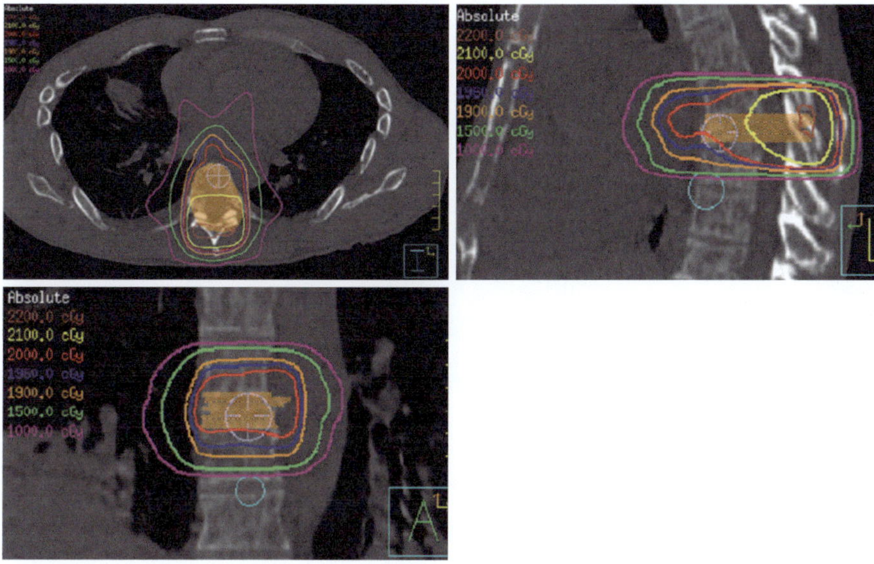

Isodose distribution. Note that for palliative treatment for MM, only the vertebral body in question needs to be treated—there is no need to treat one vertebral body above and below.

Case 6: MM of Skull

A 45-year-old female with history of MM s/p autologous stem cell transplant who had enlarging masses on the forehead and posterior skull. Biopsy revealed plasma cells. Imaging showed a destructive subgaleal mass with extension into the frontal sinus without intracranial extension. Plan to treat definitively with 2400 cGy in 12 fractions using IMRT with 6MV photons.

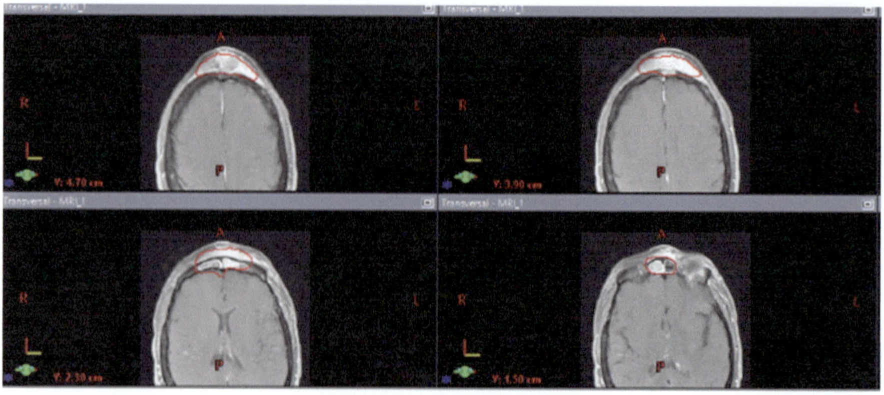

GTV contoured in red on MRI fusion.

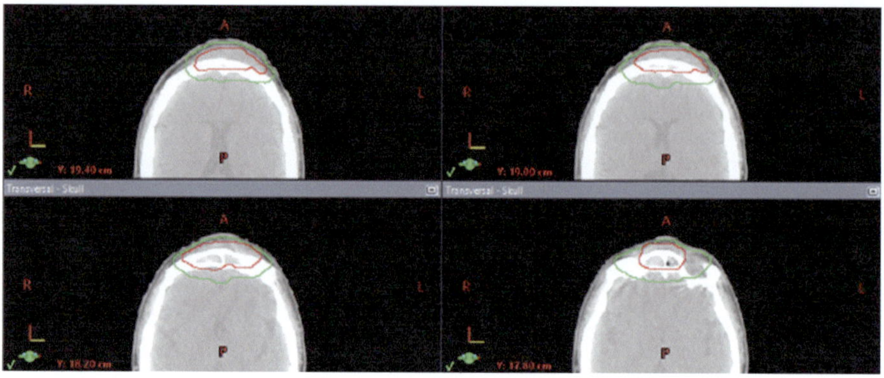

GTV (red) to PTV (green) expansion of 1 cm accounting for CTV expansion of 0.7 cm and an additional 0.3 cm CTV to PTV expansion.

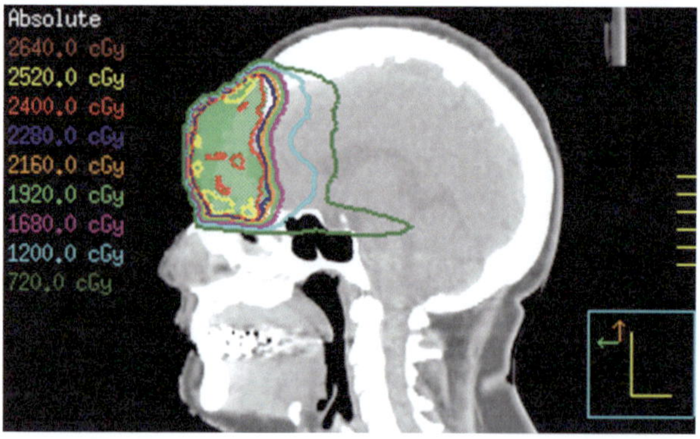

Isodose distribution (patient had second site on scalp also seen here).

References

1. Halperin EC. Perez & Brady's principles and practice of radiation oncology. 7th ed. Philadelphia, PA: Wolters Kluwer; 2019.
2. The Surveillance, Epidemiology, and End Results (SEER) program of the National Cancer Institute. Cancer stat facts: myeloma. 2020. https://seer.cancer.gov/statfacts/html/mulmy.html. Accessed 21 May 2020.
3. Society AC. Key statistics about multiple myeloma. Published 2020. https://www.cancer.org/cancer/multiple-myeloma/about/key-statistics.html. Accessed 19 May 2020.
4. Kyle RA, Therneau TM, Rajkumar SV, et al. A long-term study of prognosis in monoclonal gammopathy of undetermined significance. N Engl J Med. 2002;346(8):564–9.
5. Landgren O, Kyle RA, Pfeiffer RM, et al. Monoclonal gammopathy of undetermined significance (MGUS) consistently precedes multiple myeloma: a prospective study. Blood. 2009;113(22):5412–7.
6. Weiss BM, Abadie J, Verma P, Howard RS, Kuehl WM. A monoclonal gammopathy precedes multiple myeloma in most patients. Blood. 2009;113(22):5418–22.
7. Ozsahin M, Tsang RW, Poortmans P, et al. Outcomes and patterns of failure in solitary plasmacytoma: a multicenter Rare Cancer Network study of 258 patients. Int J Radiat Oncol Biol Phys. 2006;64(1):210–7.
8. Knowling MA, Harwood AR, Bergsagel DE. Comparison of extramedullary plasmacytomas with solitary and multiple plasma cell tumors of bone. J Clin Oncol. 1983;1(4):255–62.
9. Tsang RW, Campbell BA, Goda JS, et al. Radiation therapy for solitary plasmacytoma and multiple myeloma: guidelines from the International Lymphoma Radiation Oncology Group. Int J Radiat Oncol Biol Phys. 2018;101(4):794–808.
10. Schirrmeister H, Buck AK, Bergmann L, Reske SN, Bommer M. Positron emission tomography (PET) for staging of solitary plasmacytoma. Cancer Biother Radiopharm. 2003;18(5):841–5.
11. Martin MA, Howley PM, Byrne JC, Garon CF. Characterization of supercoiled oligomeric SV40 DNA molecules in productively infected cells. Virology. 1976;71(1):28–40.
12. Dimopoulos M, Kyle R, Fermand JP, et al. Consensus recommendations for standard investigative workup: report of the International Myeloma Workshop Consensus Panel 3. Blood. 2011;117(18):4701–5.
13. Dimopoulos MA, Hillengass J, Usmani S, et al. Role of magnetic resonance imaging in the management of patients with multiple myeloma: a consensus statement. J Clin Oncol. 2015;33(6):657–64.
14. Cavo M, Terpos E, Nanni C, et al. Role of 18F-FDG PET/CT in the diagnosis and management of multiple myeloma and other plasma cell disorders: a consensus statement by the International Myeloma Working Group. Lancet Oncol. 2017;18(4):e206–17.
15. Catell D, Kogen Z, Donahue B, Steinfeld A. Multiple myeloma of an extremity: must the entire bone be treated? Int J Radiat Oncol Biol Phys. 1998;40(1):117–9.
16. Townsend PW, Smalley SR, Cozad SC, Rosenthal HG, Hassanein RE. Role of postoperative radiation therapy after stabilization of fractures caused by metastatic disease. Int J Radiat Oncol Biol Phys. 1995;31(1):43–9.
17. Townsend PW, Rosenthal HG, Smalley SR, Cozad SC, Hassanein RE. Impact of postoperative radiation therapy and other perioperative factors on outcome after orthopedic stabilization of impending or pathologic fractures due to metastatic disease. J Clin Oncol. 1994;12(11):2345–50.
18. Elhammali A, Milgrom SA, Amini B, et al. Postoperative radiotherapy for multiple myeloma of long bones: should the entire rod be treated? Clin Lymphoma Myeloma Leuk. 2019;19(8):e465–9.
19. Mendel E, Bourekas E, Gerszten P, Golan JD. Percutaneous techniques in the treatment of spine tumors: what are the diagnostic and therapeutic indications and outcomes? Spine (Phila Pa 1976). 2009;34(22 Suppl):S93–100.

20. Kyriakou C, Molloy S, Vrionis F, et al. The role of cement augmentation with percutaneous vertebroplasty and balloon kyphoplasty for the treatment of vertebral compression fractures in multiple myeloma: a consensus statement from the International Myeloma Working Group (IMWG). Blood Cancer J. 2019;9(3):27.
21. Lutz S, Balboni T, Jones J, et al. Palliative radiation therapy for bone metastases: update of an ASTRO evidence-based guideline. Pract Radiat Oncol. 2017;7(1):4–12.
22. Wolanczyk MJ, Fakhrian K, Adamietz IA. Radiotherapy, bisphosphonates and surgical stabilization of complete or impending pathologic fractures in patients with metastatic bone disease. J Cancer. 2016;7(1):121–4.
23. Mendenhall CM, Thar TL, Million RR. Solitary plasmacytoma of bone and soft tissue. Int J Radiat Oncol Biol Phys. 1980;6(11):1497–501.
24. Liebross RH, Ha CS, Cox JD, Weber D, Delasalle K, Alexanian R. Solitary bone plasmacytoma: outcome and prognostic factors following radiotherapy. Int J Radiat Oncol Biol Phys. 1998;41(5):1063–7.
25. Mayr NA, Wen BC, Hussey DH, et al. The role of radiation therapy in the treatment of solitary plasmacytomas. Radiother Oncol. 1990;17(4):293–303.
26. Tsang RW, Gospodarowicz MK, Pintilie M, et al. Solitary plasmacytoma treated with radiotherapy: impact of tumor size on outcome. Int J Radiat Oncol Biol Phys. 2001;50(1):113–20.
27. Mignot F, et al. Solitary plasmacytoma treated by lenalidomide-dexamethasone in combination with radiation therapy: clinical outcomes. Int J Radiat Oncol Biol Phys. 2020;106(3):589–96. https://doi.org/10.1016/j.ijrobp.2019.10.043. Epub 2019 Nov 7.Int J Radiat Oncol Biol Phys. 2020. PMID: 31707123.
28. Rades D, Hoskin PJ, Stalpers LJ, et al. Short-course radiotherapy is not optimal for spinal cord compression due to myeloma. Int J Radiat Oncol Biol Phys. 2006;64(5):1452–7.
29. Rudzianskiene M, Inciura A, Gerbutavicius R, et al. Single vs. multiple fraction regimens for palliative radiotherapy treatment of multiple myeloma: a prospective randomised study. Strahlenther Onkol. 2017;193(9):742–9.

Further Reading

Rajkumar SV, Dimopoulos MA, Palumbo A, et al. International Myeloma Working Group updated criteria for the diagnosis of multiple myeloma. Lancet Oncol. 2014;15:e538–48.

Terpos E, Morgan G, Dimopoulos MA, et al. International Myeloma Working Group recommendations for the treatment of multiple myeloma-related bone disease. J Clin Oncol. 2013;31:2347–57.

Tsang RW, Campbell BA, Goda JS, Kelsey CR, Kirova YM, Parikh RR, Ng AK, Ricardi U, Suh CO, Mauch PM, Specht L, Yahalom J. Radiation therapy for solitary plasmacytoma and multiple myeloma: guidelines from the International Lymphoma Radiation Oncology Group. Int J Radiat Oncol Biol Phys. 2018;101(4):794–808. PMID: 29976492.

Primary Central Nervous System Lymphoma

13

Dodul Mondal and Rahul R. Parikh

Contents

Part 1: Background and Epidemiology

- Lymphomas involving the central nervous system (CNS) may be primary CNS lymphoma (PCNSL) that is restricted to the CNS, or secondary CNS lymphoma that disseminates from a systemic site. This chapter focuses on PCNSL.
- PCNSL can involve the brain, eyes, spinal cord, and leptomeninges.
- PCNSL is a rare aggressive variant of non-Hodgkin Lymphoma (NHL) that represents approximately 4% of all intracranial neoplasms in immunocompetent

D. Mondal
Department of Oncology/Radiation Oncology, Max Institute of Cancer Care, Max Super Speciality Hospital, New Delhi, India

R. R. Parikh (✉)
Department of Radiation Oncology, Rutgers Cancer Institute of New Jersey, New Brunswick, NJ, USA
e-mail: parikhrr@cinj.rutgers.edu

C. Pinnix et al. (eds.), *Target Volume Delineation in Hematologic Malignancies*, Practical Guides in Radiation Oncology,
https://doi.org/10.1007/978-3-031-67722-9_13

patients. However, in recent years, a rising incidence has been recognized, particularly in people over 60 years of age. Approximately 1500 new cases are diagnosed annually in the USA [1].

- Immunodeficiency is a risk factor for PCNSL, which can be seen in patients who are on long-term immunosuppressive therapy or have human immunodeficiency virus/acquired immunodeficiency syndrome (HIV/AIDS).
- Immunocompetent people are typically affected during the sixth or seventh decade of life, whereas immunocompromised people may be affected at younger ages.
- More than 90% of PCNSL cases are intermediate- to high-grade diffuse large B-cell lymphoma (DLBCL) [2]. Most are non-germinal center subtype and have activating mutations of MYD88 and CD79B that lead to BTK-mediated NFkB pathway activation [3]. Common antigenic markers include pan B-cell markers (CD19, CD20, CD22, CD79a), MUM1, BCL2, and BCL6. Rarer histologies include low-grade B-cell, Burkitt, or T-cell lymphomas.
- Presenting symptoms of PCNSL may include:
  - Cognitive impairment.
  - Personality and behavior change.
  - Headache.
  - Nausea.
  - Focal neurological symptoms.
  - Visual changes, including blurred vision and/or floaters with ocular involvement.
  - Seizures.
- Ocular involvement is common in PCNSL; however, isolated ocular lymphoma without brain involvement is rare and known as primary intraocular, or vitreoretinal, lymphoma. Orbital, or ocular adnexal, lymphoma is a different entity that is typically an indolent NHL and may involve the conjunctiva, lacrimal gland, or soft tissues of the orbit without intraocular involvement.

Part 2: Management and Treatment of PCNSL

- Staging, work-up, and response assessment [4]:
  - Baseline workup should include:

    Clinical assessments:
    - Physical examination with attention to lymphatic regions, including Waldeyer's ring.
    - Performance status and age (have prognostic implications).
    - Neurological examination.
    - Testicular examination in males.
    - Cognitive function with mini-mental status examination or formal neuro-psychological testing.

    Corticosteroid use should be recorded, if applicable. When possible, corticosteroids should be avoided until the diagnosis has been established.

Laboratory tests:

- Serum LDH.
- Hepatic and renal function.
- HIV serology.

Disease extent evaluation: An evaluation for systemic disease is necessary. It is also critical to establish the extent of CNS disease (focal, diffuse cranial, craniospinal), which can impact the radiation treatment plan significantly.

- MRI of the brain and whole spine. Brain imaging should include a gadolinium-enhanced MRI scan. Involvement of the spinal cord is sufficiently rare that a gadolinium-enhanced spine MRI is necessary only in the presence of spinal symptoms.
- Contrast-enhanced CT may be performed if MRI is contraindicated or not feasible.
- Cerebrospinal fluid (CSF) cytology and total protein levels should be obtained unless a lumbar puncture is contraindicated. Other CSF studies that may be useful include cell count, β2 microglobulin, immunoglobulin H gene rearrangement, and flow cytometry.
- Ophthalmologic examination, including dilated fundus examination, to assess for vitreous, retinal, or optic nerve involvement.
- Whole body 18F-FDG PET-CT scan to assess for systemic disease (contrast-enhanced CT scan of the neck, chest, abdomen, pelvis is an acceptable alternative).
- Consider bone marrow biopsy with aspirate.
- Consider testicular ultrasound.

Testicular evaluation with an examination +/− ultrasound is vital, because primary testicular lymphoma has a predilection for metastasis to the CNS.

– International Workshop recommendations for response assessment are summarized in Table 13.1 [4].

- There are two prognostic models in PCNSL. Of note, survival outcomes have improved since these models were established. The first one was proposed by researchers at Memorial Sloan Kettering Cancer Center (MSKCC) and the second by the International Extranodal Lymphoma Study Group (IELSG) [4, 5].
  – MSKCC prognostic model [4]: Incorporates age and Karnofsky performance status (KPS), and divides patients into three prognostic classes as shown in Table 13.2.
  – IELSG prognostic model [5]: incorporates age, Eastern Cooperative Oncology Group (ECOG) performance score, tumor involvement of deep brain structures, LDH serum level, and CSF protein concentration, and divides patients into three groups based on a prognostic score as shown in Table 13.3.

- **Overview of standard treatment:**

Table 13.1 Response criteria in PCNSL (Modified from International PCNSL Lymphoma Collaborative Group)

Response type	Findings on contrast-enhanced brain MRI	Steroid use	Ophthalmic evaluation	CSF results
CR	No enhancing lesion	None	Normal finding	Negative cytology
CRu	No enhancing lesion	Any	Normal finding	Negative cytology
	Minor changes noted	Any	Minor changes on RPE	Negative cytology
PR	50% reduction in enhancing component	Not relevant	Minor changes/normal	Negative cytology
	No enhancing lesion	Not relevant	Reduction in vitreous cells or retinal infiltrate	Persistent or suspicious cytology
PD	25% or more increase in size of enhancing tumor	Not relevant	Recurrent or new ocular disease	Recurrent or positive cytology
	New site of disease	–		

CR complete response; CRu unconfirmed complete response; RPE retinal pigment epithelium; PR partial response; PD progressive disease

Table 13.2 MSKCC prognostic classes and survival in PCNSL

Prognostic class	Age	KPS	Median survival (years)
Class 1	<50 years	–	8.5
Class 2	≥50 years	KPS >70	3.2
Class 3	≥50 years	KPS <70	1

Table 13.3 IELSG prognostic score and survival

Prognostic score	2-year survival rate (%)
0–1	80
2–3	48
4–5	15

- The optimal treatment strategy in PCNSL includes high-dose methotrexate (HD-MTX). Other systemic agents with CNS activity are also used to treat PCNSL, such as rituximab, procarbazine, vincristine, cytarabine, thiotepa, carmustine, temozolomide, etoposide, and ifosfamide.
- The role of surgery is limited to biopsy to establish the diagnosis and shunt placement if needed to relieve elevated intracranial pressure. The risk of diffuse, deep brain infiltration is very high, even in radiographically localized disease; thus, there is no convincing evidence to support surgical resection in PCNSL.
- The role of radiation therapy has evolved over the years. Historically, whole brain radiotherapy (WBRT) was associated with favorable response rates, but poor long-term disease control. Furthermore, when radiation was used as the only modality, a high dose was necessary so there was a risk of significant neurocognitive impairment, particularly in elderly patients. Over the years, the use of radiation therapy in PCNSL has evolved. Currently, reduced-dose WBRT is used in combination with MTX-based chemotherapy.

- Recently, high-dose chemotherapy with autologous stem cell transplant (HDC-ASCT) has been investigated as an alternative consolidation strategy that may allow omission of WBRT in patients who are sufficiently fit to receive this intensive systemic therapy.

Pre-radiotherapy Imaging and Evaluation

- Any investigations and imaging studies that showed evidence of PCNSL at initial diagnosis should be repeated before radiation to assess disease response to chemotherapy and to establish a new, pre-radiation baseline.

Principles of Management

- **Upfront treatment of newly diagnosed PCNSL**: Initial treatment is systemic therapy based on a HD-MTX backbone due to its ability to penetrate the blood–brain barrier. Upfront chemotherapy is followed by consolidation in patients who have achieved a disease response. The modalities that are used for consolidation include radiation therapy and HDC-ASCT.
  - Induction therapy: HD-MTX is an effective chemotherapeutic agent for PCNSL and is used with variable doses (3–8 g/m^2).

    When used alone, HD-MTX has been associated with a complete response (CR) rate of 52%, median progression-free survival (PFS) of 12.8 months, and median overall survival (OS) of 55 months [6].

    HD-MTX has been used in combination with other agents, such as rituximab, procarbazine, vincristine, cytarabine, thiotepa, carmustine, temozolomide, etoposide, and ifosfamide, with select results described below.

    - On RTOG 9310, 102 patients were treated with 5 cycles of combination chemotherapy administered at 2 weekly intervals consisting of methotrexate 2.5 g/m^2, vincristine 1.4 mg/m^2 (maximum 2.8 mg/m^2), and procarbazine 100 mg/m^2/day (D1–D7) in cycles 1, 3, and 5. Intravenous methotrexate was followed in the next week by administration of 12 mg of methotrexate via an Ommaya reservoir. Chemotherapy was followed by consolidation with WBRT. Initially, all patients received WBRT with a dose of 45 Gy in 25 fractions. Patients with ocular involvement also received radiation to the eyes with 36 Gy in 20 fractions. Subsequently, the radiation dose was modified in patients who achieved a CR to chemotherapy, to reduce the risk of CNS toxicity; these patients were treated with a hyperfractionated regimen using 36 Gy in 30 fractions, 1.2 Gy per fraction, with 2 fractions daily at 6-h intervals. Patients with less than a CR to initial chemotherapy were treated with the original dose and fractionation scheme of 45 Gy in 25 fractions administered daily. WBRT was followed by two additional cycles of high-dose cytarabine. The median survival of all patients was 36.9 months. The median

OS in the conventional and hyperfractionated WBRT arms were 37 months and 47.9 months, respectively. Almost 10% of patients had grade 5 neurotoxicity [7].

- On IELSG32, thiotepa and rituximab were added to HD-MTX and cytarabine (MATRix). In this phase II study, 219 patients received induction chemotherapy with either HD-MTX and Cytarabine, or HD-MTX, Cytarabine, and Rituximab, or HD-MTX, Cytarabine, rituximab, and thiotepa. Patients with responsive or stable disease were further randomized to receive either WBRT (36 Gy +/− 9 Gy tumor boost) or HDC-ASCT. In this study, the addition of rituximab and thiotepa improved complete response rates (49% vs. 23%), 2-year PFS (61% vs. 36%), and 2-year OS (69% vs. 42%) [8]. At a median follow-up of 88 months, patients treated with MATRix and either consolidation strategy had a 7-year overall survival rate of 70%, with comparable efficacy of WBRT and ASCT but greater neurocognitive impairment associated with WBRT [9].

To reduce the risk of neurotoxicity, studies have explored lowering the dose of WBRT after a complete response to induction chemotherapy. In a multicenter phase II trial, 52 patients with PCNSL were treated with 5–7 cycles of induction rituximab, HD-MTX, procarbazine, and vincristine (R-MPV). Patients with CSF-positivity also received inter-cycle 12 mg MTX via an Ommaya reservoir. Patients with a CR were treated with reduced-dose consolidation WBRT (23.4 Gy at 1.8 Gy per fraction). Patients with residual disease received the historical standard WBRT dose of 45 Gy in 25 fractions. All patients received consolidation high-dose cytarabine after radiation. The median PFS was 7.7 years and median OS was not reached (3-year OS was 87%). Neurotoxicity after reduced-dose WBRT was minimal [10].

Studies have also explored lower dose WBRT with a boost to persistent sites of disease after an incomplete response to MTX-based induction chemotherapy. For example, in the prospective IELSG32 study, patients with a partial response received 36 Gy WBRT with an additional 9 Gy focal tumor-directed boost [8]. On the HOVON 105/ALLG NHL 24 study, patients with a partial response to induction chemotherapy were treated with a simultaneous integrated boost technique; the whole brain received 30 Gy (1.5 Gy/fraction) and the residual disease received 40 Gy (2.0 Gy/fraction) delivered in 20 fractions [11]. Additionally, retrospective data support the use of 23.4–36 Gy WBRT with a tumor-directed boost to persistent sites of disease [12].

Studies have explored omitting WBRT from upfront therapy and reserving it for salvage if needed. In a multicenter randomized phase 3 study (G-PCNSL-SG-1), patients received 6 cycles of induction chemotherapy with HD-MTX and ifosfamide and were randomized to subsequently receive immediate WBRT versus deferred WBRT at the time of relapse. The WBRT dose was 45 Gy delivered in 30 fractions. In the chemotherapy alone arm, patients were treated with additional high-dose cytarabine if they did not achieve a complete response. There was no statistically significant difference in OS or PFS (although median PFS was 18.3 months in the WBRT arm vs. 11.9 months in the chemotherapy alone arm, $p = 0.14$). There was an increased risk of neurotoxicity in the WBRT arm [13]. That said, there were multiple limitations to this study [14]. Furthermore, preliminary results from the randomized study RTOG1114 demonstrate that the addition of reduced-dose WBRT to MTX-based chemotherapy is associated with superior PFS in newly diagnosed PCNSL [15].

Other studies have explored replacing WBRT with HDC-ASCT. With this approach, initial induction chemotherapy is followed by CNS-active HDC, followed by ASCT. Initial results are encouraging, with high response rates and limited neurotoxicity [16].

Other studies have explored the use of partial brain RT, instead of WBRT. In a retrospective analysis, patterns of failure were assessed in 38 patients who were treated with partial brain RT. The out-of-field recurrence rate was 49% at 5 years (45% in patients with unifocal disease and 67% in patients with multifocal disease). In-field recurrence was high (83%) when a margin of less than 4 cm around the tumor was used, but lower (22%) when a margin of more than 4 cm was used [17]. The high rates of relapse after focal RT suggested that WBRT should be used. Of note, however, only a small minority of patients in this study received HD-MTX. Future study may better elucidate the role of partial brain RT after treatment with HD-MTX in PCNSL. In the meantime, partial brain RT may be considered in patients at high risk of toxicity from WBRT.

CSI is not routinely used in PCNSL. In a historical Japanese series, a small percentage of patients with meningeal deposits were treated with CSI without significant benefit [18].

- **Treatment of Recurrence/Relapse:** For recurrent PCNSL, HD-MTX-based chemotherapy or other CNS-active systemic regimens, with or without HDC-ASCT, should be considered. WBRT should be considered in patients who did not receive it as a part of the initial treatment. Partial brain RT may be considered in patients at high risk of toxicity from WBRT.

General Considerations for Radiotherapy

- Radiation is usually given as consolidation after induction chemotherapy for PCNSL.
- Traditionally, opposed lateral beams with a "German Helmet" shape have been used to deliver WBRT. With this approach, equally weighted opposed lateral beams are used to treat the whole brain and posterior orbits. Ideally, CT-based planning should be used to ensure adequate coverage of the frontal lobes and cribriform plate. The inferior border can be placed at the bottom of C1 or C2. In patients who do not have upfront ocular involvement, the posterior aspect of the

globes should be included (Fig. 13.1f). In patients with ocular involvement at diagnosis, the entire globes should be included in the treatment field without lens sparing (Fig. 13.2e). Field-in-field techniques may be used to improve dose uniformity (Fig. 13.1g).

- Conformal radiation techniques, such as intensity modulated or volumetric arc therapy, are an alternative that may improve OAR sparing. For radiation that is delivered using advanced techniques, the target volumes are described in Table 13.4 and shown in Figs. 13.1 and 13.2. The target is the whole brain and

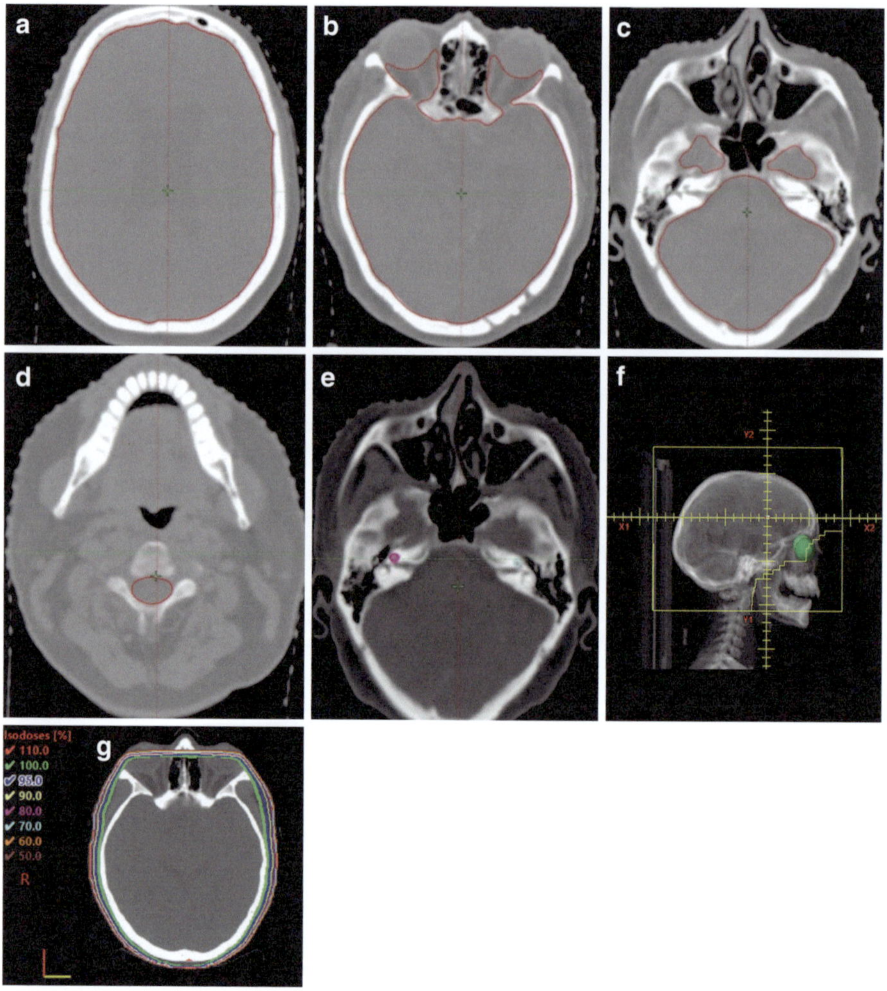

Fig. 13.1 (**a–e**) shows axial images of contouring for IMRT planning. Contouring is performed using bone windows to optimize visualization of the inner table of the skull. In (**a–d**), the CTV is shown in red. (**e**) Shows the contours for the cochleae. (**f**) Shows the beam's eye view for treatment using 3D-CRT with opposed lateral beams. (**g**) Shows that hot spots were minimized in the 3D-CRT parallel opposed WBRT plan using a field-in-field approaches

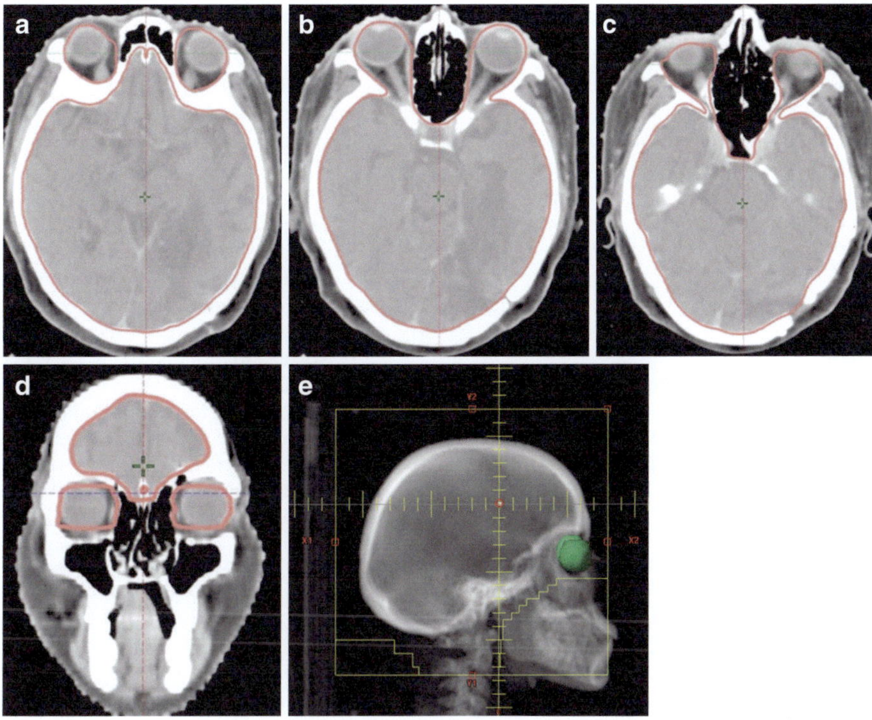

Fig. 13.2 (**a–d**) shows axial images of contouring for IMRT planning. The CTV is shown in pink. (**e**) Shows the beam's eye view for treatment with 3D-CRT using opposed lateral beams

posterior orbits in the absence of upfront ocular involvement. The target is the whole brain and bilateral globes in the presence of upfront ocular involvement.

- If persistent disease is present at the time of radiation therapy, it may be treated with a focal, tumor-directed boost. This boost may be given simultaneously or sequentially. It is typically delivered using conformal radiation techniques, such as intensity modulated or volumetric arc therapy.
- Hippocampal avoidance is not recommended with WBRT in PCNSL, unlike in metastatic disease of brain, because it may result in inadequate treatment of areas involved by PCNSL and thus may compromise disease control. It must be demonstrated that PFS is non-inferior using hippocampal avoidance-WBRT compared to standard WBRT, before this approach is recommended.
- Patients should be simulated supine with their arms by their sides. A headrest and thermoplastic mask should be used for immobilization.
- If focal RT is planned (i.e. a boost or partial brain irradiation), fusing the simulation CT with a contrast-enhanced MRI scan is recommended to improve delineation of the enhancing tumor. Although deformable registration software is available, rigid registration is adequate for brain radiation planning (Table 13.5).

Table 13.4 Recommended target volume definition in PCNSL [19]

Volume	Description	
Gross tumor volume (GTV)	The GTV should be contoured on a fused image set with a contrast-enhanced MRI. $\text{GTV}_{\text{pre-chemotherapy}}$ represents all disease that was present at diagnosis. $\text{GTV}_{\text{post-chemotherapy}}$ represents any persistent disease at the time of radiation, if applicable	
Whole brain clinical target volume (CTV_{WBRT})	Without ocular involvement	• Entire brain parenchyma with meningeal coverings • Care should be exercised to include the meningeal reflection near the cribriform plate • Inferiorly, the CTV should extend to lower border of the C1 or C2 vertebra • The posterior orbit including the optic nerves should be included, extending to the posterior globe • All sites of intracranial CSF flow should be included. Fusion with a T2 or FIESTA sequence MRI, which clearly demonstrates CSF extension is ideally recommended
	With ocular involvement	• As above, but the bilateral globes should be included in the CTV
Boost clinical target volume ($\text{CTV}_{\text{boost}}$)	Consider adding a 5–10 mm margin to the $\text{GTV}_{\text{pre-chemotherapy}}$ or $\text{GTV}_{\text{post-chemotherapy}}$. The $\text{GTV}_{\text{pre-chemotherapy}}$ should be expanded if it is small enough that it can be boosted without excess toxicity risk. If the $\text{GTV}_{\text{pre-chemotherapy}}$ is too extensive to boost, then the $\text{GTV}_{\text{post-chemotherapy}}$ should be expanded	
Planning target volume (PTV)	Depending on institutional protocol, a 3–5 mm PTV margin can be added to the CTV_{WBRT} and $\text{CTV}_{\text{boost}}$ to create a PTV_{WBRT} and $\text{PTV}_{\text{boost}}$, respectively	
Organs at risk (OAR)	Cochleae, lenses, spinal cord, oropharyngeal and nasopharyngeal mucosa, pinnae, parotid glands, lacrimal glands	

Table 13.5 Radiation dose and fractionations [19]

Situation	Recommended dose
Radiation alone (in patients not fit for chemotherapy)	• WBRT 24–36 Gy with a boost to gross disease for a total dose of 45 Gy
Palliative	• 25–36 Gy to the whole brain. 1.8–2.5 Gy/fraction is recommended. 3 Gy/fraction may be considered depending on the clinical scenario, but larger dose per fraction is associated with a higher risk of neurotoxicity that may be observed soon after RT. Partial brain RT may be considered depending on the clinical scenario
Radiation as consolidation	• 23.4 Gy in 13 fractions if in CR after R-MPV chemotherapy • 23.4–36 Gy in 13–20 fractions to the whole brain and a focal boost to a total of 40–45 Gy to persistent disease at the time of radiation, if not in CR after MTX-based chemotherapy

Part 3: Cases

Case 1

A 55-year-old immunocompetent female with recent onset forgetfulness was diagnosed with PCNSL, DLBCL-type, CD20-positive. She did not have ocular involvement at initial diagnosis. She underwent induction with R-MVP chemotherapy and achieved a CR. She presents for consolidation radiation.

The recommendation was for reduced-dose WBRT to a dose of 23.4 Gy in 13 fractions. The CTV included the entire brain and posterior orbits, extending inferiorly to the lower border of C2, as in Fig. 13.1.

Case 2

A 52-year-old immunocompetent gentleman with a history of headaches and occasional floaters in both eyes was diagnosed with primary CNS lymphoma, DLBCL-type, CD20-positive. His initial evaluation did not include an ophthalmic examination. He underwent induction chemotherapy with R-MVP. After completion of chemotherapy, there was no evidence of disease in the brain by MRI or the eyes by ophthalmological examination. He presents for consolidation radiation.

For PCNSL with bilateral ocular involvement suggestive from clinical history, the recommendation was for reduced-dose WBRT including the eyes. The CTV included the brain and the bilateral globes, extending to the lower border of C2, as in Fig. 13.2.

References

1. Grommes C, DeAngelis LM. Primary CNS lymphoma. J Clin Oncol. 2017;35(21):2410–8.
2. Camilleri-Broet S, Martin A, Moreau A, Angonin R, Henin D, Gontier MF, et al. Primary central nervous system lymphomas in 72 immunocompetent patients: pathologic findings and clinical correlations. Groupe Ouest Est d'etude des Leucenies et Autres Maladies du Sang (GOELAMS). Am J Clin Pathol. 1998;110(5):607–12.
3. Nakamura T, Tateishi K, Niwa T, Matsushita Y, Tamura K, Kinoshita M, et al. Recurrent mutations of CD79B and MYD88 are the hallmark of primary central nervous system lymphomas. Neuropathol Appl Neurobiol. 2016;42(3):279–90.
4. Abrey LE, Batchelor TT, Ferreri AJ, Gospodarowicz M, Pulczynski EJ, Zucca E, et al. Report of an international workshop to standardize baseline evaluation and response criteria for primary CNS lymphoma. J Clin Oncol. 2005;23(22):5034–43.
5. Ferreri AJ, Blay JY, Reni M, Pasini F, Spina M, Ambrosetti A, et al. Prognostic scoring system for primary CNS lymphomas: The International Extranodal Lymphoma Study Group experience. J Clin Oncol. 2003;21(2):266–72.
6. Gerstner ER, Carson KA, Grossman SA, Batchelor TT. Long-term outcome in PCNSL patients treated with high-dose methotrexate and deferred radiation. Neurology. 2008;70(5):401–2.

7. Fisher B, Seiferheld W, Schultz C, DeAngelis L, Nelson D, Schold SC, et al. Secondary analysis of Radiation Therapy Oncology Group study (RTOG) 9310: an intergroup phase II combined modality treatment of primary central nervous system lymphoma. J Neuro-Oncol. 2005;74(2):201–5.
8. Ferreri AJ, Cwynarski K, Pulczynski E, Ponzoni M, Deckert M, Politi LS, et al. Chemoimmunotherapy with methotrexate, cytarabine, thiotepa, and rituximab (MATRix regimen) in patients with primary CNS lymphoma: results of the first randomisation of the International Extranodal Lymphoma Study Group-32 (IELSG32) phase 2 trial. Lancet Haematol. 2016;3(5):e217–27.
9. Ferreri AJM, Cwynarski K, Pulczynski E, Fox CP, Schorb E, Celico C, et al. Long-term efficacy, safety and neurotolerability of MATRix regimen followed by autologous transplant in primary CNS lymphoma: 7-year results of the IELSG32 randomized trial. Leukemia. 2022;36(7):1870–8.
10. Morris PG, Correa DD, Yahalom J, Raizer JJ, Schiff D, Grant B, et al. Rituximab, methotrexate, procarbazine, and vincristine followed by consolidation reduced-dose whole-brain radiotherapy and cytarabine in newly diagnosed primary CNS lymphoma: final results and long-term outcome. J Clin Oncol. 2013;31(31):3971–9.
11. Bromberg JEC, Issa S, Bakunina K, Minnema MC, Seute T, Durian M, et al. Rituximab in patients with primary CNS lymphoma (HOVON 105/ALLG NHL 24): a randomised, open-label, phase 3 intergroup study. Lancet Oncol. 2019;20(2):216–28.
12. Sheu T, Milgrom SA, Andraos TY, Gunther JR, Chi L, Nastoupil L, et al. Response-adapted radiation therapy for newly diagnosed primary diffuse large B-cell lymphoma of the CNS treated with methotrexate-based systemic therapy. Adv Radiat Oncol. 2018;3(4):639–46.
13. Thiel E, Korfel A, Martus P, Kanz L, Griesinger F, Rauch M, et al. High-dose methotrexate with or without whole brain radiotherapy for primary CNS lymphoma (G-PCNSL-SG-1): a phase 3, randomised, non-inferiority trial. Lancet Oncol. 2010;11(11):1036–47.
14. Milgrom SA, Yahalom J. The role of radiation therapy in the management of primary central nervous system lymphoma. Leuk Lymphoma. 2015;56(5):1197–204.
15. Omuro A. Randomized phase II study of rituximab, methotrexate (MTX), procarbazine, vincristine, and cytarabine (R-MPV-A) with and without low-dose whole-brain radiotherapy (LD-WBRT) for newly diagnosed primary CNS lymphoma (PCNSL). ASCO. 2020;38:2501.
16. Seidel S, Schlegel U. Have treatment protocols for primary CNS lymphoma advanced in the past 10 years. Expert Rev Anticancer Ther. 2019;19(10):909–15.
17. Shibamoto Y, Hayabuchi N, Hiratsuka J, Tokumaru S, Shirato H, Sougawa M, et al. Is whole-brain irradiation necessary for primary central nervous system lymphoma? Patterns of recurrence after partial-brain irradiation. Cancer. 2003;97(1):128–33.
18. Shibamoto Y. Radiation therapy for primary central nervous system lymphoma. Oncol Rev. 2013;7(1):e4.
19. Yahalom J, Illidge T, Specht L, Hoppe RT, Li YX, Tsang R, et al. Modern radiation therapy for extranodal lymphomas: field and dose guidelines from the International Lymphoma Radiation Oncology Group. Int J Radiat Oncol Biol Phys. 2015;92(1):11–31.

Target Volume Delineation for Extramedullary Leukemia

14

Richard Bakst

Contents

Introduction

Leukemias are liquid tumors of the hematopoietic and lymphoid tissues that are classified by the cell type (i.e. monocytes or lymphocytes) and maturation (i.e. acute or chronic). Extramedullary (EM) manifestations of leukemia are most commonly seen in acute leukemias and occur when tumor cells extravasate from the bone marrow or vasculature, resulting in seeding of tissues to form solid tumors. The two

R. Bakst (✉)
Department of Radiation Oncology, Icahn School of Medicine at Mount Sinai, New York, NY, USA
e-mail: Richard.Bakst@mountsinai.org

C. Pinnix et al. (eds.), *Target Volume Delineation in Hematologic Malignancies*, Practical Guides in Radiation Oncology,
https://doi.org/10.1007/978-3-031-67722-9_14

most common EM manifestations are myeloid sarcoma (MS) and leukemia cutis (LC). In this chapter, we provide an update on the radiation strategies to treat MS.

Myeloid Sarcoma (MS)

MS, also known as granulocytic sarcoma or chloroma due to its green color change in the presence of myeloperoxidase (MPO) [1], is a rare extramedullary tumor of immature myeloid cells. MS was first described in 1811 [2], and its relationship with acute leukemia was identified five decades later [3]. The term granulocytic sarcoma was introduced by Rappapport to describe tumors of granulocytic origin [4]; however, the term is currently applied to any tumor related to acute leukemia or myelodysplastic syndrome (MDS). MS is reported in up to 10% of patients with AML and can occur concomitantly, following, or rarely, antedating the onset of systemic bone marrow leukemia [5–7]. While MS most frequently develops in patients with AML, it has been associated with an accelerated phase of CML and MDS. Isolated MS, defined by the absence of a history of leukemia, MDS, or myeloproliferative neoplasm and a negative bone marrow biopsy, has been described in limited case reports [8]; however, it is worth noting that many of these patients are often misdiagnosed with lymphoma. MS can also develop at relapse following systemic treatment with or without bone marrow involvement. The incidence of patients developing MS after allogeneic hematopoietic cell transplantation (HCT) has been reported to be approximately 1% and is associated with poor overall survival [9, 10].

Clinical Presentation and Work-Up of MS

The clinical manifestations of MS are diverse, given the various sites of occurrence with signs and symptoms determined by its specific location and size. The most common locations include the soft tissue, bone, periosteum, and lymph nodes; however, several other sites have been described such as the orbit, central nervous system, gallbladder, and gonads [11, 12]. The diagnosis of MS in patients with a known leukemia diagnosis is relatively straightforward, and MS should always be included in the differential diagnosis of patients with AML who develop a soft tissue mass.

Radiographic Features

Given the wide variety of sites in which MS develops, proper imaging is critical for diagnosis. MS often appears as a soft-tissue mass and is best suited for computed tomography (CT) imaging [13]. The addition of 18FDG-PET to CT scan is a very effective screening modality to detect MS in patients presenting with bone-marrow AML. Based on 18FDG-PET imaging, Stolzel et al. demonstrated a 19% incidence of MS in a prospective study of 93 patients [14]. In terms of detection of MS, the use of 18FDG-PET resulted in sensitivity of 77% and specificity of 97%, indicating that a small percentage of EM disease sites will be PET-negative. Additionally, MRI with and without gadolinium contrast is routinely employed for MS involving brain, spine, and orbit to better define the impact of the tumor on these structures.

The diagnosis of MS is confirmed by tissue sampling, typically by fine needle aspirate, if the risks of biopsy are reasonable. The morphology of MS on hematoxylin-eosin can vary according to the degrees of myeloid differentiation. MS typically consists of a diffuse and infiltrative population of myeloblasts and granulocytic cell components (Fig. 14.1) with the malignant cells appearing large with abundant cytoplasm and large nuclei. In addition, immunohistochemistry (IHC) can be performed on tissue samples, and, when feasible, samples are sent for flow cytometry, fluorescence in situ hybridization, and molecular analysis. In the absence of a clinical history of leukemia, a histologic diagnosis of MS can be difficult. It is important to make every effort to obtain tissue for accurate diagnosis. MS can often be misdiagnosed, typically as non-Hodgkin lymphoma (NHL), in up to 46% of patients [11]. Misdiagnosis occurs most commonly with poorly differentiated MS, in which the morphology may resemble large-cell NHL when the cells are MPO-negative and weakly stained [15]. The differential diagnosis of MS includes other forms of NHL, lymphoblastic leukemia, melanoma, Ewing's sarcoma, blastic plasmacytoid dendritic cell neoplasm, and EM hematopoiesis [16].

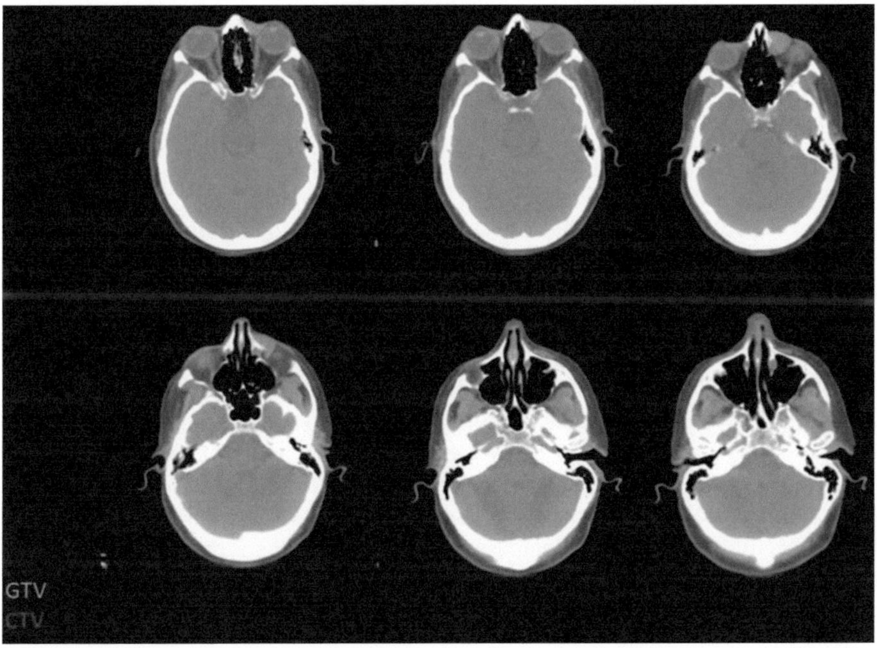

Fig. 14.1 Radiation target volumes to treat a myeloid sarcoma developing in the orbit of a 37-year-old female with AML undergoing induction chemotherapy. GTV is shown in blue; CTV is shown in red

Cytogenetic Abnormalities

A variety of chromosomal abnormalities have been reported in patients with AML with EM involvement. The t(8;21) is the most commonly reported cytogenetic abnormality associated with EM involvement [17, 18]. It occurs most often in childhood and has frequently been detected in orbital MS [19, 20]. The inv(16) is another cytogenetic abnormality with a high incidence of EM involvement, particularly in the CNS [21] and abdomen [22]. Increased risk in cases of t(8;21) and inv(16) may be related to the deregulation of transcription factors involved in cell recognition and adhesion. Specifically, inv(16) results in the CBFβ/MYH11 fusion gene [23] and carries a relatively favorable prognosis [24]. EM involvement in infants has been associated with 11q23 [25], which has a characteristic *MLL* rearrangement [26]. EM involvement has also been associated with t(9;11) [27], del(16q) [28], t(8;17) [29], t(8;16) [30, 31], and t(1;11) [32]. Recent systematic fluorescence in situ hybridization analysis on MS samples detected several chromosomal aberrations including monosomy 7, trisomy 4, trisomy 8, trisomy 11, del(5q), and del(20q), among others previously mentioned [33]. In this series, chromosomal aberrations were detected in over half of cases, suggesting an overall high prevalence. The genes or epigenetic changes impacted by these cytogenetic abnormalities that predispose patients to EM involvement are not all known at this time.

Prognostic Significance of EM Disease

Data on the prognostic significance of MS are limited. AML with both bone marrow involvement and MS is associated with a poor prognosis, resulting in 5-year survival rates between 20% and 30%. This survival rate is similar to that of AML without EM involvement [12, 34, 35]. The prognostic impact of cytogenetic alterations in the presence of EM disease has not been clearly delineated in the literature. Byrd et al. reported a series of 84 patients with AML that was associated with a t(8,21) translocation. In this series, patients harboring MS had a worse survival. This study was potentially biased due to a high percentage of MS patients having CNS disease. At present, EM disease is considered to be a poor prognostic indicator, but isolated MS may be favorable. A study by Tsimberidou et al. compared outcomes of 16 patients with isolated MS to a large cohort of AML patients who underwent standard treatment. Patients were matched for age and cytogenetics. The results showed improved event-free and overall survival in those harboring isolated MS when treated with anti-AML chemotherapy [36]. Moyassahghian et al. confirmed this finding in a SEER database review of 345 patients, demonstrating 3-year survival rates were 31.9% and 17.2% for isolated EM disease compared to bone-marrow AML, respectively ($p < 0.0001$) [37].

Systemic Treatment

MS that presents either concurrently with bone marrow involvement or in isolation always warrants systemic treatment directed at the underlying leukemia. Isolated MS with delayed or inadequate systemic treatment will almost always progress to AML [38], with a median time to development of AML ranging from 5 to 12 months [6, 35, 39]. Typically, MS is treated with remission-induction chemotherapy regimens similar to those used for AML [12, 35, 39–42]. The chemotherapy regimen choice and dosing follow standard age and cytogenetic-based risk profiling [43–45].

To date, the role of post-remission HCT remains unclear, as there have been no randomized trials addressing the optimal treatment for patients with EM involvement. Two retrospective studies have supported the use of allogeneic or autologous HCT [33, 46]. Chevallier et al. assessed the outcome of 51 patients with MS who underwent allogeneic HCT and demonstrated that 5-year overall survival was 47% [46]. Remission status at the time of HCT was an important prognostic consideration [46]. Kaur et al. reported a retrospective review of 23 patients with MS. Overall survival was significantly improved for patients who achieved a complete response to induction chemotherapy (25.7 vs. 0.8 months, $p < 0.001$). All patients who underwent allogeneic HCT achieved long-term remission at a median follow-up of 54 months [47]. Given these favorable results, treatment intensification with allogeneic HCT should be considered for patients with MS and concurrent marrow involvement, taking into consideration other patient-related factors.

Radiation Therapy

Radiation therapy (RT) can be used to treat MS and should be considered in selected cases. Current indications include isolated MS at presentation or at recurrence after HCT, residual disease after chemotherapy, or circumstances requiring symptomatic relief such as with orbital involvement (Fig. 14.1), head-and-neck involvement (Fig. 14.2), or compression of the spinal cord or other vital structures. RT can also be used for durable pain control, for example for symptomatic bony disease (Fig. 14.3). RT has been used as a consolidation treatment for isolated MS; however, there is no evidence that this combined approach is superior to aggressive chemotherapy alone [48]. RT may be used to treat MS following an incomplete response to chemotherapy in an attempt to reduce the significant risk of early bone marrow relapse due to re-seeding.

Low-dose radiation (20–24 Gy in 2 Gy/fraction) is very effective in achieving durable local tumor control, with response rates up to 97% [48]. Even lower doses such as 12 Gy in 3 fractions can be considered in a palliative setting when life expectancy is particularly poor. Low-dose radiation is well tolerated, and it does not preclude total body irradiation in preparation for HCT if it is indicated later during the treatment course. For treatment planning, the gross tumor volume (GTV) is contoured, and a 3–5 mm expansion for a clinical target volume (CTV) may be included, if appropriate, based on concern for microscopic disease depending on the

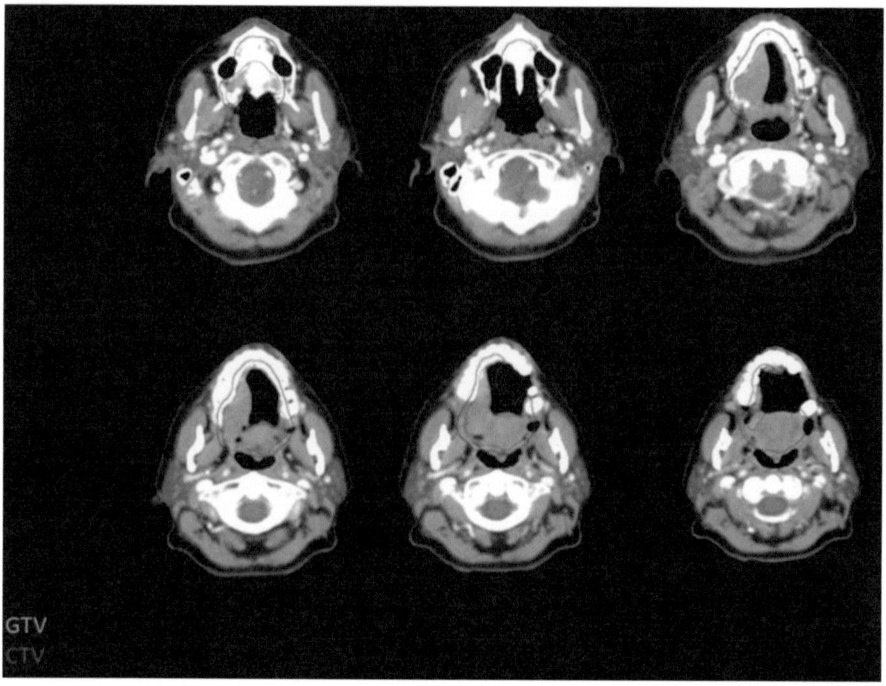

Fig. 14.2 Radiation target volumes to treat a myeloid sarcoma involving the hard palate of a 57-year-old male with AML, 6 months after allogeneic transplant. GTV is shown in blue; CTV is shown in red

anatomic site. A planning target volume (PTV) is added, as appropriate for the disease site and technique.

Follow-Up and Prognosis

After treatment, patients with MS should have careful physical examinations, repeat diagnostic imaging, and routine peripheral blood and/or bone marrow analyses to confirm remission. If the follow-up scan is negative, further scans do not need to be performed. Patients with a history of EM involvement have a predisposition to EM relapses; therefore, any new or suspicious soft tissue or skin abnormality should always be biopsied [49].

The prognostic significance of EM disease is not fully understood. In some series, the presence of EM disease has been associated with a poor prognosis [12]. However, in others, the presence of EM disease has not been found to adversely affect prognosis [50]. Further, 5-year survival rates for patients with MS range between 20% and 30%, which is comparable to AML in general [35, 51]. Given the conflicting reports, the presence of MS may be considered an additional poor prognostic factor until more definitive data are available.

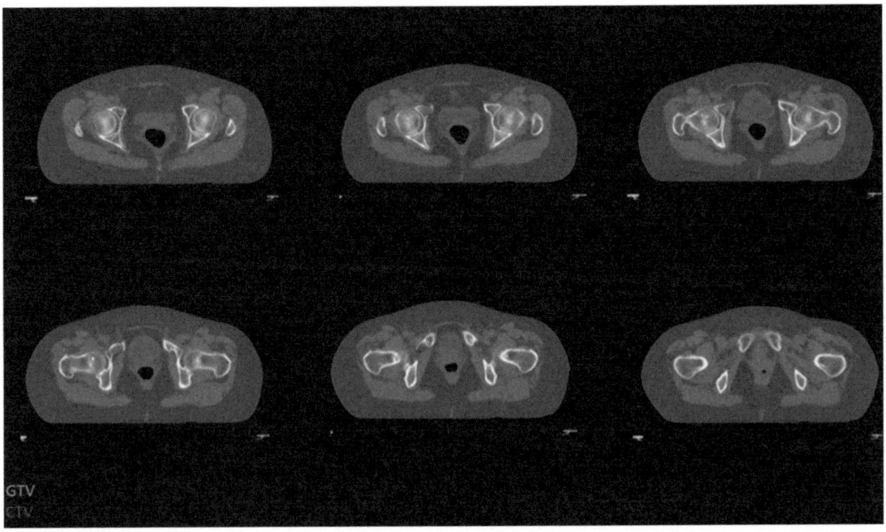

Fig. 14.3 Radiation target volumes to treat a painful myeloid sarcoma developing in the pelvis of a 63-year-old female with AML at initial diagnosis. GTV is shown in blue; CTV is shown in red

Conclusion

Myeloid sarcoma (MS) is a manifestation of extramedullary leukemia. It is seen most commonly in the context of AML; however, EM disease may present in patients with other forms of leukemia and may present antedating the onset of leukemia or in isolation. The existing literature on MS as a prognostic indicator is limited and conflicting. Diagnosis of MS requires biopsy. Imaging may be useful, especially 18FDG-PET, which improves detection of occult MS lesions. The t(8;21) translocation is the most commonly reported cytogenetic abnormality associated with EM involvement, but several other cytogenetic abnormalities have been reported. Treatment of MS involves systemic chemotherapy and/or HCT. RT can provide meaningful palliation of symptomatic lesions utilizing low doses.

References

1. Reardon G, Moloney WC. Chloroma and related myeloblastic neoplasms. JAMA Intern Med. 1961;108(6):864–71.
2. Burns A, Pattison GS. Observations on the surgical anatomy of the head and neck, illustrated by cases and engravings. Baltimore/Philadelphia: F. Lucas, jr., E.J. Coale, and Cushing & Jewett/H Carey & I Lea; 1823.
3. Dock G, Warthin A. A new case of chloroma with leukemia. Trans Assoc Am Phys. 1904;19:64–115.
4. Rappaport H. Tumors of the hematopoietic system. Atlas of tumor pathology. Washington, DC: Armed Forces Institute of Pathology; 1966.

5. Liu PI, et al. Autopsy study of granulocytic sarcoma (chloroma) in patients with myelogenous leukemia, Hiroshima-Nagasaki 1949-1969. Cancer. 1973;31(4):948–55.
6. Neiman RS, et al. Granulocytic sarcoma: a clinicopathologic study of 61 biopsied cases. Cancer. 1981;48(6):1426–37.
7. Wiernik PH, Serpick AA. Granulocytic sarcoma (chloroma). Blood. 1970;35(3):361–9.
8. Eshghabadi M, Shojania AM, Carr I. Isolated granulocytic sarcoma: report of a case and review of the literature. J Clin Oncol. 1986;4(6):912–7.
9. Szomor A, et al. Myeloid leukemia and myelodysplastic syndrome relapsing as granulocytic sarcoma (chloroma) after allogeneic bone marrow transplantation. Ann Hematol. 1997;75(5–6):239–41.
10. Bekassy A, et al. Granulocytic sarcoma after allogeneic bone marrow transplantation: a retrospective European multicenter survey. Acute and Chronic Leukemia Working Parties of the European Group for Blood and Marrow Transplantation. Bone Marrow Transplant. 1996;17(5):801–8.
11. Byrd JC, et al. Extramedullary myeloid cell tumors in acute nonlymphocytic leukemia: a clinical review. J Clin Oncol. 1995;13(7):1800–16.
12. Paydas S, Zorludemir S, Ergin M. Granulocytic sarcoma: 32 cases and review of the literature. Leuk Lymphoma. 2006;47(12):2527–41.
13. Pui MH, Fletcher BD, Langston JW. Granulocytic sarcoma in childhood leukemia: imaging features. Radiology. 1994;190(3):698–702.
14. Stölzel F, et al. The prevalence of extramedullary acute myeloid leukemia detected by 18FDG-PET/CT: final results from the prospective PETAML Trial. Haematologica. 2020;105(6):1552–8.
15. Breccia M, et al. Clinico-pathological characteristics of myeloid sarcoma at diagnosis and during follow-up: report of 12 cases from a single institution. Leuk Res. 2004;28(11):1165–9.
16. Ngu IW, et al. Unusual presentation of granulocytic sarcoma in the breast: a case report and review of the literature. Diagn Cytopathol. 2001;24(1):53–7.
17. Tallman MS, et al. Granulocytic sarcoma is associated with the 8;21 translocation in acute myeloid leukemia. J Clin Oncol. 1993;11(4):690–7.
18. Sugimoto Y, et al. Acute myeloid leukemia with t(8;21)(q22;q22) manifesting as granulocytic sarcomas in the rhinopharynx and external acoustic meatus at relapse after high-dose cytarabine: case report and review of the literature. Hematol J. 2004;5(1):84–9.
19. Schwyzer R, et al. Granulocytic sarcoma in children with acute myeloblastic leukemia and t(8;21). Med Pediatr Oncol. 1998;31(3):144–9.
20. Bonig H, Gobel U, Nurnberger W. Bilateral exopthalmus due to retro-orbital chloromas in a boy with t(8;21)- positive acute myeloblastic acute leukemia. Pediatr Hematol Oncol. 2002;19(8):597–600.
21. Holmes R, et al. A unique pattern of central nervous system leukemia in acute myelomonocytic leukemia associated with inv(16)(p13q22). Blood. 1985;65(5):1071–8.
22. Zhang XH, Zhang R, Li Y. Granulocytic sarcoma of abdomen in acute myeloid leukemia patient with inv(16) and t(6;17) abnormal chromosome: case report and review of literature. Leuk Res. 2010;34(7):958–61.
23. Xavier SG, et al. Granulocytic sarcoma of the small intestine with CBFbeta/MYH11 fusion gene: report of an aleukaemic case and review of the literature. Leuk Res. 2003;27(11):1063–6.
24. Bloomfield CD, et al. Frequency of prolonged remission duration after high-dose cytarabine intensification in acute myeloid leukemia varies by cytogenetic subtype. Cancer Res. 1998;58(18):4173–9.
25. Park KU, et al. Granulocytic sarcoma in MLL-positive infant acute myelogenous leukemia: fluorescence in situ hybridization study of childhood acute myelogenous leukemia for detecting MLL rearrangement. Am J Pathol. 2001;159(6):2011–6.
26. Leblanc T, et al. An interstitial 11q23 deletion proven to be a rearrangement interrupting the MLL gene in an infant with acute myeloblastic leukemia. Leukemia. 1996;10(11):1844–6.
27. Hagemeijer A, et al. Translocation (9;11)(p21;q23) in three cases of acute monoblastic leukemia. Cancer Genet Cytogenet. 1982;5(2):95–105.

28. Dachary D, et al. Acute myeloid leukemia with marrow hypereosinophilia and chromosome 16 abnormality. Cancer Genet Cytogenet. 1986;20(3–4):241–6.
29. Miura I, et al. Translocation (8;17)(p21;q21), a possible variant of t(15;17), in acute promyelocytic leukemia. Cancer Genet Cytogenet. 1994;72(1):75–7.
30. Bernstein R, et al. A unique 8;16 translocation in two infants with poorly differentiated monoblastic leukemia. Cancer Genet Cytogenet. 1987;24(2):213–20.
31. Diab A, et al. Acute myeloid leukemia with translocation t(8;16) presents with features which mimic acute promyelocytic leukemia and is associated with poor prognosis. Leuk Res. 2012;37:32.
32. Douet-Guilbert N, et al. Rearrangement of MLL in a patient with congenital acute monoblastic leukemia and granulocytic sarcoma associated with a t(1;11)(p36;q23) translocation. Leuk Lymphoma. 2005;46(1):143–6.
33. Pileri SA, et al. Myeloid sarcoma: clinico-pathologic, phenotypic and cytogenetic analysis of 92 adult patients. Leukemia. 2007;21(2):340–50.
34. Lan T-Y, et al. Prognostic factors of treatment outcomes in patients with granulocytic sarcoma. Acta Haematol. 2009;122(4):238–46.
35. Tsimberidou AM, et al. Outcome in patients with nonleukemic granulocytic sarcoma treated with chemotherapy with or without radiotherapy. Leukemia. 2003;17(6):1100.
36. Tsimberidou AM, et al. Myeloid sarcoma is associated with superior event-free survival and overall survival compared with acute myeloid leukemia. Cancer. 2008;113(6):1370–8.
37. Movassaghian M, et al. Presentation and outcomes among patients with isolated myeloid sarcoma: a Surveillance, Epidemiology, and End Results database analysis. Leuk Lymphoma. 2015;56(6):1698–703.
38. Meis JM, et al. Granulocytic sarcoma in nonleukemic patients. Cancer. 1986;58(12):2697–709.
39. Yamauchi K, Yasuda M. Comparison in treatments of nonleukemic granulocytic sarcoma: report of two cases and a review of 72 cases in the literature. Cancer. 2002;94(6):1739–46.
40. Imrie KR, et al. Isolated chloroma: the effect of early antileukemic therapy. Ann Intern Med. 1995;123(5):351–3.
41. Reinhardt D, Creutzig U. Isolated myelosarcoma in children—update and review. Leuk Lymphoma. 2002;43(3):565–74.
42. Döhner H, et al. Diagnosis and management of acute myeloid leukemia in adults: recommendations from an international expert panel, on behalf of the European LeukemiaNet. Blood. 2010;115(3):453–74.
43. Löwenberg B, et al. Cytarabine dose for acute myeloid leukemia. N Engl J Med. 2011;364(11):1027–36.
44. Burnett A, Wetzler M, Lowenberg B. Therapeutic advances in acute myeloid leukemia. J Clin Oncol. 2011;29(5):487–94.
45. Fernandez HF, et al. Anthracycline dose intensification in acute myeloid leukemia. N Engl J Med. 2009;361(13):1249–59.
46. Chevallier P, et al. Allogeneic hematopoietic stem-cell transplantation for myeloid sarcoma: a retrospective study from the SFGM-TC. J Clin Oncol. 2008;26(30):4940–3.
47. Kaur V, et al. Clinical characteristics, molecular profile and outcomes of myeloid sarcoma: a single institution experience over 13 years. Hematology. 2018;23(1):17–24.
48. Bakst RL, et al. Use of radiation in extramedullary leukemia/chloroma: guidelines from the International Lymphoma Radiation Oncology Group. Int J Radiat Oncol Biol Phys. 2018;102(2):314–9.
49. Michel G, et al. Risk of extramedullary relapse following allogeneic bone marrow transplantation for acute myelogenous leukemia with leukemia cutis. Bone Marrow Transplant. 1997;20(2):107–12.
50. Bisschop MM, et al. Extramedullary infiltrates at diagnosis have no prognostic significance in children with acute myeloid leukaemia. Leukemia. 2001;15(1):46–9.
51. Lan TY, et al. Prognostic factors of treatment outcomes in patients with granulocytic sarcoma. Acta Haematol. 2009;122(4):238–46.

Radiation Therapy for Relapsed and Refractory Hodgkin Lymphoma and Non-Hodgkin Lymphoma

15

Andrea K. Ng, Andrew Wirth, and Sandy Constine

Contents

A. K. Ng (✉)
Radiation Oncology, Boston, MA, USA
e-mail: Andrea_Ng@dfci.harvard.edu

A. Wirth
Peter MacCallum Cancer Centre, Melbourne, VIC, Australia
e-mail: Andrew.wirth@petermac.org

S. Constine
Radiation Oncology, Cancer, Strong Memorial Hospital, Rochester, NY, USA
e-mail: louis_constine@urmc.rochester.edu

C. Pinnix et al. (eds.), *Target Volume Delineation in Hematologic Malignancies*, Practical Guides in Radiation Oncology,
https://doi.org/10.1007/978-3-031-67722-9_15

Part 1: Background and Epidemiology

Relapsed/Refractory Hodgkin Lymphoma

- Hodgkin Lymphoma (HL) is an uncommon hematological malignancy with an incidence of approximately 80,000 new cases per year worldwide, and 8500 in the United States [1].
- HL has a bimodal age distribution with a large peak in the adolescent-young adult age group and a second, smaller peak in later life. There is a slight male predominance.
- Classical HL is a considered an aggressive lymphoma and constitutes approximately 90% of cases. Nodular lymphocyte predominant HL typically behaves as an indolent B-cell lymphoma.
- Just over half of patients with HL present with stage I–II and have a treatment failure rate of under 10%. In contrast, 20–30% of patients with advanced disease have persistent disease, or relapse, after first-line therapy. Approximately 970 deaths from HL are expected for the year 2020.

Relapsed/Refractory Non-Hodgkin Lymphoma

- Non-Hodgkin lymphoma (NHL) is the most common hematologic malignancy with an annual incidence of greater than 385,000 worldwide. In the United States, the annual incidence of NHL is over 77,000, with an estimated number of deaths from NHL of almost 20,000 each year [1].
- Diffuse large B-cell lymphoma (DLBCL) is the most common type of NHL, accounting for approximately 30% of all cases.
- Although the majority of patients with DLBCL are cured with immunochemotherapy, approximately 30% of patients will have refractory or relapsed disease. The outcome with conventional-dose salvage therapy in these patients is extremely poor, with an overall response rate of 26% and complete response rate of 7%, and a median survival of well under 1 year [2].

Part 2: Management and Treatment

Relapsed/Refractory Hodgkin Lymphoma

- Following failure of first-line chemotherapy, conventional-dose second-line chemotherapy achieves long-term survival in less than 20% of patients [3, 4].
- For selected patients with limited extent relapse, salvage radiotherapy achieves durable remissions in less than a third of patients with chemotherapy failure [5–10].

- For fit patients with relapsed/refractory disease, high-dose chemotherapy and stem cell transplantation, often given with peri-transplant radiotherapy, results in a cure rate of approximately 50% [11–16].
- Several novel treatments, including Brentuximab Vedotin and immune check point inhibitors, show promise for relapsed/refractory HL [17].
- Patients who relapse or progress do so in sites of disease prior to high-dose chemotherapy, and the risk of local relapse after high-dose chemotherapy is significantly lower in patients who receive radiation as a component of the therapy for relapsed/refractory disease [18].

Relapsed/Refractory Non-Hodgkin Lymphoma

- Based on results of landmark Phase III trials, chimeric antigen receptor (CAR) T-cell therapy has replaced salvage chemotherapy and autologous stem cell transplantation in patients with refractory large B-cell lymphoma or relapsed disease within 1 year post-treatment [19–21].
- Patterns of failure analysis after CAR-T cell therapy have shown that over 80% of progression occurred in preexisting sites [22], therefore supporting the role of radiation therapy in the peri-CAR-T therapy setting.
- Multiple studies have addressed the role of radiation therapy as bridging therapy to CAR-T cell therapy [23–31], showing that it is well tolerated.
- Increasing data are also available on the use of radiotherapy as salvage for post-CAR-T therapy failure [27, 32, 33] and as consolidation to high-risk sites after CAR-T therapy [34].
- A trend toward better outcome with use of comprehensive treatment volume has been demonstrated.
- Optimal bridging radiation dose is unclear, with doses of 20–30 Gy in 3–4 Gy per fraction being the most commonly used fractionation scheme. Ongoing trials are evaluating differential dosing, split course, and hypofractionation. In the consolidation and salvage setting, doses of 35–40 Gy in conventional fractionation have been used.

Part 3: General Considerations for Radiotherapy

- Key indications for radiotherapy in relapsed HL or NHL are as follows:
  - Localized relapsed/refractory disease: local radiation therapy should be considered if sites of concern than be safely encompassed.
  - Disseminated relapsed refractory disease: local radiation should be considered for bulky areas (>5 cm), dominant skeletal involvement, incomplete response in a locoregionally confined site, or an area of involvement where local control is critical e.g., cord compression and at symptomatic sites for palliation.

- Patient positioning and immobilization depend on the site(s) of radiotherapy. In general, thermoplastic masks are used for head and neck and mediastinal sites. Breath-hold techniques should be used, whenever feasible, for mediastinal, chest wall, and upper abdominal sites to minimize cardiac and pulmonary exposures.
- Target volume definitions are outlined in Table 15.1. Intravenous contrast can be helpful for target and organ-at-risk (OAR) definitions, especially for head and neck and mediastinal sites.
- Target volumes may be treated with 3D conformal radiation, intensity-modulated radiotherapy (IMRT), or proton therapy. Beam arrangements should be chosen to minimize doses to OAR.
- Radiation doses for relapsed/refractory HL and NHL are summarized in Tables 15.2 and 15.3, respectively.

Table 15.1 Planning target definitions for treatment of relapsed/refractory HL and NHL

Volume	Description
Gross tumor volume (GTV)	• Sites of active disease—generally FDG avid and/or biopsy proven sites. Where the GTV is present within a larger FDG negative mass, the whole mass may be regarded as the GTV, or alternatively the mass may be included in the CTV and treated to a lower dose
Clinical target volume (CTV)	• Nodal disease: include nodal sites involved at relapse; may consider including adjacent nodal sites that were involved at diagnosis, or at a prior relapse, if such inclusion is not expected to cause significant toxicity • Extranodal disease: include entire organ for extranodal sites such as orbits, salivary glands, thyroid, breast, and stomach; otherwise limit the CTV to area of relapse • Boost volume: residual FDG-avid sites
Internal target volume (ITV)	• Contains the CTV plus an internal margin that accounts for variation in CTV shape, size, and position, but is generally not indicated for head and neck sites which are subject to minimal motion, or when breath-hold technique is used
Planning target volume (PTV)	• Contains CTV or ITV plus a margin to account for setup uncertainties associated with patient position and beam alignment • CTV-to-PTV expansions are patient- and institution-specific; any recommendations in this chapter or elsewhere must be adjusted to reflect factors unique to the patient and institution
Organs at risk (OAR)	• Includes uninvolved normal structures at risk of RT-related toxicity for which RT planning or dose may be altered • Key OARs for: – Head and neck: lens, optic nerves, retina, lacrimal glands, salivary glands, thyroid – Mediastinum: lungs, heart, cardiac substructures (LAD, left ventricle, cardiac valves), breasts in young women – Abdomen/pelvis: liver, kidneys, small bowel, spleen, bone marrow

Table 15.2 Radiation dose for relapsed/refractory HL

Scenario	Radiation dose
Complete response to salvage chemotherapy (Deauville 1–3), peri-transplant RT	30–30.6 Gy in 1.8–2 Gy/fraction
Partial response to salvage chemotherapy with residual FDG avid foci (Deauville 4–5), peri-transplant RT	36–45 Gy in 1.8–2 Gy/fraction
Localized refractory disease to primary or salvage chemotherapy, pre-transplant RT	36–45 Gy in 1.8–2 Gy/fraction
Localized relapsed/refractory disease, not a candidate for further chemotherapy or transplant	36–45 Gy in 1.8–2 Gy/fraction

Table 15.3 Radiation dose for relapsed/refractory NHL

Scenario	Radiation dose
Complete response to salvage chemotherapy (Deauville 1–3), peri-transplant RT	30–36 Gy in 1.8–2 Gy/fraction
Partial response to salvage chemotherapy with residual FDG avid foci (Deauville 4–5), peri-transplant RT	36 Gy with either sequential or simultaneous integrated boost to a final dose of 40–45 Gy in 1.8–2 Gy/fraction
Localized refractory disease to primary or salvage chemotherapy, pre-transplant RT	40–50 Gy in 1.8–2 Gy per fraction, or consider 35–40 Gy in 1.3–1.5 Gy per fraction BID if rapidly progressive disease
Localized relapsed/refractory disease, not a candidate for further chemotherapy or transplant	Curative intent (based on age, PS, co-morbidities, life expectancy): 45–55 Gy in 1.8–2 Gy/fraction Palliative intent: hypofractionated schedule of 8–30 Gy

Part 4: Pre-radiotherapy Imaging and Evaluation

- PET-CT and diagnostic CT with IV contrast (if available) performed at the time of initial diagnosis, at relapse, and immediately prior to radiotherapy after salvage chemotherapy are essential for target volume delineation and radiation dose prescription.
- It is important that imaging be available from each point in the patient's trajectory and that the imaging studies are carefully reviewed by the radiation oncologist. This will include imaging performed at initial diagnosis, interim scans during first-line therapy, and imaging at each relapse and during salvage therapies. Creating contours representing disease locations at prior time points allows the identification and potential inclusion of previously involved sites adjacent to known relapse sites.
- Relevant organ function in the area to be treated should be assessed prior to therapy.

Cases

See Figs. 15.1, 15.2, 15.3, 15.4, and 15.5.

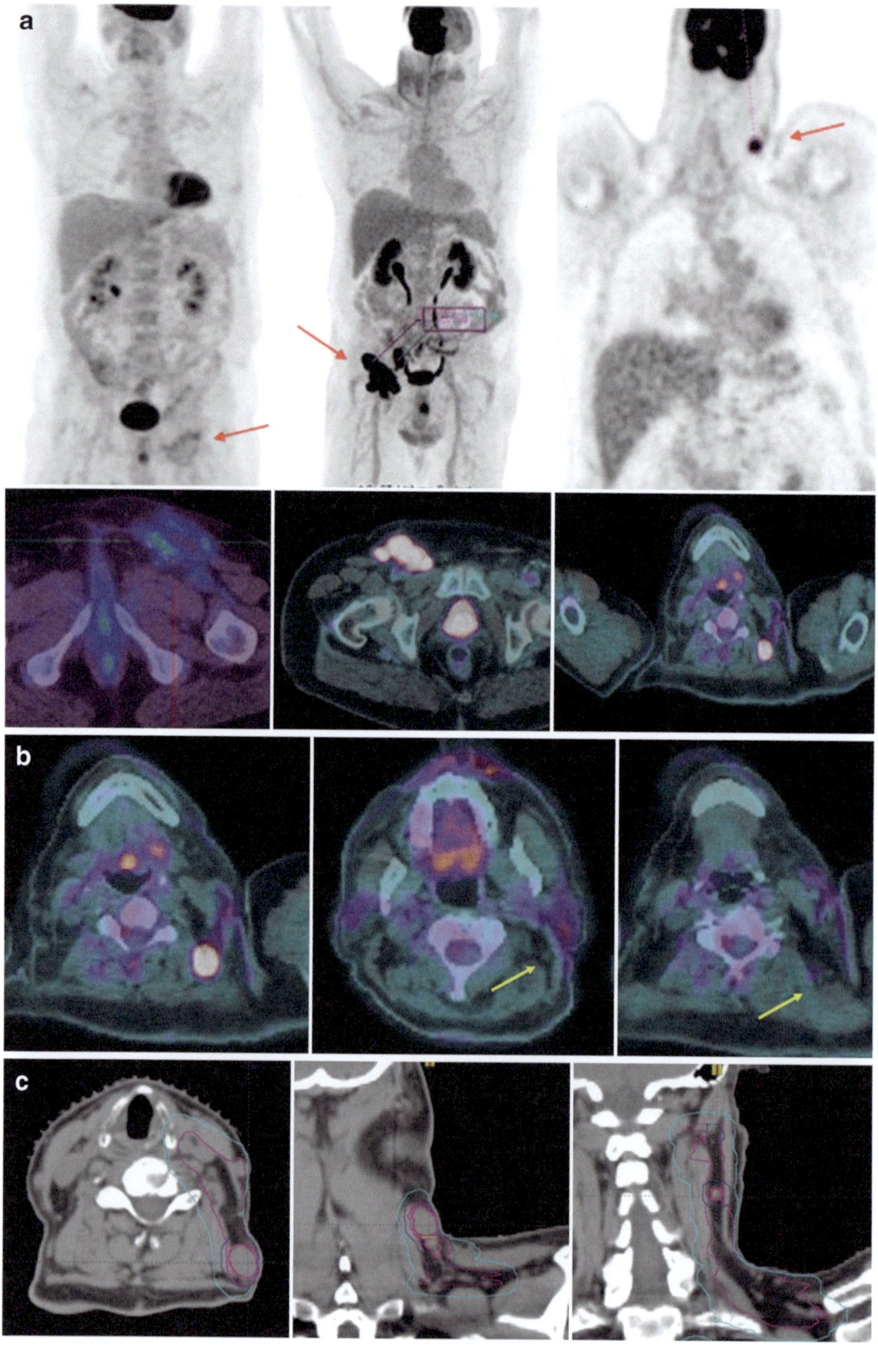

Fig. 15.1 (**a–e**) A 73-year-old male with stage I classical HL of the L groin s/p ABVD (Doxorubicin, Bleomycin, Vinblastine, Dacarbazine) and ISRT presents with R groin relapse 3 years later s/p PACEBOM (prednisolone, doxorubicin, cyclophosphamide, etoposide, bleomycin, vincristine, and methotrexate) and ISRT. He then presented with a second relapse 5 years later in the L neck. Plan: ISRT alone as salvage given limited nodal relapse and long remission duration. (**a**) PET-CT of initial L groin disease, right groin disease at first relapse, and left neck disease at second relapse. (**b**) Axial images of PET-CT showing intensely FDG-avid left posterior neck, and sub-centimeter FDG-negative upper neck, and lower neck nodes. (**c**) The patient was simulated with chin extended. As the patient was to be treated with RT alone, a generous ISRT approach was taken to encompass both the FDG avid node and most of the cervical nodal chain, in case there was occult disease in these nearby nodes. The GTV in bold red, included both the FDG avid node (left panel) as well as prominent FDG negative nodes immediately below (mid panel) and in the upper neck (right panel). The GTV was treated to 36 Gy with a PTV expansion of 7 mm (dark blue). (**d**) A DRR image demonstrating the GTV, CTV, and PTV 30 Gy. The CTV included most of the cervical nodal compartment, to anatomic boundaries in the axial plane. The craniocaudal margins approximated a standard IFRT field, with some compromise at the upper level to reduce dose to the ipsilateral parotid gland. (**e**) A VMAT plan was used, rather than an 3D conformal technique, to reduce dose to the oral cavity

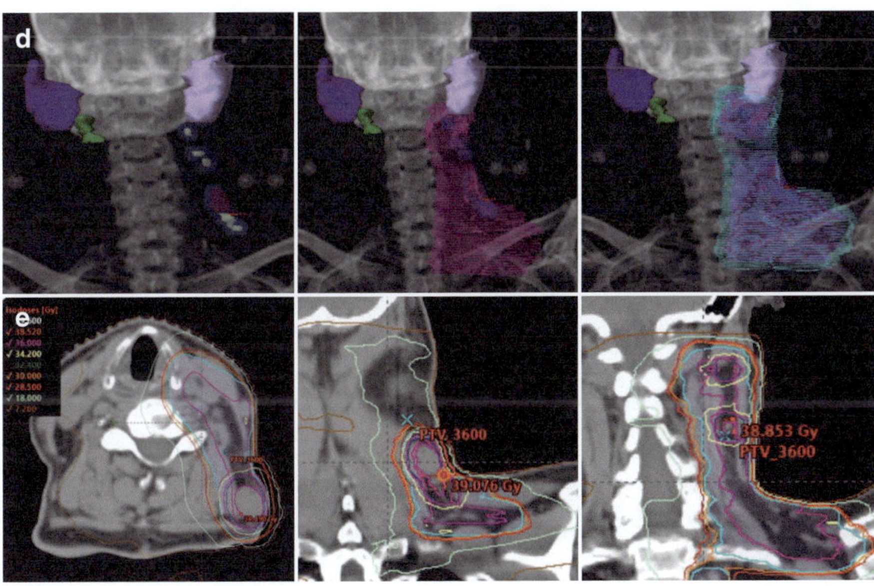

Fig. 15.1 (continued)

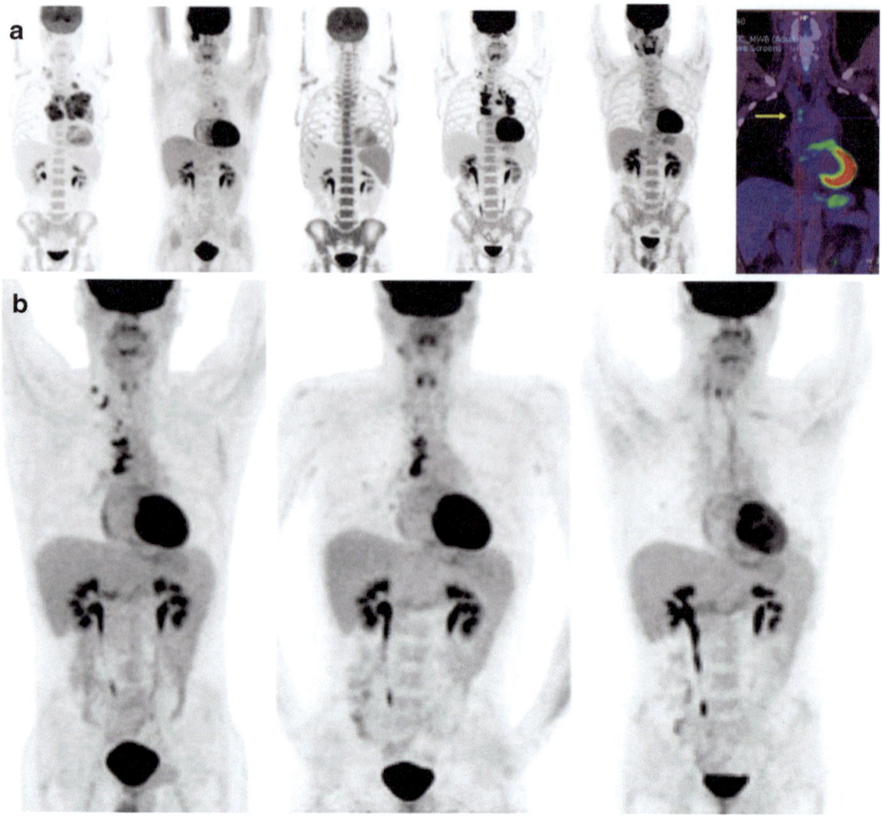

Fig. 15.2 (**a**–**d**) A 34-year-male stage IIBx classical HL involving the neck and mediastinum, with a partial metabolic response after ABVD × 2, and a complete metabolic response after escalated BEACOPP (bleomycin, etoposide, adriamycine, cyclophosphamide, vincristine, procarbazine, and prednisone) × 4. The first relapse occurred 15 months later, s/p 2 cycles of ICE with a "near complete response" with low-volume residual FDG avid disease in the mediastinum. This was followed by ASCT in May 2014. The patient was not referred for post-transplant consolidative RT. The second relapse occurred in the mediastinum and was detected on the next PET 5 months after ASCT, treated with Brentuximab with a minor response. Plan: Definitive ISRT as salvage. (**a**) Left to right: (1) PET at initial diagnosis; (2) after ABVD × 2 showing PMR; (3) after BEACOPP × 4 showing CMR; (4) first relapse at 15 months; (5) to (6) PMR after ICE, prior to transplant (left to right). (**b**) PET at relapse 5 months post-transplant (left), minor response to Brentuximab (mid), and CMR after salvage ISRT (right). (**c**) The patient was simulated with chin extended and arms akimbo. As the patient was to be treated with RT alone, a generous ISRT approach was taken to encompass residual FDG avid nodes, enlarged FDG negative nodes, previously involved nodal locations and generous expansions for potential occult disease in previously radiologically uninvolved regional nodes. The resultant ISRT volume comprised much of an old-fashioned mantle field. PET scan at relapse prior to salvage RT (left); Planning CT (mid): Planning CT with dosimetry (right). The GTV included FDG avid nodes is shown in red and the structurally abnormal, FDG negative soft tissue is shown in pink. The CTV, in pink, included sites of prior nodal involvement, extended to anatomic boundaries in the axial plane. The CTV included the

neck and supraclavicular regions, mediastinum (including hilae) down to several cm below the lowest previously involved node. The axillary apices were included to provide adequate margins on supraclavicular nodal locations. The PTV, using a 1 cm margin, is shown in blue. The CTV was treated to 36 Gy and GTV to 42 Gy. (**d**) Left to right: (1) A DRR image demonstrating the GTV (red), CTV (pink), and previous locations of involvement (brown) and the phase one field, treated to 36 Gy; (2) the reduced field covering the GTV to 42 Gy (the PTV is omitted for clarity); (3) to (4) Representative dosimetry in the coronal and sagittal planes. A 3D conformal (anterior posterior) technique was used as the coverage was intended to be comprehensive. The key organs at risk were heart and lung. The mean lung dose was 14.2 Gy with a V5 Gy of 52%. The mean heart dose was 18 Gy, which is higher than usually accepted for mediastinal radiotherapy plans. In this case, it was accepted in the interests of ensuring adequate coverage of the extensive mediastinal disease locations, given the failure of prior ASCT and the only alternative, potentially curative option being allografting. The patient will require life-long monitoring for late toxicities and optimization of any coexisting cardiac risk factors

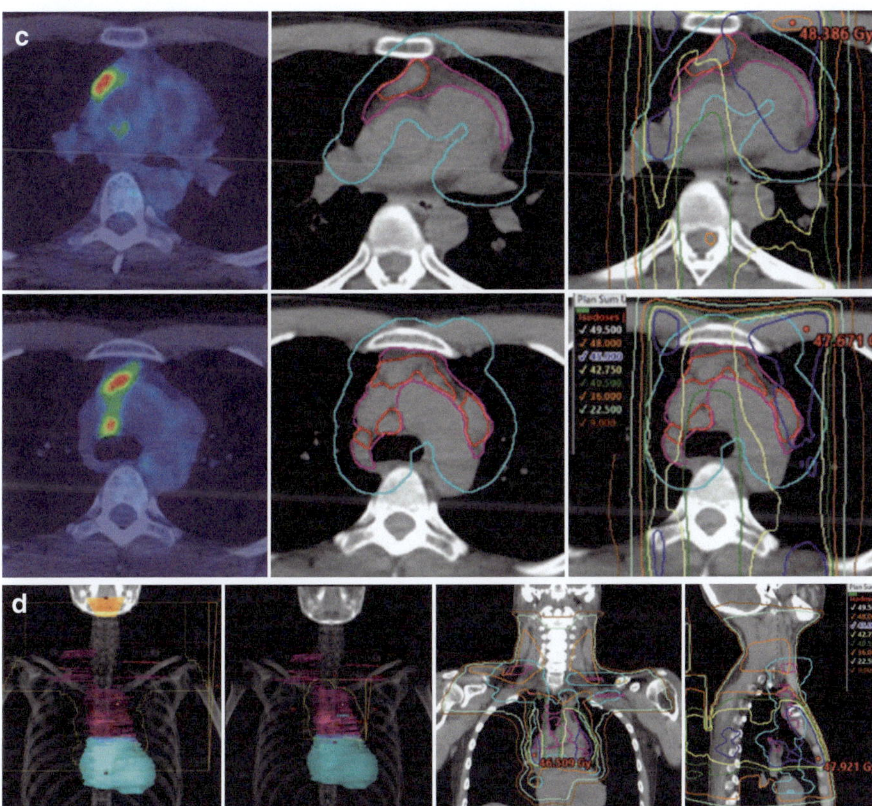

Fig. 15.2 (continued)

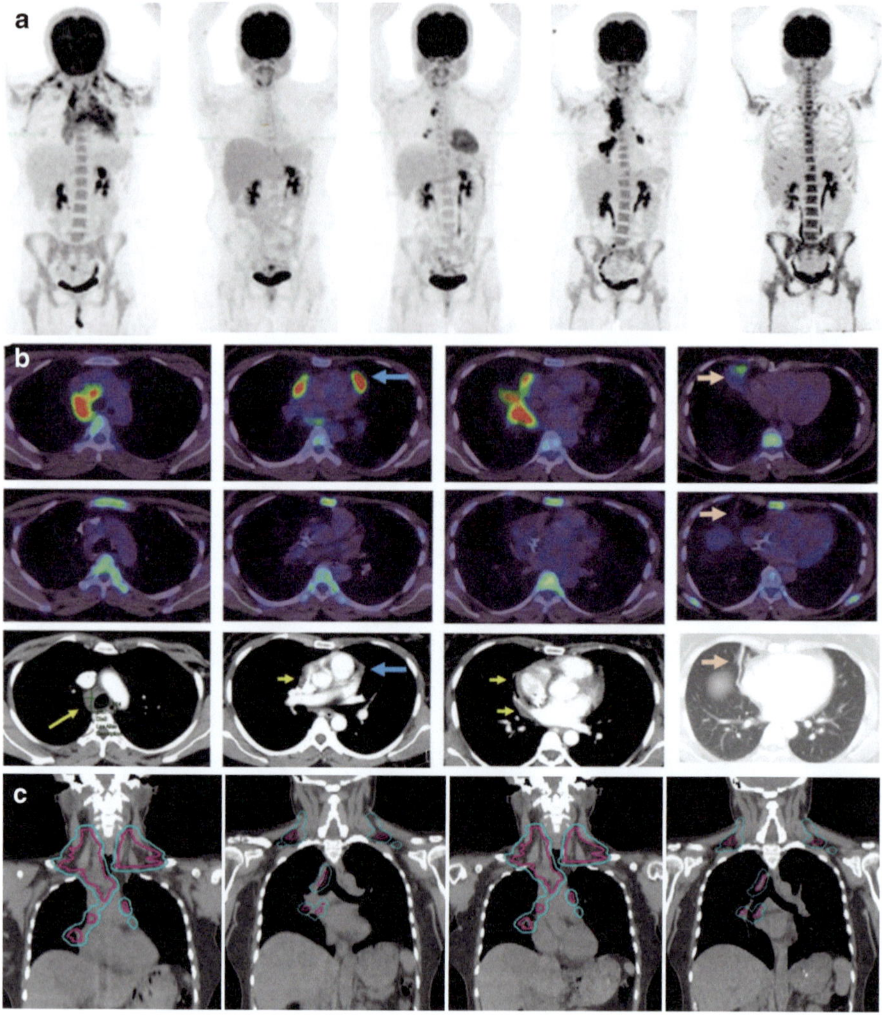

Fig. 15.3 (**a**–**e**) A 35-year-old female bulky stage II mediastinal Hodgkin lymphoma treated with 6 cycles of ABVD with a complete metabolic response. No radiation was given due to the extensive disease distribution and potential risk of late radiation toxicity. Radiological evidence of recurrence was first noted 10 months post-treatment but histological confirmation was not achieved until 3 years later. The relapse distribution partly overlapped that of the initial disease with neck, superior mediastinal, and right cardiac involvement, with a much smaller component of left-sided

mediastinal disease. Plan: Salvage chemotherapy with ICE, autologous stem cell transplantation, and post-transplant radiation therapy. A decision to offer consolidative RT was made based on: (1) the relatively early relapse (less than 12 months after first-line therapy) despite the early attainment of CMR during ABVD; (2) The presence of residual soft tissue masses post-salvage chemotherapy. (**a**) Left to right: (1) PET at initial diagnosis (note brown fat); (2) CMR after ABVD; (3) initial radiological evidence of relapse 10 months after ABVD; (4) disease extent at the time of histological confirmation of relapse prior to salvage therapy; (5) CMR after ICE, maintained after ASCT. (**b**) Top panel: Sites of relapse shown on PET-CT prior to salvage chemotherapy. The pink arrow shows an abnormality presumed to be atelectasis/inflammation rather than lymphoma; Mid panel: Post-salvage PET-CT showing CMR; Bottom panel: Planning CT with contrast showing residual soft tissue abnormality at prior sites of relapse (yellow arrows) and presumed initial atelectasis (pink arrow). Note that a relapse site overlying the left anterior descending coronary artery (blue arrow, top panel) corresponds with a small residual mass on the planning CT (blue arrow, bottom panel). (**c**) The patient was simulated in DIBH, with chin extended and arms by sides. Planning CT in free breathing (left) and in DIBH (right), which reduced the proportion of lung and heart within the planes of treatment. (**d**) Top panel: Planning CT showing CTV in pink which included all sites of nodal involvement defined at relapse. Consideration was given to including some or all of the sites involved at the initial diagnosis, but it was felt this would substantially increase cardiac and lung exposure, for a potentially small gain in tumor control. The small volume relapse site overlying the coronary artery was included in the CTV, even though it would expose a segment of the artery to the planned dose, as the presence of a residual mass was considered to increase the risk of relapse in this location. A region of pulmonary opacity noted at the right lung base at relapse was excluded from the CTV, as: (1) It was felt likely to represent atelectasis/inflammatory change and (2) Inclusion would have substantially increased lung and heart irradiation. The CTV extended to anatomic boundaries of the involved compartments in the axial plane; PTV in blue; Bottom panel: Axial images showing dosimetry. A VMAT technique was used, in particular to reduce cardiac exposure. (**e**) A DRR image demonstrates the relationship of the CTV (pink) and PTV (blue) to the heart and coronary artery (yellow). The relationship of selected sites of relapse, residual soft tissue masses on the planning CT, and the DRR is shown on the right. (**f**) A DRR image illustrates the relationship of the PTV to breast tissue (top) and representative breast tissue dosimetry (bottom). The key organs at risk were heart, breast, and lung. The mean lung dose was 7.7 Gy (V20 9% and V5 53%), the mean heart dose was 4.1 Gy, and the mean breast dose was 2.2 Gy (V4 16%). A segment of about 1–1.5 cm of the left anterior descending coronary artery received over 20 Gy

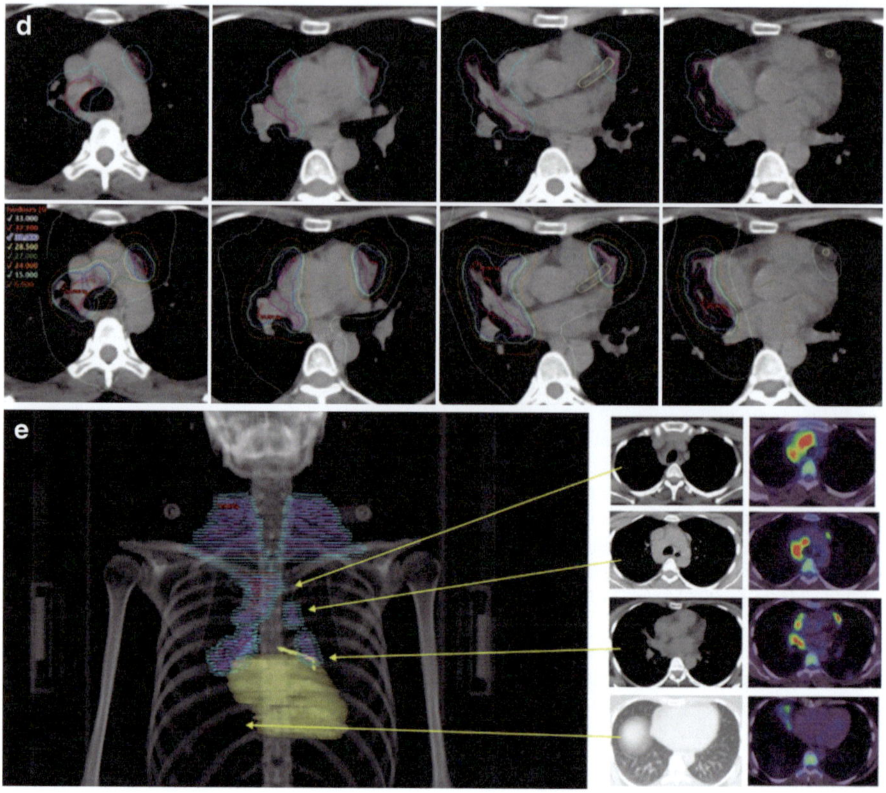

Fig. 15.3 (continued)

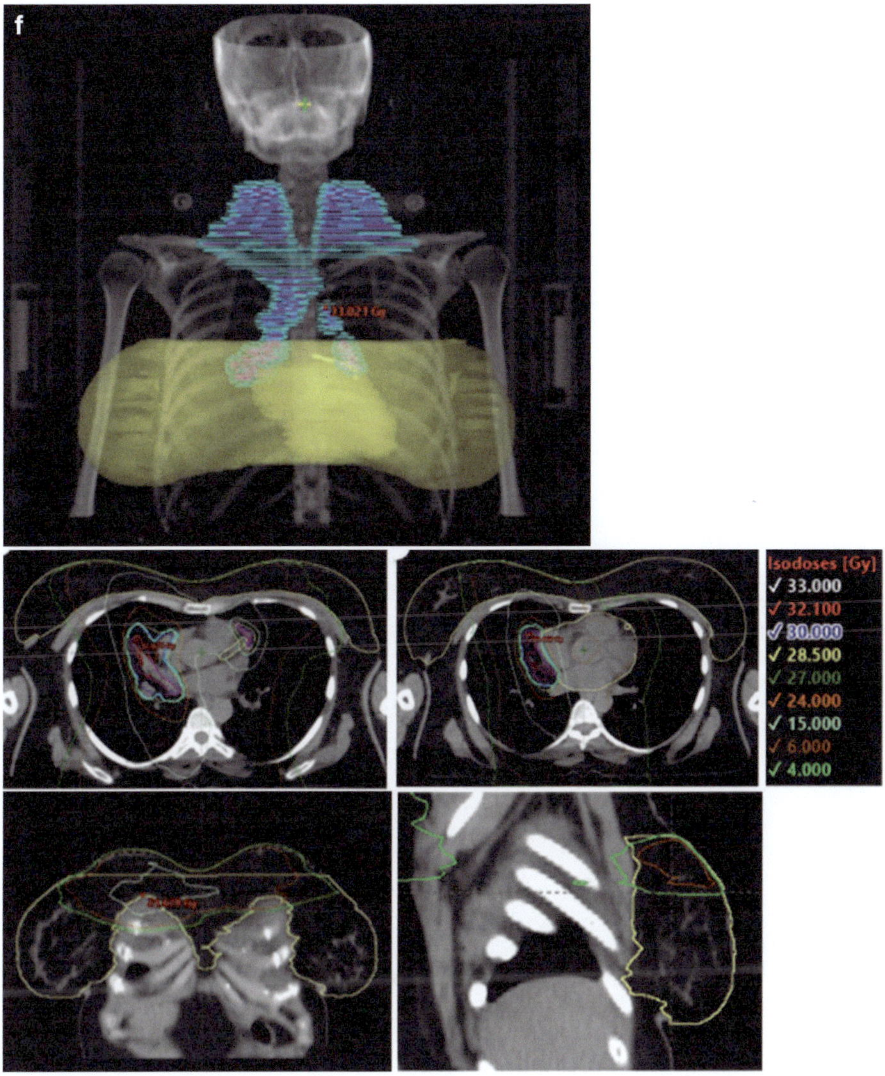

Fig. 15.3 (continued)

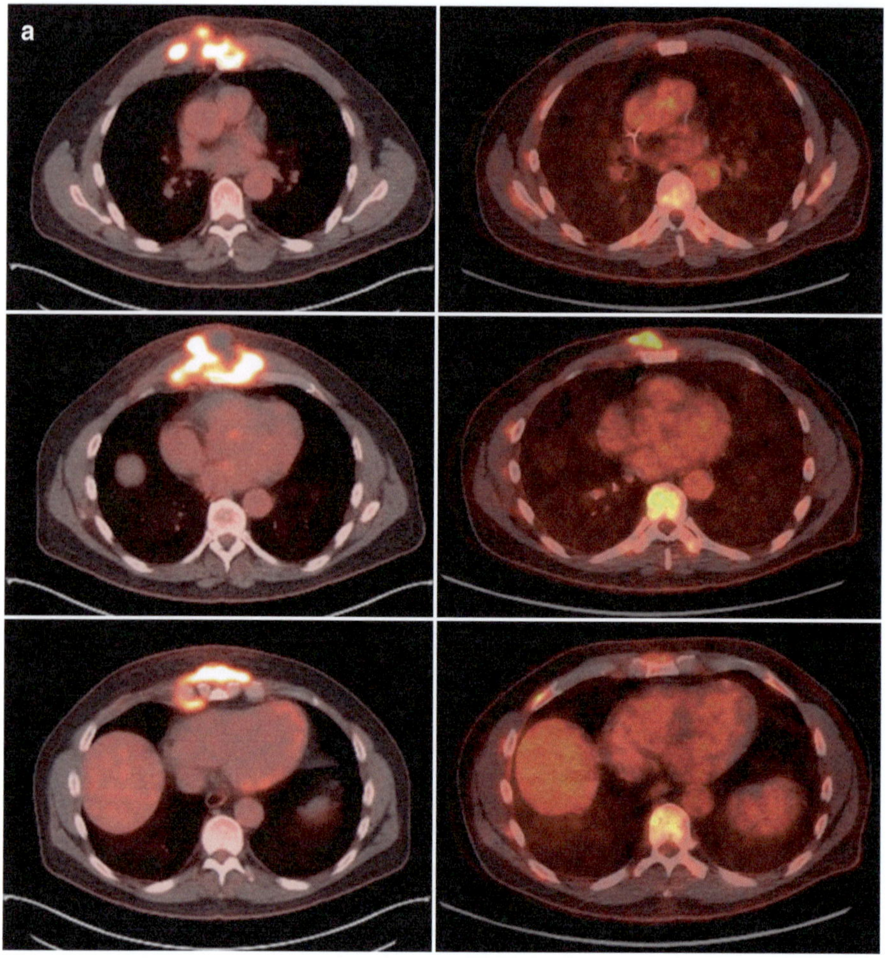

Fig. 15.4 (**a–d**) A 62-year-old man with limited-stage DLBCL with anterior chest wall involvement, s/p R-CHOP × 6 with Deauville 4 response after 6 cycles of chemotherapy. Biopsy of residual FDG-avid site showed refractory lymphoma. Plan: Bridging radiation therapy to CAR-T cell therapy. (**a**) Staging PET-CT showing anterior chest wall involvement (left) and restaging PET-CT after 6 cycles of R-CHOP showing Deauville 4 response (right). (**b**) RT Technique and Dose: Deep-inspiration breath-hold to expand lungs and reduce lung doses, and to elongate/extend the heart inferiorly away from the target volume; IMRT with simultaneous integrated boost, 3600 cGy (in 180 cGy per fraction) to original disease extent, 4400 Gy (in 220 cGy per fraction) to residual FDG-avid disease. *Planning CT in axial view*: CTV_4400 in red; CTV_3600 in magenta (left). Pre-chemotherapy PET-CT (right upper, fused with planning CT to determine CTV_3600) and post-chemotherapy PET-CT (right lower, fused with planning RT to determine CTV_4400). (**c**) *Planning CT in sagittal view*: CTV_4400 in red; CTV_3600 in magenta (left). Pre-chemotherapy PET-CT (right upper, fused with planning CT to determine CTV_3600) and post-chemotherapy PET-CT (right lower, fused with planning RT to determine CTV_4400). (**d**) *Planning CT in axial view*: CTV_4400 in red, CTV_3600 in magenta, PTV_4400 in blue, PTV_3600 in cyan, LAD in orange, left ventricle in yellow (upper); Planning CTV showing isodose distribution of IMRT plan with LAD and left ventricle as avoidance structures (lower)

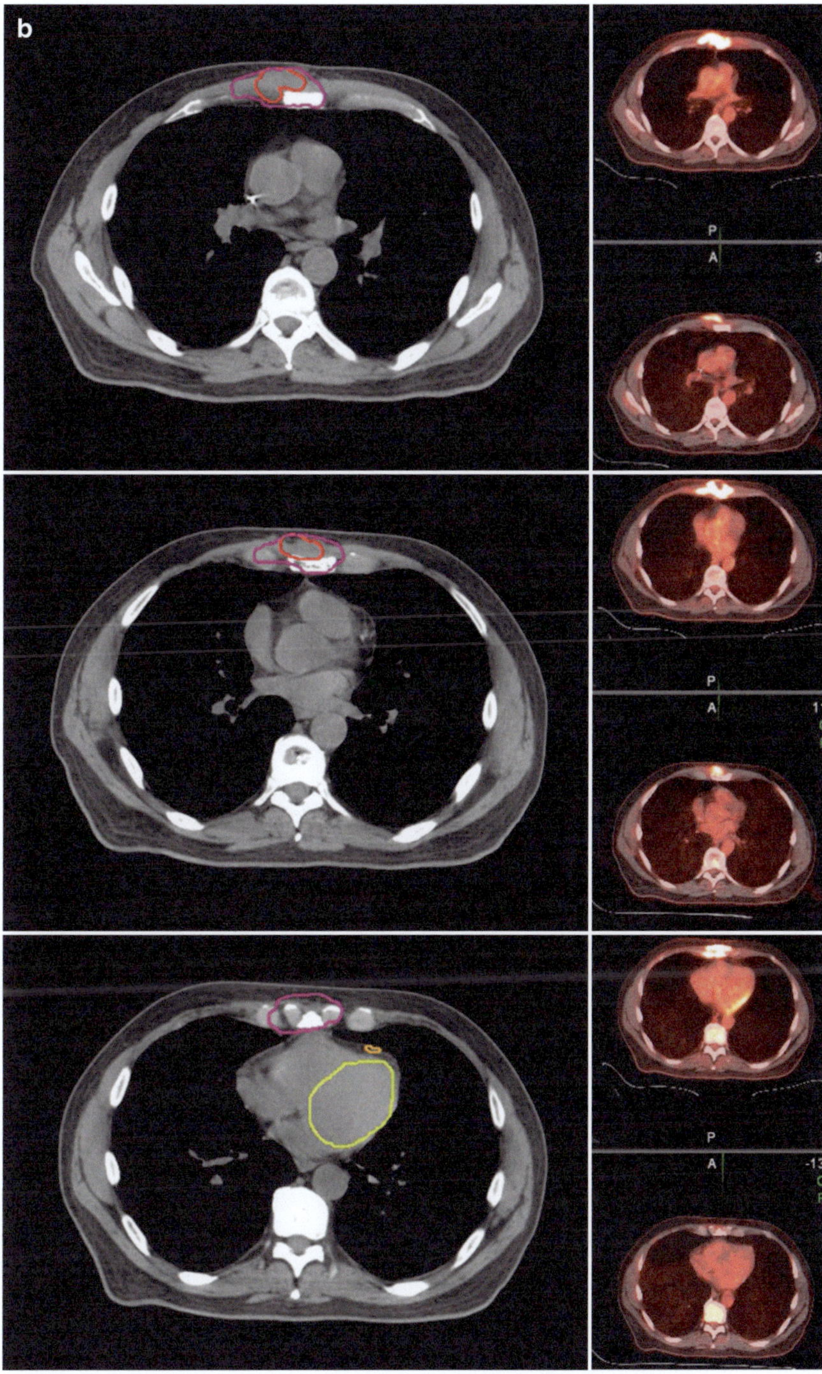

Fig. 15.4 (continued)

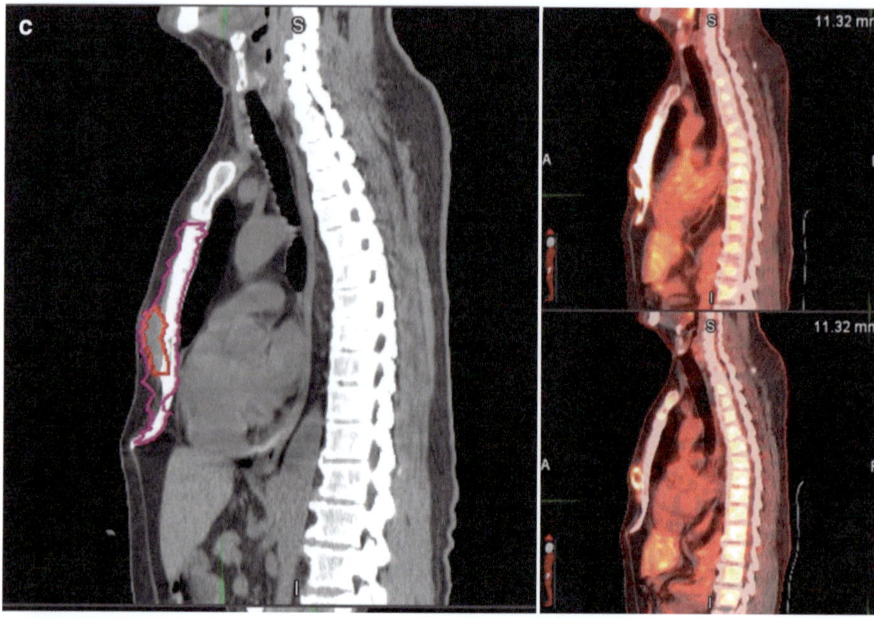

Fig. 15.4 (continued)

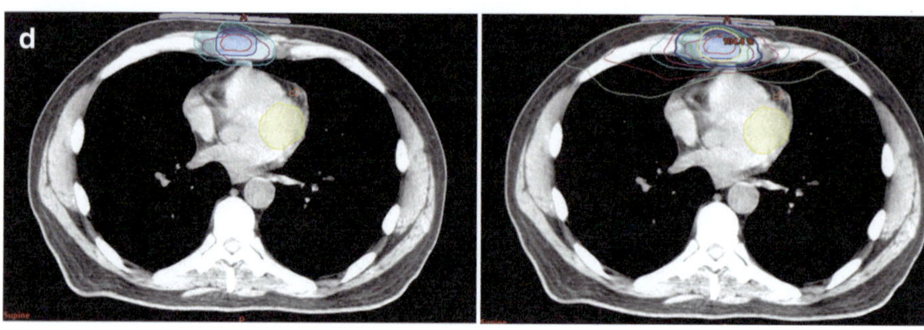

Fig. 15.4 (continued)

of most disease sites but worsening disease in the R axilla (right). (**b**) Restaging PET-CT at the time of referral (approximately 1-year post-chemotherapy) with painful right axillary disease. (**c**) Planning CT in axial view: CTV in red, PTV in blue, pacemaker in green (left), beam arrangements (mid), and isodose distribution (right). Three-field conformal (tangents and a single posterior field) technique used to limit doses to lung, and 6 MV energy to minimize neutron production to the pacemaker. (**d**) Planning CT in coronal view: CTV in red, PTV in blue, pacemaker in green (left), and isodose distribution (right)

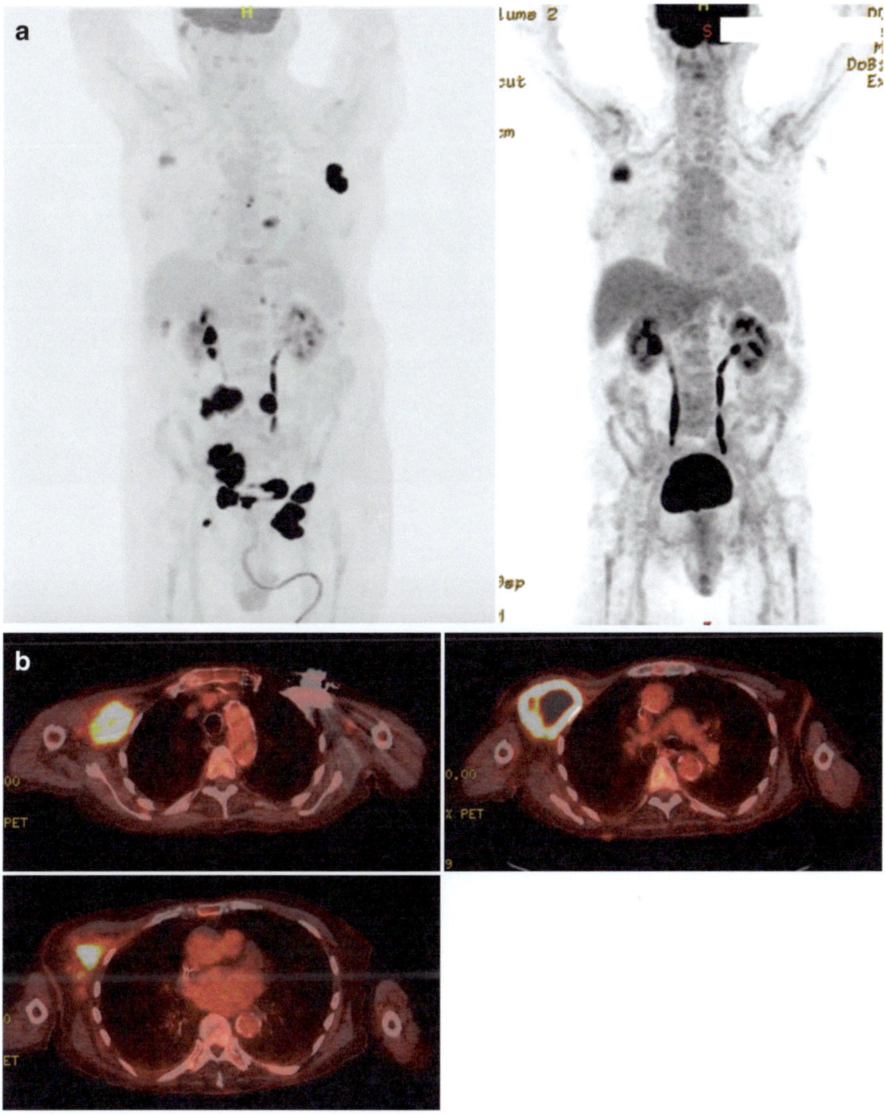

Fig. 15.5 (**a**–**d**) A 91-year-old male with advanced-stage DLBCL with bilateral axillary, abdominal, and pelvic involvement s/p mini R-CHOP × 6. Restaging PET-CT showed resolution of disease below the diaphragm but increase in size and FDG avidity of R axillary nodal disease. Post-chemotherapy course was complicated by RSV pneumonia requiring prolonged hospitalization, and atrioventricular block requiring pacemaker placement. His R axillary disease continued to progress causing local pain. The patient is not a candidate for further systemic therapy given advanced age and co-morbidities. Plan: Palliative ISRT to R axilla, 24 Gy in 6 fractions. (**a**) Staging PET-CT showing bilateral axillary, abdominal and pelvic disease at initial diagnosis (left), and restaging PET-CT after 6 cycles of mini-R-CHOP showing a mixed response with resolution

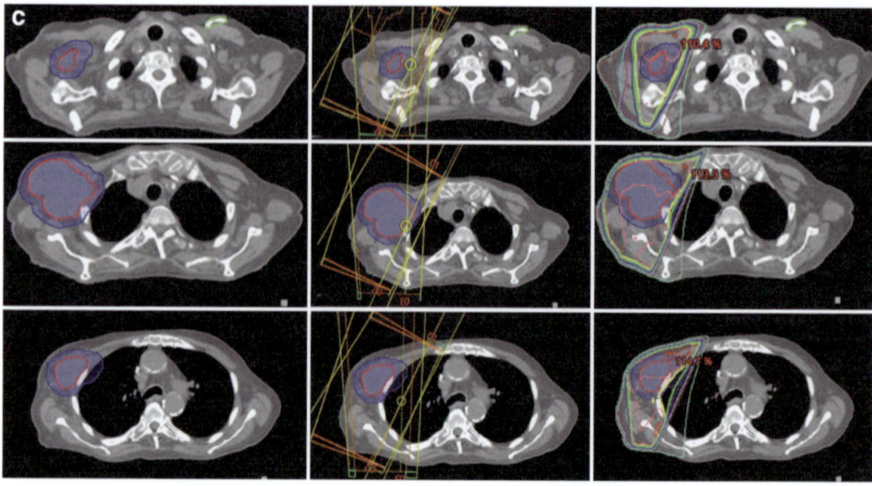

Fig. 15.5 (continued)

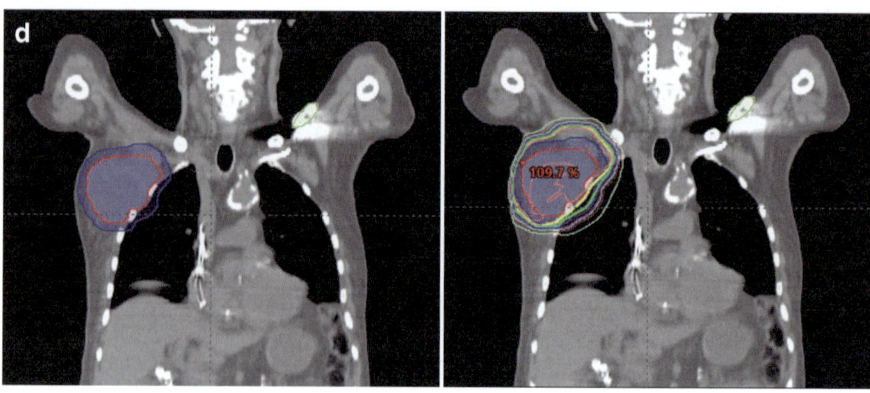

Fig. 15.5 (continued)

References

1. Siegel RL, Miller KD, Jemal A. Cancer statistics, 2020. CA Cancer J Clin. 2020;70:7–30.
2. Crump M, Neelapu SS, Farooq U, et al. Outcomes in refractory diffuse large B-cell lymphoma: results from the international SCHOLAR-1 study. Blood. 2017;130:1800–8.
3. Bonfante V, Santoro A, Viviani S, et al. Outcome of patients with Hodgkin's disease failing after primary MOPP-ABVD. J Clin Oncol. 1997;15:528–34.
4. Longo DL, Duffey PL, Young RC, et al. Conventional-dose salvage combination chemotherapy in patients relapsing with Hodgkin's disease after combination chemotherapy: the low probability for cure. J Clin Oncol. 1992;10:210–8.
5. Wirth A, Corry J, Laidlaw C, et al. Salvage radiotherapy for Hodgkin's disease following chemotherapy failure. Int J Radiat Oncol Biol Phys. 1997;39:599–607.

6. Josting A, Rueffer U, Franklin J, et al. Prognostic factors and treatment outcome in primary progressive Hodgkin lymphoma: a report from the German Hodgkin Lymphoma Study Group. Blood. 2000;96:1280–6.
7. Campbell B, Wirth A, Milner A, et al. Long-term follow-up of salvage radiotherapy in Hodgkin's lymphoma after chemotherapy failure. Int J Radiat Oncol Biol Phys. 2005;63:1538–45.
8. Josting A, Nogova L, Franklin J, et al. Salvage radiotherapy in patients with relapsed and refractory Hodgkin's lymphoma: a retrospective analysis from the German Hodgkin Lymphoma Study Group. J Clin Oncol. 2005;23:1522–9.
9. Specht L, Yahalom J, Illidge T, et al. Modern radiation therapy for Hodgkin lymphoma: field and dose guidelines from the International Lymphoma Radiation Oncology Group (ILROG). Int J Radiat Oncol Biol Phys. 2014;89:854–62.
10. Milgrom SA, Pinnix CC, Chuang H, et al. Early-stage Hodgkin lymphoma outcomes after combined modality therapy according to the post-chemotherapy 5-point score: can residual pet-positive disease be cured with radiotherapy alone? Br J Haematol. 2017;179:488–96.
11. Linch DC, Winfield D, Goldstone AH, et al. Dose intensification with autologous bone-marrow transplantation in relapsed and resistant Hodgkin's disease: results of a BNLI randomised trial. Lancet. 1993;341:1051–4.
12. Yuen AR, Rosenberg SA, Hoppe RT, et al. Comparison between conventional salvage therapy and high-dose therapy with autografting for recurrent or refractory Hodgkin's disease. Blood. 1997;89:814–22.
13. Moskowitz CH, Kewalramani T, Nimer SD, et al. Effectiveness of high dose chemoradiotherapy and autologous stem cell transplantation for patients with biopsy-proven primary refractory Hodgkin's disease. Br J Haematol. 2004;124:645–52.
14. Schmitz N, Pfistner B, Sextro M, et al. Aggressive conventional chemotherapy compared with high-dose chemotherapy with autologous haemopoietic stem-cell transplantation for relapsed chemosensitive Hodgkin's disease: a randomised trial. Lancet. 2002;359:2065–71.
15. Diehl V, Stein H, Hummel M, et al. Hodgkin's lymphoma: biology and treatment strategies for primary, refractory, and relapsed disease. Hematology Am Soc Hematol Educ Program. 2003:225–47.
16. Rancea M, Monsef I, von Tresckow B, et al. High-dose chemotherapy followed by autologous stem cell transplantation for patients with relapsed/refractory Hodgkin lymphoma. Cochrane Database Syst Rev. 2013;(6):CD009411.
17. Mina AA, Vakkalagadda C, Pro B. Novel therapies and approaches to relapsed/refractory HL beyond chemotherapy. Cancers (Basel). 2019;11:421.
18. Constine LS, Yahalom J, Ng AK, et al. The role of radiation therapy in patients with relapsed or refractory Hodgkin lymphoma: guidelines from the International Lymphoma Radiation Oncology Group. Int J Radiat Oncol Biol Phys. 2018;100:1100–18.
19. Locke FL, Miklos DB, Jacobson CA, et al. Axicabtagene ciloleucel as second-line therapy for large B-cell lymphoma. N Engl J Med. 2022;386(7):640–54. PMID: 34891224.
20. Westin JR, Oluwole OO, Kersten MJ, et al. Survival with axicabtagene ciloleucel in large B-cell lymphoma. N Engl J Med. 2023;389(2):148–57. PMID: 37272527.
21. Kamdar M, Solomon SR, Arnason J, et al. Lisocabtagene maraleucel versus standard of care with salvage chemotherapy followed by autologous stem cell transplantation as second-line treatment in patients with relapsed or refractory large B-cell lymphoma (TRANSFORM): results from an interim analysis of an open-label, randomised, phase 3 trial. Lancet. 2022;399(10343):2294–308. PMID: 35717989.
22. Saifi O, Breen WG, Lester SC, et al. Does bridging radiation therapy affect the pattern of failure after CAR T-cell therapy in non-Hodgkin lymphoma? Radiother Oncol. 2022;166:171–9. PMID: 34890736.
23. Sim AJ, Jain MD, Figura NB, et al. Radiation therapy as a bridging strategy for CAR T cell therapy with axicabtagene ciloleucel in diffuse large B-cell lymphoma. Int J Radiat Oncol Biol Phys. 2019;105(5):1012–21. PMID: 31175906.

24. Pinnix CC, Gunther JR, Dabaja BS, et al. Bridging therapy prior to axicabtagene ciloleucel for relapsed/refractory large B-cell lymphoma. Blood Adv. 2020;4(13):2871–83. PMID: 32589728.
25. Wright CM, LaRiviere MJ, Baron JA, et al. Bridging radiation therapy before commercial chimeric antigen receptor T-cell therapy for relapsed or refractory aggressive B-cell lymphoma. Int J Radiat Oncol Biol Phys. 2020;108(1):178–88. PMID: 32446950.
26. Ladbury C, Dandapani S, Hao C, et al. Long-term follow-up of bridging therapies prior to CAR T-cell therapy for relapsed/refractory large B cell lymphoma. Cancers (Basel). 2023;15(6):1747. PMID: 36980632.
27. Saifi O, Breen WG, Lester SC, et al. Don't put the CART before the horse: the role of radiation therapy in peri-CAR T-cell therapy for aggressive B-cell non-Hodgkin lymphoma. Int J Radiat Oncol Biol Phys. 2023;116(5):999–1007. PMID: 36563910.
28. Hubbeling H, Silverman EA, Michaud L, et al. Bridging radiation rapidly and effectively cytoreduces high-risk relapsed/refractory aggressive B cell lymphomas prior to chimeric antigen receptor T cell therapy. Transplant Cell Ther. 2023;29(4):259.e1–10. PMID: 36587744.
29. Ababneh HS, Ng AK, Frigault MJ, et al. Radiotherapy as a bridging strategy for patients with relapsed or refractory large B-cell lymphoma undergoing CAR T-cell therapy. Am J Hematol. 2024;99(9):1837–40. https://doi.org/10.1002/ajh.27409.
30. Roddie C, Neill L, Osborne W, et al. Effective bridging therapy can improve CD19 CAR-T outcomes while maintaining safety in patients with large B-cell lymphoma. Blood Adv. 2023;7(12):2872–83. PMID: 36724512.
31. Kuhnl A, Roddie C, Kirkwood AA, et al. Outcome and feasibility of radiotherapy bridging in large B-cell lymphoma patients receiving CD19 CAR T in the UK. Br J Haematol. 2024;205(2):483–94. https://doi.org/10.1111/bjh.19453.
32. Imber BS, Sadelain M, DeSelm C, et al. Early experience using salvage radiotherapy for relapsed/refractory non-Hodgkin lymphomas after CD19 chimeric antigen receptor (CAR) T cell therapy. Br J Haematol. 2020;190(1):45–51. PMID: 32135029.
33. Ababneh HS, Ng AK, Frigault MJ, et al. Salvage radiotherapy in relapsed/refractory large B-cell lymphoma after failure of CAR T-cell therapy. Haematologica. 2023;108(11):2972–81. PMID: 37317884.
34. Saifi O, Breen WG, Lester SC, et al. Consolidative radiotherapy for residual fluorodeoxyglucose activity on day +30 post CAR T-cell therapy in non-Hodgkin lymphoma. Haematologica. 2023;108(11):2982–92. PMID: 37317888.

The Future of RT and Immunotherapeutics (Immune Checkpoint Blockade and CAR T-Cells)

16

Carl J. DeSelm and John P. Plastaras

Contents

C. J. DeSelm
Department of Radiation Oncology, Washington University School of Medicine, St. Louis, MO, USA
e-mail: deselmc@wustl.edu

J. P. Plastaras (✉)
Department of Radiation Oncology,
Perelman School of Medicine at the University of Pennsylvania, Philadelphia, PA, USA
e-mail: plastaras@uphs.upenn.edu

C. Pinnix et al. (eds.), *Target Volume Delineation in Hematologic Malignancies*, Practical Guides in Radiation Oncology,
https://doi.org/10.1007/978-3-031-67722-9_16

Part 1: Background and Epidemiology

- Immunotherapies for cancer are on the rise. Particularly in lymphoma, it is important to distinguish between cell-based and antibody-based immunotherapy. Cell therapies rely on directly engineering anti-tumor immune cells, namely T-cells, to identify and kill targets they would not otherwise recognize. Antibody immunotherapies bind naturally expressed proteins on the surface of tumor or T-cell to facilitate T cell-mediated tumor killing.
  - Currently, US Food and Drug Administration (FDA)-approved lymphoma immunotherapies fall into two classes:
    1. Immune checkpoint inhibitor antibodies (e.g. nivolumab and pembrolizumab).
    2. Chimeric antigen receptor (CAR) T-cell therapies.
  - Other classes of molecules that similarly engage the immune response, such as bi-specific T-cell engagers, like blinatumomab are being tested in NHL [1].
  - "Immunotherapy" and "chemo-immunotherapy" have also been used to describe the use of antibodies that recognize surface proteins and engage innate immune cells, such as macrophages; however, these have multiple immune and non-immune mechanisms of action and are not included in our strict definition of immunotherapy.

    Rituximab, for example, which recognizes CD20, has been in use since the FDA approval in 1997, either alone or in combination with chemotherapy.
  - Other anti-lymphoma agents may have an immune modulation mechanism, such as lenalidomide [2], although their designed mechanism of action is not immune cell-mediated killing.
  - Because lymphoma cells arise from the immune system, classic *anti*-inflammatory molecules have also been used therapeutically, most commonly prednisone as part of CHOP combination therapy.
- The most effective immune checkpoint inhibitors tested so far in lymphoma block the PD-1 axis.
  - PD-1 is an inhibitory receptor expressed on activated T-cells that dampens further T-cell activation.
  - Blocking this interaction can "release the brakes" that tumors inevitably exert on tumor-reactive T-cells.
  - Classic Hodgkin lymphoma (cHL) is the most responsive malignancy to PD-1 inhibition compared to other solid cancers [3].

    PD-1 inhibitors have an ORR of 65–75% in refractory cHL [4, 5], with some patients experiencing long-term control of their disease, which led to the FDA approval in refractory cHL for both nivolumab and pembrolizumab in 2016 and 2017, respectively.

    Pembrolizumab was also granted approval for relapsed/refractory primary mediastinal large B-cell lymphoma (PMBCL) based on a relatively small study and somewhat less impressive ORR of ~45% [6].

- PD-1 axis inhibitors alone and in combination with other agents continue to be investigated in the lymphomas.
- CAR T cell therapies are cellular therapy agents.
  - Tumor-specific T-cells can be generated for a patient by leukapheresing and transducing their T-cells with a CAR.
  - The CAR specifies what to kill by employing an extracellular domain recognizing the tumor, an intracellular costimulatory domain (CD28 or 4-1BB), and a stimulatory (CD3 zeta) domain.
  - The first two CAR T-cell therapies approved for relapsed/refractory non-Hodgkin lymphomas differed with respect to their co-stimulatory domains. Subsequently approved CAR T-cell products have all continued to utilize one of these two co-stimulatory domains:
    - Axicabtagene ciloleucel (axi-cel) uses CD28.
    - Tisagenlecleucel uses 4-1 BB (CD137).
    - The pivotal trials supporting their FDA approvals in 2017 (axi-cel) and 2018 (tisa-cel) demonstrated ORR of 50–90% and complete response (CR) rates of 40–55% [4, 5].
- Four new immunotherapeutic agents approved for lymphomas in the span of 3 years and the role of RT combined with these agents is being explored.
  - RT was not explicitly and routinely used in the pivotal trials.
  - RT is actively being investigated with both classes of immunotherapeutics with the intent of achieving more extensive and/or longer lasting responses.
  - RT may have immune modulatory effects that may enhance the effects of immune checkpoint blockade.
    - RT has been shown to enhance the activity of molecules that target the PD-1 and CTLA4 pathways [6, 7].
    - Preclinical data have also suggested that low dose RT may enhance the activity of CAR T-cell therapy aimed at solid tumors [7].
  - Clinical experiences of CD19-directed CAR T cell therapy combined with RT have been published in the bridging setting [8–11].
  - RT after CAR T-cell therapy has suggested a potential role for RT as part of a post-CAR T cell salvage strategy [12].

Presentation and Pre-radiotherapy Imaging and Evaluation

- Since immune therapies are currently approved only for relapsed or refractory patients, the average patient is heavily pretreated with chemotherapy, with aggressive disease.
  - Prior therapies should be documented.
- See indications below for common scenarios in which radiation may benefit a patient on, or scheduled for immunotherapy.
- Genetic subtypes of lymphomas may be important for developing immune-RT strategies, including cell of origin for aggressive B cell lymphomas, myc status, and cell surface markers.

- Pre-radiation workup should include a PET/CT scan.
  - All prior imaging should be obtained to understand previous sites of disease that may have responded to prior therapies, but may be at risk for microscopic disease.
- CBC should be obtained prior to RT and monitored.
  - In particular, attention should be paid to the absolute lymphocyte count since these are the cells responsible for immune effects.

Part 2: Radiation Management and Treatment of Immunotherapy Patients

Indications

Immune Checkpoint Inhibitors

- Pembrolizumab is approved for refractory cHL, or who have relapsed after three or more prior lines of therapy, and for PMBCL or who have relapsed after two or more prior lines of therapy.
- Nivolumab is approved for adult patients with cHL that has relapsed or progressed after autologous HSCT and brentuximab vedotin, or three or more lines of systemic therapy that includes autologous HSCT.
- The decision of which agent to use may depend on the preferred dosing interval, which has evolved over time for both approved agents.
  - Pembrolizumab can be given every 3 weeks or every 6 weeks in adults.
    Or every 3 weeks in children.
  - Nivolumab can be given every 2 weeks or every 4 weeks.
  - The long half-life of these antibody-based therapies should be recognized when "sequencing" with RT, since the drugs remain after for weeks after the last dose.

Radiation with Immune Checkpoint Inhibitors

- Justifications for adding RT to immune checkpoint inhibitors include:
  - Targeting limited sites of persistent disease.
  - Targeting limited sites of progressing disease while others are stable or resolved.
  - Targeting sites of previous or current bulky disease.
  - Extended fields to include previously involved sites of disease can be considered when using a "definitive" approach (see Case 1).
  - Palliation of pain, bleeding, dysphagia, SVC syndrome, or other symptoms.
  - Controlling growth in particularly problematic or dangerous areas, such as around the great vessels, esophagus, biliary tree, major nerves, the CNS, or spinal cord.
- Although the "abscopal effect" appears to be reliably induced in some animal studies [13–17], it is not consistently elicited in humans, and thus adding radiation to immune checkpoint inhibitor therapy with the primary rationale of induc-

ing an abscopal effect or enhancing the immune therapy is still under investigation.

CAR T-Cells

- KYMRIAH™ (tisagenlecleucel or "tisa-cel") is FDA-approved for adults with relapsed or refractory diffuse large B-cell lymphoma (DLBCL), and young adult patients up to age 25 with relapsed or refractory acute lymphoblastic leukemia (ALL).
- YESCARTA™ (axicabtagene ciloleucel or "axi-cel") is FDA-approved for the following adult patients who have progressed or relapsed following two or more lines of systemic therapy:
  - DLBCL.
  - Primary mediastinal B-cell lymphoma.
  - High grade B-cell lymphoma.
  - DLBCL resulting from transformed follicular lymphoma.
- BREYANZI™ (lisocabtagene maraleucel) is FDA-approved for adult patients with relapsed or refractory large B-cell lymphoma after two or more lines of systemic therapy.
- TECARTUS™ (brexucabtagene autoleucel) is FDA-approved for patients with relapsed or refractory mantle cell lymphoma, or adult patients with relapsed or refractory B-cell precursor acute lymphoblastic leukemia (ALL).

Radiation with CAR T-Cells

- Radiation with CAR T-cell therapy may be used prior to CAR T-cells as "bridging" therapy [8, 9, 11] or in the post-CAR T-cell relapse salvage setting [12] to:
  - Target limited sites of persistent or progressive disease, or areas at high risk for recurrence or progression.
  - Palliate pain, bleeding, dysphagia, SVC syndrome, or other symptoms.
  - Control growth in particularly problematic or dangerous areas, such as around the great vessels, esophagus, biliary tree, major nerves, the CNS, or spinal cord.
- Potential other uses, demonstrated and/or suggested by retrospective reports but requiring prospective confirmation, include:
  - Improve systemic disease control through debulking [10], since overall disease burden is associated with poor lasting response to CAR T-cell therapy.
  - Decreasing post-CAR T-cell hospitalization [9].
  - Debulking disease to minimize CAR T-cell side effects [10], since disease burden is often correlated with cytokine release syndrome (CRS) and neurotoxicity.
  - Increasing the likelihood of receiving CAR T-cells by decreasing the chance of progression between leukapheresis and CAR T-cell delivery [11].

General Considerations for Radiotherapy

Target Volume

- Radiotherapy is generally delivered only to sites with pathologic, radiographic, or clinically active disease, while minimizing radiation dose to normal surrounding tissues.
- If initial sites of disease have resolved and are not suspicious for residual disease, they do not in principle need to be targeted. However, recognizing that initial sites of disease are the most common areas of recurrence, including them may be indicated depending on the perceived risk of recurrence versus additional toxicity.
- Patients should be simulated as appropriate for the treatment site and dose, with thermoplastic mask and/or custom immobilization used if delivering higher doses, head and neck treatments, reirradiation, or if the target site has nearby critical avoidance structures that would benefit from greater precision.
- IV contrast should be used if the tumor is not easily distinguished from normal tissues.
- Axial CT images should be acquired with slice thickness of 2–10 mm, depending on the level of anatomic detail desired. CT slice thickness of 2–5 mm yield excellent quality and are generally preferred. For larger fields up to 40 cm in length, a 5 mm slice is commonly used; for patients who struggle to stay in position, a 10-mm slice is generally adequate for target volumes in the bone, or for simple treatment set-ups.
- Deep inspiration breath hold (DIBH) should be considered for all sites in the thorax to minimize dose to the heart and lungs.
- For the area of active disease being targeted, creation of three target volumes are generally useful for radiation planning:
  - Currently active Gross tumor volume (GTV) as assessed by physical exam, PET, and CT, with other imaging if performed and informative.
  - Clinical target volume (CTV) which takes into consideration pre-chemotherapy GTV and assesses possible subclinical disease extension.
  - Internal target volume (ITV) which takes into account target motion and/or imprecision in breath-hold positions.
  - Planning target volume (PTV). These volumes are further described in Table 16.1.
- In certain circumstances in which the CTV includes an organ at risk, such as brainstem, optic chiasm, heart, or kidneys and in which the treating physician intends to deliver a prescription dose that exceeds the constraint for that OAR, a "boost" or "conedown" CTV may be utilized.
- Target volumes may be treated with non-planned 2D beams, 3D conformal radiation, intensity-modulated radiotherapy (IMRT), *en face* electrons, or proton therapy. Beam arrangements should be chosen to minimize dose to organs at risk.

Dose

- RT may be combined with CAR T-cells to achieve various goals:

Table 16.1 Planning target definitions for treatment of patients on immunotherapies

Volume	Description	
Gross tumor volume (GTV)	• Contains gross tumor volume as identified on diagnostic imaging (generally PET with CT) obtained within the last month	
Clinical target volume (CTV)	CTV	• Generally, 0.5–1 cm expansion from the active GTV • Excludes adjacent normal organs, bone, or anatomically contained tissues that are displaced by tumor • Should be further expanded to include adjacent tissue that previously harbored active disease, if doing so does not significantly increase toxicity • Includes consideration of the following: – Image accuracy and quality. CTV should be increased in size to account for uncertainties such as suboptimal fusion of PET or other diagnostic images to planning images – Changes in volume since the time of imaging – Adjacent organ dose constraints
	Boost or conedown CTV	• In certain circumstances in which the CTV includes an organ at risk, such as brainstem, optic chiasm, kidney, heart, etc., and in which the treating physician intends to deliver a prescription dose that exceeds the constraint for that OAR, a "boost" or "conedown" CTV may be constructed • This volume should include the initial CTV, but exclude the OARs in question, and may be prescribed to receive a higher radiation dose than the initial CTV
Internal target volume (ITV)	• In areas with internal movement such as the thorax, the ITV contains the CTV plus an internal margin that accounts for variation in CTV shape, size, and position. Reproducibility of breath-hold position can also be accounted for in an ITV	
Planning target volume (PTV)	• Contains CTV or ITV plus a margin to account for setup uncertainties associated with patient position and beam alignment • PTV expansions are patient- and institution-specific, adjusted to reflect factors unique to the patient, immobilization techniques, image guidance, and institution, but are generally 3–7 mm	
Organs at risk (OAR)	• Includes uninvolved normal nearby structures at risk of RT-related toxicity for which RT planning or dose may be altered	

– Tumor elimination, generally in higher doses, to eliminate sites of gross disease.

These may include conventional fractionation or hypofractionation approaches.

  - Conditioning, generally in lower doses, in order to help control disease burden while CAR T-cells are being manufactured or to facilitate CAR T-cell engraftment.
  - Tumor sensitization or priming, for example doses that do not eliminate disease but modulate the tumor or immune system in ways that facilitate CAR T-cell mediated tumor elimination.
- Dose regimens that may result in delay of CAR T cell delivery should be avoided.
- Although mouse models suggest hypofractionated radiation leads to more immune activation than conventional fractionation, human studies have not confirmed this, particularly in the CAR T cell scenario, so doses and fractionations most appropriate for the tumor type and goals of therapy should be used regardless of immune therapy combination.
- Common regimens for both immune checkpoint inhibitor and CAR T-cell patients range from 4 to 45 Gy in 2–25 fractions (for example, 2 Gy × 2, 4 Gy × 5 fractions, 3 Gy × 10 fractions, or 36–45 Gy conventionally fractionated).
  - The best dosing regimens for RT combined with immunotherapeutics is still evolving. Unlike SBRT for solid tumors where "ablative" doses are often used, lower BED approaches are often effective in hematologic malignancies.
  - Patient-specific considerations, such as how sensitive the patient's tumor histology is to RT, the location of disease and likelihood of future morbidity or mortality if it progressed locally, and the local organs at risk and potential toxicity of the particular regimen, and the goals of therapy, should be considered in choosing a regimen.

Timing

- Animal studies and case reports have suggested synergy between radiation and checkpoint inhibitors when the radiation is delivered, before, during, or even after the immune checkpoint inhibitor.
  - FDA-approved checkpoint inhibitors have a long half-life as they are antibodies.
- As a bridge to CAR T-cells, the most established time to treat patients with radiation is after leukapheresis and before CAR T-cell delivery, which typically provides a 2–4 week interval.
  - Radiation before leukapheresis may deplete T-cells to be collected for CAR T-cell generation.
  - Radiation after CAR T-cell delivery risks destroying the cytotoxic cells, which accumulate in tumor sites after days to weeks and persist for weeks to months, depending on the patient and CAR type.

    Tisa-cel persists longer than axi-cel due to differences in the costimulatory domains.

RT Volume

- Various RT target volumes may be employed, with the intent to treat:
  - Focal areas of gross disease.
  - Bulky sites of disease.
  - All gross disease.
  - All gross disease plus an elective volume.

- The optimal volume, and dose associated with each volume, is an active area of investigation.

Toxicity

- Immune checkpoint blockade can induce a range of autoimmune toxicities, including pneumonitis, colitis, myocarditis, hypophysitis, hepatitis, rash, acute kidney injury, and radiation recall reactions. Many of these can clinically mimic direct radiation side effects, but the mechanism is different.
- Radiation does not appear to increase the risk of immunotherapy toxicities; however, if organ damage has occurred from a checkpoint inhibitor, specific care should be taken to avoid further damage from radiation.
  - For example, radiation pneumonitis rates may be higher in patients who have had immune-related adverse events from checkpoint inhibitor treatment [18].
- Radiation before CD19 targeting CAR T-cell therapy has not increased toxicity in clinical series thus far, and radiation does not appear to affect CD19 expression levels.
  - Future CAR targets will need to be evaluated independently, particularly when expression of the target surface antigens *is* modulated by radiation.

Part 3: Cases

Case 1: Classical Hodgkin Lymphoma Patient Treated with PD-1 Inhibitor and Radiation

A 20-year old man was diagnosed with Stage IVB classical Hodgkin lymphoma, nodular sclerosis subtype with a bulky mediastinal mass and disease in the left axilla, bilateral hila, neck, and bilateral lungs. His ESR was 37 and albumin was 3.5. His international prognostic score was 3 (male, stage IV, albumin <4). His pretreatment ECHO was normal and his DLCO was 80% predicted. He underwent sperm banking. He was treated with ABVD and his PET/CT after the second cycle showed a Deauville Score 4 response. His lung lesions had completely resolved and his lymphadenopathy was much smaller but with residual uptake. Repeat PET/CT after a fourth cycle of ABVD showed increased uptake in right paratracheal and left hilar nodes as well as persistent FDG uptake in the left supraclavicular, left axillary, right hilum, and mediastinum. Biopsy of the right paratracheal node showed persistent classic Hodgkin lymphoma. He was treated with brentuximab vedotin as monotherapy salvage for two cycles. He had a Deauville Score 2 response and he underwent autologous stem cell transplant, and PET/CT showed continued complete response. He started brentuximab maintenance; however, 4 months later a PET/CT showed progressive disease in a previously involved paratracheal node and new disease in a left subpectoral and internal mammary node. He was treated with pembrolizumab and 2 months later had a complete metabolic response. He was then treated with definitive intent radiotherapy to two dose levels in 20 fractions: 30 and 36 Gy. He resumed pembrolizumab and was treated with an additional 2 years of therapy. Clinically he had remained asymptomatic until he took a 2 month break from pembrolizumab when he tested positive for SARS-Cov2. His follow-up PET/

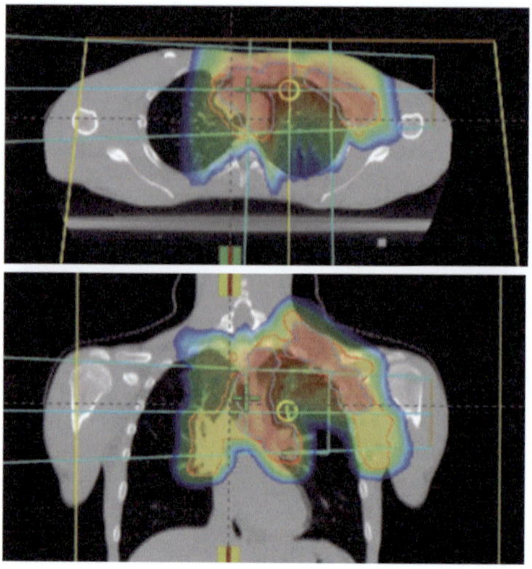

Fig. 16.1 Radiotherapy planning for Stage IVB cHL treated with multiple lines of chemotherapy and ASCT with locoregional recurrence. Diagnostic PET/CT scans from initial presentation, initial relapse, and second relapse were fused to a simulation CT to delineate all previously and recently active disease. A CTV_3600 was created by expanding the recently avid disease by 1 cm, cropping adjacent uninvolved bone, heart, and lungs. A CTV_3000 was created to include previously PET-avid disease at the time of pre-brentuximab relapse to account for potential subclinical involvement. A 5 mm margin was used to create the PTV, and the patient was treated to 30 and 36 Gy in 20 fractions using proton radiotherapy

CT scans have shown only a stable small FDG avid node in the right paratracheal region that was infield, but he has been considered in remission (Fig. 16.1).

Case 2: Stage IV DLBCL Patient with Recurrent, Metastatic Disease Post Multiple Lines of Chemotherapy, Treated with RT to a Dominant Persistent Lesion Prior to CAR T-Cells

A 77-year-old female presented with stage IV DLBCL, with features of high-risk disease including elevated Ki-67 of 95%, and non-GCB by Hans algorithm. She completed R-CHOP × 6 and intrathecal methotrexate × 4. She experienced a biopsy-proven relapse in the right femur/pelvis and left neck, and underwent R-gemcitabine/oxaliplatin with intrathecal methotrexate prophylaxis, and high-dose systemic methotrexate. After two doses of R-gemcitabine/oxaliplatin, the patient had no response and developed worsening right leg/pelvic pain with associated further local disease progression on imaging. She was then treated with high-dose cytarabine and dexamethasone with a partial response and was consented for CAR T-cells on clinical trial. Prior to CAR T-cell infusion, she was treated with consolidation RT to the dominant pelvic mass invading the sciatic nerve to 20 Gy in 5 fractions using IMRT. Ten days post radiation, CAR T-cells were delivered. Two months later, PET scan was obtained and showed a complete systemic response (Figs. 16.2 and 16.3).

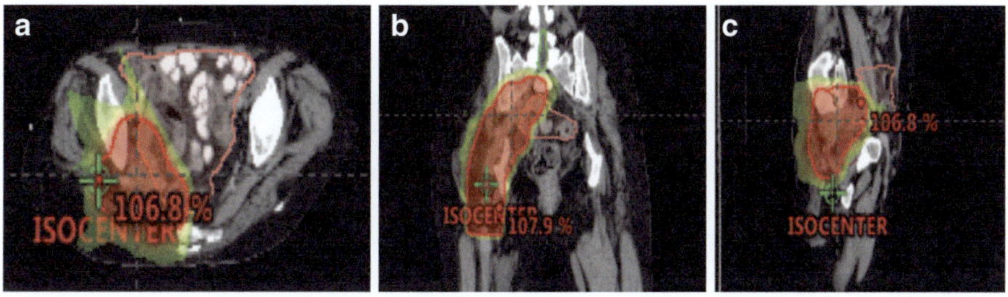

Fig. 16.2 Radiation planning for recurrent DLBCL patient with a dominant, symptomatic right pelvic/femur mass. A GTV was created to include all tumor with hypermetabolic activity, with precise borders defined by CT-defined extent of disease. A CTV was created by expanding 0.5 cm, and shaving off uninvolved bone, bowel, and muscle. A PTV (red) was created by expanding the remaining CTV 0.5 cm, and treated to 20 Gy in 5 fractions using IMRT

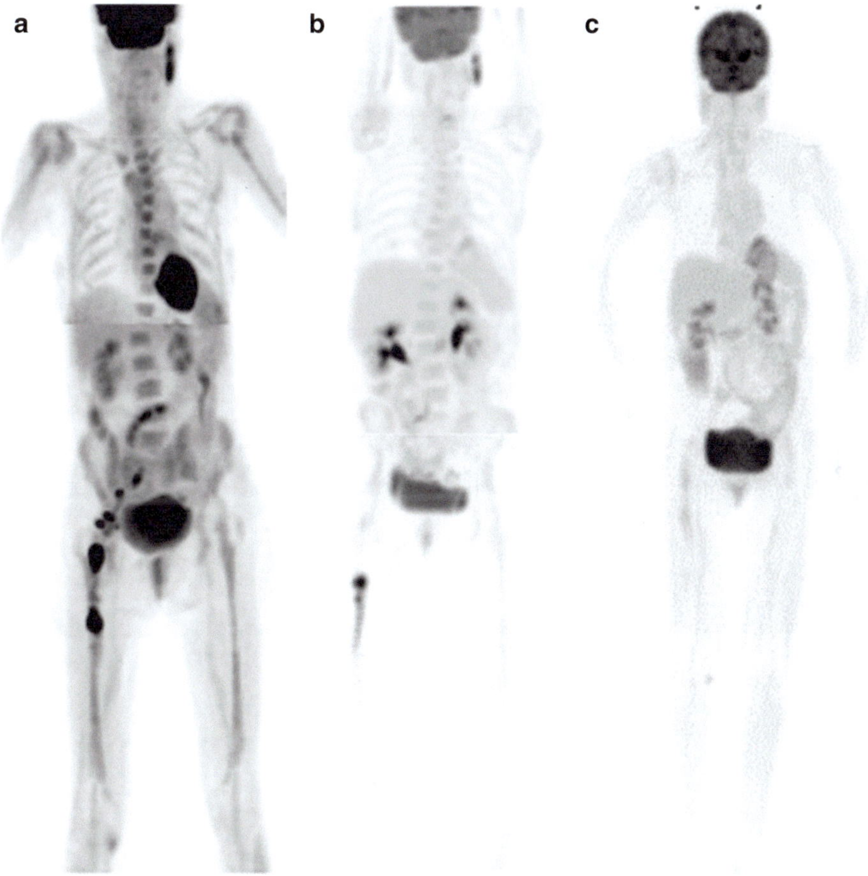

Fig. 16.3 Disease assessment before and after RT, and after CAR T-cells in relapsed, refractory DLBCL patient. After multiple chemotherapy regimens, biopsy and PET scan demonstrated disease in the right pelvis and femur, and left neck (**a**). PET scan was repeated 1 week after RT to the right pelvis/femur disease demonstrating persistent disease (**b**), then 2 months post CAR T-cells (**c**) demonstrating a complete systemic response

Part 4: Areas of Future Investigation

- Why rare patients exhibit a significant abscopal response after radiation and immune checkpoint blockade, and how to more consistently evoke such response, is unclear and remains under intense investigation.
- The optimal target volume (bulky sites of disease, all sites of disease, elective volume, total lymphoid irradiation, etc.) remains to be determined.
- Draining lymph nodes have numerous potential functions, including orchestrating an anti-tumor immune response, as well as harboring tumor cells in transit to metastasizing. The long-term systemic effects of targeting draining nodes, especially in patients receiving immune therapies, remain to be determined.
- Radiation may affect the two approved CAR T-cell products differently, given potential differences in radiation's downstream effect on CD28 or 4-1BB pathways.
- CAR T-cell patients receiving radiation may benefit from bone marrow constraints to improve hematopoietic reserve after leukapheresis, while some dose to the bone marrow may improve CAR T-cell engraftment—bone marrow constraints in CAR T-cell patients are yet to be established.
- The optimal dose and timing of radiation before CAR T-cells in humans in the context of potentially improving systemic control and decreasing CAR toxicity needs further investigation.

References

1. Goebeler ME, Knop S, Viardot A, Kufer P, Topp MS, Einsele H, et al. Bispecific T-cell engager (BiTE) antibody construct blinatumomab for the treatment of patients with relapsed/refractory non-Hodgkin lymphoma: final results from a phase I study. J Clin Oncol. 2016;34(10):1104–11.
2. Li S, Gill N, Lentzsch S. Recent advances of IMiDs in cancer therapy. Curr Opin Oncol. 2010;22(6):579–85.
3. LaRiviere MJ, Pinnix CC, Plastaras JP. Immune therapies for lymphomas: a disruptive technology with opportunities for radiation. Int J Radiat Oncol Biol Phys. 2018;102(5):1396–9.
4. Ansell SM, Lesokhin AM, Borrello I, Halwani A, Scott EC, Gutierrez M, et al. PD-1 blockade with nivolumab in relapsed or refractory Hodgkin's lymphoma. N Engl J Med. 2015;372(4):311–9.
5. Armand P, Shipp MA, Ribrag V, Michot JM, Zinzani PL, Kuruvilla J, et al. Programmed death-1 blockade with pembrolizumab in patients with classical Hodgkin lymphoma after brentuximab vedotin failure. J Clin Oncol. 2016;34(31):3733–9.
6. Dangaj D, Lanitis E, Zhao A, Joshi S, Cheng Y, Sandaltzopoulos R, et al. Novel recombinant human B7-H4 antibodies overcome tumoral immune escape to potentiate T-cell antitumor responses. Cancer Res. 2013;73(15):4820–9.
7. DeSelm C, Palomba ML, Yahalom J, Hamieh M, Eyquem J, Rajasekhar VK, et al. Low-dose radiation conditioning enables CAR T cells to mitigate antigen escape. Mol Ther. 2018;26(11):2542–52.
8. Sim AJ, Jain MD, Figura NB, Chavez JC, Shah BD, Khimani F, et al. Radiation therapy as a bridging strategy for CAR T cell therapy with axicabtagene ciloleucel in diffuse large B-cell lymphoma. Int J Radiat Oncol Biol Phys. 2019;105(5):1012–21.
9. Wright CM, LaRiviere MJ, Baron JA, Uche C, Xiao Y, Arscott WT, et al. Bridging radiation therapy prior to commercial chimeric antigen receptor T-cell therapy for relapsed/refractory aggressive B-cell lymphoma. Int J Radiat Oncol Biol Phys. 2020;108:178.

10. Qu C, Ping N, Kang L, Liu H, Qin S, Wu Q, et al. Radiation priming chimeric antigen receptor T-cell therapy in relapsed/refractory diffuse large B-cell lymphoma with high tumor burden. J Immunother. 2020;43(1):32–7.
11. Pinnix CC, Gunther JR, Dabaja BS, Strati P, Fang P, Hawkins MC, et al. Bridging therapy prior to axicabtagene ciloleucel for relapsed/refractory large B-cell lymphoma. Blood Adv. 2020;4(13):2871–83.
12. Imber BS, Sadelain M, DeSelm C, Batlevi C, Brentjens RJ, Dahi PB, et al. Early experience using salvage radiotherapy for relapsed/refractory non-Hodgkin lymphomas after CD19 chimeric antigen receptor (CAR) T cell therapy. Br J Haematol. 2020;190:45.
13. Dovedi SJ, Adlard AL, Lipowska-Bhalla G, McKenna C, Jones S, Cheadle EJ, et al. Acquired resistance to fractionated radiotherapy can be overcome by concurrent PD-L1 blockade. Cancer Res. 2014;74(19):5458–68.
14. Honeychurch J, Glennie MJ, Johnson PW, Illidge TM. Anti-CD40 monoclonal antibody therapy in combination with irradiation results in a CD8 T-cell-dependent immunity to B-cell lymphoma. Blood. 2003;102(4):1449–57.
15. Twyman-Saint Victor C, Rech AJ, Maity A, Rengan R, Pauken KE, Stelekati E, et al. Radiation and dual checkpoint blockade activate non-redundant immune mechanisms in cancer. Nature. 2015;520(7547):373–7.
16. Dovedi SJ, Melis MH, Wilkinson RW, Adlard AL, Stratford IJ, Honeychurch J, et al. Systemic delivery of a TLR7 agonist in combination with radiation primes durable antitumor immune responses in mouse models of lymphoma. Blood. 2013;121(2):251–9.
17. Dovedi SJ, Lipowska-Bhalla G, Beers SA, Cheadle EJ, Mu L, Glennie MJ, et al. Antitumor efficacy of radiation plus immunotherapy depends upon dendritic cell activation of effector CD8+ T cells. Cancer Immunol Res. 2016;4(7):621–30.
18. Shaverdian N, Beattie J, Thor M, Offin M, Shepherd AF, Gelblum DY, et al. Safety of thoracic radiotherapy in patients with prior immune-related adverse events from immune checkpoint inhibitors. Ann Oncol. 2020;31(12):1719–24.

MIX
Papier aus verantwortungsvollen Quellen
Paper from responsible sources
FSC® C105338

If you have any concerns about our products,
you can contact us on
ProductSafety@springernature.com

In case Publisher is established outside the EU,
the EU authorized representative is:
Springer Nature Customer Service Center GmbH
Europaplatz 3, 69115 Heidelberg, Germany

Printed by Libri Plureos GmbH
in Hamburg, Germany

SpringerBriefs in Mathematical Physics

Volume 55

SpringerBriefs are characterized in general by their size (50–125 pages) and fast production time (2–3 months compared to 6 months for a monograph).

Briefs are available in print but are intended as a primarily electronic publication to be included in Springer's e-book package.

Typical works might include:

- An extended survey of a field
- A link between new research papers published in journal articles
- A presentation of core concepts that doctoral students must understand in order to make independent contributions
- Lecture notes making a specialist topic accessible for non-specialist readers.

SpringerBriefs in Mathematical Physics showcase, in a compact format, topics of current relevance in the field of mathematical physics. Published titles will encompass all areas of theoretical and mathematical physics. This series is intended for mathematicians, physicists, and other scientists, as well as doctoral students in related areas.

Tamiaki Yoneya

Introduction to Nambu's Generalized Hamiltonian Dynamics

Springer

Tamiaki Yoneya
Institute of Physics
The University of Tokyo
Komaba, Meguro-ku, Tokyo, Japan

ISSN 2197-1757 ISSN 2197-1765 (electronic)
SpringerBriefs in Mathematical Physics
ISBN 978-981-95-7029-4 ISBN 978-981-95-7030-0 (eBook)
https://doi.org/10.1007/978-981-95-7030-0

Mathematics Subject Classification: 70, 34, 37, 76, 49, 81

This Springer imprint is published by the registered company Springer Nature Singapore Pte Ltd.
The registered company address is: 152 Beach Road, #21-01/04 Gateway East, Singapore 189721, Singapore

Preface

In a remarkable paper published in 1973, Nambu proposed generalization of Hamiltonian dynamics to extended phase spaces of arbitrary dimensions including odd dimensions. Though Nambu had not participated in developing this work further, several important works appeared following his inspiring proposal. It also gradually turned out that structures similar to that of Nambu dynamics could play roles in various areas of theoretical physics: for instance, in theoretical particle physics, the relativistic theories of strings and higher-dimensional objects such as membranes naturally led us to the Nambu-bracket structure, an extension of the usual Poisson-bracket structure, in formulating dynamics and underlying symmetries. In other areas such as fluid or plasma physics in which various vortical structures are ubiquitous, the Nambu-bracket, being closely connected with vorticity, has also been recognized similarly to be a useful concept.

Nobody would deny the significance of Nambu dynamics in that, at the very least, it exhibits a characteristic possibility of extended dynamical systems equipped with more than one conserved quantity in such a way that they govern the time evolution of systems on an equal footing. It also suggests, as Nambu himself had anticipated in his original paper, an extended framework for statistical mechanics in which statistical ensembles are characterized in equilibrium by many temperatures. Such structures might become important in some unexpected manner in both micro and macro domains of the natural world. We should not dismiss such intriguing possibilities.

The purpose of this small monograph is, firstly, to introduce the reader to Nambu dynamics by providing a pedagogical account on the principal aspects of *classical* Nambu dynamics and, secondly, to scrutinize and hopefully develop it further from a coherent and unified standpoint: in particular, a special emphasis will be put on the role of the underlying symmetries. To facilitate understanding of the main contents for a broad spectrum of the readers, I use plain technical notations and terminologies, being familiar in traditional theoretical physics, and emphasize analogies with some key elements of conventional Hamiltonian dynamics in order to motivate corresponding developments for Nambu dynamics. Whenever use is made of unfamiliar mathematical nomenclatures for the sake of convenience, explanation of their meanings will be added appropriately.

Chapter 1 is devoted to a historical overview, summarizing the main streams of developments from Hamiltonian dynamics to Nambu dynamics. The Chaps. 2 and 3 constitute the core of this monograph, for which I take a constructive approach in a self-contained manner consistently, starting anew with basic elements and developing them gradually in accord with naturally emerging logical steps; in particular, preference is given to clarity in the sense of physics rather than mathematical rigor and completeness, and, of course, effort will also be made to maintain balance with the latter aspects as far as possible. By so doing, I hope that some interesting new perspectives, physical pictures, and novel interpretations may be gained even though sometimes the final formulae themselves might not be new.

Reflecting these features, no reference to the literature is given in the main text; instead, the final Chap. 4, 'Bibliographical Remarks', is devoted to a brief guide to selected references. Needless to say, the literature is vast, and the selection is necessarily subjective. My intention in adding this chapter is also to make some brief comments, situating the position of Nambu dynamics and Nambu brackets in a historical but broader perspective through the literature, on various interconnections among various different areas of research as a complement to the description given in the first chapter.

Another somewhat unusual feature of the present exposition, from a stylistic viewpoint, is that figures and tables are treated as cousins to equations and are immersed harmoniously as such in the text with only minimal captions, so that the readers will be able to integrate them with the main text and the equations.

Thus from the viewpoints of both contents and style, this book is *not* intended to be a status report or review in any sense. The requirements for the readers are a reasonable mastery of conventional classical analytical dynamics, and working knowledge of basic physics and standard mathematical methods of analysis, algebra, and geometry, etc. at a level of first-year graduate students in theoretical physics. For deeper understanding of some aspects of applications and extensions, experience and knowledge of some elementary aspects of quantum field theory might also be helpful.

I wish to thank Spenta Wadia for reading through the manuscript and making valuable comments and also to the referees for pointing out many typos as well as for useful and supportive suggestions.

Finally, I would like to dedicate this book to the memory of Yoichiro Nambu, from whom I constantly received precious inspiration and stimulation.

Komaba, Meguro-ku, Japan Tamiaki Yoneya
July 2025

Contents

Chapter 1
Introduction: Historical Overview and Basic Concepts

1.1 Hamiltonian Dynamics: Its Origin and the Basic Properties

Hamiltonian dynamics is the most advanced form of classical dynamics. It was introduced by William Rowan Hamilton in the mid 1830s. The equations of motion in Lagrangian dynamics are expressed in general as differential equations of second order,

$$\frac{d}{dt}\Big(\frac{\partial L}{\partial \dot{q}_i}\Big) - \frac{\partial L}{\partial q_i} = 0 \quad (i = 1, 2, \ldots, n),$$

in n-dimensional configuration space with the generalized coordinates $(q_1, q_2, \ldots, q_n)$. The Lagrangian $L = L(\dot{q}_1, \dot{q}_2, \ldots, \dot{q}_n, q_1, q_2, \ldots, q_n)$ is a function of the generalized coordinates q_i and the corresponding velocities $\dot{q}_i \equiv \frac{dq_i}{dt}$ as independent variables.[1] In ordinary Hamiltonian dynamics starting with a given Lagrangian, one defines generalized momentum variables p_i by $p_i \equiv \frac{\partial L}{\partial \dot{q}_i}$, and the Hamilton equations of motion take a particular form of $2n$ differential equations of first order as

$$\frac{dq_i}{dt} = \frac{\partial H}{\partial p_i}, \quad \frac{dp_i}{dt} = -\frac{\partial H}{\partial q_i}.$$

The space of $2n$ dimensions where the independent dynamical coordinates consist of $(p_1, p_2, \ldots, p_n, q_1, q_2, \ldots, q_n)$ is called phase space. The Hamilton function (or Hamiltonian) H as a function on phase space is derived from the Lagrangian $L(\dot{q}, q)$ by applying a Legendre transformation:

$$H = \sum_{i=1}^{n} p_i \dot{q}_i - L = H(p_1, p_2, \ldots, p_n, q_1, q_2, \ldots, q_n),$$

[1] Here and in what follows we use the symbol '≡' for equality which itself gives a definition.

T. Yoneya, *Introduction to Nambu's Generalized Hamiltonian Dynamics*,
SpringerBriefs in Mathematical Physics 55,
https://doi.org/10.1007/978-981-95-7030-0_1

where the velocity variables $\{\dot{q}_i\}$ are solved in terms of $\{q_i\}$ and $\{p_i\}$. In this formalism, the Hamiltonian is manifestly a constant of motion:

$$\frac{dH}{dt} = \sum_{i=1}^{n} \left[\frac{dq_i}{dt}\frac{\partial H}{\partial q_i} + \frac{dp_i}{dt}\frac{\partial H}{\partial p_i} \right] = 0.$$

Thus the trajectory of a particle obeying the Hamilton equations of motion always lies on the hyper-surface (called the *level surface*) of $2n-1$ dimensions defined by $H(p, q) = E$ with a constant E, 'energy', which is determined by the initial values with respect to the phase space coordinates at $t = 0$. It is also possible to reverse the role of the Lagrangian and Hamiltonian: starting with the Hamiltonian and the Hamilton equations of motion, we can just define a Lagrangian $L = \sum_{i=1}^{n} p_i \dot{q}_i - H$. Provided that the velocity variables are solvable in terms of the generalized coordinates and momenta, both formalisms are completely equivalent.

Jacobi developed Hamiltonian dynamics into the canonical formalism in which the time evolution of a dynamical system is formulated in terms of canonical transformations of $2n$ coordinates

$$(p_1, p_2, \ldots, p_n, q_1, q_2, \ldots, q_n) \rightarrow (P_1, P_2, \ldots, P_n, Q_1, Q_2, \ldots, Q_n)$$

in phase space, which preserve the form of the Hamilton equations of motion. A canonical transformation in general is characterized by the requirements

$$\{P_i, Q_j\} = \delta_{ij}, \quad \{Q_i, Q_j\} = 0 = \{P_i, P_j\}, \tag{1.1}$$

where

$$\{A, B\} \equiv \sum_{i=1}^{n} \left(\frac{\partial A}{\partial p_i}\frac{\partial B}{\partial q_i} - \frac{\partial B}{\partial p_i}\frac{\partial A}{\partial q_i} \right) = -\{B, A\}$$

is the Poisson bracket. By definition, the Poisson bracket satisfies the Jacobi identity

$$\{\{A, B\}, C\} + \{\{B, C\}, A\} + \{\{C, A\}, B\} = 0,$$

for three arbitrary functions, A, B and C, of the canonical variables.

Using the Poisson bracket, the equations of motion for an arbitrary function $F = F(p, q)$ in phase space are expressed succinctly as

$$\dot{F} = \sum_i \left(\frac{\partial F}{\partial p_i}\dot{p}_i + \frac{\partial F}{\partial q_i}\dot{q}_i \right) = \{H, F\}. \tag{1.2}$$

In general, any infinitesimal canonical transformation, $F \rightarrow F + \delta F$, takes the form

$$\delta F = \delta_G F \equiv \{G, F\} \tag{1.3}$$

with a corresponding infinitesimal generating function $G = G(q, p)$. Thus the equations of motion are indeed a special case of infinitesimal canonical transformations with H being the generating function.

Now, considering the time derivative of the Poisson bracket of two arbitrary functions F_1 and F_2, we have

$$\frac{d}{dt}\{F_1, F_2\} = \{H, \{F_1, F_2\}\}.$$

If we assume that the derivation with respect to time is commutative with the Poisson bracket operation, the left-hand side of this equation can also be written using the Leibniz rule of the time derivative as

$$\frac{d}{dt}\{F_1, F_2\} = \{\dot{F}_1, F_2\} + \{F_1, \dot{F}_2\} = \{\{H, F_1\}, F_2\} + \{F_1, \{H, F_2\}\}.$$

Identifying the results of these two expressions, we observe conversely that the Jacobi identity ensures the commutativity of time evolution and Poisson bracket operation. In particular, applying the Jacobi identity to (1.1), we have

$$\begin{aligned}\frac{d}{dt}\{P_i, Q_j\} &= \{\{H, P_i\}, Q_j\} + \{P_i, \{H, Q_j\}\} \\ &= \{H, \{P_i, Q_j\}\} = 0, \quad \text{similarly for } \{Q_i, Q_j\} \text{ and } \{P_i, P_j\}.\end{aligned}$$

Hence, the canonical Poisson brackets are consistently preserved under the time evolution.

An infinitesimal canonical transformation in the above form can also be interpreted as a specific linear differential operator D_G acting on the space of arbitrary functions in phase space:

$$\delta_G F = D_G F, \quad D_G \equiv \sum_{i=1}^{n} \left(\frac{\partial G}{\partial p_i} \frac{\partial}{\partial q_i} - \frac{\partial G}{\partial q_i} \frac{\partial}{\partial p_i} \right). \tag{1.4}$$

The Jacobi identity for the Poisson bracket is then equivalent to that of the Lie algebra satisfied by commutators $[\cdot, \cdot]$ among these linear differential operators:

$$[D_A, D_B] = D_{\{A,B\}}, \tag{1.5}$$

since by definition we have $D_A D_B C = D_A\{B, C\} = \{A, \{B, C\}\}$ for three arbitrary functions A, B and C, and

$$[D_A, [D_B, D_C]] + [D_B, [D_C, D_A]] + [D_C, [D_A, D_B]] = 0.$$

The canonical formalism culminated in the Hamilton-Jacobi theory, where dynamics is reduced to a non-linear partial differential equation of first order

$$\frac{\partial S}{\partial t} = -H\left(\frac{\partial S}{\partial q_1}, \frac{\partial S}{\partial q_2}, \ldots, \frac{\partial S}{\partial q_n}, q_1, q_2, \ldots, q_n\right) \tag{1.6}$$

for a single time-dependent function $S = S(q_1, q_2, \ldots, q_n, t)$ of the generalized coordinates. This is called the Hamilton–Jacobi equation. The function S was originally called the Hamilton's *principal function*, and, in modern terminology, the action function, since it can be defined as the action integral, $S(q, t) = \int_{t_0}^{t} L(\dot{q}(s), q(s))ds$, along the trajectory $q_i(s)$ which is uniquely determined as a function of (q, t) by the condition that it satisfies the equations of motion and ends at $q_i = q_i(t)$ with a *fixed* initial condition $q_i(t_0) \equiv Q_i$. The momentum variables are then given by

$$p_i = \frac{\partial S}{\partial q_i}. \tag{1.7}$$

When time dependence is separated by setting $S(q, t) = \bar{S}(q) - E(t - t_0)$ with a constant energy E and $\bar{S}(q) = \int_Q^q \sum_i p_i(s)dq_i(s)$, the Hamilton–Jacobi equation takes a time-independent form,

$$H\left(\frac{\partial \bar{S}}{\partial q_1}, \ldots, \frac{\partial \bar{S}}{\partial q_n}, q_1, \ldots, q_n\right) = E. \tag{1.8}$$

This particular form, together with the fact that ordinarily $H\ (= \frac{|\boldsymbol{p}|^2}{2m} + V)$ is quadratic in p_i, suggests a geometrical interpretation that the paths of motions are something like light rays traversing wave surfaces. In the so-called 'geometrical optics', the wave surfaces are characterized by a function $W(\boldsymbol{x})$ in real 3-dimensional space ($(q_1, q_2, q_3) = \boldsymbol{x}$): its gradient ∇W gives the tangent vectors along light rays, expressing Huygens' principle, and satisfies the analog of (1.8),

$$(\nabla W)^2 = 1/v_w^2, \tag{1.9}$$

where $v_w = c/n$ is the light velocity in the medium with $n = n(\boldsymbol{x})$ being its refractive index. Historically, Hamilton conceived of his theory on the basis of this analogy and developed geometrical treatments of both optical rays and mechanics in parallel. The optical analogy also played a primordial role in developing variational principles in classical dynamics. In fact, the historical origin of the variational principles goes back to Fermat's principle that amounts to minimizing the integral $\int n(\boldsymbol{x})d|\boldsymbol{x}|$ along light paths. In the realm of dynamics, Fermat's principle was transformed into the principle of least action (also known as Maupertuis' principle) most notably by Jacobi.

The action function $S(q, t; Q)$, dependent on n independent parameters Q_i ($i = 1, \ldots, n$), can be interpreted as a generating function of *finite* time-dependent canonical transformations $(q, p) \to (Q, P)$ which unfold the time evolution in reverse (i.e., $\dot{Q}_i = 0 = \dot{P}_i$), sending the Hamiltonian function H to zero:

$$\sum_{i=1}^{n} p_i dq_i - H dt = \sum_{i=1}^{n} P_i dQ_i - H' dt + dS, \quad H' = 0, \tag{1.10}$$

yielding the Hamilton–Jacobi Eqs. (1.7) + (1.6), and also

$$\frac{\partial S}{\partial Q_i} = -P_i, \tag{1.11}$$

which we call the 'Jacobi condition', for convenience, since the differential relation (1.10) is often called Jacobi's theorem. Conversely, finding a *complete solution*

$$S = S(q_1, q_2, \ldots, q_n, t; Q_1, Q_2, \ldots, Q_n) \tag{1.12}$$

of the Hamilton–Jacobi equation with n integration constants Q_i amounts to solving the equations of motion. Namely, we regard (1.11) as n independent algebraic equations which implicitly determine the generalized coordinates q_i as the general solution of the Hamilton equations of motion, $q_i = q_i(t; Q_1, Q_2, \ldots, Q_n, P_1, P_2, \ldots, P_n)$, with $2n$ arbitrary integration constants (Q_i, P_i) under the condition

$$\det\left(\frac{\partial^2 S}{\partial Q_i \partial q_j}\right) \neq 0. \tag{1.13}$$

Through (1.7), the generalized momenta p_i are then given also as functions of time $p_i = p_i(t; Q_1, Q_2, \ldots, Q_n, P_1, P_2, \ldots, P_n)$.

Here, we briefly recapitulate how the equations of motion follow from the Hamilton–Jacobi equation *under* the Jacobi condition: since (1.11) must be valid independently of time, we have

$$\begin{aligned} 0 = \frac{d}{dt}\frac{\partial S}{\partial Q_i} &= \frac{\partial^2 S}{\partial t \partial Q_i} + \sum_{j=1}^{n} \frac{\partial^2 S}{\partial Q_i \partial q_j}\frac{dq_j}{dt} \\ &= -\frac{\partial H}{\partial Q_i} + \sum_{j=1}^{n} \frac{\partial^2 S}{\partial Q_i \partial q_j}\frac{dq_j}{dt} \\ &= -\sum_{j=1}^{n}\left(\frac{\partial H}{\partial p_j}\frac{\partial S}{\partial q_j \partial Q_i} - \frac{\partial^2 S}{\partial Q_i \partial q_j}\frac{dq_j}{dt}\right), \end{aligned}$$

which yields, under the condition (1.13),

$$\dot{q}_i = \frac{\partial H}{\partial p_i}. \tag{1.14}$$

On the other hand, due to (1.7), we also have

$$\dot{p}_i = \frac{\partial p_i}{\partial t} + \sum_{j=1}^{n} \frac{\partial p_i}{\partial q_j}\frac{dq_i}{dt} = \frac{\partial^2 S}{\partial q_i \partial t} + \sum_{j=1}^{n} \frac{\partial^2 S}{\partial q_j \partial q_i}\frac{dq_i}{dt}$$

$$= -\frac{\partial H}{\partial q_i} - \sum_{j=1}^{n} \frac{\partial H}{\partial p_j}\frac{\partial^2 S}{\partial q_i \partial q_j} + \sum_{j=1}^{n} \frac{\partial^2 S}{\partial q_j \partial q_i}\frac{dq_i}{dt} = -\frac{\partial H}{\partial q_i},$$

where in the last equality use has been made of (1.14).

1.2 From Hamiltonian Dynamics to Quantum Mechanics and Statistical Mechanics

The canonical formalism prepared the foundations for developing quantum mechanics in 1925–1926: Hamilton's equations of motion in terms of Poisson brackets led to 'Matrix' mechanics (Heisenberg, Born–Jordan–Heisenberg, ...), while the Hamilton-Jacobi equation in terms of the action function to 'Wave' mechanics (de Broglie, Schrödinger, ...). These two approaches were soon unified by Dirac's 'transformation' theory.

In quantum mechanics, the classical (finite) canonical transformations are turned into unitary transformations in an infinite-dimensional (Hilbert) space of all possible quantum states. The Hilbert space may be regarded as an extension of an infinite-dimensional space of functions on the classical phase space, at least in a partial sense. In this framework, a dynamical variable in classical theory becomes a Hermitian operator, which, upon exponentiation, generate a unitary transformation. Thus the time evolution (Heisenberg equation or Schrödinger equation) in quantum mechanics is also a unitary transformation. The Heisenberg equation is obtained by replacing the Poisson brackets (multiplied by $i/\hbar$) between the dynamical variables and the Hamiltonian with the commutators of the corresponding operators. Similarly, the Schrödinger equation is obtained by replacing the role of action function $S(q,t)$ with wave function $\Psi(q,t)$ which, in the limit of vanishing Planck constant $\hbar \to 0$, is approximated as $\Psi(q,t) \simeq e^{iS(q,t)/\hbar} = e^{i(\bar{S}(q)-Et)/\hbar}$. Thus, the action function $S(q,t)$ now becomes literally the phase function for the 'matter wave'.

Furthermore, Feynman proposed the path-integral formulation in 1948 as yet another possible approach to quantum mechanics in a rather intuitive fashion. A precursor to Feynman's path-integral was Dirac's observation, made much earlier in 1932, that a generic short-time transition amplitude in quantum mechanics can be expressed approximately in the form $\langle q(t+\Delta t)|q(t)\rangle \simeq \exp iL(q,\dot{q})\Delta t/\hbar$. Both in Lagrangian and Hamiltonian approaches, path integrals can be regarded as an extended version of classical variational principles: in the limit $\hbar \to 0$, path integrals invariably reduce to the evolutions along classical paths characterized by the variational equations corresponding to

$$\delta \int L(\dot{q}, q)dt = 0, \quad \text{or,} \quad \delta \int \big(p\dot{q} - H(p, q)\big)dt = 0,$$

yielding directly the Lagrangian or Hamiltonian equations of motion, respectively.

On the other hand, we should also remember that Hamiltonian formalism provides a crucial conceptual foundation of statistical mechanics, both classically and quantum mechanically, through Liouville's theorem. At the beginning of the twentieth century, the standard framework of statistical mechanics was formulated in a general way by Gibbs, and independently by young Einstein, on the basis of Hamiltonian formalism by extending various results which Maxwell and Boltzmann previously had achieved in the latter half of the nineteenth century. They focused their considerations on ensembles consisting of a large number of identical Hamiltonian systems with $2n$ degrees of freedom. The physical quantities of interests are then the statistical distributions of states of member systems in the ensemble. They are described by a density function $\rho(q, p, t)$ in phase space. If we follow the trajectories of phase points in time evolution, Liouville's theorem says that the density function $\rho\big(q, p, t\big)$ satisfies $\frac{\partial\rho}{\partial t} + \{H, \rho\} = 0$. Given a distribution function, any macroscopic observable F is described by the expectation value of an appropriate function $F(q, p)$ on phase space corresponding to the observable F: it is expressed as a statistical average (usually called the ensemble average) over all possible states in phase space, using the density function,

$$\langle F\rangle(t) = \int F(p, q)\rho(p, q, t)d^n q d^n p$$

under the normalization condition $1 = \int \rho(p, q, t)d^n q d^n p$. In statistical equilibrium, a macroscopic states correspond to a stationary density function satisfying $\frac{\partial\rho}{\partial t} = 0$, and hence must obey $\{H, \rho\} = 0$. In quantum statistical mechanics, the Poisson bracket here is replaced by the commutator between the corresponding operators.

Provided that the *average* energy of the whole systems constituting an ensemble is fixed to be a given numerical value E, the most probable distribution with maximum entropy is given by the canonical (or generalized Maxwell–Boltzmann) distribution

$$\rho(p, q) = \exp\big(\alpha - H(p, q)/T\big)$$

with α being fixed by the normalization condition, and the absolute temperature T is determined such that $\langle H\rangle = E$ holds.

We have now essentially finished giving a minimum overview of the historical backgrounds for Nambu's proposal of generalized Hamiltonian formalism.

1.3 Nambu's Generalized Hamiltonian Dynamics

1.3.1 Notational Preparation

As a preparation for proceeding to Nambu's proposal, we update our notations of the phase-space coordinates by defining

$$\{x^i\,;\,(x^1,\ldots,x^{2n})\equiv(p_1,q_1,p_2,q_2\ldots,p_n,q_n)\},$$

namely, $2n$ phase-space coordinates x^i with upper indices. Using the traditional language of differential geometry that is familiar in general relativity theory, we treat these coordinates as the components of a *contravariant* vector which transform as $\tilde{x}^i=\sum_{j=1}^{2n}A^i{}_j x^j$ under a linear coordinate transformation $x^i\to\tilde{x}^i=\tilde{x}^i(x)$, or more generally

$$d\tilde{x}^i=\sum_{j=1}^{2n}\frac{\partial\tilde{x}^i}{\partial x^j}dx^j$$

under a general coordinate transformation $x^i\to\tilde{x}^i(x)$. Note here that both x^i and $\tilde{x}^i$ physically represent one and the same point in phase space. In other words, the transformation changes only the coordinate frames. By this convention we can express the differential operator (1.4) in the form

$$D_H\equiv\sum_{i=1}^{2n}X^i(x)\frac{\partial}{\partial x^i},\tag{1.15}$$

where we introduced the abbreviations

$$X^{2i-1}(x)=-\frac{\partial H}{\partial q_i},\quad X^{2i}(x)=\frac{\partial H}{\partial p_i},\quad (i=1,\ldots,n).$$

The coefficient functions $X^i(x)$'s as the components of a contravariant vector field give the Hamilton equations of motion

$$\frac{dx^i}{dt}=X^i(x),\quad (i=1,\ldots,2n).$$

Geometrically, the vector $X^i(x)$ is tangent to the trajectory of a particle at each point x^i in the $2n$-dimensional phase space. With a generic vector function $X^i(x)$, this is a general form of first-order differential equations for the phase coordinates.

As we shall discuss later in detail, Liouville's theorem is equivalent to the divergence-less condition for the coefficient functions $X^i(x)$,

$$\sum_{i=1}^{2n} \frac{\partial X^i(x)}{\partial x^i} = \sum_{i=1}^{n} \left[\frac{\partial}{\partial q_i} \frac{\partial H}{\partial p_i} - \frac{\partial}{\partial p_i} \frac{\partial H}{\partial q_i} \right] = 0. \tag{1.16}$$

For partial derivatives with respect to the phase-space coordinates x^is, we often use a familiar abbreviation as $\partial_i \equiv \frac{\partial}{\partial x^i}$. In dealing with the products of any generic vectors or tensors, Einstein's summation convention for repeated indices is assumed, such as $\partial_i X^i \equiv \sum_i \partial_i X^i$, $D_H = X^i \partial_i$, etc., in what follows. The lower indices in general indicate that they transform as a *covariant* vector, $\tilde{\partial}_i = \frac{\partial x^j}{\partial \tilde{x}^i} \partial_j$. The contraction of a pair of upper and lower indices automatically gives a scalar as in these examples. It is to be noted that in classical Hamiltonian dynamics, the phase space is assumed geometrically to be an ordinary flat Euclidean space with metric $ds^2 = dx_i dx^i$, the metric tensor being the Kronecker's delta symbol, $g_{ij} = g^{ij} = \delta^i_j$ in terms of the Cartesian coordinates $\{x^i\}$.

1.3.2 The Nambu Equations of Motion

In the simplest nontrivial case of 3-dimensional phase space $\left(x^1(t), x^2(t), x^3(t)\right)$, the Nambu equations of motion take the form

$$\frac{dx^i(t)}{dt} = X^i\bigl(x(t)\bigr), \quad X^i(x) = \epsilon^{ijk} \frac{\partial K}{\partial x^j} \frac{\partial H}{\partial x^k}, \tag{1.17}$$

being equipped with two 'Hamiltonians' $H = H(x^1, x^2, x^3)$, $K = K(x^1, x^2, x^3)$, where the symbol ϵ^{ijk} is the Levi–Civita tensor in three dimensions, which is completely antisymmetric (or often termed, *skew* symmetric) under any permutations of indices $(1 = \epsilon^{123} = \epsilon^{231} = \epsilon^{312} = -\epsilon^{213} = -\epsilon^{132} = -\epsilon^{321})$. Obviously, the coefficient functions X^i identically satisfy the condition $\partial_i X^i = 0$. We called both the functions H and K 'Hamiltonians', since they together describe the motion of a particle on an equal footing and both are conserved: $\dot{H} = \dot{K} = 0$.

In what follows, for convenience, we call any degrees of freedom obeying the equations of the type (1.17) a *Nambu particle*. A Nambu particle moves along a fixed curve which is the intersection of two level surfaces defined by $H = c$ and $K = c'$ with two independent constants c and c' determined by the initial condition $\bigl(x^1(0), x^2(0), x^3(0)\bigr)$.

To explain the motivation behind his proposal, it is perhaps best to quote his own words verbatim in the very beginning of his original paper :

> A notable feature of the Hamiltonian description of classical dynamics is the Liouville theorem which states that the volume of phase space occupied by an ensemble of systems is conserved. The theorem plays, among others, a fundamental role in statistical mechanics. On the other hand, Hamiltonian dynamics is not the only formalism that makes a statistical mechanics possible. Any set of equations which lead to a Liouville theory in a suitably defined phase space will do (provided of course that ergodicity may be assumed).

Thus his main motivation was to seek a new generalized dynamical system satisfying Liouville's theorem. His hope was that it might be a natural starting point for constructing a generalized statistical mechanics which involves two or more Hamiltonians, and correspondingly two or more temperatures, on an equal footing.

In fact, the above form of the equations of motion can be generalized immediately to phase spaces $(x^1, x^2, \ldots, x^n)$ of *any* dimensions n by introducing $n-1$ independent Hamiltonians, $H_1, H_2, \ldots, H_{n-1}$:

$$\frac{dx^i}{dt} = X^i(x), \quad X^i(x) = \epsilon^{ij_1 j_2 \ldots j_{n-1}} \frac{\partial H_1}{\partial x^{j_1}} \frac{\partial H_2}{\partial x^{j_2}} \cdots \frac{\partial H_{n-1}}{\partial x^{j_{n-1}}}, \tag{1.18}$$

satisfying $\partial_i X^i = 0$ and $\dot{H}_i = 0$, where $\epsilon^{ij_1 j_2 \ldots j_{n-1}}$ is the n-dimensional Levi–Civita tensor. The trajectory of a Nambu particle then lies on an intersection of $n-1$ level hyper-surfaces defined by $H_i = E_i$ $(i = 1, \ldots, n-1)$, always resulting in a one-dimensional curve embedded in n-dimensional phase space.

As a justification of his proposal, Nambu pointed out that the familiar Euler equations of motion,

$$\begin{aligned}
\frac{dL_1}{dt} &= -\left(\frac{1}{I_2} - \frac{1}{I_3}\right) L_2 L_3, \\
\frac{dL_2}{dt} &= -\left(\frac{1}{I_3} - \frac{1}{I_1}\right) L_3 L_1, \\
\frac{dL_3}{dt} &= -\left(\frac{1}{I_1} - \frac{1}{I_2}\right) L_1 L_2,
\end{aligned}$$

for a free rigid rotator with a single fixed point, using the body-fixed coordinates, indeed take the form (1.17) with

$$K = \frac{1}{2}(L_1^2 + L_2^2 + L_3^2), \tag{1.19}$$

$$H = \frac{1}{2}\left(\frac{L_1^2}{I_1} + \frac{L_2^2}{I_2} + \frac{L_3^2}{I_3}\right), \tag{1.20}$$

provided that the components L_i of the angular momentum as the collective coordinates for a rigid body are identified *effectively* with the phase-space coordinates x^i of a Nambu particle. In the ordinary approach to canonical formalism for a rotating rigid body, we construct the Hamiltonian (H), starting with the Euler angles as the generalized coordinates and the corresponding generalized momenta, while the additional conserved quantity (K) exists as a consequence of rotation symmetry for which K plays the role of a Casimir invariant. It is indeed remarkable and amazing that the resulting equations of motion can be reformulated neatly such that both H

and K (and more generally $n-1$ Hamiltonians $H_1, \ldots, H_{n-1}$ in (1.18)) appear in a completely 'democratic' manner in time evolution, by adopting the components of the angular momentum itself as canonical coordinates in Nambu's generalized Hamiltonian dynamics.

1.3.3 Nambu Brackets

It is convenient to define a generalized Poisson bracket, or the *Nambu bracket* of order n for an arbitrary set of n different functions F_i, $i \in (1, 2, \ldots, n)$, by

$$\{F_1, F_2, \ldots, F_n\} \equiv \epsilon^{i_1 i_2 \ldots i_n} \frac{\partial F_1}{\partial x^{i_1}} \frac{\partial F_2}{\partial x^{i_2}} \cdots \frac{\partial F_n}{\partial x^{i_n}} = \frac{\partial(F_1, F_2, \ldots, F_n)}{\partial(x^1, x^2, \ldots, x^n)},$$

which, being totally skew symmetric under permutations of any pair of entities in $(F_1, F_2, \ldots, F_n)$, is nothing but the n-dimensional Jacobian corresponding to a transformation of the phase-space coordinates $(x^1, x^2, \ldots, x^n)$ to $(F_1, F_2, \ldots, F_n)$. Using this notation, (1.17) with $n = 3$ is

$$\dot{x}^i = \{K, H, x^i\} = \frac{1}{2} \epsilon^{ijk} \frac{\partial(K, H)}{\partial(x^j, x^k)}.$$

For a generic function $F = F(x)$, we have

$$\dot{F} = \partial_i F \dot{x}^i = \{K, H, x^i\} \partial_i F = \{K, H, F\},$$

as the analog of (1.2). The conservations of K and H are then obvious consequences of $\{K, H, K\} = 0 = \{K, H, H\}$.

Clearly, the Nambu bracket for the phase-space coordinates takes the form

$$\{x^i, x^j, x^k\} = \epsilon^{ijk}, \tag{1.21}$$

which is the analog to the conventional canonical Poisson bracket $\{p, q\} = 1$ $(\{q, q\} = 0 = \{p, p\})$ in the primitive 2-dimensional phase space (p, q). Therefore, Nambu justifiably called a mapping $(x^1, x^2, x^3) \to (x'^1, x'^2, x'^3)$ a canonical transformation when the Nambu bracket is preserved,

$$\{x'^i, x'^j, x'^k\} = \epsilon^{ijk},$$

or equivalently,

$$\frac{\partial(x'^i, x'^j, x'^k)}{\partial(x^1, x^2, x^3)} = \epsilon^{ijk}.$$

In the present exposition, to discriminate from the ordinary canonical transformation of conventional Hamiltonian dynamics, we shall call such transformations *generalized canonical transformations*.

The equation of motion is form-invariant against the generalized canonical transformation:

$$\dot{F} = \{K, H, F\} = \frac{\partial(K, H, F)}{\partial(x^1, x^2, x^3)} \frac{\partial(x^1, x^2, x^3)}{\partial(x'^1, x'^2, x'^3)} = \frac{\partial(K, H, F)}{\partial(x'^1, x'^2, x'^3)}. \tag{1.22}$$

Nambu studied only the special case of linear generalized canonical transformations $x'^i_a = \sum_b (A_{ab})^i{}_j x^j_b$ in detail by assuming that there are two or more independent triplets (x^1_a, x^2_a, x^3_a) in $3n$-dimensional phase space $(a, b, \ldots = 1, \ldots, n)$ and that the canonical Nambu brackets are given as $\{x^i_a, x^j_a, x^k_a\} = \epsilon^{ijk}$ (no summation over a) for each single triplet suffixed with a. The brackets with mixed a indices are set to zero by definition, in analogy with the conventional Poisson bracket. He then arrived at a "rather unexciting result that the only continuous canonical transformations consist of independent transformations of the individual triplets", quoting again his own words. Namely, the transformation matrix A works consistently only for $a = b$.

He also mentioned an interesting class of 'gauge' symmetry of the equations of motion with respect to the choice of the pair of Hamiltonians under the transformation $(K, H) \to \big(K'(K, H), H'(K, H)\big)$ such that

$$\frac{\partial(K', H')}{\partial(K, H)} = 1.$$

This condition guarantees that the equations of motion is invariant, since

$$\{K', H', x^i\} = \frac{1}{2}\epsilon^{ijk} \frac{\partial(K', H')}{\partial(K, H)} \frac{\partial(K, H)}{\partial(x^j, x^k)} = \{K, H, x^i\}.$$

Let us call this symmetry 'N-gauge symmetry'. For a justification of the naming *gauge* symmetry, see the next chapter.

Another suggestion Nambu himself made for possible extensions of his equations of motion was to introduce a multiple pair $(K_a(x), H_a(x))$ of Hamiltonians, keeping the 3 dimensions of phase-space coordinates such that the equations of motion are

$$\dot{x}^i = \sum_a \{K_a, H_a, x^i\} = \epsilon^{ijk} \sum_a \partial_j K_a \partial_k H_a. \tag{1.23}$$

The Liouville condition $\partial_i \dot{x}^i = 0$ is satisfied. However, now none of the Hamiltonians $(K_1, H_1, K_2, H_2, \ldots)$ as themselves is conserved. Therefore, the attractive higher symmetries attained in the above simplest case for generalizing Hamiltonian dynamics are largely lost by extensions of this type; though we can conceive of some systems which are represented in this way it seems difficult to attach particular merits to them more than to conventional Hamiltonian dynamics. Furthermore, obviously, his motivation concerning extended statistical mechanics with multiple temperatures cannot be realized in this direction. For these reasons, we will not pursue such possibilities in the present exposition.

He finally proceeded to investigate the quantization of the system, assuming a plausible candidate, a *triple commutator*,

$$[A, B, C] \equiv ABC + BCA + CAB - BAC - ACB - CBA, \qquad (1.24)$$

as a quantized version for the bracket for operators $A, B, C, \ldots$ etc., that satisfies the same skew symmetry as the classical Nambu bracket ($n = 3$) under the permutations of operators. As a further condition in order to restrict the nature of these operators and their triple commutator, he required the 'derivation' law,

$$[A_1 A_2, B, C] = [A_1, B, C]A_2 + A_1[A_2, B, C], \quad \text{etc.}$$

Unfortunately, to his disappointment, he could not find any satisfactory solution.

In the present monograph, we restrict ourselves to the classical theory of Nambu dynamics, except for making some short and sporadic remarks related to quantum theory. The literature on quantization are briefly mentioned in Chap. 4.

In fact, attempts toward quantized Nambu dynamics have been constituting one of the main impetus for studying Nambu dynamics and Nambu brackets, inspired often by some developments in string theory (as in the case of the present author himself). Notwithstanding such history, the author believes that, even restricted within the realm of classical theory, Nambu dynamics has significant and useful implications which are worthy of investigation in depth. Remember that the present quantum theory, essentially due to its probability interpretation, still depends basically on classical Hamiltonian formalism. In view of this, any truly serious pursuits of the extension of classical Hamiltonian formalism to various directions before delving into quantum theory would be sufficiently interesting and valuable by themselves. It may even be possible that they help to deepen our understanding on the nature of quantum theory itself. Besides, from a broader and long-term perspective, the main motif for the present author to study and develop Nambu dynamics is to seek for new structures and symmetries in formulating physical dynamics extending conventional ones, aiming to construct or uncover possible new frameworks associated with such extended scheme of dynamics; a hope is that they may play useful roles someday in some unexpected way in exploring new territories of physical nature. In principle, that could happen both in fundamental and effective theories.

Chapter 2
The Construction of Generalized Canonical Structure for Nambu Dynamics

2.1 Liouville's Theorem and the Nambu Equations of Motion

Let us begin with a general form of the first-order differential equations of motion of a particle in phase space of 3 dimensions,

$$\frac{dx^i}{dt} = X^i(x), \quad (i = 1, 2, 3). \tag{2.1}$$

Remember that geometrically the phase space is simply treated as an ordinary flat Euclidean space as we have already emphasized in the case of conventional Hamiltonian dynamics. If we consider an ensemble consisting of a large number N of *non-interacting* particles obeying these same equations with different initial conditions, their trajectories in phase space never cross each other, since each trajectory is uniquely determined by the values of phase-space coordinates imposed at any one time as initial conditions.

We define the density of particles in the ensemble $\rho(x, t)$ (≥ 0) as a function of phase-space coordinates and time: within a sufficiently small volume element $\Delta^3 v \equiv \Delta x^1 \Delta x^2 \Delta x^3$ around the coordinates x^i the number of particles is given by $\rho(x, t)\Delta^3 v$. By definition, we then have

$$N = \int \rho(x, t)\, d^3x.$$

Consider a set of particles contained in a given (connected) domain V_0 of an arbitrary shape at initial time $t = 0$. The number of particles inside V_0 is

$$N(V_0) \equiv \int_{V_0} \rho(x, 0) d^3x.$$

T. Yoneya, *Introduction to Nambu's Generalized Hamiltonian Dynamics*, SpringerBriefs in Mathematical Physics 55,
https://doi.org/10.1007/978-981-95-7030-0_2

When we follow the time development of this set of particles, the shape and position of the domain in general change during time evolution, and therefore, we have to regard the domain as a function of time, $V(t) : V(0) = V_0$. Since the number of particles inside the domain $V(t)$ remains constant under time evolution, we have

$$0 = \frac{d}{dt}N(V_0) = \frac{d}{dt}\int_{V(t)} \rho(x,t)d^3x.$$

The right-hand side of this equation can be expressed as

$$\frac{d}{dt}\int_{V(t)} \rho(x,t)d^3x = \int_{\partial V(t)} \rho(x,t)X^i(x)dS_i + \int_{V(t)} \frac{\partial \rho(x,t)}{\partial t}d^3x,$$

where the first term on the right is the contribution from the change of the shape of the domain $V(t)$ which can be expressed as integral over the boundary surface denoted by $\partial V(t)$. Note that $X^i(x)dS_i = \dot{x}^i dS_i$ is the infinitesimal volume swept out by the infinitesimal area element dS_i (including sign measured along the direction from inside to outside)

$$d\boldsymbol{S} = (dx^2dx^3, dx^3dx^1, dx^2dx^3).$$

Applying the Gauss theorem for the first term, the right-hand side equals to

$$\int_{V(t)} \left[\frac{\partial}{\partial x^i}(\rho X^i) + \frac{\partial \rho}{\partial t}\right]d^3x.$$

Since this is valid for arbitrary choice of V_0, we can conclude that

$$\frac{\partial}{\partial x^i}(\rho X^i) + \frac{\partial \rho}{\partial t} = 0,$$

which can be rewritten as

$$\frac{d\rho}{dt} = -\rho \partial_i X^i \tag{2.2}$$

by defining

$$\frac{d\rho}{dt} \equiv \frac{\partial \rho}{\partial t} + X^i \frac{\partial \rho}{\partial x^i}.$$

The derivative $\frac{d\rho}{dt}$, usually called the *Lagrange derivative*, describes the change of density function relative to the flow of particles in phase space. In the following, the equations of the type $\frac{d\rho}{dt} = 0$ will be called *Liouville equation* for convenience.

The result (2.2) is well known as the equation of continuity in hydrodynamics. Thus the condition $\frac{d\rho}{dt} = 0$ is equivalent to

$$\partial_i X^i = 0. \tag{2.3}$$

This is a general form of Liouville's theorem. Using the terminology of hydrodynamics, fluids characterized by this condition are called incompressible, since the density is constant along the flow lines of fluid. With a broader geometric terminology, the (infinitesimal) transformations $x^i \to x'^i(x) = x^i + \varepsilon X^i(x)$ induced by (2.1) satisfying (2.3) are often called (infinitesimal) *volume-preserving diffeomorphism.* To avoid possible confusion, it should be kept in mind that we always treat these transformations as the *real physical movements of phase points* in phase space, not mere changes of coordinate frames as in the case of general relativity theory. Whenever we consider the transformation in the latter sense, we will use the different notation, $x^i \to \tilde{x}^i(x)$, as we have done so in the previous chapter. This critical difference arises because we are dealing with the dynamics of *particles* obeying the Nambu equations of motion. In general relativity, in contrast, basic dynamical variables are *fields* (such as the space-time metric) which are defined at each space-time point.

Now going back to the original definition of the density function, we can express the density function $\rho(x,t)$ for an aggregate of N point particles more concretely as

$$\rho(x,t) = \sum_{a=1}^{N} \delta^3\big(x - x_a(t)\big), \tag{2.4}$$

using Dirac's δ-function, where $x_a^i(t)$ describes the trajectory of the a-th particle in phase space. In order to satisfy the Liouville equation with this particular form, the functions $x_a(t)$ must obey the equations of motion $\dot{x}_a(t) = X^i\big(x_a(t)\big)$ for each a separately, which indeed guarantee the validity of

$$\left(\frac{\partial}{\partial t} + X^i(x)\frac{\partial}{\partial x^i}\right)\delta^3\big(x - x_a(t)\big) = 0,$$

because

$$\begin{aligned}\partial_t \delta^3\big(x - x_a(t)\big) &= -\dot{x}_a^i(t)\partial_i\delta^3\big(x - x_a(t)\big) = -X^i\big(x_a(t)\big)\partial_i\delta^3\big(x - x_a(t)\big)\\ &= -X^i(x)\partial_i\delta^3\big(x - x_a(t)\big),\end{aligned}$$

where the last equality is due to $\partial_i X^i = 0$: for an arbitrary function $f(x)$, we have

$$\begin{aligned}\int f(x)X^i(x_a(t))\partial_i\delta^3\big(x - x_a(t)\big)d^3x &= -\int (\partial_i f(x))X^i(x)\delta^3\big(x - x_a(t)\big).\\ &= -\int \partial_i(f(x)X^i(x))\delta^3\big(x - x_a(t)\big)d^3x\\ &= \int X^i(x)f(x)\partial_i\delta^3\big(x - x_a(t)\big)d^3x.\end{aligned}$$

Thus we can legitimately say that the Liouville equation

$$\left(\frac{\partial}{\partial t} + X^i(x)\frac{\partial}{\partial x^i}\right)\rho(x,t) = 0 \tag{2.5}$$

is essentially equivalent to the equations of motion themselves if we assume the above discretized form for $\rho(x,t)$.

Furthermore, concentrating our attention to a particular trajectory satisfying the initial conditions $x^i(0) = x_0^i$ with a given vector x_0^i, the equations $x^i = x^i(t)$ are inverted uniquely, as $x_0^j = g^j(x,t)$, which *implicitly* gives $x^i = x^i(t)$. Using the fact that

$$0 = \frac{d}{dt}g^j(x(t),t) = \left(\frac{\partial}{\partial t} + X^i(x(t))\frac{\partial}{\partial x^i}\right)g^j(x,t)\Big|_{x=x(t)}$$

is valid for arbitrary t, the vector function $g^j(x,t)$ satisfies in general

$$(\partial_t + X^i(x)\partial_i)g^j = 0, \quad g^j(x,0) = x^j, \tag{2.6}$$

where the second condition follows from $x_0^i = g^i(x(0),0) = x^i(0)$ for any initial values of coordinates x_0^i.

Then, returning to the aggregate of particles, we can write using $\frac{\partial(x^1,x^2,x^3)}{\partial(x_a^1,x_a^2,x_a^3)} = 1$,

$$\delta^3\big(x - x_a(t)\big) = \delta^3\big(x_a - g(x,t)\big),$$

which implies another equivalent expression for the density function,

$$\rho(x,t) = \sum_{a=1}^{N}\delta^3\big(x_a - g(x,t)\big),$$

satisfying the Liouville Eq. (2.5).

In fact, we can extend this form of the solution of the Liouville equation to a still more general form: since the Liouville equation is linear, we can superpose any solutions with arbitrary constant weights. Applying this procedure to a solution with a single δ-function, we get using an arbitrary function $F(x)$,

$$G_F(x,t) \equiv \int F(x_0)\,\delta^3\big(x_0 - g(x,t)\big)d^3x_0 = F\big(g(x,t)\big), \tag{2.7}$$

whose initial condition is $G_F(x,0) = F(x)$. It is easy to confirm directly using (2.6) that this expression indeed satisfies the Liouville equation:

$$(\partial_t + X^i(x)\partial_i)G_F(x,t) = \frac{\partial F}{\partial g^j}(\partial_t + X^i\partial_i)g^j = 0.$$

The foregoing discussions are given for flows in three-dimensional phase space. It must be fairly clear to reader that all the arguments can be straightforwardly extended to arbitrary dimensions by simply extending the spatial indices to n-dimensions. The reader should remember here that, as a matter of fact, an ensemble in the conventional Hamiltonian dynamics can also be regarded similarly as an incompressible fluid in $2n$-dimensional phase space.

Now, returning to 3 dimensions, the condition (2.3) implies that we can represent X^i by introducing the vector potential A_i such that

$$X^i = \epsilon^{ijk}\partial_j A_k. \tag{2.8}$$

The Nambu equations of motion (1.17) amount to *restricting* ourselves to a special choice of the vector potential which is given by two independent scalar functions K and H as

$$A_i = K\partial_i H + \partial_i \Lambda \tag{2.9}$$

with an arbitrary scalar function Λ. Note that the last term on the right-hand side does not contribute to X^i because of the identity $\epsilon^{ijk}\partial_j\partial_k\Lambda = 0$, namely, gauge invariance. Then X^i takes the Jacobian form,

$$X^i = \frac{1}{2}\epsilon^{ijk}\frac{\partial(K, H)}{\partial(x^j, x^k)}$$

as given in the previous chapter. This particular form of X^i is known as *Clebsch's transformation* in hydrodynamics. In the context of hydrodynamics, the vector potential A_i and its *rotation* X^i are the *velocity* field and *vorticity* field, respectively.

Thus what Nambu proposed was a new kind of dynamics generalizing the structure of conventional Hamiltonian dynamics in the sense that the velocity of a particle, a Nambu particle, in phase space is given directly by the vorticity of a Clebsch form, $\dot{x}^i = X^i(x) = \{K, H, x^i\}$. This suggests naturally that we should proceed to construct a generalized canonical formalism in extended phase spaces of arbitrary dimensions n as (1.18), in which there exist $n-1$ conserved 'Hamiltonians' participating equally in the time evolution. The flow lines in this dynamics form a set of curves which are lying along the intersections of $n-1$ different level (hyper) surfaces defined by $H_i(x) = E_i$ $(i = 1, \ldots, n-1)$ with E_i's being fixed by initial conditions. It is the main purpose of this chapter to construct the generalized canonical structure by fully taking into account this characteristic feature, and to develop tools necessary for such discussions by extending or reformulating appropriately the usual apparatus of classical analytical dynamics.

Remark 2.1 From a general viewpoint of hydrodynamics, we can imagine a special compressive flow for which the density function is continuous and steady, satisfying

$$\frac{\partial\rho}{\partial t} = 0,$$

instead of the incompressibility condition $\frac{d\rho}{dt} = 0$. In this case, the equation of continuity, (2.2) is equivalent to

$$\partial_i(\rho X^i) = 0$$

replacing (2.3). This is satisfied identically by setting

$$X^i = \frac{1}{2\rho(x)}\epsilon^{ijk}\frac{\partial(K, H)}{\partial(x^j, x^k)}.$$

The conservation law of (K, H) is still valid since $\partial_i K X^i = 0 = \partial_i H X^i = 0$.

Historically, the equations of motion (2.1) with this particular form was already touched upon by Jacobi in the early 1840s (relevant references are given in Chap. 4). Jacobi called such a factor $\rho(x)$ for a given system of the general first-order differential equations of the general form (2.1), *Last Multiplier*. But his work went unnoticed for a long time. The Nambu equations of motion are in fact a special case where the Last Multiplier is identically 1. In this sense, Jacobi predated Nambu's proposal almost 130 years. This is remarkable but is understandable if we remember that Jacobi's works on this particular subject had almost never been cited in most of familiar textbooks and even in well-known treatises on the history of classical dynamics.

2.2 N-Gauge Symmetry

The fact that two (or more) conserved Hamiltonians play equal roles in Nambu dynamics implies new symmetries which are not present in the conventional Hamiltonian dynamics. We have already mentioned in the previous chapter that the Jacobian form of the equations of motion is invariant under a map from a pair (K, H) to another pair $(K', H') = \big(K'(K, H), H'(K, H)\big)$, when

$$\frac{\partial(K', H')}{\partial(K, H)} = 1 \tag{2.10}$$

is satisfied. This condition is equivalent to, for any pair of different indices (i, j),

$$\partial_i K' \partial_j H' - \partial_j K' \partial_i H' = \partial_i K \partial_j H - \partial_j K \partial_i H.$$

As we have proposed in the previous chapter, this type of the transformations of a set of Hamiltonians is to be called the 'N-gauge transformations'. We now explain in what sense they are 'gauge' transformations.

Since one condition is imposed on two variables K', H', one degree of freedom remains for such transformations. If we regard four variables (K, H, K', H') as functions of phase coordinates, there must exist some function $F = F(x)$ such that

$$K'\partial_i H' - K\partial_i H = \partial_i F. \tag{2.11}$$

In terms of the vector potential for the vector field $X^i = \epsilon^{ijk}\partial_j A_k$,

$$A'_i = K'\partial_i H' + \partial_i \Lambda'$$

gives the same X^i and therefore A'_i must be obtained from A_i by a gauge transformation. This immediately leads to the above relation between (K', H') and (K, H) with a function F. It implies that F can be regarded as the one degree of freedom characterizing the map $(K, H) \to (K', H')$. As a consequence, Clebsch's form for the gauge field can represent only *one* true physical degree of freedom, in spite of the fact that there are two independent Hamiltonian functions (K, H): in other words, the number of 'true' degrees of freedom of the Hamiltonian functions by which the time evolution of the system is governed is actually one.

In three dimensions, the number of physical degrees of freedom of a vector potential (or 'gauge field') is *two* in general. In other words, we can eliminate one degree of freedom out of the three components of A_i by gauge transformations. From this point of view, an extension of the equations of motion exemplified in (1.23) would serve to recover full physical degrees of freedom for the gauge field by representing the gauge field as $A_i = K_1\partial_i H_1 + K_2\partial_i H_2 + \partial_i \Lambda$. Indeed, two (or more) pairs of the functions (K_1, H_1) and (K_2, H_2) are sufficient for providing full degrees of freedom for the gauge field. But as has been emphasized before, this extension in our case would cost a high price of losing conservation laws for these Hamiltonian functions.

On the other hand, the Eq. (2.11) indicates that we should treat F as a function, $F = F(H', H)$, of two independent variables (H', H), instead of the original variables (K, H). Then (2.11) is equivalent to

$$\frac{\partial F}{\partial H'} = K', \quad \frac{\partial F}{\partial H} = -K. \tag{2.12}$$

The readers who are familiar with the conventional canonical formalism in classical analytical dynamics would recognize that this form is identical with the general form of a finite canonical transformation $(p, q) \to (p', q')$. In fact, the condition in that case is $\{p', q'\} = 1$, which coincides with (2.10) by the correspondence $(p, q) \leftrightarrow (K, H)$ and $(p', q') \leftrightarrow (K', H')$. If we choose (p', p) as independent variables, there is a generating function $f(p', p)$ satisfying

$$\frac{\partial f}{\partial p'} = q', \quad \frac{\partial f}{\partial p} = -q.$$

In analogy with this, it is appropriate to call the function $F(H', H)$ the generating function for the N-gauge transformation $(K, H) \to (K', H')$, satisfying

$$K'\delta H' - K\delta H = \delta F$$

with arbitrary infinitesimal variations, δK and $\delta K'$, of the independent variables.

When we consider Nambu dynamics in higher dimensions, the vector gauge field and its gauge transformation must be extended appropriately to higher-form gauge fields and associated higher-form gauge transformations. Such extensions will be introduced later (Sect. 2.5) by developing our formulation using the apparatus of differential forms.

Example 2.1 Consider a linear N-gauge transformation

$$\begin{pmatrix} K' \\ H' \end{pmatrix} = \begin{pmatrix} a & b \\ c & d \end{pmatrix} \begin{pmatrix} K \\ H \end{pmatrix}$$

with real constants (a, b, c, d). The condition (2.10) gives $ad - bc = 1$. Thus the set of the linear N-gauge transformations consists of 2×2 real matrices of unit determinant, which form the group $SL(2, \mathbb{R})$ under the matrix products: for instance, the inverse is,

$$\begin{pmatrix} K \\ H \end{pmatrix} = \begin{pmatrix} d & -b \\ -c & a \end{pmatrix} \begin{pmatrix} K' \\ H' \end{pmatrix}.$$

Because of the linearity of transformations, the generating function is a bilinear form. After some calculations, we obtain

$$F = F(H', H) = \frac{1}{2c}\left(aH'^2 - 2H'H + dH^2\right).$$

The reader should check that this indeed satisfies (2.12). The last expression looks rather peculiar in that it apparently diverges when $c = 0$. However, as a function of K, H, it is

$$F = F\big(H'(K, H), H\big) = \frac{1}{2}\left(acK^2 + 2bcKH + bdH^2\right),$$

which does not diverge. This expression shows that, in the limit of the identity transformation with vanishing b and c, F actually approaches zero, provided that it is regarded as a function of (K, H), even though it must be non-zero in the limit as a function of (H', H). Otherwise, the second relation of (2.12) could not be valid.

Let us next study an infinitesimal form of a general N-gauge transformation briefly. In order to represent the identity transformation, it is more convenient to choose the independent variables (H', K), instead of (H', H) as being suggested in the above example. By rewriting (2.11) as

$$K'\partial_i H' + H\partial_i K = \partial_i G, \quad G \equiv HK + F,$$

the function $G = G(H', K)$ can now be treated as the generating function,

$$\frac{\partial G}{\partial H'} = K', \quad \frac{\partial G}{\partial K} = H. \tag{2.13}$$

For an infinitesimal transformation, we define

$$H' = H + \delta H, \quad K' = K + \delta K, \quad G = KH' + \delta G, \tag{2.14}$$

where the variations δH, δK and δG are regarded as infinitesimal quantities of order ϵ ($|\epsilon| \ll 1$). By substituting (2.14) into (2.13), we have

$$\delta K = \frac{\partial \delta G}{\partial H}, \quad \delta H = -\frac{\partial \delta G}{\partial K}, \tag{2.15}$$

to the same accuracy of order ϵ. The identity transformation $\delta G = 0$ corresponds to $G = KH' = KH$. The relation (2.15) indeed coincides with the familiar form of a general infinitesimal canonical transformation in the simplest case of 2-dimensional phase space in the conventional canonical formalism.

2.3 The Properties of Nambu Brackets

2.3.1 *Skew Symmetry and Derivation Property*

We now enumerate the general properties of Nambu brackets for generic functions $F_i(x)$ ($i = 1, 2, 3$). First it is skew symmetric (or totally anti-symmetric) under permutations of F_is:

$$\{F_1, F_2, F_3\} = (-1)^{\epsilon(P)}\{F_{P(1)}, F_{P(2)}, F_{P(3)}\},$$

where $P(i)$ denotes the permutation of indices i and $\epsilon(P)$ is the parity of the permutation ($\epsilon(P) = 0$ if P is an even permutation and $\epsilon(P) = 1$ if P is an odd permutation). Secondly, it has a derivation property:

$$\{F_1 F_2, F_3, F_4\} = \{F_1, F_3, F_4\}F_2 + F_1\{F_2, F_3, F_4\}.$$

Both of these properties are obvious from the definition $\{F_1, F_2, F_3\} = \frac{\partial(F_1, F_2, F_3)}{\partial(x^1, x^2, x^3)}$ and the Leibniz rule of the first derivative, $\partial_i(F_1 F_2) = (\partial_i F_1)F_2 + F_1(\partial_i F_2)$. These two properties are the generalizations of the relations, $\{F_1, F_2\} = -\{F_2, F_1\}$ and $\{F_1 F_2, F_3\} = \{F_1, F_3\}F_2 + F_1\{F_2, F_3\}$, respectively, satisfied by the conventional Poisson brackets.

2.3.2 Generalized Jacobi Identity

An important question is now what is, if any, the property corresponding to the Jacobi identity of Poisson brackets? As explained in the first chapter, the Jacobi identity of Poisson brackets ensures consistency of the Hamilton equations of motion with the canonical Poisson brackets. Similarly, we study how consistency of the Nambu equations of motion with the Nambu brackets is achieved. Consider the time development of generic Nambu brackets. By definition that is given by

$$\frac{d}{dt}\{F_1, F_2, F_3\} = \epsilon^{ijk}\partial_j K \partial_k H \partial_i \{F_1, F_2, F_3\} = \{K, H, \{F_1, F_2, F_3\}\}.$$

On the other hand, *if* we assume that the Nambu bracket is commutative with the derivation with respect to time just as in the case of the conventional Poisson brackets, we should have also

$$\begin{aligned}\frac{d}{dt}\{F_1, F_2, F_3\} &= \{\dot{F}_1, F_2, F_3\} + \{F_1, \dot{F}_2, F_3\} + \{F_1, F_2, \dot{F}_3\} \\ &= \{\{K, H, F_1\}, F_2, F_3\} + \{F_1, \{K, H, F_2\}, F_3\} \\ &\quad + \{F_1, F_2, \{K, H, F_3\}\},\end{aligned} \tag{2.16}$$

in order to satisfy the Leibniz rule of the time derivative. To be consistent, we must have

$$\begin{aligned}\{\{K, H, F_1\}, F_2, F_3\} + \{F_1, \{K, H, F_2\}, F_3\} + \{F_1, F_2, \{K, H, F_3\}\} \\ = \{K, H, \{F_1, F_2, F_3\}\},\end{aligned} \tag{2.17}$$

for an arbitrary set of five functions (K, H, F_1, F_2, F_3). This is an analog of the Jacobi identity of the conventional Hamiltonian dynamics. If the identity (2.17) is satisfied, the canonical Nambu bracket relation (1.21), for instance, is also guaranteed to be preserved under the time evolution consistently, $\frac{d}{dt}\{x^i, x^j, x^k\} = 0$.

Historically, (2.17) has often been called the 'fundamental identity'. In fact, however, as we shall see below, it is an immediate consequence of invariance under the generalized canonical transformation of the Nambu bracket, which is *more* fundamental to the Nambu dynamics than (2.17) from our viewpoint. In other words, the above assumption of the commutativity of the time derivative with the Nambu bracket is valid, *provided* that the process of constructing the Nambu bracket is invariant under a general infinitesimal volume-preserving diffeomorphism,

$$x^i \to x'^i = x^i + \varepsilon X^i(x), \quad \partial_i X^i = 0.$$

Note that the time derivative for any functions of the phase coordinates is only a special case of infinitesimal volume-preserving transformations under the assumption of the Clebsch form $X^i = \epsilon^{ijk}\partial_j K \partial_k H$. In point of fact, we have tacitly confirmed the corresponding property of the Nambu bracket for the generalized canonical transformation in (1.22) in the previous chapter, and that was already mentioned by Nambu himself in his original paper. In order to make this crucial property manifest in a more explicit form, it is convenient, albeit somewhat unusual, to express the Jacobian introducing a special symbol as

$$\frac{\partial \times \partial \times \partial}{\partial(x^1, x^2, x^3)}(A, B, C) \equiv \{A, B, C\} = \frac{\partial(A, B, C)}{\partial(x^1, x^2, x^3)},$$

where the linear operator symbolized as '$\frac{\partial\times\partial\times\partial}{\partial(x^1,x^2,x^3)}$' on the left-hand side is placed separately, acting to the right on a triplet (A, B, C) which is the operand consisting of three independent arbitrary functions. Let us call, for convenience, the differential operator $\frac{\partial\times\partial\times\partial}{\partial(x^1,x^2,x^3)}$ the 'Jacobian operator'. Owing to the identity

$$\frac{\partial(x'^1, x'^2, x'^3)}{\partial(x^1, x^2, x^3)} = 1,$$

which is valid for arbitrary volume-preserving diffeomorphism, the Jacobian operator, $\frac{\partial\times\partial\times\partial}{\partial(x^1,x^2,x^3)}$, is invariant under *arbitrary* generalized canonical transformations:

$$\frac{\partial \times \partial \times \partial}{\partial(x^1, x^2, x^3)} \to \frac{\partial \times \partial \times \partial}{\partial(x'^1, x'^2, x'^3)} = \frac{\partial(x^1, x^2, x^3)}{\partial(x'^1, x'^2, x'^3)} \frac{\partial \times \partial \times \partial}{\partial(x^1, x^2, x^3)} = \frac{\partial \times \partial \times \partial}{\partial(x^1, x^2, x^3)}.$$

For infinitesimal transformations, we can express this identity as

$$\mathcal{D}_X \frac{\partial \times \partial \times \partial}{\partial(x^1, x^2, x^3)} = \frac{\partial \times \partial \times \partial}{\partial(x^1, x^2, x^3)} \mathcal{D}_X,$$

in terms of a first-order differential operator $\mathcal{D}_X \equiv X^i \partial_i$ that represents the action of any infinitesimal generalized canonical transformation to an arbitrary function of coordinates with a vector field X^i satisfying $\partial_i X^i = 0$. The commutativity of $\mathcal{D}_X$ with the Jacobian operator expressed in this form immediately yields (2.16), since we have the following identity,

$$\begin{aligned}\mathcal{D}_X \frac{\partial \times \partial \times \partial}{\partial(x^1, x^2, x^3)}(A, B, C) &= \frac{\partial \times \partial \times \partial}{\partial(x^1, x^2, x^3)} \mathcal{D}_X(A, B, C) \\ &= \frac{\partial \times \partial \times \partial}{\partial(x^1, x^2, x^3)} \big[(\mathcal{D}_X A, B, C) + (A, \mathcal{D}_X B, C) + (A, B, \mathcal{D}_X C)\big],\end{aligned}$$

or equivalently,

$$\mathcal{D}_X\{A, B, C\} = \{\mathcal{D}_X A, B, C\} + \{A, \mathcal{D}_X B, C\} + \{A, B, \mathcal{D}_X C\}. \tag{2.18}$$

It is straightforward to extend the above discussions to higher-dimensional Nambu brackets. The identity (2.17) is generalized to

$$\begin{aligned}&\{\{H_1, H_2, \ldots, H_{n-1}, F_1\}, F_2, \ldots, F_n\} + \{F_1, \{H_1, H_2, \ldots, H_{n-1}, F_2\}, F_3, \cdots, F_n\} \\ &\quad + \cdots + \{F_1, F_2, \ldots, \{H_1, H_2, \ldots, H_{n-1}, F_n\}\} \\ &\quad = \{H_1, H_2, \ldots, H_{n-1}, \{F_1, F_2, \ldots, F_n\}\},\end{aligned} \tag{2.19}$$

for two sets, $(H_1, H_2, \ldots, H_{n-1})$ and $(F_1, F_2, \ldots, F_n)$, of n arbitrary functions. This is again a consequence of the commutativity

$$\left[\mathcal{D}_X, \frac{\overbrace{\partial \times \partial \times \cdots \times \partial}^{n}}{\partial(x^1, x^2, \ldots, x^n)}\right] = 0, \tag{2.20}$$

with any X^i satisfying $\partial_i X^i = 0$, of which $X^i = \epsilon^{ij_1\cdots j_{n-1}}(\partial_{j_1} H_1)\cdots(\partial_{j_{n-1}} H_{n-1})$ is only a special case. The n-dimensional Jacobian operator is defined such that

$$\frac{\overbrace{\partial \times \partial \times \cdots \times \partial}^{n}}{\partial(x^1, x^2, \ldots, x^n)}(F_1, \ldots, F_n) = \{F_1, \ldots, F_n\}.$$

To conclude, the identity

$$\begin{aligned}\mathcal{D}_X\{F_1, \ldots, F_n\} &= \{\mathcal{D}_X F_1, F_2, \ldots, F_n\} + \{F_1, \mathcal{D}_X F_2, \ldots, F_n\} \\ &\quad + \cdots + \{F_1, \ldots, F_{n-1}, \mathcal{D}_X F_n\}\end{aligned} \tag{2.21}$$

is *more fundamental* than (2.19), since we have only used the property $\partial_i X^i = 0$. Let us call (2.21), including (2.18) as a special case, the 'generalized Jacobi identity'.

Exercise 2.1 For appreciating the significance of the above discussion leading to (2.21), it is instructive to give a direct proof of (2.17) for $n = 3$ by a brute force calculation. First we directly compute $X^\ell \partial_\ell \{F_1, F_2, F_3\}$ with a generic form $X^\ell = \epsilon^{\ell pq}\partial_p A_q$, satisfying $\partial_i X^i = 0$:

$$\begin{aligned}&\epsilon^{ijk} X^\ell \partial_\ell(\partial_i F_1 \partial_j F_2 \partial_k F_3) \\ &\quad = \epsilon^{ijk} X^\ell \big[(\partial_\ell \partial_i F_1)\partial_j F_2 \partial_k F_3 + \partial_i F_1 (\partial_\ell \partial_j F_2)\partial_k F_3 + \partial_i F_1 \partial_j F_2 (\partial_\ell \partial_k F_3)\big] \\ &\quad = \epsilon^{ijk}\big[\partial_i (X^\ell \partial_\ell F_1)\partial_j F_2 \partial_k F_3 + \partial_i F_1 \partial_j (X^\ell \partial_\ell F_2)\partial_k F_3 + \partial_i F_1 \partial_j F_2 \partial_k (X^\ell \partial_\ell F_3)\big] \\ &\quad - \epsilon^{ijk}\big[\partial_i X^\ell \partial_\ell F_1 \partial_j F_2 \partial_k F_3 + \partial_i F_1 \partial_j X^\ell \partial_\ell F_2 \partial_k F_3 + \partial_i F_1 \partial_j F_2 \partial_k X^\ell \partial_\ell F_3\big].\end{aligned}$$

The first line alone of the last equality gives the desired result:

$$\epsilon^{ijk}\big[\partial_i(\mathcal{D}_X F_1)\partial_j F_2 \partial_k F_3 + \partial_i F_1 \partial_j (\mathcal{D}_X)\partial_k F_3 + \partial_i F_1 \partial_j F_2 \partial_k (\mathcal{D}_X F_3)\big].$$

Hence we have to check that the second line is zero identically. Evidently, the latter vanishing property precisely amounts to the invariance of the Jacobian operator against the infinitesimal generalized canonical transformation $\mathcal{D}_X$, since it involves only first derivatives of F_is with no direct operations of $\mathcal{D}_X$ itself to $F_i s$. Let us rewrite that expression by a rearrangement of indices as

$$\begin{aligned}
&\epsilon^{ijk}\big[\partial_i X^\ell \partial_\ell F_1 \partial_j F_2 \partial_k F_3 + \partial_i F_1 \partial_j X^\ell \partial_\ell F_2 \partial_k F_3 + \partial_i F_1 \partial_j F_2 \partial_k X^\ell \partial_\ell F_3\big] \\
&\quad = \epsilon^{\ell jk}\partial_\ell X^i \partial_i F_1 \partial_j F_2 \partial_k F_2 + \epsilon^{i\ell k}\partial_\ell X^j \partial_i F_1 \partial_j F_2 \partial_k F_3 + \epsilon^{ij\ell}\partial_\ell X^k \partial_i F_1 \partial_j F_2 \partial_k F_3 \\
&\quad = \big[\epsilon^{\ell jk}\partial_\ell X^i + \epsilon^{i\ell k}\partial_\ell X^j + \epsilon^{ij\ell}\partial_\ell X^k\big]\partial_i F_1 \partial_j F_2 \partial_k F_3.
\end{aligned}$$

Now consider the expression in the bracket of the last line,

$$\begin{aligned}
&\epsilon^{\ell jk}\partial_\ell X^i + \epsilon^{i\ell k}\partial_\ell X^j + \epsilon^{ij\ell}\partial_\ell X^k \\
&\quad = \big(\epsilon^{\ell jk}\epsilon^{ipq} + \epsilon^{i\ell k}\epsilon^{jpq} + \epsilon^{ij\ell}\epsilon^{kpq}\big)\partial_\ell(\partial_p A_q).
\end{aligned} \tag{2.22}$$

By construction, the tensor coefficient appearing on the right-hand side

$$\epsilon^{\ell jk}\epsilon^{ipq} + \epsilon^{i\ell k}\epsilon^{jpq} + \epsilon^{ij\ell}\epsilon^{kpq}$$

must be completely anti-symmetric with respect to permutations of the set (ijk): indeed it gives, under the permutation $i \leftrightarrow j$,

$$\epsilon^{\ell ik}\epsilon^{jpq} + \epsilon^{j\ell k}\epsilon^{ipq} + \epsilon^{ji\ell}\epsilon^{kpq} = -\epsilon^{i\ell k}\epsilon^{jpq} - \epsilon^{\ell jk}\epsilon^{ipq} - \epsilon^{ij\ell}\epsilon^{kpq};$$

similarly, under $i \leftrightarrow k$,

$$\epsilon^{\ell ji}\epsilon^{kpq} + \epsilon^{k\ell i}\epsilon^{jpq} + \epsilon^{kj\ell}\epsilon^{ipq} = -\epsilon^{\ell jk}\epsilon^{ipq} - \epsilon^{i\ell k}\epsilon^{jpq} - \epsilon^{ij\ell}\epsilon^{kpq};$$

and under $j \leftrightarrow k$,

$$\epsilon^{\ell kj}\epsilon^{ipq} + \epsilon^{i\ell j}\epsilon^{kpq} + \epsilon^{ik\ell}\epsilon^{jpq} = -\epsilon^{\ell jk}\epsilon^{ipq} - \epsilon^{i\ell k}\epsilon^{jpq} - \epsilon^{ij\ell}\epsilon^{kpq}.$$

Thus we can set $i = 1,\ j = 2,\ k = 3$ without losing generality. It is then easy to check that only non-zero contributions with respect the configurations of the set $(\ell,\ p, q)$ are

$$\epsilon^{\ell jk}\epsilon^{ipq} = 1 \times (\pm 1): \quad \ell = 1,\ \ p = 2,\ \ q = 3 \ or\ \ p = 3,\ \ q = 2,$$

$$\epsilon^{i\ell k}\epsilon^{jpq} = 1 \times (\pm 1): \quad \ell = 2,\ \ p = 3,\ \ q = 1 \ or\ \ p = 1,\ \ q = 3,$$

$$\epsilon^{ij\ell}\epsilon^{kpq} = 1 \times (\pm 1): \quad \ell = 3,\ \ p = 1,\ \ q = 2,\ \ or\ \ p = 2\ ,q = 1.$$

This establishes the identity,

$$\epsilon^{\ell jk}\epsilon^{ipq} + \epsilon^{i\ell k}\epsilon^{jpq} + \epsilon^{ij\ell}\epsilon^{kpq} = \epsilon^{ijk}\epsilon^{\ell pq}.$$

Consequently, the right-hand side of (2.22) vanishes owing to $\epsilon^{\ell pq}\partial_\ell(\partial_p A_q) = \partial_\ell X^\ell = 0$. We stress that the explicit (Clebsch) form of the vector potential field A_i is not used, as it is also the case in the above derivation of invariance of the Jacobian operator under the general infinitesimal canonical transformations given in the text, which is based only on $\partial_i X^i = 0$. By putting $X^i = \epsilon^{ijk}\partial_j K \partial_k H$ as a special case we have (2.17).

2.3.3 Rigidity

As we have mentioned briefly in the previous chapter, Nambu has suggested in his original paper to generalize the system to those with multiple canonical triplets (x_a^1, x_a^2, x_a^3) $(a = 1, \ldots, n)$ which form a $3n$-dimensional phase space, in analogy with the $2n$-dimensional phase space (q_a, p_a) in conventional Hamiltonian dynamics. The equations of motion would then be replaced by

$$\dot{F} = \sum_{a=1}^{n} \frac{\partial(K, H, F)}{\partial(x_a^1, x_a^2, x_a^3)},$$

because the Hamiltonians $K(x)$ and $H(x)$ in general should depend on all the variables x_a^i of the $3n$-dimensional phase space according to this extension.

Obviously, if K and H are given as

$$K = \sum_{a=1}^{n} K_a(x_a^1, x_a^2, x_a^3), \quad H = \sum_{a=1}^{n} H_a(x_a^1, x_a^2, x_a^3), \tag{2.23}$$

where K_a and H_a depend only on the single triplet x_a^i, the equations of motion are also a direct sum of separated Jacobians

$$\dot{F} = \sum_{a=1}^{n} \frac{\partial(K_a, H_a, F)}{\partial(x_a^1, x_a^2, x_a^3)}, \tag{2.24}$$

and hence the dynamics itself is separated into each triplet

$$\dot{x}_a^i = \frac{\partial(K_a, H_a, x_a^i)}{\partial(x_a^1, x_a^2, x_a^3)} = \epsilon^{ijk} \frac{\partial K_a}{\partial x_a^j} \frac{\partial H_a}{\partial x_a^k}.$$

This simply amounts to considering a collection of completely independent motions of Nambu particles within these triplets.

Let us next consider the case where K and H involve terms that depend on different triplets simultaneously such as two-body interactions, $K_{ab}(x_a, x_b)$ and $H_{ab}(x_a, x_b)$ with $a \neq b$. Then the equations of motion involve also interaction terms,

$$\dot{x}_a^i = \frac{\partial(K_a, H_a, x_a^i)}{\partial(x_a^1, x_a^2, x_a^3)} + \sum_{b=1}^{n} \epsilon^{ijk} \frac{\partial K_{ab}}{\partial x_a^j} \frac{\partial H_{ab}}{\partial x_a^k}.$$

The differential operator corresponding to time evolution now takes the form

$$\mathcal{D}_X = \sum_{a=1}^{n} X_a^i \frac{\partial}{\partial x_a^i}, \quad X_a^i = \epsilon^{ijk} \frac{\partial K_a}{\partial x_a^j} \frac{\partial H_a}{\partial x_a^k} + \sum_{b=1}^{n} \epsilon^{ijk} \frac{\partial K_{ab}}{\partial x_a^j} \frac{\partial H_{ab}}{\partial x_a^k}. \tag{2.25}$$

Note that the condition of incompressibility is satisfied for each a separately, $\partial X_a^i / \partial x_a^i = 0$. However, owing to the second term in X_a^i of (2.25), all of the $3n$ coordinates are mixed together during the time evolution: by abbreviating as $x_a^i(t') = x_a'^i$, $x_a^i(t) = x_a^i$, we have

$$x_a'^i = f_a^i(x_1, x_2, \ldots, x_n), \quad x_a^i = (f^{-1})_a^i(x_1', x_2', \ldots, x_n').$$

In the presence of mixing among different triplets as exhibited in (2.25), the requirement of commutativity of $\mathcal{D}_X$ with the Jacobian operators associated with such brackets cannot be maintained since the action of $\mathcal{D}_X$ induces the transformations of partial differential operators of the coordinates x_a^i as

$$\frac{\partial}{\partial x_a^i} \to \frac{\partial}{\partial x_a'^i} = \sum_{b=1}^{n} \frac{\partial x_b^j}{\partial x_a'^i} \frac{\partial}{\partial x_b^j},$$

which mixes different triplets with respect to the a-index. It is also easy to check that the commutativity is not satisfied by a direct computation in the manner of Exercise 2.1. A closely related discussion to confirm this property by explicit calculations will be given later (see Sect. 2.5.3, Exercise 2.3).

Therefore we can conclude that, for Nambu systems with multiple triplets, (2.18) is valid only when triplets are completely separable as in (2.23). It is clear that the same conclusion holds equally for higher n-dimensional Nambu systems of (1.18) with multiple n-tuple brackets instead of triple brackets.

That the *generalized* canonical structure governing Nambu dynamics has a kind of *rigidity* in the sense explained is in stark contrast to the situation in conventional Hamiltonian dynamics, where the canonical structure is extended to any even-dimensional phase space in which the Hamiltonian can be an arbitrary function that mixes $2n$ canonical coordinates $(p_1, q_1, \ldots, p_n, q_n) = (x^1, \ldots, x^{2n})$. Using the differential operator (1.15) corresponding to the infinitesimal canonical transformation with the generating function H, the invariance of the Poisson-bracket under canonical transformations in general $2n$ dimensions can also be expressed as the commutativity of the Jacobian-like differential operator in the same spirit as in (2.20) against D_H defined in (1.15),

$$D_H\Big(\sum_{i,j=1}^{2n} J^{ij}\frac{\partial\times\partial}{\partial(x^i,x^j)}\Big)=\Big(\sum_{i,j=1}^{2n} J^{ij}\frac{\partial\times\partial}{\partial(x^i,x^j)}\Big)D_H, \tag{2.26}$$

where J_{ij} is the $2n\times 2n$ skew-symmetric (block) matrix with only non-zero matrix elements

$$J^{2i-1,2i}=1=-J^{2i,2i-1}. \tag{2.27}$$

for all i. Using this notation, the Poisson bracket of two arbitrary functions $F(x)$ and $G(x)$ takes the following form,

$$\{F,G\}\equiv\sum_{i,j=1}^{2n} J^{ij}\frac{\partial\times\partial}{(x^i,x^j)}(F,G)\equiv\sum_{i,j=1}^{2n} J^{ij}\frac{\partial F}{\partial x^i}\frac{\partial G}{\partial x^j}.$$

The commutativity relation (2.26) yields

$$\begin{aligned}D_H\{F,G\}&=\sum_{i,j=1}^{2n} J^{ij}\frac{\partial\times\partial}{(x^i,x^j)}\big((D_HF,G)+(F,D_HG)\big)\\&=\{D_HF,G\}+\{F,D_HG\},\end{aligned}$$

which is equivalent to the Jacobi identity $\{H,\{F,G\}\}=\{\{H,F\},G\}+\{F,\{H,G\}\}$.

2.4 Nambu Brackets and Generalized Poisson Brackets

Let us next examine whether there exist connections among the Poisson and Nambu systems of various different dimensions. To motivate our discussion, we start with a trivial case where $K=x^3$ in the Nambu equations of motion in three dimensions. Then, we have $\dot{x}^3=0$ and for $i\in(1,2)$, $\dot{x}^i=\{x^3,H,x^i\}=-\epsilon^{ij}\partial_jH$ ($\epsilon^{12}=-\epsilon^{21}=1$ and zero otherwise), which is the simplest 2-dimensional Hamilton equations of motion. The Poisson bracket $\{x^i,x^j\}=\epsilon^{ij}$ corresponding to this case is therefore directly related to the Nambu bracket: $\{p,q\}=\{x^1,x^2\}=\{K,x^1,x^2\}=1$, $\dot{x}^i=\{H,x^i\}$. In this sense, the Nambu system reduces to a conventional Hamilton system with a special choice of the conserved quantities. It is easy to check similarly that the n-dimensional Nambu system reduces to the $(n-1)$-dimensional Nambu system with a special choice $H_{n-1}\propto x^n$ for general $n\geq 3$. Geometrically, this method of reduction amounts to restricting the dynamics in n-dimensional phase space to a $(n-1)$-dimensional flat hyper-plane.

More generally, we can introduce similar kinds of reduction by imposing a constraint that one of the Hamiltonian functions $K(x^1,x^2,x^3)$ of an arbitrary given form is equal to a fixed numerical constant, and hence the dynamics is restricted to a two-dimensional curved surface from the outset. Then, we reinterpret the Nambu bracket $\{K, F_1, F_2\}$ with two arbitrary other functions (F_1, F_2) as a '*generalized* Poisson bracket' by defining

$$\{F_1, F_2\}_K \equiv \{K, F_1, F_2\} = -\{K, F_2, F_1\} = -\{F_2, F_1\}_K.$$

It is easy to check that the identity (2.17) indeed reduces to the Jacobi identity for the generalized Poisson bracket by fixing $F_3 = K$:

$$\{\{H, F_1\}_K, F_2\}_K + \{\{F_2, H\}_K, F_1\}_K + \{\{F_1, F_2\}_K, H\}_K = 0.$$

Also, the equations of motion become $\dot{F} = \{H, F\}_K$.

The fact that this reformulation of Nambu dynamics in terms of the generalized Poisson bracket is indeed a realization of the above picture of reducing the dynamics on a fixed curved surface associated with K can be formulated in a more concrete manner as follows. Let us interpret the generalized Poisson bracket between the phase coordinates with an arbitrary function F as the action of a corresponding differential operator on F, in analogy with the case of the ordinary Poisson bracket,

$$\{x^i, F\}_K = \{K, x^i, F\} = -\epsilon^{ijk}\partial_j K \partial_k F \equiv -\Delta^i_K F,$$

where $\Delta^i_K \equiv \epsilon^{ijk}\partial_j K \partial_k$, satisfying obviously $\Delta^i_K K = 0$. The last equation indicates that the action of the differential operator Δ^i_K is restricted such that it preserves a curved level-surface defined by $K =$ constant. Since

$$\{H, F\}_K = \{K, H, F\} = \epsilon^{ijk}\partial_i K \partial_j H \partial_k F = -\partial_i H \Delta^i_K F,$$

the time evolution is generated wholly by the differential operators Δ^i_K. It is straightforward to check that Δ^i_K form a closed algebra

$$[\Delta^i_K, \Delta^j_K] = f^{ij}_\ell(K)\Delta^\ell_K, \tag{2.28}$$

where $f^{ij}_\ell(K) \equiv -\epsilon^{ijk}\partial_k\partial_\ell K = -f^{ji}_\ell(K)$. When the coefficients f^{ij}_ℓ are all constants, the closed algebra (2.28) is a Lie algebra with f^{ij}_ℓ being the structure constant. This is the case when K is a quadratic form ($c_{ij} = c_{ji}$ =constants) $K = \frac{1}{2}c_{ij}x^i x^j$, yielding $f^{ij}_\ell = -\epsilon^{ijk}c_{k\ell} = -f^{ji}_\ell$. The generalized Poisson bracket then takes the form

$$\{H, F\}_K = -x^k f^{ij}_k \partial_i H \partial_j F.$$

This particular type of generalized Poisson brackets associated with a Lie algebra is often called a *Lie-Poisson* bracket.

The emergence of generalized Poisson brackets suggests itself a possible but rather trivial approach to quantization through a replacement of them by some appropriate commutation relations. However, such a simple-minded procedure would violate the N-gauge symmetry, though at least apparently there seems nothing wrong in principle in setting up such a system. A relevant issue is then to what extent, in general, the classical symmetries should be kept for claiming a quantized Nambu dynamics.

Example 2.2 Let us take the case of the Euler equation where the components $x^i = L_i$ of the angular momentum constitute the 3-dimensional Nambu phase space (x^1, x^2, x^3). Owing to Eq. (1.19), L_i satisfy

$$\{L_i, L_j\}_K \equiv \{K, L_i, L_j\} = \epsilon_{ijk} L_k, \tag{2.29}$$

which is a simplest nontrivial example of the Lie-Poisson bracket. Correspondingly, since $\partial_k \partial_\ell K = \delta_{k\ell}$ and $f_k^{ij} = -\epsilon^{ijk}$, we have the commutation relation for the differential operators $L_K^i \equiv -i\epsilon^{ijk} x^j \partial_k = -i\Delta_K^i$, with which the reader is familiar in quantum mechanics,

$$[L_K^i, L_K^j] = i\epsilon^{ijk} L_K^k. \tag{2.30}$$

The differential operator $\omega_i L_K^i$ acting on wave functions (as the functions of the phase coordinates) generates an infinitesimal rotation of the phase space coordinates $\delta x^i = \epsilon^{ijk}\omega_j x^k$ around the axis defined by a vector ω_i, under which the K-sphere, the level surface of K, is invariant. The equations of motion $\{H, F\}_K = i\partial_i H L_K^i F$ then describe an infinitesimal rotation with $\omega_i = \partial_i H = x_i/I_i$ at each point on the K-sphere. Since this motion itself conserves H, the trajectory lies on an intersection of the two level surfaces corresponding to K and H. This curve essentially coincides with what is called the *polhode* traditionally in conventional classical mechanics.

Now let us confirm how the above reduction of the Nambu bracket to generalized Poisson brackets is extended to higher-dimensional cases. If we choose one, H_1, out of the $(n-1)$ conserved Hamiltonians in n-dimensions and set $F_n = H_1$, the identity (2.19) is reduced to

$$\begin{aligned}
&\{\{H_2, \ldots, H_{n-1}, F_1\}_{H_1}, F_2, \ldots, F_{n-1}\}_{H_1} \\
&\quad + \{F_1, \{H_2, \ldots, H_{n-1}, F_2\}_{H_1}, F_3, \cdots, F_{n-1}\}_{H_1} \\
&\quad + \cdots + \{F_1, F_2, \ldots, \{H_2, \ldots, H_{n-1}, F_{n-1}\}_{H_1}\}_{H_1} \\
&= \{H_2, \ldots, H_{n-1}, \{F_1, F_2, \ldots, F_{n-1}\}_{H_1}\}_{H_1},
\end{aligned}$$

where

$$\{G_1, \ldots, G_{n-1}\}_{H_1} \equiv \{H_1, G_1, \ldots, G_{n-1}\}$$

is reinterpreted as a *generalized* $(n-1)$-dimensional *Nambu* bracket for arbitrary $n-1$ functions $(G_1, \ldots, G_{n-1})$, in the same sense as $\{H, F\}_K = \{K, H, F\}$ is reinterpreted as the generalized Poisson bracket in the foregoing arguments. By repeating this procedure until we reach three dimensions, we come to a 'generalized Nambu bracket', $\{x_i, x_j, x_k\}_{(H_1, H_2, H_3, \ldots, H_{n-3})}$, specified by a set of $n-3$ conserved Hamiltonian functions $(H_1, H_2, H_3, \ldots, H_{n-3})$ as 'passive' Hamiltonians and remaining two 'active' Hamiltonians H_{n-2} and H_{n-1}. Finally, we have the further reduction of the system to a generalized *Poisson* bracket specified by $n-2$ conserved but passive Hamiltonians $(H_1, \ldots, H_{n-3}, H_{n-2})$ with a remaining single active Hamiltonian H_{n-1}. Equation (2.19) ensures that the resulting generalized Poisson bracket $\{x_i, x_j\}_{(H_1, \ldots, H_{n-2})}$ satisfies the Jacobi identity. This series of reductions is made possible because of the fact that all higher-dimensional systems in this series describe one and the same set of one-dimensional trajectories which are intersections of the level hyper-surfaces of $n-1$ dimensions corresponding to $n-1$ conserved Hamiltonians, all playing equal roles in n-dimensional Nambu phase space.

Example 2.3 As a simple extension of Example 2.2, we can conceive of a 4-dimensional generalization of $x^i = L_i$ with the following three conserved Hamiltonians:

$$
\begin{aligned}
K &= \frac{1}{2}(L_1^2 + L_2^2 + L_3^2 + L_4^2), \\
H_1 &= \frac{1}{2}\left(\frac{L_1^2}{I_1} + \frac{L_2^2}{I_2} + \frac{L_3^2}{I_3} + \frac{L_4^2}{I_4}\right), \\
H_2 &= \frac{1}{2}\left(\frac{L_1^2}{J_1} + \frac{L_2^2}{J_2} + \frac{L_3^2}{J_3} + \frac{L_4^2}{J_4}\right).
\end{aligned}
$$

If we choose the passive conserved Hamiltonian to be K, the 4-dimensional brackets of phase coordinates L_i constitute a closed algebra of the generalized 3-dimensional Nambu bracket,

$$
\{L_i, L_j, L_k\}_K \equiv \{K, L_i, L_j, L_k\} = \epsilon_{ijk\ell} L_\ell, \tag{2.31}
$$

which is a natural 4-dimensional extension of the Lie Poisson bracket (2.29). The equations of motion $\frac{dL_i}{dt} = \{H_1, H_2, L_i\}_K$ yield an extension of the Euler equations,

$$
\frac{dL_1}{dt} = \left[-\frac{1}{I_2}\left(\frac{1}{J_3} - \frac{1}{J_4}\right) + \frac{1}{I_3}\left(\frac{1}{J_2} - \frac{1}{J_4}\right) - \frac{1}{I_4}\left(\frac{1}{J_2} - \frac{1}{J_3}\right)\right] L_2 L_3 L_4, \quad \text{etc.}
$$

It would be an interesting problem to explore whether there exists a realistic physical system, a 'generalized Euler top', effectively obeying these equations with two independent sets (I_i, J_i) of the moments of inertia. In view of the correspondence between the generalized Poisson bracket (2.29) and the commutation relation (2.30), another related question is whether there exist any concrete realizations of closed operator algebra which precisely correspond to the generalized Nambu bracket (2.31), in terms of e.g., matrices, or differential operators. It might also provide us a suggestive test case when we make an attempt toward quantized Nambu dynamics.

On the other hand, if we apply a further reduction to the generalized Poisson bracket by defining $\{L_i, L_j\}_{(K,H_1)} \equiv \{K, H_1, L_i, L_j\}$, we find

$$\{L_i, L_j\}_{(K,H_1)} = \epsilon_{ijkl}\partial_k K \partial_\ell H_1 = \frac{1}{2}\epsilon_{ijk\ell}\left(\frac{1}{I_\ell} - \frac{1}{I_k}\right)L_k L_\ell.$$

Since the right-hand side is not linear in L_i, it is necessary to consider an infinite set of polynomial functions of L_i if we wish to obtain a closed algebra with respect to the generalized Poisson bracket. Let $f(L) = f(L_1, \ldots, L_4)$ and $g(L) = g(L_1, \ldots, L_4)$ be two arbitrary polynomials. Then we have

$$\{f(L), g(L)\}_{(K,H_1)} = h_{[f,g]}(L),$$

where

$$h_{[f,g]}(L) = -h_{[g,f]}(L) \equiv \frac{1}{2}\epsilon_{ijkl}L_k L_\ell\left(\frac{1}{I_\ell} - \frac{1}{I_k}\right)\partial_i f \partial_j g.$$

In terms of this strange algebra, the equations of motion take a simple form, $\dot{L}_i = \{H_2, L_i\}_{(K,H_1)}$.

2.5 Generalized Canonical Transformations and Higher-Form Gauge Symmetries

2.5.1 Generalized Canonical Transformations and Jacobian

We have seen from the foregoing discussions, especially in Sect. 2.3.2, that the invariance of the Jacobian under generalized canonical transformations is crucial in characterizing the structure of Nambu dynamics. Let us now begin to investigate the generalized canonical transformations in general n-dimensions. In n-dimensional Nambu phase space, the generalized canonical transformation is defined as the mapping of phase space onto itself $x^i \to x'^i(x)$ such that

$$\frac{\partial(x'^1, x'^2, \ldots, x'^n)}{\partial(x^1, x^2, \ldots, x^n)} = 1. \tag{2.32}$$

The set of all generalized canonical transformations form a group, since

$$\frac{\partial(x'^1, x'^2, \ldots, x'^n)}{\partial(x^1, x^2, \ldots, x^n)} \frac{\partial(x^1, x^2, \ldots, x^n)}{\partial(x'^1, x'^2, \ldots, x'^n)} = 1,$$

$$\frac{\partial(x''^1, x''^2, \dots, x''^n)}{\partial(x'^1, x'^2, \dots, x'^n)} \frac{\partial(x'^1, x'^2, \dots, x'^n)}{\partial(x^1, x^2, \dots, x^n)} = \frac{\partial(x''^1, x''^2, \dots, x''^n)}{\partial(x^1, x^2, \dots, x^n)}$$

are identically satisfied for three arbitrary transformations ($x^i \to x'^i, x^i \to x''^i, x'^i \to x''^i$) and are consistent with the requirement (2.32): the first and the second of these identities show the existence of the inverse transformation and that the resultant of two generalized canonical transformations in succession is again a generalized canonical transformation. Other requirements to be a group, the existence of the identity element and the associativity law, are also derived from these identities trivially.

The general Nambu equations of motion $\dot{F} = \{H_1, \dots, H_{n-1}, F\}$ in n dimensions are clearly form-invariant under the generalized canonical transformations. To motivate the following discussions, we note that solving the Nambu equations of motion actually amounts to performing a special finite generalized canonical transformation such that $x^i \to x'^i = H_i$ for $i = 1, \dots, n-1$: by definition we then have

$$\{H_1, \dots, H_{n-1}, x'^n\} = 1, \tag{2.33}$$

which, for transformed variables, implies the equations of motion $\dot{H}_1 = \cdots = \dot{H}_{n-1} = 0$ and $\dot{x}'^n = 1$. The last equation allows us to identity $x'^n = t + c_n$ with an arbitrary constant c_n. Therefore, this special generalized canonical transformation $x'^i = x'^i(x^1, \dots, x^n)$ implicitly gives the general solution of the Nambu equations of motion with n integration constants consisting of the initial conditions, $H_i = c_i$ and $x'^n(0) = c_n$.

Let us here briefly recall the origin of the Jacobian, the determinant of the coefficient matrix of the transformation of infinitesimal differentials dx^i,

$$dx'^i = \frac{\partial x'^i}{\partial x^j} dx^j, \qquad \frac{\partial(x'^1, \dots, x'^n)}{\partial(x^1, \dots, x^n)} = \det\left(\frac{\partial x'^i}{\partial x^j}\right).$$

Each component dx^i of the differentials corresponds to an infinitesimal line element directed positively along the i-th coordinate axis. A pair of two differentials dx^i and dx^j with different directions i and j corresponds to an infinitesimal rectangle lying in the plane spanned by the i-th and j-th axes. In three dimensions $n = 3$, in particular, this infinitesimal plane can be represented by the infinitesimal area vector in terms of the familiar notations of vector analysis ($d\mathbf{x}^i \times d\mathbf{x}^j = -d\mathbf{x}^j \times d\mathbf{x}^i$),

$$d\mathbf{S} = (dx^2dx^3, dx^3dx^1, dx^1dx^2) = d\mathbf{x}^1 \times d\mathbf{x}^2 + d\mathbf{x}^2 \times d\mathbf{x}^3 + d\mathbf{x}^3 \times d\mathbf{x}^1,$$
$$d\mathbf{x}^1 \equiv (dx^1, 0, 0), \;\; d\mathbf{x}^2 \equiv (0, dx^2, 0), \;\; d\mathbf{x}^3 \equiv (0, 0, dx^3),$$

already being used in discussing Liouville's theorem in Sect. 2.1. The triple of three differentials corresponds to an infinitesimal cube and their product gives an infinitesimal volume as a scalar,

$$dV = \frac{1}{6}\epsilon_{ijk}d\mathbf{x}^i \cdot (d\mathbf{x}^j \times d\mathbf{x}^k) = d\mathbf{x}^1 \cdot (d\mathbf{x}^2 \times d\mathbf{x}^3) = -d\mathbf{x}^1 \cdot (d\mathbf{x}^3 \times d\mathbf{x}^2),$$

satisfying

$$dV' = \frac{1}{6}\epsilon_{ijk}\frac{\partial x'^i}{\partial x^p}\frac{\partial x'^j}{\partial x^q}\frac{\partial x'^k}{\partial x^\ell}d\mathbf{x}^p \cdot (d\mathbf{x}^q \times d\mathbf{x}^\ell) = \frac{\partial(x'^1, x'^2, x'^3)}{\partial(x^1, x^2, x^3)}dV.$$

The sign changes under permutations of vector differentials $d\mathbf{x}^i$ reflect that these infinitesimal geometrical objects have their own orientations. If we continue to use vector notations, however, the extension to phase spaces with arbitrary dimensions becomes increasingly cumbersome. To facilitate our work toward this direction, it is suitable to adopt the notion of differential forms. That will play useful roles in developing the physics of Nambu dynamics with a clear geometrical picture.

2.5.2 *Differential Forms and Exterior Differentiation*

We start with summarizing briefly the definition and the properties of differential forms to a minimal extent needed for later developments. The partial differentiation of an arbitrary scalar function $f(x)$ gives

$$df = \frac{\partial f}{\partial x^i}dx^i.$$

This is a special (and the simplest) case of general *1-form* $\omega^{(1)}$ which is defined as a linear combination of the differentials dx^i (a *contravariant* vector) ,

$$\omega^{(1)} \equiv \omega_i dx^i$$

with arbitrary coefficient functions $\omega_i = \omega_i(x)$ constituting the components of a *covariant* vector. A scalar function f itself can be regarded as a 'zero' form, $\omega^{(0)}(x) = f(x)$. The derivation (*exterior differentiation*) of the 1-form is defined by

$$d\omega^{(1)} \equiv d\omega_i \wedge dx^i \equiv \frac{1}{2}(\partial_i\omega_j - \partial_j\omega_i)dx^i \wedge dx^j$$

where the product symbol '$\wedge$' of two differentials dx^i and dx^j is called the *exterior* product and, by definition satisfies $dx^i \wedge dx^j = -dx^j \wedge dx^i$, which represents the infinitesimal area element lying in the ij-plane with orientation, corresponding to dS of the previous subsection. Just as df is a special case of $\omega^{(1)}$, $d\omega^{(1)}$ is a special case of the general *2-form* $\omega^{(2)}$:

$$\omega^{(2)} \equiv \frac{1}{2}\omega_{ij}dx^i \wedge dx^j,$$

where $\omega_{ij}(x) = -\omega_{ji}(x)$ is an arbitrary covariant skew-symmetric tensor field.

Remark 2.2 Let us here consider the above definitions from the viewpoint of the change of coordinate frames $x^i \to \tilde{x}^i$. Since we can write

$$\omega^{(1)}(x) = \omega_i(x)\frac{\partial x^i}{\partial \tilde{x}^j}d\tilde{x}^j = \tilde{\omega}_j(\tilde{x})d\tilde{x}^j, \quad \tilde{\omega}_j(\tilde{x}) \equiv \omega_i(x)\frac{\partial x^i}{\partial \tilde{x}^j},$$

the components field $\omega_i(x)$ can be regarded as a covariant vector. Furthermore, this immediately yields

$$\begin{aligned}\tilde{\partial}_k\tilde{\omega}_j - \tilde{\partial}_j\tilde{\omega}_k &= \frac{\partial x^\ell}{\partial \tilde{x}^k}\partial_\ell\left(\omega_i(x)\frac{\partial x^i}{\partial \tilde{x}^j}\right) - \frac{\partial x^\ell}{\partial \tilde{x}^j}\partial_\ell\left(\omega_i(x)\frac{\partial x^i}{\partial \tilde{x}^k}\right)\\ &= \frac{\partial x^\ell}{\partial \tilde{x}^k}\frac{\partial x^i}{\partial \tilde{x}^j}(\partial_\ell\omega_i - \partial_i\omega_\ell),\end{aligned}$$

using $\frac{\partial x^\ell}{\partial \tilde{x}^k}\partial_\ell\frac{\partial x^i}{\partial \tilde{x}^j} = \frac{\partial^2 x^i}{\partial \tilde{x}^k\partial \tilde{x}^j} = \frac{\partial^2 x^i}{\partial \tilde{x}^j\partial \tilde{x}^k} = \frac{\partial x^\ell}{\partial \tilde{x}^j}\partial_\ell\frac{\partial x^i}{\partial \tilde{x}^k}$. This shows that $\partial_i\omega_j - \partial_j\omega_i$ can be regarded as a second-rank tensor which is antisymmetric with respect to the two indices (i, j). Thus, the definition of the exterior differentiation automatically keeps the covariance property for the components fields with respect to the change of coordinate frames.

Extending the procedures given above, we are naturally led to a general definition of the exterior product of higher differentials as a totally skew-symmetric product of k $(k \geq 2)$ differentials:

$$dx^{i_1} \wedge dx^{i_2} \wedge \cdots \wedge dx^{i_k} = (-1)^{\epsilon(P)}dx^{i_{P(1)}} \wedge dx^{i_{P(2)}} \wedge \cdots \wedge dx^{i_{P(k)}},$$

where, as we have already used in defining the Nambu bracket, $P(i)$ denotes the permutation of indices i and $\epsilon(P)$ is its parity ($\epsilon(P) = 0$ if P is an even permutation and $= 1$ if P is an odd permutation). This product geometrically corresponds to an *oriented* infinitesimal k-dimensional hyper-parallelepiped of which the faces consist of $k(k-1)/2$ pairs of infinitesimal parallel rectangles $dx^{i_p} \wedge dx^{i_q}$: its orientation is reversed whenever the ordering of a pair (i_p, i_q) is replaced with (i_q, i_p) $(p, q \in (1, \ldots, k))$. Obviously, in n-dimensional phase space, we have $0 \leq k \leq n$.

We can now define a general *k-form* by

$$\omega^{(k)} \equiv \frac{1}{k!}\omega_{i_1\ldots i_k}dx^{i_1} \wedge \cdots \wedge dx^{i_k},$$

where $\omega_{i_1\cdots i_k} = \omega_{i_1\cdots i_k}(x)$ is an arbitrary totally skew-symmetric covariant k-tensor field. This is equivalently written $\omega_{i_1\ldots i_k}dx^{i_1} \wedge \cdots \wedge dx^{i_k}$, *with the proviso* that we impose the ordering condition $i_1 < i_2 < \ldots < i_k$ for the summations with respect to k contracted indices; by contrast, in the above expression, no ordering condition is assumed and hence we need the pre-factor $1/k!$. Both conventions will be used in what follows depending on situations at hand.

The basic k-forms $dx^{i_1} \wedge \cdots dx^{i_k}$ in terms of coordinate differentials dx^i thus constitute a basis for general k-forms. Furthermore, given arbitrary p-form and q-form ($i_1 < \cdots < i_p$, $j_1 < \cdots < j_q$),

$$\alpha^{(p)} = \alpha_{i_1 \ldots i_p} dx^{i_1} \wedge \cdots \wedge dx^{i_p}, \quad \beta^{(q)} = \beta_{j_1 \ldots j_q} dx^{j_1} \wedge \cdots \wedge dx^{j_q},$$

we can construct their exterior product $\alpha^{(p)} \wedge \beta^{(q)}$,

$$(dx^{i_1} \wedge \cdots \wedge dx^{i_p}) \wedge (dx^{j_1} \cdots \wedge dx^{j_q}) \equiv dx^{i_1} \wedge \cdots \wedge dx^{i_p} \wedge dx^{j_1} \wedge \cdots \wedge dx^{j_q}.$$

By definition, the product of the base differential forms vanishes whenever there exist common indices among the two sets $(i_1, \ldots, i_p)$ and $(j_1, \ldots, j_q)$. It follows immediately that

$$\alpha^{(p)} \wedge \beta^{(q)} = (-1)^{pq} \beta^{(q)} \wedge \alpha^{(p)}.$$

The associativity of exterior products is also obvious from the above definition and hence we can write the exterior products of any numbers of differential forms without using parentheses simply as $\alpha^{(p)} \wedge \beta^{(q)} \wedge \gamma^{(r)} \wedge \cdots$.

The exterior derivation of a general $(k-1)$-form is given by

$$\begin{aligned} d\omega^{(k-1)} &= d\omega_{i_1 \ldots i_{k-1}} \wedge dx^{i_1} \wedge \cdots \wedge dx^{i_{k-1}} \quad (i_1 < i_2 < \ldots < i_{k-1}) \\ &= \partial_{[i_1} \omega_{i_2 \ldots i_k]} dx^{i_1} \wedge dx^{i_2} \wedge \cdots \wedge dx^{i_k} \quad (i_1 < i_2 < \ldots < i_k), \end{aligned}$$

where the symbol $[i_1, \ldots, i_k]$ indicates total skew symmetrization with respect to the ordering among the set $(i_1, i_2, \ldots, i_k)$ of the k indices enclosed in $[\ldots]$:

$$\partial_{[i_1} \omega_{i_2]} \equiv \partial_{i_1} \omega_{i_2} - \partial_{i_2} \omega_{i_1}, \quad \partial_{[i_1} \omega_{i_2 i_3]} \equiv \partial_{i_1} \omega_{i_2 i_3} + \partial_{i_2} \omega_{i_3 i_1} + \partial_{i_3} \omega_{i_1 i_2}, \quad \text{etc.}$$

It is evident that in n-dimensional space, the highest form possible is the n-form. We also see immediately that for an arbitrary k-form $\omega^{(k)}$

$$dd\omega^{(k)} = 0, \tag{2.34}$$

since $\partial_{[i_1} \partial_{i_2} \omega_{i_3 \cdots i_n]} = 0$, because of the commutativity of partial derivatives $\partial_{i_1} \partial_{i_2} = \partial_{i_2} \partial_{i_1}$. If a k-form satisfies $d\omega^{(k)} = 0$, we say that $\omega^{(k)}$ is a *closed* k-form. If a k-form is given as $\omega^{(k)} = d\omega^{(k-1)}$ with some $(k-1)$-form, we say that it is an *exact* k-form. The 'nilpotency' property $d^2 = 0$ exhibited in (2.34) implies that an exact k-form necessarily gives a closed $(k+1)$-form $d\omega^{(k)}$.

It is also not difficult to verify that the exterior differentiation of exterior product of two differential forms is given by

$$d(\alpha^{(p)} \wedge \beta^{(q)}) = d\alpha^{(p)} \wedge \beta^{(q)} + (-1)^p \alpha^{(p)} \wedge d\beta^{(q)}. \tag{2.35}$$

Indeed, by direct calculation, the left-hand side gives

$$\begin{aligned}
d(\alpha^{(p)} \wedge \beta^{(q)}) &= \frac{1}{p!}\frac{1}{q!} d(\alpha_{i_1 \ldots i_p} \beta_{j_1 \ldots j_q} dx^{i_1} \wedge \cdots \wedge dx^{i_p} \wedge dx^{j_1} \wedge \cdots \wedge dx^{j_q}) \\
&= \frac{1}{p!}\frac{1}{q!}\big[(\partial_k \alpha_{i_1 \ldots i_p} \beta_{j_1 \ldots j_q} + \alpha_{i_1 \ldots i_p} \partial_k \beta_{j_1 \ldots j_p}) dx^k \wedge dx^{i_1} \wedge \cdots \wedge dx^{i_p} \\
&\qquad \wedge dx^{j_1} \wedge \cdots \wedge dx^{j_q}\big] \\
&= \frac{1}{p!}\frac{1}{q!}\big[(\partial_k \alpha_{i_1 \ldots i_p} dx^k \wedge dx^{i_1} \wedge \cdots \wedge dx^{i_p}) \wedge (\beta_{j_1 \ldots j_q} dx^{j_1} \wedge \cdots \wedge dx^{j_q}) \\
&\quad + (-1)^p (\alpha_{i_1 \ldots i_p} dx^{i_1} \wedge \cdots \wedge dx^{i_p}) \wedge (\partial_k \beta_{j_1 \ldots j_q} dx^k \wedge dx^{j_1} \wedge \cdots \wedge dx^{j_q}\big] \\
&= d\alpha^{(p)} \wedge \beta^{(q)} + (-1)^p \alpha^{(p)} \wedge d\beta^{(q)}.
\end{aligned}$$

Example 2.4 We here exemplify exterior differentiations in a completely explicit manner in three dimensions:

$$\begin{aligned}
\omega^{(1)} &= \omega_1 dx^1 + \omega_2 dx^2 + \omega_3 dx^3, \\
d\omega^{(1)} &= (\partial_1 \omega_2 - \partial_2 \omega_1) dx^1 \wedge dx^2 + (\partial_2 \omega_3 - \partial_3 \omega_2) dx^2 \wedge dx^3 \\
&\quad + (\partial_1 \omega_3 - \partial_3 \omega_1) dx^1 \wedge dx^3, \\
d^2\omega^{(1)} &= \big[\partial_3(\partial_1 \omega_2 - \partial_2 \omega_1) + \partial_1(\partial_2 \omega_3 - \partial_3 \omega_2) + \partial_2(\partial_3 \omega_1 - \partial_1 \omega_3)\big] dx^1 \wedge dx^2 \wedge dx^3 \\
&= 0, \\
\omega^{(2)} &= \omega_{12} dx^1 \wedge dx^2 + \omega_{23} dx^2 \wedge dx^3 + \omega_{13} dx^1 \wedge dx^3, \\
d\omega^{(2)} &= (\partial_3 \omega_{12} + \partial_1 \omega_{23} + \partial_2 \omega_{31}) dx^1 \wedge dx^2 \wedge dx^3, \\
d^2\omega^{(2)} &= \partial_i (\partial_3 \omega_{12} + \partial_1 \omega_{23} + \partial_2 \omega_{31}) dx^i \wedge dx^1 \wedge dx^2 \wedge dx^3 = 0, \\
\omega^{(3)} &= \omega_{123} dx^1 \wedge dx^2 \wedge dx^3, \\
d\omega^{(3)} &= \partial_i \omega_{123} dx^i \wedge dx^1 \wedge dx^2 \wedge dx^3 = 0.
\end{aligned}$$

Just as $\omega^{(1)}$ corresponds to a generic covariant vector with a general direction, $\omega^{(2)}$ represents a generic covariant oriented area 2-tensor with a general direction.

Examples of the exterior product of differential forms are as follows:

$$\begin{aligned}
\alpha^{(1)} \wedge \beta^{(1)} &= (\alpha_1 dx^1 + \alpha_2 dx^2 + \omega_3 dx^3) \wedge (\beta_1 dx^1 + \beta_2 dx^2 + \beta_3 dx^3) \\
&= (\alpha_1 \beta_2 - \alpha_2 \beta_1) dx^1 \wedge dx^2 + (\alpha_2 \beta_3 - \alpha_3 \beta_2) dx^2 \wedge dx^3 \\
&\quad + (\alpha_1 \beta_3 - \alpha_3 \beta_1) dx^1 \wedge dx^3, d(\alpha^{(1)} \wedge \beta^{(1)}) \\
&= \big[\partial_3(\alpha_1 \beta_2 - \alpha_2 \beta_1) + \partial_1(\alpha_2 \beta_3 - \alpha_3 \beta_2) + \partial_2(\alpha_3 \beta_1 - \alpha_1 \beta_3)\big] dx^1 \wedge dx^2 \wedge dx^3.
\end{aligned}$$

It is easy to check that the last expression is equal to $d\alpha^{(1)} \wedge \beta^{(1)} - \alpha^{(1)} \wedge d\beta^{(1)}$, using the above formula for $d\omega^{(1)}$. Note also that

$$d(d\alpha^{(1)} \wedge \beta^{(1)} - \alpha^{(1)} \wedge d\beta^{(1)}) = d\alpha^{(1)} \wedge d\beta^{(1)} - d\alpha^{(1)} \wedge d\beta^{(1)} = 0.$$

To help an intuitive grasp of exterior differentiation, we give below graphical images in the case of the 1-form $\omega^{(1)}$ (Fig. 2.1):

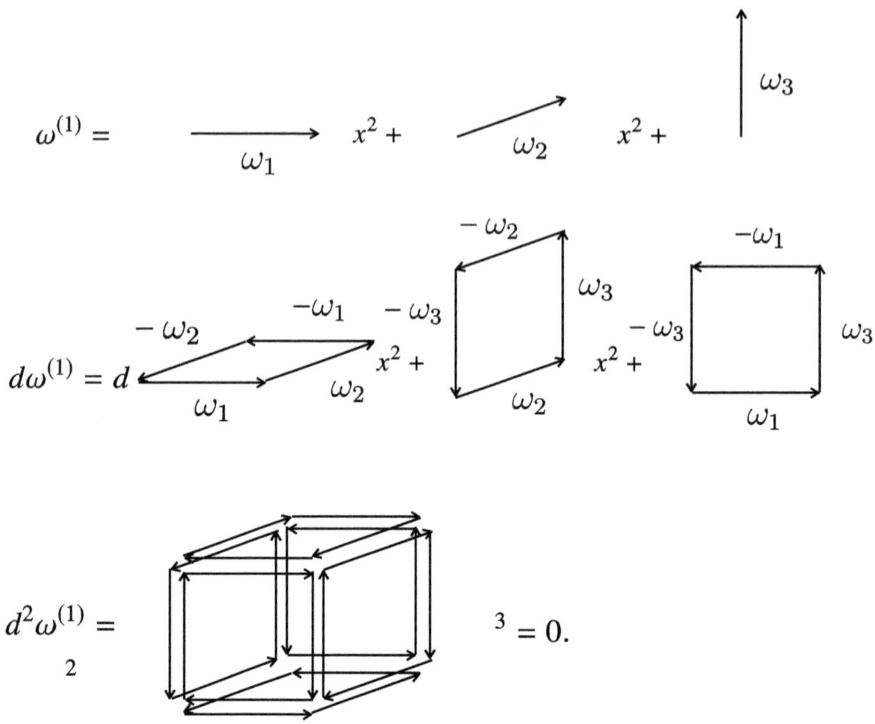

Fig. 2.1 The exterior derivatives of a 1-form

Note that the vanishing of $d^2\omega^{(1)}$, namely the nilpotency $d^2 = 0$, in the last line occurs through the cancellation of the pairs of edges with opposite orientations, ω_i and $-\omega_i$, at the same positions, that are created from the exact 1-form $d\omega^{(1)}$ by the operation of the second exterior differentiation. The reader should endeavor to imagine the generalization of these graphical pictures for higher forms.

2.5.3 *Finite Generalized Canonical Transformations*

The exterior product naturally yields the Jacobian for an arbitrary coordinate transformation $x^i \to x'^i(x)$ in n dimensions, using the 1-form relation $dx'^i = \frac{\partial x'^i}{\partial x^j} dx^j$:

$$dx'^1 \wedge dx'^2 \wedge \cdots \wedge dx'^n = \frac{\partial(x'^1, x'^2, \ldots, x'^n)}{\partial(x^1, x^2, \ldots, x^n)} dx^1 \wedge dx^2 \wedge \cdots \wedge dx^n. \quad (2.36)$$

Thus, in terms of differential forms, the condition for a finite generalized canonical transformation in n-dimensional Nambu phase space is given by

$$dx'^1 \wedge dx'^2 \wedge \cdots \wedge dx'^n = dx^1 \wedge dx^2 \wedge \cdots \wedge dx^n. \tag{2.37}$$

It should be noted here that if we rename the transformed coordinates x'^i by identifying them with a set of n arbitrary functions $F_i = F_i(x)$, the exterior product in (2.36) just amounts to defining the n-dimensional Nambu bracket

$$dF_1 \wedge dF_2 \wedge \cdots \wedge dF_n \equiv \{F_1, F_2, \ldots, F_n\} dx^1 \wedge dx^2 \wedge \cdots \wedge dx^n. \tag{2.38}$$

For simplicity and definiteness, let us now specialize to the case $n = 3$. We have

$$dx'^1 \wedge dx'^2 \wedge dx'^3 = dx^1 \wedge dx^2 \wedge dx^3, \tag{2.39}$$

and

$$dx^1 \wedge dx^2 \wedge dx^3 = d(x^1 dx^2 \wedge dx^3) = d(x^2 dx^3 \wedge dx^1) = d(x^3 dx^1 \wedge dx^2)$$

and similarly for transformed coordinates (x'^1, x'^2, x'^3), which yield

$$d(x'^{i'} dx'^{j'} \wedge dx'^{k'} - x^i dx^j \wedge dx^k) = 0 \tag{2.40}$$

for any pair of two triplets (i', j', k') and (i, j, k) of indices, being obtained by cyclic permutation of $(1, 2, 3)$. If any 2-form $S^{(2)} = S_{ij} dx^i \wedge dx^j$, $(i < j)$ is closed, namely if $dS^{(2)} = 0$, or $\epsilon^{ijk}\partial_i S_{jk} = \partial_i v^i = 0$, where $v^i \equiv \epsilon^{ijk} S_{jk}$, we can introduce a vector potential S_i whose rotation gives $v^i = \epsilon^{ijk}\partial_j S_k$ by an elementary theorem (known as Helmholtz's theorem) of vector analysis. This is equivalent to the property that, if a 2-form $S^{(2)}$ is closed, $dS^{(2)} = 0$, then there is a 1-form $S^{(1)} = S_i dx^i$ satisfying $S^{(2)} = \frac{1}{2}(\partial_i S_j - \partial_j S_i) dx^i \wedge dx^j = dS^{(1)}$. Namely, any closed 2-form is necessarily exact. Equivalently, $S_{ij} = \partial_i S_j - \partial_j S_i$.

Therefore, using this property in (2.40), we can set

$$x'^{i'} dx'^{j'} \wedge dx'^{k'} - x^i dx^j \wedge dx^k = dS^{(1)} = \frac{1}{2}(\partial_a S_b - \partial_b S_a) dx^a \wedge dx^b, \tag{2.41}$$

which, by equating the coefficients of $dx^a \wedge dx^b$ on both sides, is equivalent to

$$x'^{i'} \left(\frac{\partial x'^{j'}}{\partial x^a} \frac{\partial x'^{k'}}{\partial x^b} - \frac{\partial x'^{j'}}{\partial x^b} \frac{\partial x'^{k'}}{\partial x^a} \right) - x^i (\delta^j_a \delta^k_b - \delta^j_b \delta^k_a) = \partial_a S_b - \partial_b S_a, \tag{2.42}$$

where (a, b) is an arbitrary pair of two different indices a and b. Since the right-hand side is invariant under gauge transformation $S_a \to S_a + \partial_a \Lambda$ with an arbitrary scalar function Λ, the number of true degrees of freedom contributing to the right is two, which coincides with that of generalized canonical transformations for

$n = 3$. This agreement guarantees the general validity of (2.42). Thus, the 1-form $S^{(1)}$ plays a role of generating function for finite generalized canonical transformations in 3-dimensional Nambu phase space.

In fact, the structure of finite generalized canonical transformations in Nambu dynamics revealed here has an aspect which is more intricate than finite canonical transformations in conventional Hamiltonian dynamics: in the conventional case, *once* the generating (0-form) function S as a function of independent variables is given explicitly, canonical transformation is reduced to algebraic relations between the original and transformed variables, as exemplified in the last line of the table below for the choice of $2n$ independent variables (q, q'). This is made possible because obtaining the generating function S amounts to integrating the [1-form relation]. Other choices of independent variables such as (q, p'), (q', p) and (p, p') can be expressed similarly by redefining S appropriately, using $p'dq' + q'dp' = d(p'q')$ and $pdq + qdp = d(pq)$.

Nambu dynamics	Hamiltonian dynamics
(2.39) [3-form relation]	$dp'_i \wedge dq'_i = dp_i \wedge dq_i$ [2-form relation]
(2.40) [closed 2-form]	$d(p'_i dq'_i) = d(p_i dq_i)$ [closed 1-form]
(2.41) [2-form relation]	$p'_i dq'_i - p_i dq_i = dS$ [1-form relation]
(2.42)	$p'_i = \frac{\partial S}{\partial q'_i}, \quad p_i = -\frac{\partial S}{\partial q_i}$

In the case of Nambu dynamics, by contrast, a similar reduction to completely algebraic relations is, *in general,* not possible. The reason is that the left-hand side of (2.41) involves *four* differentials $(dx'^{j'}, dx'^{k'}, dx^j, dx^k)$: any one choice of four directions (j', k', j, k) involves one dependent directions because we can only have *three* independent variables in 3 dimensions. Therefore *at least* one of these four differentials must be expressed in terms of three independent differentials implicitly, which necessarily makes those relations differential equations. This is so even if these relations themselves have already been integrated once from the original Jacobian relation $\frac{\partial(x'^1, x'^2, x'^3)}{\partial(x^1, x^2, x^3)} = 1$ or (2.39) that involves three derivatives. Thus, from a practical point of view, the usefulness of the generating function is somewhat limited compared with that in the conventional Hamiltonian formalism. Fortunately, however, for *infinitesimal* generalized canonical transformations, the situation will be simplified since we can explicitly integrate out some of the differentiations in the Jacobian, as we shall see in the next section.

Now let us extend the above discussions to higher dimensions. In n-dimensional phase space, we have for any fixed pair of two n-plets $(i'_1, \ldots, i'_n)$ and $(i_1, \ldots, i_n)$ obtained by cyclic permutations from $(1, \ldots, n)$,

$$
\begin{aligned}
x'^{i'_1} dx'^{i'_2} \wedge \cdots \wedge dx'^{i'_n} - x^{i_1} dx^{i_2} \wedge \cdots \wedge dx^{i_n} &= dS^{(n-2)} \\
&= \partial_{[a_1} S_{a_2 \cdots a_{n-1}]} dx^{a_1} \wedge \cdots \wedge dx^{a_{n-1}}, \quad (a_1 < \ldots < a_{n-1}) \qquad (2.43)
\end{aligned}
$$

with some generating $(n-2)$-form $S^{(n-2)} = S_{i_1 \ldots i_{n-2}} dx^{i_1} \wedge \cdots \wedge dx^{i_{n-2}}$, $(i_1 < \ldots < i_{n-2})$. The number of degrees of freedom of $S^{(n-2)}$ is $\binom{n}{2=n(n-1)/2}$, while the degrees of freedom of the generalized gauge transformation

$$S_{i_1 \cdots i_{n-2}} \to S_{i_1 \cdots i_{n-2}} + \partial_{[i_1} \Lambda_{i_2 \ldots i_{n-2}]} \tag{2.44}$$

under which (2.43) is invariant is $(n-1)(n-2)/2$, as we prove below. Thus the number of true degrees of freedom contributing the right-hand side of (2.43) is $n(n-1)/2 - (n-1)(n-2)/2 = n-1$ in conformity with the number of degrees of freedom of the generalized canonical transformations in n-dimensional phase space. We call such a gauge transformation for $n > 3$ a *higher-form* gauge transformation.

Exercise 2.2 (Higher-form gauge transformations) Using the language of differential forms, the gauge transformation (2.44) is nothing but $S^{(n-2)} \to S^{(n-2)} + d\Lambda^{(n-3)}$, where $\Lambda^{(n-3)}$ is an arbitrary $(n-3)$ form,

$$\Lambda^{(n-3)} = \Lambda_{i_1 \cdots i_{n-3}} dx^{i_1} \wedge \cdots \wedge dx^{i_{n-3}}, \qquad (i_1 < \ldots < i_{n-3}).$$

When $n > 3$, owing to the nilpotency $d^2 = 0$, there are further degrees of freedom of gauge transformation for $(n-3)$-form

$$\Lambda^{(n-3)} \to \Lambda^{(n-3)} + d\Lambda^{(n-4)}.$$

Note that the additional higher-form gauge transformation plays the role of lessening the effective number of gauge degrees of freedom carried by $d\Lambda^{(n-3)}$. But if $n > 4$ we have yet another gauge symmetry for the latter in the form $\Lambda^{(n-4)} \to \Lambda^{(n-4)} + d\Lambda^{(n-5)}$. This continues until we finally arrive at 1-form gauge transformation for which the gauge degrees of freedom become minimum, namely, one 0-form $\Lambda^{(n-n)} = \Lambda^{(0)} = \Lambda$. Taking into account such series of *nested* multiple gauge transformations, the number of the total gauge degrees of freedom for the $(n-2)$-form $S^{(n-2)}$ is calculated as

$$\binom{n}{3} - \binom{n}{4} + \left[\binom{n}{5} - \left[\binom{n}{6} - \left[\cdots - \binom{n}{n}\underbrace{\right]\right]\cdots\right]}_{n-4}$$

$$= \sum_{r=3}^{n} (-1)^{r+1} \binom{n}{r} = \frac{(n-1)(n-2)}{2},$$

which is equivalent to the familiar identity $\sum_{r=0}^{n} (-1)^r \binom{n}{r} = (1-1)^n = 0$, because

$$\sum_{r=0}^{2} (-1)^r \binom{n}{r} = 1 - n + \frac{n(n-1)}{2} = \frac{(n-1)(n-2)}{2}.$$

This is what we have promised to prove.

Mathematically, the fact that there exists some $(k-1)$-form which allows us to write a k-form as an exact form $\omega^{(k)} = d\omega^{(k-1)}$, when $\omega^{(k)}$ is closed $d\omega^{(k)} = 0$, is known as *Poincaré's lemma*. The fact that the degrees of freedom are correctly accounted for as demonstrated here is sufficient for validating this lemma.

Exercise 2.3 Suppose we could have six independent coordinates $(z_1, \ldots, z_6)$ with a generalized canonical structure associated with a 3-form, $dz_1 \wedge dz_2 \wedge dz_3 + dz_4 \wedge dz_5 \wedge dz_6$. Consider linear coordinate transformations by constant 6×6 matrices, $z_i \to z'_i = b_{ij} z_j$, such that this 3-form is kept invariant, namely,

$$dz_1 \wedge dz_2 \wedge dz_3 + dz_4 \wedge dz_5 \wedge dz_6 = dz'_1 \wedge dz'_2 \wedge dz'_3 + dz'_4 \wedge dz'_5 \wedge dz'_6.$$

Expanding the right-hand side in terms of dz_i, we first find two conditions for the coefficients of $dz_1 \wedge dz_2 \wedge dz_3$ and $dz_4 \wedge dz_5 \wedge dz_6$, which read

$$\frac{1}{3!} \sum_{(i,j,k)=(1,2,3)}^{3} \epsilon_{ijk}(b_{1i}b_{2j}b_{3k} + b_{4i}b_{5j}b_{6k}) = 1,$$

$$\frac{1}{3!} \sum_{(i,j,k)=(4,5,6)}^{6} \epsilon_{ijk}(b_{1i}b_{2j}b_{3k} + b_{4i}b_{5j}b_{6k}) = 1,$$

where summations on the left-hand side with the condition $(i, j, k) = (1, 2, 3)$ are done over different permutations (including both cyclic and anti-cyclic permuations) of the set of indices $(1, 2, 3)$, etc. All other combinations involving mixing between (dz_1, dz_2, dz_3) and (dz_4, dz_5, dz_6) such as, e.g. (dz_1, dz_4, dz_5), (dz_1, dz_5, dz_6) etc. must be equal to zero, giving conditions in the following manner:

$$\frac{1}{3!} \sum_{(i,j,k)=(1,4,5)} \epsilon_{ijk}(b_{1i}b_{2j}b_{3k} + b_{4i}b_{5j}b_{6k}) = 0,$$

$$\frac{1}{3!} \sum_{(i,j,k)=(1,5,6)} \epsilon_{ijk}(b_{1i}b_{2j}b_{3k} + b_{4i}b_{5j}b_{6k}) = 0, \qquad \text{etc.}$$

By enumerating all possible combinations of the indices of this type, it is not difficult to convince oneself that there are 18 independent conditions of this type.[1] Thus in total we have $18 + 2 = 20$ conditions for the matrix elements b_{ij} which have $6 \times 6 = 36$ degrees of freedom. There remain $36 - 20 = 16$ free parameters. Obviously, if we restrict the transformations within each triplet (z_1, z_2, z_3) and (z_4, z_5, z_6) without mixing among them, we have $9 - 1 = 8$ degrees of freedom for each case, and therefore $2 \times 8 = 16$ free parameters, exhausting the remaining freedom. This means that only allowed coordinate transformations satisfying the present requirement are, in fact, those which are separated into linear generalized canonical transformations in each 3-dimensional system. This conforms also to our conclusion of Sect. 2.3.3

---

1 $(i, j, k) = (1, 4, 5), (1, 5, 6), (1, 4, 6), (2, 4, 5), (2, 5, 6), (2, 4, 6), (3, 4, 5), (3, 5, 6), (3, 4, 6), (4, 1, 2), (4, 2, 3), (4, 1, 3), (5, 1, 2), (5, 2, 3), (5, 1, 3), (6, 1, 2), (6, 2, 3), (6.1, 3)$..

on the *rigidity* of the Nambu-bracket structure, and explains the difficulties which Nambu was faced with in his original paper.

In the conventional Hamiltonian formalism, by contrast, the canonical structure governed by a fundamental 2-form in $2n$-dimensional phase space $(x^1, \ldots, x^{2n}) = (p_1, q_1, p_2, q_2, \ldots, p_n, q_n)$:

$$J_{ij}dx^i \wedge dx^j \equiv dp_k \wedge dq_k, \qquad (J = \{J_{ij}\} = \{J^{ij}\} = -J^T)$$

is invariant under linear canonical transformations $x^i \to x'^i = a^i{}_j x^j$ with $2n \times 2n$ matrices $A = \{a^i{}_j\}$ satisfying $J_{ij}a^i{}_k a^j{}_\ell = J_{k\ell}$ or $A^T J A = J$. These transformations in general give rise to mixing among n canonical coordinates (p_k, q_k) $(k = 1, 2, \ldots, n)$, with the number of total degrees of freedom being given by $(2n)^2 - \frac{1}{2}2n(2n-1) = n(2n+1)$. The group of such linear transformations is known as the *symplectic group*, Sp($2n$). The differential operators D_G with an arbitrary function G already introduced in Sect. 1.1 is the infinitesimal generator of this group as discussed in (2.26).

2.6 Infinitesimal Generalized Canonical Transformations

2.6.1 The Generators of Infinitesimal Transformations

We now restrict ourselves to infinitesimal generalized canonical transformations, $x'^i(x) = x^i + \varepsilon X^i(x)$, $|\varepsilon| \ll 1$, with a vector field $X^i(x)$ in n-dimensional phase space. Substituting this form into (2.37), its left-hand side is given, to the order $O(\varepsilon)$,

$$\begin{aligned} dx'^1 \wedge dx'^2 \wedge \cdots \wedge dx'^n - dx^1 \wedge dx^2 \wedge \cdots \wedge dx^n \\ = \varepsilon(\partial_i X^1 dx^i \wedge dx^2 \wedge \cdots \wedge dx^n + dx^1 \wedge \partial_i X^2 dx^i \wedge \cdots \wedge dx^n \\ + \cdots dx^1 \wedge dx^2 \wedge \cdots \wedge \partial_i X^n dx^i) = \varepsilon \partial_i X^i dx^1 \wedge dx^2 \wedge \cdots \wedge dx^n. \end{aligned} \tag{2.45}$$

Therefore we must have $\partial_i X^i = 0$. This is equivalently written

$$\begin{aligned} 0 = d\big(X^1 dx^2 \wedge \cdots \wedge dx^n - X^2 dx^1 \wedge dx^3 \wedge \cdots \wedge dx^n \\ + \ldots + (-1)^{n-1} X^n dx^1 \wedge \cdots \wedge dx^{n-1}\big). \end{aligned}$$

Then we can set

$$\begin{aligned} X^1 dx^2 \wedge \cdots \wedge dx^n - X^2 dx^1 \wedge dx^3 \wedge \cdots \wedge dx^n \\ + \cdots + (-1)^{n-1} X^n dx^1 \wedge \cdots \wedge dx^{n-1} = d\tilde{S}^{(n-2)} \end{aligned} \tag{2.46}$$

with some $(n-2)$-form $\tilde{S}^{(n-2)} = \frac{1}{(n-2)!}\tilde{S}_{i_1 \dots i_{n-2}} dx^{i_1} \wedge \dots \wedge dx^{i_{n-2}}$, yielding

$$X^i = \epsilon^{i i_1 i_2 \dots i_{n-1}} \partial_{[i_1} \tilde{S}_{i_2 \dots i_{n-1}]}, \qquad (i_1 < \dots < i_{n-1}). \tag{2.47}$$

Obviously, this is a generalization of (2.8). Thus the infinitesimal variation X^i is directly (namely *algebraically* without involving its derivatives) expressed in terms of the generating $(n-2)$-form $\tilde{S}^{(n-2)}$. It is to be noted, however, that the present $(n-2)$-form $\tilde{S}^{(n-2)}$ does not coincide with the $S^{(n-2)}$ of the previous section, though apparently we are performing conceptually the same manipulation. This originates from the difference between the left-hand side of (2.43) and that of (2.46).

Exercise 2.4 To understand more about the difference just mentioned, let us study the limit of infinitesimal generalized canonical transformation from finite transformations characterized by (2.41) $(n = 3)$ of the previous section and derive their relationship. Choosing $i' = i = 1$, $j' = j = 2$, $k' = k = 3$, we first obtain, to the first order in ε,

$$x'^1 dx'^2 \wedge dx'^3 - x^1 dx^2 \wedge dx^3 = X^1 dx^2 \wedge dx^3$$
$$+ x^1(\partial_1 X^2 dx^1 \wedge dx^3 + \partial_2 X^2 dx^2 \wedge dx^3 + \partial_1 X^3 dx^2 \wedge dx^1 + \partial_3 X^3 dx^2 \wedge dx^3).$$

By equating this expression with $dS^{(1)}$, $S^{(1)} = S_i dx^i$, we find

$$X^1 + x^1(\partial_2 X^2 + \partial_3 X^3) = \partial_2 S_3 - \partial_3 S_2,$$
$$-x^1 \partial_1 X^2 = \partial_3 S_1 - \partial_1 S_3,$$
$$-x^1 \partial_1 X^3 = \partial_1 S_2 - \partial_2 S_1.$$

As we have stressed in the previous section, these relations are indeed a set of differential equations for X^i's, involving X^2 and X^3 through their derivatives. However, in comparison with the case of a finite canonical transformation, a simplification occurs in that the differential equations are completely linearized with respect to X^i due to the limit $\varepsilon \to 0$. We can confirm that $\partial_i X^i = 0$ holds, by applying the identity $\epsilon^{ijk}\partial_i(\partial_j S_k - \partial_k S_j) = 0$ to the right-hand sides of these three equations.

Then, the second relation shows that using (2.47), these relations can be used in order to express the relationship of $\tilde{S}_i$ to S_i in a gauge-invariant manner as a set of differential equations:

$$\tilde{F}^1 + x^1(\partial_2 \tilde{F}^2 + \partial_3 \tilde{F}^3) = F^1, \quad -x^1 \partial_1 \tilde{F}^2 = F^2, \quad -x^1 \partial_1 \tilde{F}^3 = F^3,$$

where F^i and $\tilde{F}^i$ are gauge-invariant 'field strengths' of S_i and $\tilde{S}_i$, namely, $F^i = \epsilon^{ijk}\partial_j S_k$, $\tilde{F}^i = \epsilon^{ijk}\partial_j \tilde{S}_k$, respectively. It is straightforward to integrate these equations conversely expressing $\tilde{S}^i$'s in terms of S^i's. In other words, (2.47) is indeed an integrated form of (2.41) in the limit of infinitesimal transformations.

2.6.2 The Characteristic Properties of Infinitesimal Generalized Canonical Transformations

We next investigate the properties of infinitesimal generalized canonical transformations acting on an arbitrary scalar function $F(x)$ in Nambu phase space:

$$\delta F(x) \equiv F(x') - F(x) = X^i(x)\partial_i F(x) = \mathcal{D}_X F(x), \quad \mathcal{D}_X \equiv X^i(x)\partial_i.$$

Consider two different infinitesimal transformations whose actions are represented by the vector differential operators $\mathcal{D}_X$ and $\mathcal{D}_Y$ with corresponding vector fields $X^i(x)$ and $Y^i(x)$. If we perform these two infinitesimal transformations successively, reverse the order and take the difference of the results, we obtain a commutation relation

$$[\mathcal{D}_X, \mathcal{D}_Y]F = (X^i\partial_i Y^j - Y^i\partial_i X^j)\partial_j F \equiv \mathcal{D}_{[X,Y]}F,$$

where we have defined

$$[X, Y]^k \equiv X^i\partial_i Y^k - Y^i\partial_i X^k, \tag{2.48}$$

which is usually called the *Lie bracket* of two vector fields X^i and Y^i. The reader should not confuse this symbol with the commutators for differential operators themselves. Note that the conditions $\partial_i X^i = 0 = \partial_i Y^i$ lead automatically to $\partial_i[X, Y]^i = 0$ and hence $\mathcal{D}_{[X,Y]}$ also induces an infinitesimal generalized canonical transformation, as it should be because of the group property of generalized canonical transformations. Using this notation, we can write

$$[\mathcal{D}_X, \mathcal{D}_Y] = \mathcal{D}_{[X,Y]}, \tag{2.49}$$

analogously as (1.5) in Sect. 1.1, where the Poisson bracket takes the role of the Lie bracket in the above relation.

In fact, using the present notation, the differential operator defined in (1.4) associated with the conventional Hamiltonian flow takes the following form,

$$D_H = \mathcal{D}_{X(H)}, \quad X^i(H) \equiv -J^{ij}\partial_j H,$$

where $J^{ij} = -J^{ji}$ is the symplectic matrix introduced for expressing the Poisson bracket [see (2.27)]. It is not difficult to check (see Exercise 2.6 below) that

$$[X(H), X(K)]^i = X^i(\{H, K\}) \tag{2.50}$$

for two arbitrary functions H and K. Therefore, with the 'Hamiltonian vector field' $X^i(H) = -J^{ij}\partial_j H$, satisfying

$$X^i(H)\partial_i K = -J^{ij}\partial_j H\partial_i K = -\{H, K\},$$

the algebra (2.49) of vector-differential operators $\mathcal{D}_X$ is equivalent to that of D_H,

$$[D_H, D_K] = D_{\{H,K\}}.$$

Because of (2.49), given three different arbitrary vector fields A^i, B^i and C^i, the Jacobi identity which is automatically satisfied by their definition for commutators among the corresponding vector-differential operators $\mathcal{D}_A$, $\mathcal{D}_B$ and $\mathcal{D}_C$,

$$[\mathcal{D}_A, [\mathcal{D}_B, \mathcal{D}_C]] + [\mathcal{D}_B, [\mathcal{D}_C, \mathcal{D}_A]] + [\mathcal{D}_C, [\mathcal{D}_A, \mathcal{D}_B]] = 0,$$

immediately implies the Jacobi-identity for Lie bracket

$$[A, [B, C]]^i + [B, [C, A]]^i + [C, [A, B]]^i = 0,$$

(and *vice versa*) .

Exercise 2.5 Let us confirm (2.50). By direct calculation, we have

$$\begin{aligned}[X(H), X(K)]^i &= X^j(H)\partial_j X^i(K) - X^j(K)\partial_j X^i(H) \\ &= J^{jk}\partial_k H \partial_j (J^{i\ell}\partial_\ell K) - J^{jk}\partial_k K \partial_j (J^{i\ell}\partial_\ell H) \\ &= \partial_j (J^{jk} J^{i\ell} \partial_k H \partial_\ell K - J^{j\ell} J^{ik} \partial_k H \partial_\ell K).\end{aligned}$$

Now the symplectic matrix J satisfies the identity, $J^{jk}J^{i\ell} - J^{j\ell}J^{ik} = -J^{ij}J^{k\ell}$. For instance, in the simplest case of 2-dimensional phase space $(x^1, x^2) = (p, q)$, J^{ij} is equal to the two-dimensional Levi–Civita tensor ϵ^{ij}, it is trivially satisfied. In higher $2n$ dimensions, the $2n \times 2n$ matrix J^{ij}, (2.27), is block-diagonal with diagonal elements being all equal to 2×2 matrices of the same form as ϵ^{ij}, and hence the above identity is maintained also in higher dimensions. This yields

$$[X(H), X(K)]^i = -J^{ij}\partial_j (J^{k\ell}\partial_k H \partial_\ell K) = X^i(\{H, K\}),$$

as promised.

Let us here recall that in conventional Hamiltonian dynamics an arbitrary infinitesimal canonical transformation is generated by a corresponding generating function $H(x)$ by

$$\delta_H F = \{H, F\} = D_H F.$$

The generating function H itself is automatically preserved ($D_H H = 0$) under the corresponding canonical transformation. In the present case of generalized infinitesimal canonical transformations in Nambu dynamics, a similar phenomenon happens if there is a function H satisfying

$$\mathcal{D}_X H = X^i \partial_i H = 0.$$

Conversely, given an arbitrary function H, we can restrict ourselves to consider only generalized canonical transformations which preserve H. Evidently, the set of all such transformations also forms a group, which is a subgroup of all possible generalized canonical transformations. Infinitesimally, this is confirmed by checking that $[X,Y]^i\partial_i H=0$ if $X^i\partial_i H=0=Y^i\partial_i H$. Indeed, using $\partial_i[X,Y]^i=0$ and $\partial_i X^i=0=\partial_i Y^i$, we have

$$\begin{aligned}[X,Y]^i\partial_i H &= \partial_i([X,Y]^i H)=\partial_i\big(H(\partial_j Y^i)X^j-H(\partial_j X^i)Y^j\big)\\ &=\partial_i\big(H\partial_j(Y^iX^j-Y^jX^i)\big)\\ &=\partial_i\partial_j\big(H(Y^iX^j-Y^jX^i)\big)=0.\end{aligned}$$

In n dimensions, the maximum number of such conserved quantities is $n-1$, since if there were n *independent* such conserved functions there could not be any nontrivial transformation in phase space. Denoting them as $(H_1,H_2,\ldots,H_{n-1})$, we can express X^i, without losing generality, in the form

$$\begin{aligned}X^i &= f(H_1,\ldots,H_{n-1})\epsilon^{j_1\ldots j_{n-1}i}\partial_{j_1}H_1\partial_{j_2}H_2\cdots\partial_{j_{n-1}}H_{n-1},\\ &= f(H_1,\ldots,H_{n-1})\{H_1,H_2,\ldots,H_{n-1},x^i\},\end{aligned}$$

where f is an arbitrary function of $n-1$ variables $(H_1,H_2,\ldots,H_{n-1})$, such that both $X^i\partial_i H_j=0$ $(j=1,2,\ldots,n-1)$ and $\partial_i X^i=0$ are satisfied, since we have $df=\sum_{j=1}^{n-1}\frac{\partial f}{\partial H_j}\partial_i H_j dx^i$. Actually, however, f can be eliminated by redefining one of H_is, say, H_1, as $H_1\to H_1'=\int^{H_1} f(H_1,\ldots,H_n)dH_1$. This is because we can write $f\{H_1,H_2,\ldots,H_{n-1}\}=\{H_1',H_2,\ldots,H_{n-1}\}$. Thus the expression of X^i without f is the most general form for systems with $n-1$ independent conserved functions.

Remark 2.3 (An electromagnetic analogy) In the simplest non-trivial case $n=3$, the conservation condition $\partial_i HX^i=0$ allows us to write a general form $X^i=\epsilon^{ijk}b_k\partial_j H$ of X^i with some vector field $b_k=b_k(x)$. To maintain the condition $\partial_i X^i=0$, $b_i(x)$ must satisfy $\epsilon^{ijk}\partial_i H\partial_j b_k=0$. For an intuitive understanding, let us think of $H=H(x)$ as an electrostatic potential $\phi(x)=H(x)$ for a static electric field $\boldsymbol{E}=-\nabla\phi$, and b_i as the vector potential for magnetic field $\boldsymbol{B}=\nabla\times\boldsymbol{b}$. Then, this condition shows that $\boldsymbol{E}\cdot\boldsymbol{B}=0$. In other words, given an electric potential ϕ, the lines of allowed magnetic fields lie on the equipotential surfaces of $\phi=H$. A typical example of such situations is the configuration of electric and magnetic fields around a straight and uniform electric wire along which a steady current is flowing, where the non-vanishing Poynting vector $\boldsymbol{E}\times\boldsymbol{B}$ expresses the energy propagating along the wire. The totality of vector potentials giving such magnetic fields comprises a subgroup, which we symbolize CT_H^3 for convenience, of the total group CT^3 of generalized canonical transformations.

Now this subgroup has a special class of group elements with vanishing magnetic field $\boldsymbol{B}=0$, corresponding to 'pure gauge' $\epsilon^{ijk}\partial_j b_k=0$, in which case we have $\boldsymbol{b}=\nabla b$, with some scalar function $b=b(x)$. Using the above analogy with a straight electric wire, no current is flowing, and hence wire has only static electric charges. We then have a Clebsch form $X^i = \epsilon^{ijk}\partial_j H \partial_k b$, which generates a special class of infinitesimal generalized canonical transformations whose action is given by a generalized Poisson bracket $\delta_G F = \{G, F\}_H = \{H, G, F\}$ with $b = G$, discussed before in Sect. 2.1. The validity of Jacobi identity with arbitrary scalar functions G_1 and G_2,

$$\{G_1, \{G_2, F\}_H\}_H - \{G_2, \{G_1, F\}_H\}_H = \{\{G_1, G_2\}_H, F\}_H$$

assures us that this *special* class of generalized canonical transformations generated by the totality of G form a subgroup, denoted by $speCT^3_H$: $speCT^3_H \subset CT^3_H \subset CT^3$.

Exercise 2.6 Let us study the explicit form of $[X, Y]^i$ for CT^3_H. Set $X^i = \epsilon^{ijk}\partial_j H a_k$ and $Y^i = \epsilon^{ijk}\partial_j H b_k$. We find after some rearrangements

$$\begin{aligned}
[X, Y]^i &= X^j \partial_j Y^i - Y^j \partial_j X^i \\
&= \epsilon^{jkj_1}\partial_k H a_{j_1} \partial_j (\epsilon^{i\ell j_2}(\partial_\ell H) b_{j_2}) - \epsilon^{jkj_1}\partial_k H b_{j_1} \partial_j (\epsilon^{i\ell j_2}(\partial_\ell H) a_{j_2}) \\
&= \epsilon^{i\ell j_2}\partial_\ell H \epsilon^{jkj_1}(\partial_k H a_{j_1}\partial_j b_{j_2} - \partial_k H b_{j_1}\partial_j a_{j_2}) \\
&\quad + (\epsilon^{jkj_1}\epsilon^{i\ell j_2} - \epsilon^{jkj_2}\epsilon^{i\ell j_1})\partial_k H \partial_j \partial_\ell H a_{j_1} b_{j_2}.
\end{aligned}$$

If we multiply $\partial_i H$ on the right-hand side of this equation, the first term of the last equality manifestly vanishes. On the other hand, the second term itself before the multiplication of $\partial_i H$, can further be rearranged by noticing the following identity,

$$(\epsilon^{jkj_1}\epsilon^{i\ell j_2} - \epsilon^{jkj_2}\epsilon^{i\ell j_1})\partial_k H \partial_j \partial_\ell H = \epsilon^{ikj}\epsilon^{j_1 j_2 \ell}\partial_k H \partial_j \partial_\ell H, \tag{2.51}$$

with two free indices j_1 and j_2. In fact, if we consider the case $j_1 = 1$ and $j_2 = 2$, the right-hand side is equal to $\epsilon^{ikj}\partial_k H \partial_j \partial_3 H$. The left-hand side yields for each case of $i = 1, i = 2$ and $i = 3$,

$$\begin{aligned}
i = 1: \quad & (\epsilon^{jk1}\epsilon^{i\ell 2} - \epsilon^{jk2}\epsilon^{i\ell 1})\partial_k H \partial_j \partial_\ell H = -\partial_3 H \partial_2 \partial_3 H + \partial_2 H \partial_3 \partial_3 H, \\
i = 2: \quad & (\epsilon^{jk1}\epsilon^{i\ell 2} - \epsilon^{jk2}\epsilon^{i\ell 1})\partial_k H \partial_j \partial_\ell H = -\partial_1 H \partial_3 \partial_3 H + \partial_3 H \partial_1 \partial_3 H, \\
i = 3: \quad & (\epsilon^{jk1}\epsilon^{i\ell 2} - \epsilon^{jk2}\epsilon^{i\ell 1})\partial_k H \partial_j \partial_\ell H = \epsilon^{jk1}\partial_k H \partial_j \partial_1 H + \epsilon^{jk2}\partial_k H \partial_j \partial_2 H \\
& \qquad = -\partial_2 H \partial_1 \partial_3 H + \partial_1 H \partial_2 \partial_3 H,
\end{aligned}$$

respectively, which as a whole are identical with $\epsilon^{ikj}\partial_k H \partial_j \partial_3 H$. By cyclic permutations of indices, (2.51) follows immediately. Then, after renaming the indices suitably, we have $[X, Y]^i = \epsilon^{ikj}\partial_k H c_j$, where

$$c_j = \epsilon^{j_1 j_2 \ell}(\partial_{j_1} H a_{j_2} \partial_\ell b_j - \partial_{j_1} H b_{j_2} \partial_\ell a_j + \partial_j \partial_\ell H a_{j_1} b_{j_2}).$$

This shows that the second term also vanishes after the contraction with $\partial_i H$, as it should.

Furthermore, for the infinitesimal transformations belonging to the subgroup $speCT_H^3$, we set $a_i = \partial_i a$ and $b_i = \partial_i b$ with scalar functions $a = a(x)$ and $b = b(x)$. We then obtain

$$\begin{aligned} c_j &= \epsilon^{j_1 j_2 \ell}(\partial_{j_1} H \partial_{j_2} a \partial_\ell \partial_j b - \partial_{j_1} H \partial_{j_2} b \partial_\ell \partial_j a + \partial_j \partial_\ell H \partial_{j_1} a \partial_{j_2} b) \\ &= \partial_j \left(\epsilon^{j_1 j_2 \ell} \partial_{j_1} H \partial_{j_2} a \partial_\ell b\right) = \partial_j \{H, a, b\} = \partial_j \{a, b\}_H, \end{aligned}$$

satisfying $\partial_i c_j - \partial_j c_i = 0$. As discussed in Remark 2.2 above , this is what we should expect for the commutation relation for the infinitesimal generalized canonical transformations belonging to the subgroup $speCT_H^3$.

As an interesting example corresponding to CT_H^3 (not belonging to $speCT_H^3$), let us examine the case where the vector fields a_i and b_i are given in Clebsch's form as

$$a_i = f(H)\partial_i a, \quad b_i = g(H)\partial_i b,$$

where f and g are arbitrary functions of a single variable H. They have non-vanishing field strengths, $\partial_i a_j - \partial_j a_i = f'(\partial_i H \partial_j a - \partial_j H \partial_i a) \neq 0$ and $\partial_i b_j - \partial_j b_i = g'(\partial_i H \partial_j b - \partial_j H \partial_i b \neq 0)$, but yield X_i and Y_i that automatically satisfy $\partial_i X^i = 0 = \partial_j Y^j$. After straightforward calculations, we obtain

$$\begin{aligned} c_j &= f(H) g(H) \partial_j \{H, a, b\}, \\ \partial_i c_j - \partial_j c_i &= \partial_i (fg) \partial_j \{H, a, b\} - \partial_j (fg) \partial_i \{H, a, b\} \neq 0. \end{aligned}$$

Thus, the resultant vector c_i has a *new* Clebsch form $fg\partial_i c, c = \{H, a, b\}$.

2.6.3 *The Infinitesimal Generalized Canonical Transformations of General Differential Forms*

Let us now study the action of an infinitesimal transformation $x^i \to x'^i = x^i + \varepsilon X^i(x)$ on a general k-form $\omega^{(k)}(x) = \omega_{i_1 i_2 \ldots i_k}(x) dx^{i_1} \wedge dx^{i_2} \wedge \cdots \wedge dx^{i_k}$ $(i_1 < \ldots < i_k, k \leq n)$. We have to calculate

$$\omega_{i_1 i_2 \ldots i_k}(x') dx'^{i_1} \wedge dx'^{i_2} \wedge \cdots \wedge dx'^{i_k} - \omega_{i_1 i_2 \ldots i_k}(x) dx^{i_1} \wedge dx^{i_2} \wedge \cdots \wedge dx^{i_k}.$$

The result can be expressed in the form,

$$\lim_{\varepsilon \to 0} \frac{1}{\varepsilon} \left(\omega^{(k)}(x') - \omega^{(k)}(x)\right) \equiv \mathcal{L}_X \omega^{(k)}.$$

We find, *keeping the ordering* $i_1 < \ldots < i_k$ of indices,

$$\begin{aligned}
\mathcal{L}_X\omega^{(k)} &= X^i \partial_i \omega_{i_1 i_2 \ldots i_k}(x) dx^{i_1} \wedge dx^{i_2} \cdots \wedge dx^{i_k} \\
&\quad + \omega_{i_1 \ldots i_k}\big(\partial_i X^{i_1} dx^i \wedge dx^{i_2} \wedge \cdots \wedge dx^{i_k} + \partial_i X^{i_2} dx^{i_1} \wedge dx^i \wedge \cdots \wedge dx^{i_k} + \ldots \\
&\quad + \partial_i X^{i_k} dx^{i_1} \wedge dx^{i_2} \wedge \cdots \wedge dx^{i_{k-1}} \wedge dx^i\big), \\
&= X^i \partial_i \omega_{i_1 i_2 \ldots i_k}(x) dx^{i_1} \wedge dx^{i_2} \cdots \wedge dx^{i_k} \\
&\quad + \omega_{i_1 \ldots i_k}\big(\partial_i X^{i_1} dx^i \wedge dx^{i_2} \wedge \cdots \wedge dx^{i_k} - \partial_i X^{i_2} dx^i \wedge dx^{i_1} \wedge dx^{i_3} \wedge \cdots \wedge dx^{i_k} + \ldots \\
&\quad + (-1)^{k-1} \partial_i X^{i_k} dx^i \wedge dx^{i_1} \wedge dx^{i_2} \wedge \cdots \wedge dx^{i_{k-1}}\big) \qquad (2.52)
\end{aligned}$$

which we call the *Lie derivative* of a k-form $\omega^{(k)}$. For $k = 0$, $\mathcal{L}_X = X^i \partial_i = \mathcal{D}_X$, and for $k = n$,

$$\mathcal{L}_X \omega^{(n)} = \partial_i(\omega_{12\ldots n} X^i) dx^1 \wedge dx^2 \wedge \cdots \wedge dx^n.$$

It should be noted that the present definition of Lie derivative for general k-form is *valid for arbitrary infinitesimal coordinate transformations* $x^i \to x^i + \varepsilon X^i(x)$ not necessarily satisfying $\partial_i X^i = 0$. When $k = n$ and $\omega_{12\ldots n} = 1$ this reduces to (2.45) of the previous section and gives the condition $\partial_i X^i = 0$ corresponding to the requirement for the generalized canonical transformation.

By definition, the Leibniz rule is guaranteed to be valid for Lie derivative: namely

$$\mathcal{L}_X(\alpha^{(p)} \wedge \beta^{(q)}) = (\mathcal{L}_X \alpha^{(p)}) \wedge \beta^{(q)} + \alpha^{(p)} \wedge (\mathcal{L}_X \beta^{(q)}).$$

This shows that how Lie derivative acts on a general higher form is essentially governed by the case of 1-form:

$$\mathcal{L}_X \omega^{(1)} = (X^i \partial_i \omega_j + \partial_j X^i \omega_i) dx^j = \big[X^i(\partial_i \omega_j - \partial_j \omega_i) + \partial_j (X^i \omega_i)\big] dx^j. \quad (2.53)$$

For example, we can obtain the commutation relation of two Lie derivative operators for general differential forms on the basis of this fact, since non-vanishing contributions for the commutator come only when they operate on one and the same constituent 1-form of a given exterior product. Using

$$\mathcal{L}_X \mathcal{L}_Y \omega^{(1)} = [X^i \partial_i (Y^k \partial_k \omega_j + \partial_j Y^k \omega_k) + \partial_j X^i (Y^k \partial_k \omega_i + \partial_i Y^k \omega_k)] dx^j,$$

we obtain, after a straightforward calculation,

$$\begin{aligned}
\mathcal{L}_X \mathcal{L}_Y \omega^{(1)} - \mathcal{L}_Y \mathcal{L}_X \omega^{(1)} &= \big[(X^i \partial_i Y^k - Y^i \partial_i X^k) \partial_k \omega_j + \partial_j (X^i \partial_i Y^k - Y^i \partial_i X^k) \omega_k\big] dx^j \\
&= \mathcal{L}_{[X,Y]} \omega^{(1)}.
\end{aligned}$$

We already know that the Lie derivative for zero forms coincide with the vector derivative $\mathcal{D}_X$ satisfying $[\mathcal{D}_X, \mathcal{D}_Y] = \mathcal{D}_{[X,Y]}$: we have thus established

$$[\mathcal{L}_X, \mathcal{L}_Y] = \mathcal{L}_{[X,Y]}$$

for all k (≥ 0) forms.

A characteristic feature of the formula (2.53) is that it consists of two parts: the first part $X^i(\partial_i\omega_j - \partial_j\omega_i)dx^j$ is gauge invariant under $\omega^{(1)} \to \omega^{(1)} + d\Lambda$ with an arbitrary zero-form Λ, and the second part $\partial_j(X^i\omega_i)dx^j = d(X^i\omega_i)$ is not gauge-invariant, in general, and itself takes the form of a gauge transformation with a zero-form that is obtained as the scalar product $X^i\omega_i$. Let us next confirm explicitly whether and how this property be extended to Lie derivatives acting on general higher forms.

We first notice that, unlike exterior differentiation that sends a k-form to a $(k+1)$-form, Lie derivative is a derivative operation sending a k-form to another k-form. These two different derivative operations may be related in general if we introduce a suitable operation which lowers the rank of differential forms by one for arbitrary higher forms. In the case of a 1-form $\omega^{(1)} = \omega_i(x)dx^i$, we recall that the set of differentials dx^i is a basis with the covariant vector field $\omega_i(x)$ being the components of $\omega^{(1)}$ with respect to this basis. Similarly, a contravariant vector field $X^i(x)$ can be associated with the vector differential operator $\mathcal{D}_X = X^i\partial_i$, where a set of partial differential operators ∂_i forms a basis with the X^i being the components of $\mathcal{D}_X$. This suggests the introduction of a bracket symbol $< \cdot, \cdot >$ as a pairing of $\omega^{(1)}$ and $\mathcal{D}_X$ to denote the usual scalar product $X^i\omega_i$,

$$\langle \mathcal{D}_X, \omega^{(1)} \rangle \equiv X^i\omega_i, \tag{2.54}$$

which is equivalent to $\langle \partial_i, dx^j \rangle = \delta_i^j$ in terms of their bases.

In differential geometry, the vector space consisting of arbitrary vector differential operators, spanned by the basis ∂_i, is called *tangent space*, denoted by T_xM, at a point $(x^1, \ldots, x^n)$ of a manifold M, while the vector space consisting of arbitrary 1-forms, spanned by the basis dx^i, is called *cotangent space*, denoted by T_x^*M. The tangent space and the cotangent space are mutually *dual* to each other in the sense that they together allow us to define the internal product at each point of M as a bilinear product between them as in (2.54). Of course, in our case, the manifold M is globally a flat Euclidean space, and hence its tangent space TM is identical to M itself. Similarly, the cotangent space T^*M is also globally a flat Euclidean space.

Given this definition for pairing the differential operator $\mathcal{D}_X$ in T^*M with the 1-form $\omega^{(1)}$ in TM, it is natural to extend it to operations on arbitrary k-forms in $TM = M$: it is called *interior product*, which we denote by a special new symbol ι_X. It sends a k-form $\omega^{(k)}$ ($k \geq 1$) to a new $(k-1)$-form by making a contraction of a vector field X^i with each of the indices of the covariant (and totally skew symmetric) tensor field $\omega_{i_1\ldots i_k}$ successively, in analogy with the usual Leibniz rule for first-order differential operators, as

$$\begin{aligned}\iota_X\omega^{(k)} &\equiv X^j\omega_{ji_1\ldots i_{k-1}}dx^{i_1} \wedge \cdots \wedge dx^{i_{k-1}} \\ &= \omega_{i_1i_2\cdots i_k}(X^{i_1}dx^{i_2} \wedge \cdots \wedge dx^{i_k} - X^{i_2}dx^{i_1} \wedge dx^{i_3} \wedge \cdots \wedge dx^{i_k}\end{aligned}$$

$$+\ldots+(-1)^{k-1}X^{i_k}dx^{i_1}\wedge\cdots\wedge dx^{i_{k-1}}), \qquad (i_1<\ldots<i_k). \qquad (2.55)$$

Note that summations over the repeated index j without sub-indices in the first line are performed independently of the other indices $(i_1, \ldots, i_{k-1})$ with ordered sub-indices. The equality in the second line where the indices are ordered as indicated in the parentheses comes from this difference. By definition, $\iota_X\omega^{(1)} = \langle\mathcal{D}_X, \omega^{(1)}\rangle = X^i\omega_i$ for $k = 1$. If two interior products act on $\omega^{(k)}$ one after another, we have

$$\iota_X\iota_Y\omega^{(k)} = X^iY^j\omega_{jii_1\ldots i_{k-2}}dx^{i_1}\wedge\cdots\wedge dx^{i_{k-2}} = -\iota_Y\iota_X\omega^{(k)}$$

and therefore $\iota_X^2 = 0$. Also the following distribution law holds:

$$\iota_X(\alpha^{(k)}\wedge\beta^{(\ell)}) = \iota_X\alpha^{(k)}\wedge\beta^{(\ell)} + (-1)^k\alpha^{(k)}\wedge\iota_X\beta^{(\ell)}.$$

Finally, we note an obvious fact that, if $\iota_X\omega^{(k)} = 0$ for arbitrary vector field X^i, then $\omega^{(k)} = 0$, since it implies that by choosing $X^i = \delta^i_j$ with all possible $j \in (1, 2, \ldots, n)$, $\omega_{ji_1,\ldots,i_{k-1}} = 0$. On the other hand, for a special choice of X^i, a condition such as $\iota_X\omega^{(k)} = 0$ may provide an important characterization for a given differential form.

Now, let us apply an exterior differentiation to the $(k-1)$-form $\iota_X\omega^{(k)}$. Then we obtain a new k-form associated with the original k-form $\omega^{(k)}$,

$$\begin{aligned}
d(\iota_X\omega^{(k)}) = \omega_{i_1i_2\cdots i_k}(&\partial_iX^{i_1}dx^i\wedge dx^{i_2}\wedge\cdots\wedge dx^{i_k}\\
&-\partial_iX^{i_2}dx^i\wedge dx^{i_1}\wedge dx^{i_3}\wedge\cdots\wedge dx^{i_k}+\ldots\\
&+(-1)^{k-1}\partial_iX^{i_k}dx^i\wedge dx^{i_1}\wedge\cdots\wedge dx^{i_{k-1}})\\
&+\partial_i\omega_{i_1i_2\cdots i_k}(X^{i_1}dx^i\wedge dx^{i_2}\wedge\cdots\wedge dx^{i_k}-X^{i_2}dx^i\wedge dx^{i_1}\wedge dx^{i_3}\wedge\cdots\wedge dx^{i_k}\\
&+\ldots+(-1)^{k-1}X^{i_k}dx^i\wedge dx^{i_1}\wedge\cdots\wedge dx^{i_{k-1}}), \qquad (i_1<\ldots<i_k).
\end{aligned}$$

Evidently, there is another way of getting a new k-form from a given k-form $\omega^{(k)}$ by reversing the order of exterior differentiation and interior product: by using

$$d\omega^{(k)} = \partial_i\omega_{i_1\ldots i_k}dx^i\wedge dx^{i_1}\wedge\cdots\wedge dx^{i_k}, \qquad (i_1<\ldots<i_k),$$

we obtain

$$\begin{aligned}
\iota_X(d\omega^{(k)}) = X^i\partial_i\omega_{i_1i_2\ldots i_k}&dx^{i_1}\wedge\cdots\wedge dx^{i_k}\\
&-\partial_i\omega_{i_1i_2\ldots i_k}(X^{i_1}dx^i\wedge dx^{i_2}\wedge\cdots\wedge dx^{i_k}-X^{i_2}dx^i\wedge dx^{i_1}\wedge dx^{i_3}\wedge\cdots\wedge dx^{i_k}\\
&+\ldots+(-1)^{k-1}X^{i_k}dx^i\wedge dx^{i_1}\wedge\cdots\wedge dx^{i_{k-1}}), \qquad (i_1<\ldots<i_k).
\end{aligned}$$

We notice that the last two lines of the expressions for $d(\iota_X\omega^{(k)})$ and $\iota_X(d\omega^{(k)})$ have the same form but with opposite signs. Therefore, adding these two results, we find, with the same ordering $(i_1<\ldots<i_k)$,

$$\begin{aligned}\iota_X(d\omega^{(k)}) + d(\iota_X\omega^{(k)}) &= X^i\partial_i\omega_{i_1i_2\ldots i_k}dx^{i_1}\wedge\cdots\wedge dx^{i_k}\\ &+\omega_{i_1i_2\cdots i_k}(\partial_i X^{i_1}dx^i\wedge dx^{i_2}\wedge\cdots\wedge dx^{i_k}\\ &-\partial_i X^{i_2}dx^i\wedge dx^{i_1}\wedge dx^{i_3}\wedge\cdots\wedge dx^{i_k}+\ldots\\ &+(-1)^{k-1}\partial_i X^{i_k}dx^i\wedge dx^{i_1}\wedge\cdots\wedge dx^{i_{k-1}}),\end{aligned}$$

which agrees with the expression (2.52). Thus we have arrived at a general formula for Lie derivative acting on a general k-form in terms of exterior differentiation and internal product,

$$\mathcal{L}_X\omega^{(k)} = \iota_X(d\omega^{(k)}) + d(\iota_X\omega^{(k)}), \tag{2.56}$$

that naturally generalizes the structure already seen in (2.53) for 1-forms. This is known as *Cartan's relation*.

As immediate consequences of (2.56), we can easily derive, for instance,

$$[\mathcal{L}_X, d] = 0, \quad [\mathcal{L}_X, \iota_X] = 0,$$

utilizing nilpotency, $d^2 = 0 = \iota_X^2$. The former relation, in particular, reflects the fact that differential forms and their exterior differentials are concepts that are invariant under general coordinate transformations: we can apply them to arbitrary manifolds (not necessarily the Euclidean space) that are represented at least locally by (curved linear) coordinates, though we have no intention of proceeding to such extension in the present monograph. It is also instructive to check the Leibniz rule of the Lie derivative in terms of Cartan's relation; using the distribution law of interior product and exterior differentiation, we find

$$\begin{aligned}&\mathcal{L}_X(\alpha^{(k)}\wedge\beta^{(\ell)}) - \mathcal{L}_X\alpha^{(k)}\wedge\beta^{(\ell)} - \alpha^{(k)}\wedge\mathcal{L}_X\beta^{(\ell)}\\ &= (-1)^{k+1}d\alpha^{(k)}\wedge\iota_X\beta^{(\ell)} + (-1)^k\iota_X\alpha^{(k)}\wedge d\beta^{(\ell)}\\ &\quad+(-1)^{k-1}\iota_X\alpha^{(k)}\wedge d\beta^{(\ell)} + (-1)^k d\alpha^{(k)}\wedge\iota_X\beta^{(\ell)} = 0.\end{aligned}$$

Before proceeding to applications of Cartan's relation in the next section, we recapitulate some of its characteristic properties and consequences:

(i) Lie derivative for a general k-form consists of two parts ($k \geq 1$), $\iota_X(d\omega^{(k)})$ and $d(\iota_X\omega^{(k)})$. The second part takes the form of a gauge transformation with a $(k-1)$-form $\Lambda^{(k-1)} = \iota_X\omega^{(k)}$ that is itself not gauge invariant. The first term may be called the *physical part* since it is invariant under gauge transformation of $\omega^{(k)}$ and can have, in general, a non-vanishing exterior derivative or *field strength* $(k+1)$ form, $d(\iota_X(d\omega^k))$. Correspondingly, the second part may be called the *gauge part*.

(ii) For the lowest 0-form $\omega^{(0)} = f$, the Lie derivative has no gauge part since $\iota_X\omega^{(0)} = 0$, resulting in just an ordinary vector derivative $\iota_X(df) = X^i\partial_i f = \mathcal{D}_X f$. In the case of the highest form $k = n$, the situation is opposite: the Lie derivative has no physical part since $d\omega^{(n)} = 0$, and the gauge part $d\Lambda^{(n-1)}$ is given by a particular $(n-1)$-form

$$\Lambda^{(n-1)} = \iota_X \omega^{(n)} = X^i \omega_{ii_1 \dots i_{n-1}} dx^{i_1} \wedge \dots \wedge dx^{i_{n-1}}$$

$(i_1 < \dots < i_{n-1})$, yielding $d\Lambda^{n-1} = \partial_i (X^i \omega_{12\dots n}) dx^1 \wedge \cdots dx^n$.

2.7 The Equations of Motion in Terms of Differential Forms

2.7.1 Preparations for Including Time

Now we are ready to go back to our main theme, implications of generalized canonical transformations for the Nambu equations of motion. Let us start with the simplest 3-dimensional case. Of course, we already know that the Nambu equations of motion are form-invariant under the generalized canonical transformation. Also, as a matter of fact, time evolution itself is a special case of generalized canonical transformations. Consider an infinitesimal time evolution from t to $t + \delta t$ which induces an infinitesimal generalized canonical transformation ($X^i = \epsilon^{ijk} \partial_j K \partial_k H,\ \partial_i X^i = 0$)

$$\delta x^i(t) = \delta t \{K, H, x^i(t)\} = \delta t X^i\big(x(t)\big).$$

When we apply this transformation to an arbitrary scalar function $f(x, t)$ in four dimensional *phase space-time* (x^i, t), it is represented as

$$\delta f(x, t) = \delta t \big(\mathcal{D}_X + \frac{\partial}{\partial t}\big) f(x, t).$$

Clearly,

$$\mathcal{D}_X + \frac{\partial}{\partial t} = X^i \partial_i + X^0 \partial_t$$

can be regarded as a vector-differential operator extended from three to four dimensions including time. This is associated with a particular 4-vector field $(X^i(x), X^0)$, with the 4-th time component $X^0 = 1$, which is now tangent to a particle trajectory at each point in the sense of 4-dimensional phase space-time. The formulation of infinitesimal generalized canonical transformations, especially the notion of Lie derivative, can thus be immediately extended to 4 dimensions. It is sufficient simply to add time components, $dt = dx^0$ and $\partial_t = \partial_{x^0}$, to the basis of differential forms and differential operators: $(dx^1, dx^2, dx^3) \to (dx^1, dx^2, dx^3, dx^0) = (dx^1, dx^2, dx^3, dt)$, $(\partial_1, \partial_2, \partial_3) \to (\partial_1, \partial_2, \partial_3, \partial_t)$, respectively. It is then convenient to denote indices by Greek letters such as dx^μ, ∂_μ following the custom of relativity theory:

$$\begin{aligned}\omega^{(1)} &= \omega_\mu dx^\mu = \omega_i dx^i + \omega_0 dt,\\ d\omega^{(2)} &= \partial_\nu \omega_\mu dx^\nu \wedge dx^\mu\\ &= \frac{1}{2}(\partial_i \omega_j - \partial_j \omega_i) dx^i \wedge dx^j + (\partial_i \omega_0 - \partial_t \omega_i) dx^i \wedge dt, \quad \text{etc.}\end{aligned}$$

Note, however, that phase space-time is still globally Euclidean ($x^0 = x_0 = t$), because we do not require Lorentz invariance, contrary to relativity theory: in other words, we never consider any transformation mixing the time coordinate with spatial coordinates in the context of Nambu dynamics. When it becomes necessary to represent vector differential operators, interior products and Lie derivatives, in the sense of four-dimensional phase space-time, we signify them as

$$\begin{aligned}\mathcal{D}_{(X,1)} &\equiv X^\mu \partial_\mu = X^i \partial_i + \partial_t = \mathcal{D}_X + \partial_t,\\ \iota_{(X,1)}\omega^{(1)} &\equiv X^\mu \omega_\mu = X^i \omega_i + \omega_0,\\ \mathcal{L}_{(X,1)}\omega^{(k)} &\equiv \iota_{(X,1)}(d\omega^{(k)}) + d(\iota_{(X,1)}\omega^{(k)}), \qquad \text{etc.}\end{aligned}$$

It is important to keep in mind that, just as the three components of the spatial differentials dx^i are independent of each other as the basis for general spatial differential forms, the time component dt is independent of the spatial components dx^i.

In Sect. 2.1, we emphasized that the Liouville equation for the density function $\rho(x, t)$ representing an aggregate of point Nambu particles in Nambu phase space

$$0 = (\partial_t + X^i(x)\partial_i)\rho(x, t) = \mathcal{D}_{(X,1)}\rho = \mathcal{L}_{(X,1)}\rho,$$

is essentially equivalent to the equations of motion.

Namely, the Liouville equation as the equations of motion demands that the zero form ρ be invariant against a particular infinitesimal canonical transformation $\delta x^\mu = X^\mu \delta t$. In view of this, it is imperative to study how similar requirements can be satisfied for higher differential forms. That would reveal to us the nature of the Nambu equations of motion in the language of differential forms.

For that purpose, it is instructive first to recall the situation of conventional Hamiltonian dynamics in the simplest case of 2-dimensional phase space (p, q). The differential operator corresponding to the Hamilton equations of motion $\dot{q} = \partial_p H$, $\dot{p} = -\partial_q H$ with an arbitrary Hamiltonian $H = H(q, p)$ is written

$$D_H = -\partial_q H \partial_p + \partial_p H \partial_q = \mathcal{D}_X$$

with $(X^1, X^2) = (-\partial_q H, \partial_p H)$, which should be related to the Lie derivative operator $\mathcal{L}_{(X,1)}$ associated with 3(=2+1)-dimensional vector $(X^1, X^2, 1) = (X, 1)$ including the time direction. The action of this extended Lie derivative on an arbitrary form is determined by the results of acting the corresponding interior product on it.

Of particular interest to us here is the Pfaffian 1-form $\alpha^{(1)} \equiv pdq - Hdt$, which, being integrated along an arbitrary particle trajectory (*i.e.* world line) in phase space-time, gives the usual action integral. If the interior product $\iota_{(X,1)}$ acts on its exterior derivative $d\alpha^{(1)}$

$$\begin{aligned}\alpha^{(2)} &\equiv d\alpha^{(1)} = dp \wedge dq - dH \wedge dt \\ &= dp \wedge dq - \partial_q H dq \wedge dt - \partial_p H dp \wedge dt,\end{aligned}$$

we find

$$\begin{aligned}\iota_{(X,1)}\alpha^{(2)} &= -\partial_q H dq - \partial_p H dp - \partial_q H \partial_p H dt \\ &\quad + \partial_q H dq + \partial_p H \partial_q H dt + \partial_p H dp = 0,\end{aligned}$$

yielding

$$\mathcal{L}_{(X,1)}\alpha^{(2)} = \iota_{(X,1)}(d\alpha^{(2)}) + d(\iota_{(X,1)}\alpha^{(2)}) = 0.$$

This means that the vector field $(X^1, X^2, 1)$ is orthogonal to the infinitesimal rectangle corresponding to $\alpha^{(2)}$. This provides us a clear 'physico-geometrical' picture for the motion of a particle in Hamiltonian dynamics. In the figure below, the gray parallelogram represents $\alpha^{(2)}$. It is tilted toward the time direction such that it becomes orthogonal to the vector $(X, 1)$ which is tangent to a 4-dimensional particle trajectory passing the rectangle. Its two time-like components $-\partial_p H dp \wedge dt$ and $-\partial_q H dq \wedge dt$ correspond to the weighted rectangles in the (p, t)-plane and (q, t)-plane, respectively, as indicated by thin dotted lines with arrows, of an infinitesimal cube (or 3-volume) representing $dp \wedge dq \wedge dt$ in 3-dimensional phase space-time (Fig. 2.2):

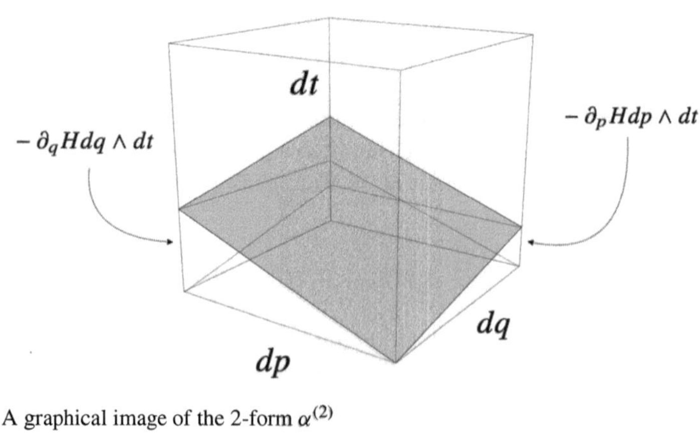

Fig. 2.2 A graphical image of the 2-form $\alpha^{(2)}$

Note that the vanishing of the Lie derivative associated with the equations of motion acting on $\alpha^{(2)}$, namely the invariance of $\alpha^{(2)}$ under infinitesimal time evolution, is due to the following two critical properties of the 2-form $\alpha^{(2)}$

$$d\alpha^{(2)} = 0 \quad \text{and} \quad \iota_{(X,1)}\alpha^{(2)} = 0.$$

The first of these two equalities is valid for each term in $\alpha^{(2)}$, namely, for the 'kinematical part' $dp \wedge dq$, and for the 'dynamical part' $-dH \wedge dt$, separately. By contrast, the second is only possible owing to the cancellation of contributions from these two parts.

On the other hand, if we apply the Lie derivative to 1-form $\alpha^{(1)}$, we find

$$\mathcal{L}_{(X,1)}\alpha^{(1)} = \iota_{(X,1)}(d\alpha^{(1)}) + d(\iota_{(X,1)}\alpha^{(1)}) = d(\iota_{(X,1)}\alpha^{(1)}), \tag{2.57}$$

using $\iota_{(X,1)}\alpha^{(2)} = 0$: thus the result is a gauge transformation with a 0-form gauge function $\Lambda^{(0)} = \iota_{(X,1)}\alpha^{(1)} = p\partial_p H - H$. We may say that the 1-form $\alpha^{(1)}$ is *quasi-invariant* under infinitesimal time evolution in the sense that the *physical part* of its Lie derivative vanishes. It is to be noted that, in a special case where H is linear in p and hence $\iota_{(X,1)}\alpha^{(1)} = 0$, $\alpha^{(1)}$ is also invariant.

2.7.2 The Nambu Equations of Motion, the Distribution of Fixed Points, and the N-Gauge Symmetry

Let us now study whether and how the structure of conventional Hamiltonian dynamics with respect to the equations of motion in terms of differential forms just discussed is generalized to Nambu dynamics. A natural candidate for the analog of the closed 2-form $\alpha^{(2)}$ is the following 3-form obtained from $dx^1 \wedge dx^2 \wedge dx^3$, which is invariant against time-independent generalized canonical transformations, by adding time components composed of dt combined with a 2-form differential form $dK \wedge dH$ that governs the time evolution of Nambu dynamics:

$$\begin{aligned}\omega^{(3)} &= dx^1 \wedge dx^2 \wedge dx^3 - dK \wedge dH \wedge dt,\\ &= dx^1 \wedge dx^2 \wedge dx^3 - (\partial_1 K \partial_2 H - \partial_2 K \partial_1 H)dx^1 \wedge dx^2 \wedge dt\\ &\quad - (\partial_2 K \partial_3 H - \partial_3 K \partial_2 H)dx^2 \wedge dx^3 \wedge dt\\ &\quad - (\partial_1 K \partial_3 H - \partial_3 K \partial_1 H)dx^1 \wedge dx^3 \wedge dt,\end{aligned}$$

where the time-like 3-forms $(\partial_i K \partial_j H - \partial_j K \partial_i H)dx^i \wedge dx^j \wedge dt$ (no summation over i and j) correspond to the three cubic-faces, wighted with the tensor coefficients $\partial_i K \partial_j H - \partial_j K \partial_i H$, of the infinitesimal 4-volume representing $dx^1 \wedge dx^2 \wedge dx^3 \wedge dt$ in phase space-time. This is manifestly closed, $d\omega^{(3)} = 0$, and is invariant under the N-gauge transformation $(K, H) \to (K', H')$, $dK' \wedge dH' = dK \wedge dH$, satisfying the Jacobian condition $\frac{\partial(K',H')}{\partial(H,K)} = 1$ (see Sect. 2.2).

Now, we have to study the interior product of $\omega^{(3)}$ with the 4-vector corresponding to the equations of motion, namely,

$$X^\mu = (X^i, 1) = (\partial_2 K \partial_3 H - \partial_3 K \partial_2 H, \partial_3 K \partial_1 H - \partial_1 K \partial_3 H, \partial_1 K \partial_2 H - \partial_2 K \partial_1 H, 1).$$

Let us consider each term of $\omega^{(3)}$, separately. The first term, the kinematical part $dx^1 \wedge dx^2 \wedge dx^3$, yields

$$\begin{aligned}\iota_{(X,1)}(dx^1 \wedge dx^2 \wedge dx^3) &= (\partial_2 K \partial_3 H - \partial_3 K \partial_2 H)dx^2 \wedge dx^3 \\ &\quad - (\partial_3 K \partial_1 H - \partial_1 K \partial_3 H)dx^1 \wedge dx^3 + (\partial_1 K \partial_2 H - \partial_2 K \partial_1 H)dx^1 \wedge dx^2 \\ &= dK \wedge dH.\end{aligned}$$

For treating the second term, the dynamical part $dK \wedge dH \wedge dt$, we first note that interior products with 1-forms $dK = \partial_i K dx^i$ and $dH = \partial_i H dx^i$ are obviously zero, because the spatial vector field $X^i = \epsilon^{ijk}\partial_j K \partial_k H$ are orthogonal to $\partial_i K$ and $\partial_i H$,

$$\iota_{(X,1)} dK = \iota_X dK = 0, \quad \iota_{(X,1)} dH = \iota_X dH = 0.$$

Therefore, only non-vanishing contribution comes from $\iota_{\hat{X}} dt = 1$, yielding

$$\iota_{(X,1)} dK \wedge dH \wedge dt = dK \wedge dH.$$

Combining these results, we indeed have

$$\iota_{(X,1)}\omega^{(3)} = 0, \tag{2.58}$$

which, together with $d\omega^{(3)} = 0$, gives $\mathcal{L}_{(X,1)}\omega^{(3)} = 0$.

Furthermore, noticing

$$\omega^{(3)} = d\omega^{(2)}, \quad \omega^{(2)} = x^1 dx^2 \wedge dx^3 - K dH \wedge dt + d\Lambda^{(1)},$$

where $\Lambda^{(1)}$ is an arbitrary 1-form, we also have

$$\mathcal{L}_{(X,1)}\omega^{(2)} = d(\iota_{(X,1)}\omega^{(2)}), \tag{2.59}$$

where

$$\iota_{(X,1)}\omega^{(2)} = x^1(X^2 dx^3 - X^3 dx^2) - K dH + \iota_{(X,1)} d\Lambda^{(1)}.$$

These results are parallel with those of conventional Hamiltonian dynamics discussed in the previous subsection: under time evolution governed by the Nambu equations of motion, $\omega^{(3)}$ or $\omega^{(2)}$ are invariant or quasi-invariant, extending $\alpha^{(2)}$ or $\alpha^{(1)}$, respectively, in the conventional Hamiltonian formalism. A crucial new element emerging from this extension is the N-gauge symmetry of the time-like parts of these forms: not only $\omega^{(3)}$ for which we have $dK' \wedge dH' = dK \wedge dH$, $\omega^{(2)}$ is also invariant under the N-gauge transformation. In fact using

$$(K'dH' - KdH) \wedge dt = dF \wedge dt = d(F \wedge dt),$$

where F is the generating function of the N-gauge transformation, we can write

$$-KdH \wedge dt + d\Lambda^{(1)} = -K'dH' \wedge dt + d\Lambda'^{(1)}$$

with $\Lambda'^{(1)} = \Lambda^{(1)} + Fdt$.

The condition (2.58) means geometrically, as is the case for $\alpha^{(2)}$, that a world line of a single particle obeying the equations of motion in 4 = 3 + 1-dimensional Nambu phase space-time is orthogonal (in the four-dimensional sense) to the infinitesimal volume elements represented by $\omega^{(3)}$ at each point along the world line. In other words, the component of $\omega^{(3)}$ projected on the world line vanishes: the motion of particles are determined by the configuration of a four-component *geometrical field* represented by $\omega^{(3)}$ in phase space-time.

For example, if a world line in phase space-time crosses a point where $dK \wedge dH = 0$, all of the three time-like components of $\omega^{(3)}$ vanish there and hence the world line is orthogonal to $dx^1 \wedge dx^2 \wedge dx^3$, implying that X^μ has only time component corresponding to vanishing velocity $\dot{x}^i = 0$. Since the configuration of $\omega^{(3)}$ is constant with respect to time, this implies that the orthogonality of the world line to $dx^1 \wedge dx^2 \wedge dx^3$ continues forever from $t = -\infty$ to $t = \infty$, namely, just a straight world line with a fixed spatial point. In general, such fixed points (or the points in equilibrium) distribute continuously along curves, since the independent components of the condition $dK \wedge dH = 0$ are only two because of the identity $d(dK \wedge dH) \equiv 0$. For this reason, the distribution of fixed points is useful as a means for characterizing the overall structure of the solutions of the Nambu equations of motion.

Example 2.5 Let us study the distribution of fixed points in the following particular case extending slightly the Euler top,

$$K = \frac{1}{2}\left((x^1)^2 + (x^2)^2 + (x^3)^2\right),$$
$$H = \frac{1}{2}\left(a(x^1 - e)^2 + b(x^2 - f)^2 + c(x^3 - g)^2\right),$$

where, for definiteness, we assume all of the coefficients (a, b, c) are positive and all different from each other. The conditions for fixed points are

$$0 = \partial_1 K \partial_2 H - \partial_2 K \partial_1 H = (b - a)x^1 x^2 - bfx^1 + aex^2, \tag{2.60}$$
$$0 = \partial_2 K \partial_3 H - \partial_3 \partial_2 H = (c - b)x^2 x^3 - cgx^2 + fbx^3, \tag{2.61}$$
$$0 = \partial_3 K \partial_1 H - \partial_1 K \partial_3 H = (a - c)x^3 x^1 - aex^3 + cgx^1. \tag{2.62}$$

The particular case with $e = f = g = 0$ corresponding to the Euler equations for a rigid rotator is very special: $x^1x^2 = x^2x^3 = x^3x^1 = 0$. There are three independent solutions, $x^1 = x^2 = 0$, $x^2 = x^3 = 0$, and $x^3 = x^1 = 0$, which coincide with the three orthogonal axes. The solutions of the equations of motion give closed curves around these axes, which are intersections of spheres, $K =$ constant, and spheroids, $H =$ constant, depending on the initial conditions, both of whose centers are at the origin, $x^1 = x^2 = x^3 = 0$.

Next, consider the case where none of the parameters (e, f, g) is zero. Although there are three conditions, it is easy to check that only two of them are independent. For example, from (2.60) and (2.61), we can express x^1 and x^3 in terms of x^2:

$$x^1 = -\frac{aex^2}{(b-a)x^2 - bf}, \quad x^3 = -\frac{cgx^2}{(b-c)x^2 - bf}.$$

The third Eq. (2.62), relating x^1 and x^3, is automatically satisfied. Therefore we can treat x^2 as an independent continuous parameter characterizing the set of all fixed points. Since there are two singularities, at $x^2 = bf/(b-a)$ and at $x^2 = bf/(b-c)$, the line of fixed points is actually separated into three different components. For concreteness, suppose that $b - a > b - c > 0$ and $e = f = g > 0$. The line of fixed points then consists of three separate connected components,

$$\text{(i) } x^2 \in \left(-\infty, \frac{bf}{b-a}\right), \quad \text{(ii) } x^2 \in \left(\frac{bf}{b-a}, \frac{bf}{b-c}\right), \quad \text{(iii) } x^2 \in \left(\frac{bf}{b-c}, \infty\right).$$

Each segmental curve corresponding to these three components comes from an infinity to an infinity, and they never cross each other, and only (i) crosses $x^1 = x^2 = x^3 = 0$ and $x^1 - e = x^2 - f = x^3 - g = 0$, centers of the spheres and the spheroids. In any case, the sets of fixed points themselves form one-dimensional continuous families.

The figure below exhibits this particular example of the separate continuous lines of fixed points:

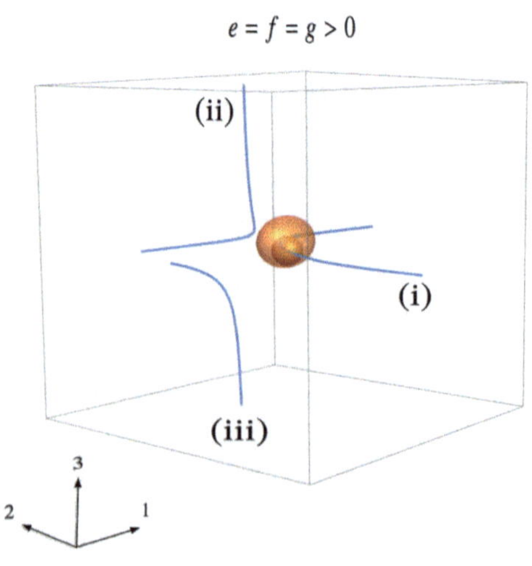

Fig. 2.3 The lines of fixed points

Only the line (i) passes through the H-spheroid contains a K-sphere tangentially inside, with the point of their contact with the K-sphere at just one of the two points crossing the H-spheroid along the component (i). We also show below the images of trajectories satisfying the equations of motion:

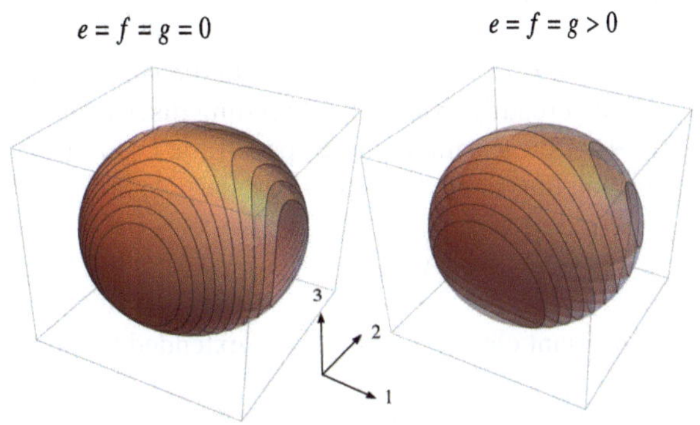

Fig. 2.4 The trajectories of the solutions of the equations of motion

The trajectories determined by the equations of motion consist of the intersections of a K-sphere of a fixed size with the H-spheroids of various different sizes; the intersections on the left figure above arise, as the spheroids of the previous figure (Fig. 2.3) are scaled down in discrete steps. On the right, the center position of the H-spheroids is shifted from the origin to a point in the positive quadrant, and hence the curves of intersections with the K-sphere are deformed from those on the left where the centers of the K-sphere and H-spheroids are both at the origin (Fig. 2.4).

In comparison with conventional Hamiltonian dynamics where the fixed points for the equations of motion coincide with the stationary points of a single Hamiltonian, the set of fixed points in Nambu dynamics in three dimensions are given by the condition that the gradient vectors of two level surfaces at the intersections become parallel to each other. The stationary points themselves of the Hamiltonian functions only form a special (ordinarily discrete) subset of points satisfying this condition along the line of fixed points: in the present example, this subset consists only of two points $x^1 = x^2 = x^3 = 0$ and $x^1 - e = x^2 - f = x^3 - g = 0$.

When $dK \wedge dH$ is not zero, the greater the magnitude of 2-form $dK \wedge dH$ is, the larger the magnitude of spatial components of X^μ is. Then the tilting, either positive or negative, of $\omega^{(3)}$ toward the time direction increases, and consequently the tangent vector, or velocity vector, of the world line gets larger magnitudes of spatial components. Thus world lines, in general, form helical lines curving around straight world lines (associated with the fixed points) which parallel the time axis.

Of course, these properties could be read off roughly from the equations of motion; the condition $\iota_{(X,1)}\omega^{(3)} = 0$ provides us a more precise mathematical representation of such a qualitative picture in terms of differential forms. Similarly, the conditions $\iota_{(X,1)}dK = 0$ and $\iota_{(X,1)}dH = 0$ express the conservation law for K and H using the language of differential forms. On the other hand, the condition of quasi-invariance

(2.59) for the 2-form $\omega^{(2)}$ is the analog of (2.57) in the case of the conventional Hamiltonian dynamics. Therefore both $\omega^{(3)}$ and $\omega^{(2)}$ are important in investigating whether and how Nambu dynamics be fitted in to the action (or variational) principle. Indeed, as we shall see in the next chapter, the conditions expressed using the operation of interior product or *contraction* for them can be regarded as a local version of extended variational principles for Nambu dynamics. Hence, it seems pertinent to call the characterization of the equations of motion using the interior product the *contraction principle* in analogy with the *variational principle*.

We can readily extend the foregoing discussions for $n = 3$ to higher dimensions. In $(n+1)$-dimensional phase space-time (x^i, t) $(i = 1, \ldots, n)$, the vector field X^μ corresponding to the trajectory of a particle is

$$X^\mu = (X^i, 1), \qquad X^i = \epsilon^{ij_1 \ldots j_{n-1}} \partial_{j_1} H_1 \partial_{j_2} H_2 \cdots \partial_{j_{n-1}} H_{n-1}.$$

The invariant closed 3-form $\omega^{(3)}$ is extended to the following n-form,

$$\omega^{(n)} = dx^1 \wedge dx^2 \wedge \cdots \wedge dx^n - dH_1 \wedge dH_2 \wedge \cdots dH_{n-1} \wedge dt,$$

satisfying $\iota_{(X,1)}\omega^{(n)} = 0$ and $d\omega^{(n)} = 0$, and hence $\mathcal{L}_{(X,1)}\omega^{(n)} = 0$. Namely, the world lines obeying the Nambu equations of motion are orthogonal to n-dimensional infinitesimal volumes represented by the n-form field $\omega^{(n)}(x)$. The conservation laws are expressed as

$$\iota_{(X,1)} dH_i = X^\mu \partial_\mu H_i = X^j \partial_j H_i = 0, \qquad (i = 1, \ldots, n-1).$$

Similarly, the quasi-invariant 2-form $\omega^{(2)}$ is extended to, with $\Lambda^{(n-2)}$ being an arbitrary $(n-2)$-form,

$$\omega^{(n-1)} = x^1 dx^2 \wedge \cdots \wedge dx^n - H_1 dH_2 \wedge \cdots \wedge dH_{n-1} \wedge dt + d\Lambda^{(n-2)},$$

satisfying $\omega^{(n)} = d\omega^{(n-1)}$ and $\mathcal{L}_{(X,1)}\omega^{(n-1)} = d\iota_{(X,1)}\omega^{(n-1)}$.

Fixed points appear whenever two out of $n-1$ gradient vectors corresponding to $n-1$ level surfaces of H_i become parallel. Hence there are $(n-1)(n-2)/2$ independent lines of fixed points. In addition, there can be much more complicated patterns of the distributions of fixed points: for $n > 3$, even if there is no pair of parallel gradient vectors, fixed points can arise when one of gradient vectors becomes linearly dependent of the other two or more gradient vectors. The distributions of such fixed points are given by two-or higher-dimensional hyper-surfaces.

Here it is perhaps useful to recall what we have mentioned about (2.33) as a motivation toward our investigations on generalized canonical transformations in n-dimensions: in terms of differential forms, (2.33) reads

$$dx^1 \wedge \cdots \wedge dx^n - dH_1 \wedge \cdots \wedge dH_{n-1} \wedge dx'^n = 0.$$

There, by the consistency with the Nambu equations of motion after making a generalized canonical transformation $x^i \to x'^i = H_i$ $(1 \le i \le n-1)$, we were led to an identification $x'^n = t + c$, and thus to $dx'^n = dt$. However, in the context of differential forms in $(n+1)$-dimensional phase space-time, such a direct identification does not make sense: it would lead to a nonsensical result that $\omega^{(n)}$ itself vanishes, which is impossible because of the independence of the bases of differential forms $(dx^1, \dots, dx^n, dt)$. What we have exhibited is that the correct formulation of the idea underlying such an identification in terms of differential forms is that the equations of motion can be expressed as $\iota_{(X,1)}\omega^{(n)} = 0$, instead of the direct vanishing of $\omega^{(n)}$.

Finally, in n dimensions, a generic N-gauge transformation $H_i \to H_i'$ is defined by the condition

$$dH_1 \wedge dH_2 \wedge \cdots \wedge dH_{n-1} = dH_1' \wedge dH_2' \wedge \cdots \wedge dH_{n-1}',$$

which is equivalent to

$$H_1' dH_2' \wedge \cdots \wedge dH_{n-1}' - H_1 dH_2 \wedge \cdots \wedge dH_{n-1} = dF^{(n-3)}$$

with some $(n-3)$-form $F^{(n-3)}$, generalizing the generating function F of $n = 3$. This shows that, by making a formal correspondence between phase space coordinates x^i and the Hamiltonians H_i, the N-gauge transformations can be treated in exactly the same way as the generalized canonical transformations. Thus we can translate all of what we have discussed on the latter also into the corresponding properties of the N-gauge transformations with suitable substitutions: e.g. the number of degrees of freedom of N-gauge transformations in n dimensions is $(n-1) - 1 = n - 2$. Hence the true physical 'Hamiltonian degrees' of freedom with $n - 1$ Hamiltonians is always one: $n - 1 - (n-2) = 1$, reflecting the fact that the time evolution of generic Nambu systems occurs always on a one-dimensional curve under a given initial condition, defined as the intersection of $n - 1$ level hyper-surfaces associated with H_i $(i = 1, \dots, n-1)$ in n-dimensional phase space.

Chapter 3
The Extension of Variational Principle and Hamilton–Jacobi Theory to Nambu Dynamics

An important and useful property in conventional Hamiltonian dynamics is that it can be formulated in terms of variational principles using action integrals. For instance, it provides a foundation for the path-integral formulation of quantum mechanics, as we have mentioned briefly in Chap. 1. The main objective of the present chapter is to formulate generalized variational principles for Nambu dynamics on the basis of geometrical apparatus hitherto developed. Then, as the final topic of the present exposition, Hamilton–Jacobi-type formulations of Nambu dynamics will be given.

3.1 Preparations

3.1.1 Integrals of Differential Forms and Stokes' Theorem

Let us first recall an elementary definition of integral of an arbitrary function $f = f(x^1, \ldots, x^n)$ in n-dimensional Euclidean space $\mathbb{R}^n \equiv (x^1, x^2, \ldots, x^n)$,

$$\int_V f(x)dx^1 \ldots dx^n \equiv \lim_{\Delta x^i \to 0} \sum_{\text{cells} \in V} f \Delta x^1 \ldots \Delta x^n, \tag{3.1}$$

where V is a connected n-dimensional region in $\mathbb{R}^n$, and Δx^is are the lengths of edges of n-dimensional rectangular cells decomposing the region V. By definition, it is obvious that the following linearity relations hold:

$$\int_V (f+g)dx^1 \ldots dx^n = \int_V f dx^1 \ldots dx^n + \int_V g dx^1 \ldots dx^n,$$

$$\int_V f dx^1 \ldots dx^n = \int_{V_1} f dx^1 \ldots dx^n + \int_{V_2} f dx^1 \ldots dx^n.$$

T. Yoneya, *Introduction to Nambu's Generalized Hamiltonian Dynamics*,
SpringerBriefs in Mathematical Physics 55,
https://doi.org/10.1007/978-981-95-7030-0_3

In the second relation, the region V is decomposed into a sum of non-intersecting connected regions V_1 and V_2 ($V_1 \cap V_2 = \varnothing$, $V = V_1 + V_2$).

The basic differential n-form $dx^1 \wedge \cdots \wedge dx^n$ can be regarded as a generalization of the volume element $d^n x \equiv dx^1 \ldots dx^n$ such that it acquires the property of *orientation*. Namely, we can naturally define an integral of a function $f(x)$ treating $dx^1 \wedge \cdots \wedge dx^n$ as an integration measure by

$$\int_V f(x) dx^{P(1)} \wedge \cdots \wedge dx^{P(n)} \equiv (-1)^{\epsilon(P)} \int_V f(x) dx^1 \ldots dx^n,$$

where $P(i)$ is a permutation of indices $(1, 2, \ldots, n)$ as before. If we perform a coordinate transformation $x^i \to x'^i$, we have

$$\int_V f dx^1 \wedge \cdots \wedge dx^n = \int_V f \frac{\partial(x^1, \ldots, x^n)}{\partial(x'^1, \ldots, x'^n)} dx'^1 \wedge \cdots \wedge dx'^n,$$

using

$$dx^1 \wedge \cdots \wedge dx^n = \frac{\partial(x^1, \ldots, x^n)}{\partial(x'^1, \ldots, x'^n)} dx'^1 \wedge \cdots \wedge dx'^n.$$

Unlike the ordinary integral (3.1) where the integration volume is always positive definite by definition and consequently the change of the integration volume obeys

$$d^n x = \left| \frac{\partial(x^1, \ldots, x^n)}{\partial(x'^1, \ldots, x'^n)} \right| d^n x',$$

the Jacobian is *not* accompanied by the absolute-value symbol in our definition.

For concreteness, take the 3-dimensional case: given an exact 3-form $d\omega^{(2)}$ with $\omega^{(2)}$ being some 2-form,

$$\begin{aligned} \omega^{(2)} &= a^3 dx^1 \wedge dx^2 + a^1 dx^2 \wedge dx^3 + a^2 dx^3 \wedge dx^1, \\ d\omega^{(2)} &= \partial_i a^i dx^1 \wedge dx^2 \wedge dx^3, \end{aligned}$$

we have, by partial integration,

$$\begin{aligned} \int_V d\omega^{(2)} &= \int_V \partial_i a^i dx^1 \wedge dx^2 \wedge dx^3 \\ &= \int_V \partial_i a^i d^3 x = \int_{\partial V} a^i d^2 S_i = \int_{\partial V} \omega^{(2)}, \end{aligned} \tag{3.2}$$

where

$$d^2S_i = (dx^2 \wedge dx^3, dx^3 \wedge dx^1, dx^1 \wedge dx^2),$$

and ∂V denotes the boundary of the region V. This is of course the well-known 'Gauss's theorem' in integral form with which the reader is familiar in elementary electromagnetism. The rule of partial integration automatically fixes the orientation of the surface integral so that the surface-element vector dS_i is directed outward normal from the boundary ∂V.

The relation (3.2) is straightforwardly extended to arbitrary dimensions as,

$$\int_V \omega^{(n)} = \int_{\partial V} \omega^{(n-1)}, \tag{3.3}$$

where

$$\omega^{(n)} = d\omega^{(n-1)} = \frac{1}{(n-1)!}\partial_i \omega_{i_1 \ldots i_{n-1}} dx^i \wedge dx^{i_1} \wedge \cdots \wedge dx^{i_{n-1}},$$
$$\omega^{(n-1)} = \frac{1}{(n-1)!}\omega_{i_1 \ldots i_{n-1}} dx^{i_1} \wedge \cdots \wedge dx^{i_{n-1}}.$$

We call this generic relation *Stokes's theorem*, for convenience. Although there exists a gauge freedom for $\omega^{(n-1)}$, $\omega^{(n-1)} \to \omega^{(n-1)} + d\Lambda^{(n-2)}$, with $\Lambda^{(n-2)}$ being an arbitrary $(n-2)$-form, we have

$$\int_{\partial V} d\Lambda^{(n-2)} = \int_{\partial\partial V} \Lambda^{(n-2)} = 0,$$

since there is no boundary for the boundary ∂V, that is, $\partial\partial V = 0$. Thus both sides of (3.3) are gauge invariant: on the left the nilpotency $d^2 = 0$ is responsible, while on the right the nilpotency $\partial^2 = 0$ is responsible for gauge invariance.

Note that in the above example (3.2), $a^i = \epsilon^{ijk}\omega_{jk}/2$. In the two-dimensional case $n = 2$, we have similarly $a^i = \epsilon^{ij}\omega_j = (\omega_2, -\omega_1)$ and

$$\omega^{(1)} = \omega_1 dx^1 + \omega_2 dx^2, \quad \omega^{(2)} = d\omega^{(1)} = (\partial_1\omega_2 - \partial_2\omega_1)dx^1 \wedge dx^2,$$
$$\int_V (\partial_1\omega_2 - \partial_2\omega_1)dx^1 \wedge dx^2 = \int_{\partial V} (a^1 dS_1 + a^2 dS_2) = \oint \omega_i dx^i.$$

The orientation of outward normal for the 2-dimensional vector $dS_i = (dx^2, -dx^1)$ corresponds to counter-clockwise direction for the line integral in the last equality, which is nothing but the elementary Stokes' theorem familiar in electromagnetism.

When the connected region V is decomposed into two parts as in (3.3), we have

$$\int_V \omega^{(n)} = \int_{V_1} \omega^{(n)} + \int_{V_2} \omega^{(n)} = \int_{\partial V_1} \omega^{(n-1)} + \int_{\partial V_2} \omega^{(n-1)} = \int_{\partial V} \omega^{(n-1)}.$$

Clearly, the orientations of two boundaries ∂V_1 and ∂V_2 are opposite in the common parts of their regions where they touch adjacent to each other, and hence cancel out, yielding $\partial V = \partial V_1 + \partial V_2$ that ensures the last equality.

We can extend the integrations of differential forms to $(n+1)$-dimensional phase space-time $x^\mu = (x^i, t)$, denoted by M_{n+1}. For differential forms, we will use the same notations and conventions that have been introduced in Sect. 2.7.1. All of the previous discussions are valid after replacing the phase space coordinates x^i to x^μ.

Now, in more general cases in which we discuss integrations of a k-form with $k \leq n$ in $(n+1)$-dimensional phase space-time, the integration region V is in general a certain k-dimensional sub-manifold M_k embedded in phase space-time. For simplicity, we assume that any parts of M_k always extends along positive time-like directions, without any hanging to negative time directions, and parametrize M_k as

$$x^\mu|_{M_k} = \left(x^i(t; \sigma^1, \ldots, \sigma^{k-1}), t\right).$$

Namely, the vector function $x^i(t; \sigma^1, \ldots, \sigma^{k-1})$ expresses the section, secM_k, of M_k in phase space-time at time t, and the spatial coordinates σ^a, $(a = 1, \ldots, k-1)$ represent points of M_k on each time slice, with their ranges depending on the shape of secM_k that can be chosen arbitrarily. The functions $x^i(t; \sigma^1, \ldots, \sigma^{k-1})$ can be interpreted as describing a continuous family (or bundle) of world lines which fill up M_k flowing without mutual intersection and being discriminated by the parameters σ^a. It should be kept in mind, as a matter of fact, for formulating variational principles that these world lines are *not in general* assumed to be the solutions of the equations of motion, contrary to the discussions in Sect. 2.7.

For M_k, $(d\sigma^1, \ldots, d\sigma^{k-1}, dt)$ is the basis for differential 1-forms: the differential basis dx^μ of phase space-time is 'projected' onto M_k by the formula $(dt|_{M_k} \equiv dt)$,

$$dx^i|_{M_k} \equiv \frac{\partial x^i}{\partial \sigma^a} d\sigma^a + \dot{x}^i dt, \qquad (\dot{x}^i = \partial_t x^i). \tag{3.4}$$

A general k-form in $(n+1)$-dimensional phase space-time M_{n+1}

$$\omega^{(k)} = \frac{1}{k!}\omega_{\mu_1,\ldots,\mu_k} dx^{\mu_1} \wedge \cdots \wedge dx^{\mu_k},$$

is then naturally projected onto M_k as

$$\begin{aligned}
\omega^{(k)}|_{M_k} &= \left[\frac{1}{k!}\omega_{i_1\ldots i_k} dx^{i_1} \wedge \cdots \wedge dx^{i_k} + \frac{1}{(k-1)!}\omega_{i_1\ldots i_{k-1}t} dx^{i_1} \wedge \cdots dx^{i_{k-1}} \wedge dt\right]_{M_k} \\
&= \frac{1}{(k-1)!}\left[\omega_{i_1\ldots i_{k-1}j}\dot{x}^j + \omega_{i_1\ldots i_{k-1}t}\right]_{M_k} \frac{\partial(x^{i_1}, \ldots, x^{i_{k-1}})}{\partial(\sigma^1, \ldots, \sigma^{k-1})} d\sigma^1 \wedge \cdots \wedge d\sigma^{k-1} \wedge dt,
\end{aligned} \tag{3.5}$$

where the coefficient tensor field $\omega_{\mu_1,\ldots,\mu_k}(x)$ is projected simply by $\omega_{\mu_1,\ldots,\mu_k}(x)|_{M_k} = \omega_{\mu_1,\ldots,\mu_k}(x(\sigma, t))$. In the mathematical literature, the formula of this type describing a k-form $\omega^{(k)}$ in M_{n+1} as a k-form $\omega^{(k)}\big|_{M_k}$ in M_k is usually called the 'pull-back' of $\omega^{(k)}$ associated with the mapping $x^\mu\big|_{M_k} : M_k \to M_{n+1}$.

In what follows, for the sake of brevity we often abbreviate the 'M_k' associated with the symbol $\cdots\big]_{M_k}$ on the right-hand side when confusion is not expected. With this convention, we can write the expression in the last equality simply as

$$\omega^{(k)}|_{M_k} = \frac{1}{(k-1)!}\big[\omega_{i_1\ldots i_{k-1}j}\dot{x}^j + \omega_{i_1\ldots i_{k-1}t}\big]dx^{i_1} \wedge \cdots \wedge dx^{i_{k-1}} \wedge dt.$$

It is easy to check that the operation of projection is commutative with exterior differentiation: e.g.,

$$\begin{aligned} d(\omega^{(1)}|_{M_k}) &= d\left(\omega_j \frac{\partial x^j}{\partial \sigma^\beta} d\sigma^\beta\right) = \partial_i \omega_j \frac{\partial x^i}{\partial \sigma^\alpha}\frac{\partial x^j}{\partial \sigma^\beta} d\sigma^\alpha \wedge d\sigma^\beta \\ &= \frac{1}{2}(\partial_i \omega_j - \partial_j \omega_i)\frac{\partial x^i}{\partial \sigma^\alpha}\frac{\partial x^j}{\partial \sigma^\beta} d\sigma^\alpha \wedge d\sigma^\beta = (d\omega^{(1)})|_{M_k}, \end{aligned}$$

where the indices α, β of the σ coordinates are extended so as to include time direction, i.e. $\sigma^\alpha = (\sigma^a, t)$, etc.

3.1.2 The Variational Principle of Conventional Hamiltonian Dynamics

Before proceeding to generalize the variational principle to Nambu dynamics, we treat, as a warm-up and also to avoid possible confusion prejudiced by the ordinary text-book formulation of variational principles, the case of conventional Hamiltonian dynamics using the general ideas and notations hitherto introduced.

The canonically invariant 2-form $\alpha^{(2)}$ is integrated over a 2-dimensional submanifold M_2 embedded in $(2n+1)$-dimensional phase space-time $(p_1, q_1, \ldots, p_n, q_n, t)$: namely, as a special case of (3.5), we write

$$\begin{aligned} \alpha^{(2)}\big|_{M_2} &= dp_i(t;\sigma) \wedge dq_i(t;\sigma) - dH(p,q) \wedge dt \\ &= \big[((\dot{q}_i - \partial_{p_i} H)\partial_\sigma p_i - (\dot{p}_i + \partial_{q_i} H)\partial_\sigma q_i\big]d\sigma \wedge dt, \end{aligned} \tag{3.6}$$

yielding

$$\int_{M_2} \alpha^{(2)} = \int_{M_2} \big[(\dot{q}_i - \partial_{p_i} H)\partial_\sigma p_i - (\dot{p}_i + \partial_{q_i} H)\partial_\sigma q_i\big]d\sigma \wedge dt.$$

Using $\alpha^{(2)} = d\alpha^{(1)}$ and $\alpha^{(1)} = p_i dq_i - H dt + d\lambda$, Stokes' theorem gives

$$\int_{M_2} \alpha^{(2)} = \int_{\partial M_2} \alpha^{(1)} = \int_{\partial M_2} (p_i dq_i - H dt). \tag{3.7}$$

Let us now assume M_2 to be an infinitesimally narrow band stretching along the time direction, such that it starts at $t = t_{\text{ini}}$ and ends at $t = t_{\text{fin}}$ where its width vanishes. The closed curve forming the boundary ∂M_2 can be decomposed into a difference, $\partial M_2 = L' - L \equiv \delta L$, of two open world lines L and L' which are infinitesimally close to each other, being oriented to positive time directions and meeting at $t = t_{\text{ini}}$ and $t = t_{\text{fin}}$, Therefore, the right-hand side of (3.7) is identical with an ordinary infinitesimal variation of the action integral,

$$\int_{\partial M_2} (p_i dq_i - H dt) = \int_{\delta L} (p_i dq_i - H dt) = \delta \int_{t_{\text{ini}}}^{t_{\text{fin}}} (p_i dq_i - H dt). \tag{3.8}$$

Note that by definition the variations of (p, q) vanish automatically at the end points. Since the Hamilton equations of motion are first-order differential equations, it is clear that boundary conditions at both ends are overspecified. Hence a unique solution exists only when we choose those conditions to be consistent with the equations of motion. We choose a representative world line, denoted by L_0 and called the *core world line* of M_2, arbitrarily among the continuous family of world lines filling up M_2, which are parametrized by σ used in (3.6). We can write

$$\int_{M_2} \alpha^{(2)} = \int_{L_0} \delta\pi_i (\dot{x}^i - X^i) dt, \tag{3.9}$$

where the notations are changed to those of Sect. 1.3.1, namely,

$$\{x^i\} = (p_1, q_1, \ldots, p_n, q_n), \quad \{X^i\} = (-\partial_{q_1} H, \partial_{p_1} H, \ldots, -\partial_{q_n} H, \partial_{p_n} H),$$

and correspondingly,

$$\{\delta\pi_i(t)\} \equiv \int_{\text{sec}M_2(t)} \Big(-\partial_\sigma q_1(t;\sigma), \partial_\sigma p_1(t;\sigma), \ldots, -\partial_\sigma q_n(t;\sigma), \partial_\sigma p_n(t;\sigma) \Big) d\sigma,$$

where 'sec$M_2(t)$' denotes the cross-section of M_2 at time t, giving an infinitesimal variation of the variables x^i at each time t, which is essentially given by the width of M_2 itself. Needless to say, arbitrariness of the infinitesimal variations is reflected in the arbitrariness of the shapes of M_2, with the core world line L_0 being fixed. The requirement of vanishing $\alpha^{(2)}$ under the restriction to infinitesimally narrow (time-like) band M_2 is when the core world line L_0 satisfies the equations of motion,

$\dot{x}^i = X^i$. This establishes our geometrical formulation of variational principle for the conventional Hamiltonian dynamics.

Example 3.1 (The case of a vibrating string): Let us briefly treat the case of a field theory, taking a vibrating string in $(1+1)$-dimensional space-time (t, s) as one of the simplest examples of such cases. The dynamical coordinates consist of a single field $q(t, s)$ and its conjugate momentum-field $p(t, s)$ where $s \in [0, 1]$ parametrizes the spatial direction with appropriate boundary conditions at the end points $s = 0, 1$. The equations of motion and Hamiltonian are

$$\dot{p} = \frac{\partial^2 x}{\partial s^2} = -\frac{\delta H}{\delta q}, \quad \dot{q} = p = \frac{\delta H}{\delta p},$$

$$H = H[p(t, s), q(t, s)] = \int_0^1 \left[p(t, s)^2 + \left(\frac{\partial q}{\partial s} \right)^2 \right] ds.$$

Note that the indices $i = 1, \ldots, n$ for canonical pair (p_i, q_i) in a $2n$-dimensional phase space are now replaced by a continuous coordinate s, and partial derivatives $\partial_{p_i}, \partial_{q_i}$ are replaced by functional derivatives $\frac{\delta}{\delta p(s)}, \frac{\delta}{\delta q(s)}$, respectively, suppressing time dependence, and the summation over i turns into integral over s. The 2-form $\alpha^{(2)}$ is then written:

$$\alpha^{(2)} = \int_0^1 \Big(dp(s) \wedge dq(s) - dH[p(s), q(s)] \wedge dt \Big) ds.$$

The infinitesimal variations are described by $p(t, s; \sigma), q(t, s; \sigma)$ with an additional parameter σ. M_2 is now a two-dimensional manifold embedded in an *infinite-dimensional* phase space-time: infinite dimensional because the phase-space coordinates are the fields on the base space-time (t, s), since the pair $(p(t, s), q(t, s))$ describes canonical coordinate and canonical moment for each s *independently*:

$$\alpha^{(2)}|_{M_2} = \int_0^1 \left\{ \left[\left(\dot{q} - \frac{\delta H}{\delta p} \right) \partial_\sigma p - \left(\dot{p} + \frac{\delta H}{\delta q} \right) \partial_\sigma q \right] d\sigma \wedge dt \right\} ds.$$

With an infinitesimally narrow M_2 as before, we finally have

$$\int_{M_2} \alpha^{(2)} = \int_{S_0} \pi_A(t, s) \big(\dot{x}^A(t, s) - X^A(t, s) \big) dt ds,$$

$$\{\pi_A(t, s)\} = \int_{\sec M_2(t)} \big(-\partial_\sigma q(t, s; \sigma), \partial_\sigma p(t, s; \sigma) \big) d\sigma, \qquad (3.10)$$

where S_0 is a core world sheet swept out by the vibrating string and x^A, $A \in (1, 2)$ denote two-dimensional vector fields on the world sheet S_0:

$$\big(x^1(t,s), x^2(t,s)\big) \equiv \big(p(t,s), q(t,s)\big),$$
$$\big(X^1(t,s), X^2(t,s)\big) \equiv \left(-\frac{\delta H}{\delta q(t,s)}, \frac{\delta H}{\delta p(t,s)}\right).$$

To avoid possible confusion, we note that it is also possible formally to treat the area element $dtds$ as the area 2-form $ds \wedge dt$, and thereby to elevate $\alpha^{(2)}$ to a 3-form, if desired, e.g. for the purpose of making the formalism to be manifestly Lorentz invariant in two-dimensional space-time (s, t) of the world sheet. We do not pursue this line of development, since there is little merit in doing this at least for the purpose of the present exposition.

Our purpose of discussing this example is to help clarify a crucial difference with respect to the nature of two continuous parameters, s and σ. The former, s, has a dynamical significance in the sense that s-derivative of the dynamical variables contribute to the Hamiltonian: in other words s describes an extended nature of the basic degrees of freedom as a vibrating string. By contrast, the latter, σ, being nothing to do with the physical extension, plays only a kinematical role to describe a continuous family of world sheets, defining the infinitesimal variation of dynamical variables: the σ-derivatives never enter into the Hamiltonian itself. In order to express this difference emphatically, we write $p(t, s; \sigma), q(t, s; \sigma)$ using the semicolon (;), instead of $p(t, s, \sigma), q(t, s, \sigma)$.

3.2 Generalized Variational Principles for Nambu Dynamics

Now we shall examine how the results of the previous section are extended to Nambu dynamics. Let us start with $n = 3$. The role of $\alpha^{(2)}$ is played by the closed 3-form,

$$\omega^{(3)} = dx^1 \wedge dx^2 \wedge dx^3 - dK \wedge dH \wedge dt,$$

introduced and studied in the previous chapter. This must be integrated over a three-dimensional sub-manifold M_3 in (3+1)-dimensional Nambu phase space-time (i.e. M_4), which is infinitesimally narrow and is parametrized by a two-dimensional family of non-intersecting world lines $x^i(t; \sigma^1, \sigma^2)$ filling up M_3 without intersection. As is the case for M_2, M_3 can take arbitrary narrow shapes, stretching to the positive time direction without hanging. Here we have to pay due attention to the difference between the variable $x^A(t, s; \sigma)$ treated in Example 3.1 and the present $x^i(t; \sigma_1, \sigma_2)$. Though both contain 3 independent variables, there is a crucial difference: s describes a physical extension, while either of σ or (σ_1, σ_2) does not, only parametrizing a one-dimensional family of string world sheets or a two-dimensional family of world lines, respectively, which are nothing to do with physical extension.

The general formula (3.5) of projection gives immediately

$$\begin{aligned}\omega^{(3)}\big|_{M_3} &= \frac{1}{2}\epsilon_{ijk}(\dot{x}^i - X^i)dx^j \wedge dx^k \wedge dt \\ &= \frac{1}{2}\epsilon_{ijk}(\dot{x}^i - X^i)\partial_a x^j \partial_b x^k d\sigma^a \wedge d\sigma^b \wedge dt,\end{aligned} \tag{3.11}$$

where $X^i = \epsilon^{ijk}\partial_j K \partial_k H$. This result makes the relation between the 3-form $\omega^{(3)}$ and the equations of motion, $\dot{x}^i = X^i$, which was formulated in the last section of the previous chapter using the interior product, into a perfectly concrete expression: The Nambu equations of motion are equivalent to the condition of vanishing $\omega^{(3)}$ *under its projection* to arbitrary infinitesimal variations expressed by M_3. Owing to this projection, the spatial differentials dx^i are *no more* independent of the time differential dt, and the vanishing becomes possible directly, as a consequence of the cancellation of contributions from the kinematical part (the first term) and the dynamical part (the second term). Similarly, for

$$\omega^{(2)} = x^1 dx^2 \wedge dx^3 - K dH \wedge dt + d\Lambda^{(1)},$$

we have

$$\begin{aligned}\omega^{(2)}\big|_{M_3} &= x^1 \partial_a x^2 \partial_b x^3 d\sigma^a \wedge d\sigma^b \\ &\quad + \left[x^1(\dot{x}^2\partial_a x^3 - \dot{x}^3\partial_a x^2) - K\partial_a x^i \partial_i H\right] d\sigma^a \wedge dt + d\Lambda^{(1)},\end{aligned}$$

satisfying $d\omega^{(2)}\big|_{M_3} = \omega^{(3)}|_{M_3}$ corresponding to the commutativity of exterior differentiation with projection.

Now for the variational principle, as is for the case of M_2 in the previous section, we assume that M_3 has an infinitesimally small spatial (two-dimensional) cross-section $\mathrm{sec}M_3(t)$ at each fixed time t for $t_{\mathrm{ini}} < t < t_{\mathrm{fin}}$ and converges to points at $t = t_{\mathrm{ini}}$ and $t = t_{\mathrm{fin}}$: $\lim_{t \to t_{\mathrm{ini}}, t_{\mathrm{fin}}} \partial_a x^i(t; \sigma_1, \sigma_2) = 0$. The area of the spatial cross-section $\mathrm{sec}M_3(t)$ is of order ϵ^2 with ϵ being a typical linear scale measuring the size of $\mathrm{sec}M_3$:

$$\int_{\mathrm{sec}M_3(t)} d\sigma^1 d\sigma^2 = O(\epsilon^2), \qquad t_{\mathrm{ini}} < t < t_{\mathrm{fin}}.$$

Then, we can write, to the leading order ϵ^2,

$$\int_{M_3} \omega^{(3)} = \int_{L_0} \delta\pi_i(\dot{x}^i - X^i)dt, \tag{3.12}$$

$$\delta\pi_i(t) \equiv \frac{1}{2}\epsilon_{ijk} \int\limits_{\sec M_3(t)} \frac{\partial\big(x^j(t;\sigma^1,\sigma^2), x^k(t;\sigma^1,\sigma^2)\big)}{\partial(\sigma^1,\sigma^2)} d\sigma^1 d\sigma^2, \tag{3.13}$$

where L_0 is the core world line, arbitrarily chosen from the family of the world lines filling up the infinitesimal variation M_3 of L_0. Evidently, (3.13) represents the area vector of $\sec M_3$ itself. As in the case of M_2, arbitrariness of infinitesimal variations $\delta\pi_i(t)$ is reflected to the arbitrariness of shapes of $\sec M_3(t)$ at each time t.

On the other hand, Stokes' theorem gives

$$\int\limits_{M_3} \omega^{(3)} = \int\limits_{\partial M_3} \omega^{(2)}.$$

The boundary ∂M_3 of M_3, which is a closed two-dimensional manifold starting at $t = t_{\text{ini}}$ and ending at $t = t_{\text{fin}}$ as points with no spatial extension, can be parametrized by introducing a new parameter θ representing the sigma-parameters $(\sigma^1,\sigma^2)|_{\partial M_3} = (\sigma^1(t;\theta), \sigma^2(t;\theta))$ on each section of the boundary ∂M_3 at time t, as $x^i(t;\sigma^1,\sigma^2)|_{\partial M_3} \equiv x^i(t;\theta)$, where the vector function $x^i(t;\theta)$ is periodic with respect to θ, satisfying $\partial_\theta x^i|_{t=t_{\text{ini}},t_{\text{fin}}} = 0$. In terms of the phase space coordinates $x^i(t;\theta)$, we have

$$\begin{aligned}
\omega^{(2)}|_{\partial M_3} &= (x^1 dx^2 \wedge dx^3 - K dH \wedge dt)|_{\partial M_3} \\
&= -\big[x^1(\dot{x}^2 \partial_\theta x^3 - \partial_\theta x^2 \dot{x}^3) + K \partial_i H \partial_\theta x^i\big] d\theta \wedge dt.
\end{aligned}$$

Consequently, the infinitesimal variation around the core world line L_0 in general takes the following form,

$$\int\limits_{\partial M_3} \omega^{(2)} = -\int\limits_{t_{\text{ini}}}^{t_{\text{fin}}} \left\{ \oint_{\partial(\sec M_3(t))} \big[x^1(\dot{x}^2\partial_\theta x^3 - \partial_\theta x^2 \dot{x}^3) + K\partial_i H \partial_\theta x^i\big] d\theta \right\} dt, \tag{3.14}$$

on the boundary of the manifold M_3. The generalized variational principle says that the integral of 2-form $\omega^{(2)}$ over any infinitesimally narrow closed 2-dimensional manifold ∂M_3 vanishes to the leading order $O(\epsilon^2)$ *if* the core world line L_0 satisfies the equations of motion.

The figure on the right below illustrates the above situation schematically, in comparison with the case of conventional Hamiltonian dynamics on the left. Note that we have shown only the small segments of M_2 and M_3 with a short time interval, the end points being far above and below them (Fig. 3.1):

Comparing with the variational Eq. (3.7) in the usual Hamiltonian dynamics, the character of the generalized variational principle is recapitulated as follows:

(i) The infinitesimal variation governed by the 3-form $\omega^{(3)} = d\omega^{(2)}$ is formulated, so to speak, as a *blowup* of a single *core* world line L_0 into a *continuous family of world lines* which together fill up an infinitesimally narrow (time-like) world

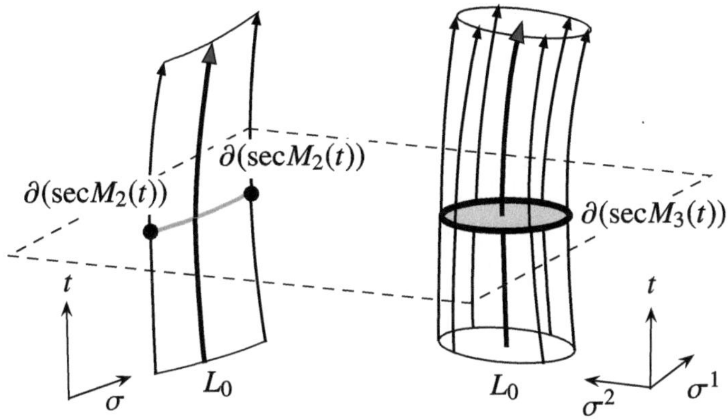

Fig. 3.1 The infinitesimal variations corresponding to M_2 (left) and M_3 (right)

volume M_3 chosen arbitrarily. Or perhaps more appropriately we may call this process *bundle-up*. On each time slice, the crossing point of the core world line describes a representative among a continuous family of the crossing points of the world lines in $\mathrm{sec}M_3(t)$ formed by blowup, constituting an infinitesimal spatial surface with its boundary $\partial(\mathrm{sec}M_3(t))$ over which $\omega^{(2)}$ is integrated. By Stokes' theorem the blowup or bundle-up is turned equivalently into a family of crossing points on the boundary $\partial(\mathrm{sec}M_3(t))$, parametrized by θ. The Eq. (3.14) is a concrete expression resulting from this mechanism.

By contrast, in the conventional case governed by the 2-form $\alpha^{(2)}$, the blowup of the core world line L_0 is a continuous family of world lines on an arbitrary infinitesimally narrow (time-like) band, M_2, which turns to a pair of two world lines on the boundary ∂M_2 of M_2; equivalently, on each time slice, the blowup is from a crossing point of L_0 to a family of crossing points on open spatial line on $\mathrm{sec}M_2(t)$. This turns into a blowup from a point to a pair of two boundary points comprising $\partial(\mathrm{sec}M_2(t))$ and hence there is *no* continuous θ-like parameter on the boundary, as expressed in (3.8). The same applies to field theories exemplified in Example 3.1.

(ii) In both cases of conventional Hamiltonian and Nambu dynamics, the details of blowups are packed, to the leading order of infinitesimally small variations, into the vector $\delta\pi_i(t)$ which is obtained by integration over spatial sections of blowup at each fixed time t. The blowup with an increased dimension 2 in Nambu dynamics arises *necessarily* and *intrinsically* from the fact that time evolution is now governed by the N-gauge invariant 2-form, $dK \wedge dH$, replacing the 1-form, dH, of conventional Hamiltonian dynamics. But it is to be noted that this does *not*, in any sense, imply the physical extension of the object we are dealing with. For instance, if a particle were extended physically to a string as in the Example 3.1, the time differential dt would be replaced by the infinitesimal surface element of the world sheet $dsdt$ (or a 2-form $ds \wedge dt$, if you like) by explicitly adding a new spatial evolution parameter s. This procedure is of course entirely different from the replacement $dH \to dK \wedge dH$, conceptually, which does not require any new evolution parameter and hence still corresponds to a particle, without physical extension, living in the phase space.

(iii) It is also appropriate here to recall the *contraction principle* stressed in Sect. 2.7.2, where we have discussed the equations of motion from a geometrical viewpoint using the interior product *without* making any projection to a submanifold. In fact, we can express the Eq. (3.11) in the following form:

$$\omega^{(3)}\big|_{M_3} = \frac{1}{2}\epsilon_{ijk}(\dot{x}^i - X^i)dx^j \wedge dx^k \wedge dt = \left(\iota_{(\dot{x},1)}\omega^{(3)}\right) \wedge dt. \tag{3.15}$$

When the equations of motion $\dot{x}^i = X^i$ are satisfied, the vanishing of the right-hand side is ensured by the orthogonality condition $\iota_{(X,1)}\omega^{(3)} = 0$, (2.58). This implies the contraction principle is indeed essentially equivalent to our generalized variational principle, despite their apparent difference in mathematical reasonings.

Finally, we summarize how the preceding results are extended to $(n+1)$-dimensional phase space-time. We consider an infinitesimally narrow n-dimensional submanifold M_n stretching along the time direction over which the n-form

$$\omega^{(n)} = dx^1 \wedge \cdots \wedge dx^n - dH_1 \wedge \cdots \wedge dH_{n-1} \wedge dt$$

is integrated. Introducing a continuous family of non-intersecting world lines that fill up M_n and are parametrized as $x^i(t; \sigma^1, \ldots, \sigma^{n-1})$, we have

$$\begin{aligned}
\omega^{(n)}\big|_{M_n} &= \frac{1}{(n-1)!}\epsilon_{ii_1\ldots i_{n-1}}(\dot{x}^i - X^i)\frac{\partial(x^{i_1}, \ldots, x^{i_{n-1}})}{\partial(\sigma^1, \ldots, \sigma^{n-1})}d\sigma^1 \wedge \cdots \wedge d\sigma^{n-1} \wedge dt, \\
X^i &= \epsilon^{ij_1\ldots j_{n-1}}\partial_{j_1}H_1 \cdots \partial_{j_{n-1}}H_{n-1},
\end{aligned}$$

yielding

$$\int_{M_n} \omega^{(n)} = \int_{L_0} \delta\pi_i(\dot{x}^i - X^i)dt, \tag{3.16}$$

$$\begin{aligned}
\delta\pi_i(t) \equiv &\frac{1}{(n-1)!}\epsilon_{ii_1\ldots i_{n-1}} \int_{\mathrm{sec}M_n(t)} d\sigma^1 \cdots d\sigma^{n-1} \\
&\times \frac{\partial\left(x^{i_1}(t; \sigma^1, \ldots, \sigma^{n-1}), \ldots, x^{i_{n-1}}(t; \sigma^1, \ldots, \sigma^{n-1})\right)}{\partial(\sigma^1, \ldots, \sigma^{n-1})},
\end{aligned} \tag{3.17}$$

to the leading order, $O(\epsilon^{n-1})$, with respect to a typical linear length scale ϵ characterizing the magnitude of the cross-section $\mathrm{sec}M_n$ being chosen arbitrarily. The blowup of the core world line L_0 to the continuous family of world lines has intrinsically

$(n-1)$-dimensional spatial time slices $\sec M_n(t)$, corresponding to the fact that time evolution is governed by the N-gauge invariant $(n-1)$-form $dH_1 \wedge \cdots \wedge dH_{n-1}$. The expression (3.17) has a definite physico-geometrical meaning that it is essentially the vector of the $(n-1)$-dimensional volume element of $\sec M_n(t)$ itself.

In terms of the interior product, we can also express the projection to M_n as

$$\omega^{(n)}\big|_{M_n} = \frac{(\dot{x}^i - X^i)}{(n-1)!}\epsilon_{ii_1\ldots i_{n-1}} dx^{i_1} \wedge \cdots dx^{i_{n-1}} \wedge dt = \left(\iota_{(\dot{x},1)}\omega^{(n)}\right) \wedge dt,$$

extending (3.15) and ensuring the equivalence of the Nambu equations of motion, $\dot{x}^i = X^i$, to the orthogonality condition $\iota_{(X,1)}\omega^{(n)} = 0$. Note also that the problem which we have discussed in connection with (2.33) is clarified further by this relation.

By Stokes' theorem, the variational equation is reduced to the integral of $\omega^{(n-1)}$ over the boundary ∂M_n:

$$\int\limits_{M_n} \omega^{(n)} = \int\limits_{\partial M_n} \omega^{(n-1)},$$

where

$$\omega^{(n-1)} = x^1 dx^2 \wedge \cdots \wedge dx^n - H_1 \wedge dH_2 \wedge \cdots \wedge dH_{n-1} \wedge dt + d\Lambda^{(n-2)},$$

which takes the following form on ∂M_n,

$$\begin{aligned}\omega^{(n-1)}\big|_{\partial M_n} = (-1)^{n-2}\Big[&x^1\Big(\dot{x}^2\partial_{b_1}x^3 \cdots \partial_{b_{n-2}}x^n - \partial_{b_1}x^2\dot{x}^3\partial_{b_2}x^4 \cdots \partial_{b_{n-2}}x^n \\ &+ \cdots + (-1)^{n-2}\partial_{b_1}x^2 \cdots \partial_{b_{n-2}}x^{n-1}\dot{x}^n\Big) \\ &- (-1)^{n-2}H_1\partial_{j_1}H_2 \cdots \partial_{j_{n-2}}H_{n-1}\partial_{b_1}x^{j_1} \cdots \partial_{b_{n-2}}x^{j_{n-2}}\Big] d\theta^{b_1} \wedge \cdots \wedge d\theta^{b_{n-2}} \wedge dt\end{aligned} \tag{3.18}$$

with $(\theta^1, \ldots, \theta^{n-2}, t)$ parametrizing the closed manifold ∂M_n of $n-1$ dimensions. It should be noted that the gauge degree of freedom $d\Lambda^{(n-2)}$ is suppressed in the last expression for brevity, since it does not contribute to the boundary integral $\int_{\partial M_n} \omega^{(n-1)}$ that cannot be reduced to integral on the core world line.

3.3 A Universal Action Integral

We have seen that, despite the difference of dimensionalities of blowups (or bundle-ups), the variational Eqs. (3.9), (3.10), (3.12) and (3.16), are always expressed in a simple and unified form

$$\int_{M_n} \omega^{(n)} = \int_{L_0} \delta\pi_i(\dot{x}^i - X^i)dt, \tag{3.19}$$

in terms of the n-form $\omega^{(n)}$ in $(n+1)$- dimensional phase space-time: all the geometrical details of blowups associated with the infinitesimal variations are completely packed into the infinitesimal vector variable $\delta\pi_i(t)$ defined along the core trajectory L_0 as (3.17), irrespective of the dimensionalities of blowups, which has a clear and definite meaning as the vector representing the infinitesimal $(n-1)$-dimensional spatial volume element, being transverse to L_0 on each time slice.

Under this circumstance, it is convenient to elevate this integral as the *universal action integral* for Nambu dynamics by reinterpreting $\delta\pi_i(t)$ as the infinitesimal variation of a new *independent* vector dynamical variable π_i defined along L_0:

$$A[x,\pi] \equiv \int_{L_0} \pi_i(\dot{x}^i - X^i)dt. \tag{3.20}$$

Namely, $\pi_i(t)$ is now treated as *momentum* conjugate to $x^i(t)$ reflecting the degrees of freedom associated with the spatial cross-sections of the infinitesimal variation M_n that are transverse to L_0. Thus π_i lives in a new vector space that is *cotangent* to Nambu phase space with coordinates x^i. The equations of motion as the variational equations for this action integral then consist of the following pair of vector equations:

$$\dot{x}^i = X^i, \qquad \dot{\pi}_i = -\pi_j\partial_i X^j. \tag{3.21}$$

This is in accord with ordinary Hamiltonian formalism with a single Hamiltonian,

$$\mathcal{H} \equiv \pi_i X^i = \epsilon^{ij_1\ldots j_{n-1}}\pi_i\partial_{j_1}H_1\cdots\partial_{j_{n-1}}H_{n-1}.$$

which is manifestly N-gauge invariant. Note that the time evolution of π_i is totally determined by that of x^i which itself is not affected in any way by π_i. The momentum π_i only plays a subsidiary and passive role as a Lagrange multiplier, not as an active dynamical variable.

From a purely formal viewpoint, (3.20) may look too trivial or simplistic, in the sense that anyone could easily conceive it without relying on any knowledge about its geometrical origin on the basis of the differential form $\omega^{(n)}$. However, from our standpoint, this form of Nambu dynamics, governed by a single Hamiltonian $\mathcal{H}$, may be interpreted as an instructive realization of the remarkable fact that there is only one invariant degree of freedom for the set of $n-1$ Hamiltonians due to the N-gauge symmetry, as we have stressed repeatedly.

It is also to be noticed that the adoption of the above universal action integral is in fact *contrary* to a seemingly natural expectation that an extended action integral would be based on $\omega^{(n-1)}$ as an apparent analog of the Pffafian 1-form $\alpha^{(1)}$ in ordinary action principles. This peculiarity arises because, for $n \geq 3$, there is a critical difference, compared with the situation in the conventional Hamiltonian dynamics: The integral $\int_{\partial M_{n-1}} \omega^{(n-1)}$ necessarily involves the integration over the continuous θ-parameters for the boundary ∂M_{n-1}. The dependence on the continuous variational parameters cannot be packed into a representative world line, in contrast to the case of the integral (3.16). As long as we wish to keep ourselves on the standpoint of our generalized variational principle, it would not be tenable to adopt any quantity that is intrinsically dependent on *unphysical* continuous parameters, which are devised only for the purpose of discussing arbitrary variations of world lines, as a *physical* action integral.

The specific Hamiltonian system described by the action integral (3.20) has the following special characteristics that are unusual but somewhat revealing. Namely, they exhibit the nature of Nambu dynamics in comparison with ordinary Hamilton systems:

(i) The Hamiltonian $\mathcal{H}$ is quite unusual or rather eccentric in the sense that it is linear in momentum variable. This implies that the momentum vector π_i *cannot* be expressed in terms of velocity vector $\dot{x}^i$, reflecting the fact that it actually encodes the degrees of freedom which are transverse to the trajectory. Hence, there is no inertial mass for this system, and the equations of motion for x^i do not involve π_i, while the equation of motion for π_i is linear and homogeneous in π_i. Since we cannot eliminate π_i, the Lagrangian $\pi_i \dot{x}^i - \mathcal{H}(x, \pi)$ cannot be expressed in the usual form $L = L(\dot{x}, x)$ without involving π_i through Legendre's *inverse* transformation.

(ii) Another evident consequence of the linearity with respect to π_i is that the Hamiltonian $\mathcal{H}$ has no bound at all. Despite that the Hamiltonian itself has no bound, the existence of the conserved quantities $(H_1, \dots, H_{n-1})$ ensures the *stability* of the system, provided at least one of them is bounded from below.

(iii) From the viewpoint of symmetry, on the other hand, the system is characterized by the existence of a gauge symmetry associated with π_i playing the role of a *gauge field in the space of Hamiltonians*. This makes it possible to interpret $n-1$ conserved quantities, $(H_1, \dots, H_{n-1})$, from the standpoint of Noether's theorem:
Consider the following transformation of π_i with an arbitrary function λ of $(n-1)$ variables,

$$\delta_\lambda \pi_i = \partial_i \lambda(H_1, \dots, H_{n-1}) = \sum_{j=1}^{n-1} \partial_i H_j \frac{\partial \lambda}{\partial H_j}. \tag{3.22}$$

Then, the action integral starting at $t = t_{\text{ini}}$ and ending at $t = t_{\text{fin}}$ transforms as

$$\delta_\lambda \int_{t_{\text{ini}}}^{t_{\text{fin}}} \pi_i (\dot{x}^i - X^i) dt = \sum_{j=1}^{n-1} \int_{t_{\text{ini}}}^{t_{\text{fin}}} \dot{x}^i \partial_i H_j \frac{\partial \lambda}{\partial H_j} dt = \lambda \Big|_{t_{\text{ini}}}^{t_{\text{fin}}},$$

because of the property

$$\partial_i H_j X^i = \epsilon^{ij_1 \dots j_{n-1}} \partial_i H_j \partial_{j_1} H_1 \cdots \partial_{j_{n-1}} H_{n-1} = 0$$

for all $j = 1, \dots, n-1$. When the equations of motion $\dot{x}^i = X^i$ are satisfied, the action integral vanishes and hence is trivially invariant under any variation of π_i. Therefore, the conservation of an arbitrary function $\lambda(H_1, \dots, H_{n-1})$ of H_j's follows, and all of H_j's are conserved as a consequence of this symmetry under the above gauge transformation (3.22). It is also easy to check directly that the equations of motion for π_i is invariant under the gauge transformation:

$$\begin{aligned} \frac{d}{dt}\delta_\lambda \pi_i &= \frac{d}{dt}\sum_{j=1}^{n-1} \partial_i H_j \frac{\partial \lambda}{\partial H_j} = \sum_{j=1}^{n-1} X^k \partial_k \partial_i H_j \frac{\partial \lambda}{\partial H_j} \\ &= -\sum_{j=1}^{n-1} \partial_i X^k \partial_k H_j \frac{\partial \lambda}{\partial H_j} = -\delta_\lambda \pi_j \partial_i X^j, \end{aligned}$$

where we have used $0 = \partial_i (X^k \partial_k H_j) = \partial_i X^k \partial_k H_j + X^k \partial_i \partial_k H_j$.

(iv) If we apply the standard Hamilton–Jacobi theory to our universal action with the 'configuration' space-time (x^i, t), the Hamilton–Jacobi equation is

$$\mathcal{H} = X^i \partial_i S = -\partial_t S, \qquad \pi_i = \partial_i S,$$

which is invariant under $\delta_\lambda S = \lambda$ that corresponds to (3.22). Owing to the linearity of the Hamiltonian with respect to π_i, this is a first-order (homogeneous) partial differential equation for S, and we immediately recognize that it coincides with the Liouville equation, $(\partial_t + X^i \partial_i)\rho = 0$, provided the action function S is identified with the density function: $S \to \rho$. Then the single-particle solution in terms of the δ-function discussed in Sect. 2.1 can be regarded as a 'complete solution' with n arbitrary constants as the initial condition $x_0^i = x^i(0)$ for the trajectory $x = x^i(t)$. On the other hand, (2.7) can be thought of as the 'general solution' , involving an arbitrary non-negative function $F(x)$ that solves the initial value problem with $\rho(x, 0) = F(x)$. Furthermore, the linearity of the Hamilton–Jacobi equation leads to a rather remarkable property that solutions for many-body configuration is simply given by a superposition of the single-particle solutions, as being exhibited in (2.4). This suggests a novel possibility that the treatment of many-body systems of Nambu particles could be based on this Hamilton–Jacobi theory.

(v) Finally, we notice that the linearity of $\mathcal{H}$ with respect to π_i renders the usual and traditional prescription for quantization almost meaningless for this Hamiltonian system; e.g., the Schrödinger equation is identical with the Hamilton–Jacobi equation itself; the Planck constant and the imaginary unit completely cancel out themselves; wave functions can be taken to be real such that the probability density coincides with the classical density function $\rho(x, t)$ obeying the Liouville equation; there is no quantum-mechanical spreading of wave packets, corresponding to the fact that x^i and $\dot{x}^i$ can be diagonalized simultaneously, but no contradiction with the uncertainly relation occurs, because the velocity $\dot{x}^i$ is *independent of* π_i. Conversely, in the sense that classical and quantum theory cannot be discriminated, we may also say that this particular Hamiltonian system is already quantized. Thus, to construct a really nontrivial quantum version of Nambu dynamics in which a minimum volume naturally exists in Nambu phase space itself, we have to recourse to some entirely different approaches or standpoints.

3.4 Generalized Hamilton–Jacobi Theory

3.4.1 A New Geometrical Picture for the Equations of Motion

In the previous section, after developing an extended variational principle for 3-dimensional Nambu dynamics by establishing the equivalence of the equations of motion to the vanishing condition $\omega^{(3)}|_{M_3} = 0$ on a 3-dimensional submanifold M_3 in $(3 + 1)$-dimensional phase space-time, we were naturally led to introduce conjugate (momentum) vector $\pi_i(t)$ as an independent dynamical variable living in the cotangent space that is dual to the tangent space associated with the Nambu phase space. Hence the dynamics is formulated in an extended phase space with $2 \times 3 = 6$ dimensions. Then its Hamilton–Jacobi theory, which is actually nothing but the Liouville equation, made it possible to reduce the dynamics back again to 3-dimensional Nambu phase space by treating π_i as a pure gauge field $\pi_i(x, t) = \partial_i S(x, t)$ on the Nambu phase space-time.

On the other hand, if we recall that one of Nambu's original motivations for his proposal was to generalize the usual $2n$-dimensional phase space (p_i, q_i) $(i = 1, \ldots, n)$, where the vector q_i describes the coordinates of a configuration space while the momentum vector p_i lives in the cotangent space dual to the configuration space, to arbitrary dimensions including odd dimensions, a natural conceptual question arises : *Is it possible to reduce the 3-dimensional Nambu dynamics to a Hamilton–Jacobi type formalism in which the 3-dimensional Nambu phase space itself is interpreted as being a combination of a configuration space and an analog to its cotangent space?* Namely, we wish to ascertain the direction reversed from what Nambu had investigated. The purpose of this final section is to examine such possibilities, which are indeed opposite to the approach pursued in the previous section. The author hopes that exploring through lower as well as higher dimensions with respect to both configuration spaces and whole phase spaces will be rewarded with a deeper grasp of Nambu dynamics.

First let us notice that nothing prevents us formally from thinking of the 3-dimensional Nambu phase space as being composed of a 2-dimensional plane, say, (x^1, x^2) as a configuration space and a continuously infinite number of orthogonal *fibres*, represented by the remaining coordinate x^3, crossing at each point of the configuration space: the Nambu phase space is now regarded as a *bundle* of continuously infinite number of fibres over the configuration space. Borrowing the terminologies of mathematical theory of *fibre bundles*, let us call our configuration space the *base space* . In analogy with the momentum in conventional Hamilton–Jacobi theory, we consider $x^3 = x^3(x^1, x^2, t)$ as a time-dependent function on the base space. Geometrically, $x^3(x^1, x^2, t)$ defines a time-dependent two-dimensional surface at each time t that represents a cross-section of this surface with the bundles of fibres. We call this process '*dynamical fibration*' for the sake of convenience.

Because of symmetrical roles played by the three coordinates, we can also choose (x^2, x^3) or (x^3, x^1) as base spaces in dynamical fibration; correspondingly, $x^1(x^2, x^3, t)$ or $x^2(x^3, x^1, t)$ describes each cross-section with the associating bundles of fibres, respectively. If we employ all of these three surfaces *simultaneously* on an equal footing in 3-dimensional Nambu phase space, each pair of these surfaces defines a curve corresponding to their intersection, and the resulting three curves intersect at a distinct point at each time as depicted in the Fig. 3.2:

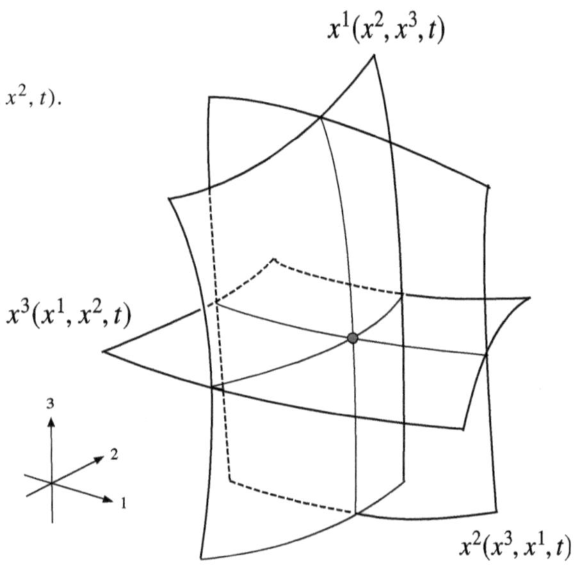

Fig. 3.2 A solution of the equations of motion as the intersection of the 3 planes, $x^1(x^2, x^3, t), x^2(x^3, x^1, t), x^3(x^1, x^2, t)$.

Providing that the motion of this distinct point obeys the Nambu equations of motion, we will arrive at an entirely new physico-geometrical picture for Nambu dynamics which is rather unfamiliar in conventional Hamiltonian dynamics. Pursuing this picture is the subject of the next subsection. Employing three moving surfaces to describe the motion of a point particle as their intersection seems a rather weird thing, but certainly provides a possible new viewpoint on the nature of Nambu dynamics as we will see.

3.4.2 *The Nambu Equations of Motion as the Intersections of Hamilton–Jacobi-Type Equations*

We can derive *partial* differential equations which govern the motion of the above surfaces, by requiring that the intersecting point indeed obeys the Nambu equations of motion. First, starting with the case of base space (x^1, x^2), we consider $x^3(x^1, x^2, t)$ and demand that it obeys the equation of motion,

$$\frac{dx^i}{dt} = \frac{1}{2}\epsilon^{ijk}\frac{\partial(K, H)}{\partial(x^j, x^k)}. \tag{3.23}$$

By this requirement, the left-hand side of this equation is rewritten as

$$\frac{dx^3}{dt} = \partial_t x^3 + \partial_1 x^3 \frac{dx^1}{dt} + \partial_2 x^3 \frac{dx^2}{dt} = \partial_t x^3 + \partial_1 x^3 \frac{\partial(K, H)}{\partial(x^2, x^3)} + \partial_2 x^3 \frac{\partial(K, H)}{\partial(x^3, x^1)}.$$

Turning our attention to the right-hand side of (3.23) with $i = 3$, we have to regard K and H also as functions of the variables $(x^1, x^2, x^3(x^1, x^2))$: we are then led to define

$$\underset{3}{K}(x^1, x^2, t) \equiv K\big(x^1, x^2, x^3(x^1, x^2, t)\big), \quad \underset{3}{H}(x^1, x^2, t) \equiv H\big(x^1, x^2, x^3(x^1, x^2, t)\big).$$

Using $\partial_i \underset{3}{K} = \partial_i K + \partial_i x^3 \partial_3 K$ for $i = 1, 2$, etc. we have, *solely* by definition,

$$\begin{aligned}
\frac{\partial(K, H)}{\partial(x^2, x^3)} &= (\partial_2 \underset{3}{K} - \partial_3 K \partial_2 x^3)\partial_3 H - (\partial_2 \underset{3}{H} - \partial_3 H \partial_2 x^3)\partial_3 K = \partial_2 \underset{3}{K} \partial_3 H - \partial_2 \underset{3}{H} \partial_3 K, \\
\frac{\partial(K, H)}{\partial(x^3, x^1)} &= \partial_3 K(\partial_1 \underset{3}{H} - \partial_3 H \partial_1 x^3) - \partial_3 H(\partial_1 \underset{3}{K} - \partial_3 K \partial_1 x^3) = \partial_3 K \partial_1 \underset{3}{H} - \partial_3 H \partial_1 \underset{3}{K}, \\
\frac{\partial(K, H)}{\partial(x^1, x^2)} &= (\partial_1 \underset{3}{K} - \partial_3 K \partial_1 x^3)(\partial_2 \underset{3}{H} - \partial_3 H \partial_2 x^3) - (\partial_1 \underset{3}{H} - \partial_3 H \partial_1 x^3)(\partial_2 \underset{3}{K} - \partial_3 K \partial_2 x^3) \\
&= \partial_1 \underset{3}{K} \partial_2 \underset{3}{H} - \partial_1 \underset{3}{H} \partial_2 \underset{3}{K} - \partial_1 x^3(\partial_3 K \partial_2 \underset{3}{H} - \partial_3 H \partial_2 \underset{3}{K}) - \partial_2 x^3(\partial_1 \underset{3}{K} \partial_3 H - \partial_1 \underset{3}{H} \partial_3 K),
\end{aligned}$$

which further yield the following identity:

$$\frac{\partial(K, H)}{\partial(x^1, x^2)} = \partial_1 \underset{3}{K} \partial_2 \underset{3}{H} - \partial_1 \underset{3}{H} \partial_2 \underset{3}{K} + \partial_1 x^3 \frac{\partial(K, H)}{\partial(x^2, x^3)} + \partial_2 x^3 \frac{\partial(K, H)}{\partial(x^3, x^1)}. \tag{3.24}$$

Putting these identities together in (3.23) with $i = 3$, we find that the coefficients of $\partial_i x^3$ $(i = 1, 2)$ cancel out between the both sides of (3.23), and obtain a desired partial differential equation for $x^3 = x^3(x^1, x^2, t)$,

$$\partial_t x^3 = \partial_1 \underset{3}{K} \partial_2 \underset{3}{H} - \partial_1 \underset{3}{H} \partial_2 \underset{3}{K}. \tag{3.25}$$

By choosing the base space (x^2, x^3) and (x^3, x^1) and repeating the same calculations, we get also

$$\partial_t x^1 = \partial_2 \underset{1}{K} \partial_3 \underset{1}{H} - \partial_3 \underset{1}{K} \partial_2 \underset{1}{H}, \tag{3.26}$$

$$\partial_t x^2 = \partial_3 \underset{2}{K} \partial_1 \underset{2}{H} - \partial_1 \underset{2}{K} \partial_3 \underset{2}{H}, \tag{3.27}$$

where

$$\underset{1}{K}(x^2, x^3, t) \equiv K\big(x^1(x^2, x^3, t), x^2, x^3\big), \quad \underset{1}{H}(x^2, x^3, t) \equiv H\big(x^1(x^2, x^3, t), x^2, x^3\big),$$
$$\underset{2}{K}(x^3, x^1, t) \equiv K\big(x^1, x^2(x^3, x^1, t), x^3\big), \quad \underset{2}{H}(x^3, x^1, t) \equiv H\big(x^1, x^2(x^3, x^1, t), x^3\big).$$

These three partial differential equations describing the cross-sections, $x^3(x^1, x^2, t)$, $x^1(x^2, x^3, t)$ and $x^2(x^3, x^1, t)$, of fibres with three different choices of base spaces treated on an equal footing, govern the motions of them in the Nambu phase space in accord with the geometrical picture introduced in the previous subsection: It is ensured by construction that, when we impose these equations together simultaneously, the intersection point of the three cross sections obeys the Nambu equations of motion.

Exercise 3.1 Let us confirm explicitly the converse of what we have exhibited above: Namely, assuming the partial differential Eqs. (3.25)–(3.27), we will be able to derive the Nambu equations of motion.

Given two surfaces $x^1 = x^1(x^2, x^3, t)$ and $x^2 = x^2(x^3, x^1, t)$, their intersection is determined by the conditions

$$x^1 = x^1(x^2(x^3, x^1, t), x^3, t), \quad x^2 = x^2(x^3, x^1(x^2, x^3, t), t),$$

which define a time-dependent one-dimensional curve, since we are imposing two conditions for three independent variables (x^1, x^2, x^3). Including the remaining surface $x^3 = x^3(x^1, x^2, t)$, we consider the intersection of all three such surfaces, determined by

$$x^1 = x^1(x^2(x^3, x^1, t), x^3(x^1, x^2, t), t),$$
$$x^2 = x^2(x^3(x^1, x^2, t), x^1(x^2, x^3, t), t),$$
$$x^3 = x^3(x^1(x^2, x^3, t), x^2(x^3, x^1, t), t).$$

Suppose that we are given a zero-dimensional point $x^i = x^i(t)$ $(i = 1, 2, 3)$ as a solution for the above conditions of intersection. Then, taking (total) time derivatives of these conditions, we have, respectively,

$$\frac{dx^1}{dt} = \partial_t x^1 + \partial_2 x^1 \frac{dx^2}{dt} + \partial_3 x^1 \frac{dx^3}{dt} = \partial_2 \underset{1}{K} \partial_3 \underset{1}{H} - \partial_3 \underset{1}{K} \partial_2 \underset{1}{H} + \partial_2 x^1 \frac{dx^2}{dt} + \partial_3 x^1 \frac{dx^3}{dt},$$

$$\frac{dx^2}{dt} = \partial_t x^2 + \partial_3 x^2 \frac{dx^2}{dt} + \partial_1 x^2 \frac{dx^1}{dt} = \partial_3 \underset{2}{K} \partial_1 \underset{2}{H} - \partial_1 \underset{2}{K} \partial_3 \underset{2}{H} + \partial_3 x^2 \frac{dx^2}{dt} + \partial_1 x^2 \frac{dx^1}{dt},$$
$$\frac{dx^3}{dt} = \partial_t x^3 + \partial_1 x^3 \frac{dx^1}{dt} + \partial_2 x^3 \frac{dx^2}{dt} = \partial_1 \underset{3}{K} \partial_2 \underset{3}{H} - \partial_2 \underset{3}{K} \partial_1 \underset{3}{H} + \partial_1 x^3 \frac{dx^1}{dt} + \partial_2 x^3 \frac{dx^2}{dt},$$

where we used the partial differential Eqs. (3.25)–(3.27) in the second equalities. Using the identity (3.24) to replace the first two terms on the right-hand side of the last equation, for instance, the latter equation takes the form

$$0 = \frac{dx^3}{dt} - \frac{\partial(K, H)}{\partial(x^1, x^2)} - \partial_1 x^3 \left(\frac{dx^1}{dt} - \frac{\partial(K, H)}{\partial(x^2, x^3)} \right) - \partial_2 x^3 \left(\frac{dx^2}{dt} - \frac{\partial(K, H)}{\partial(x^3, x^1)} \right). \tag{3.28}$$

By interchanging the combinations of the indices, we also have

$$0 = \frac{dx^1}{dt} - \frac{\partial(K, H)}{\partial(x^2, x^3)} - \partial_2 x^1 \left(\frac{dx^2}{dt} - \frac{\partial(K, H)}{\partial(x^3, x^1)} \right) - \partial_3 x^1 \left(\frac{dx^3}{dt} - \frac{\partial(K, H)}{\partial(x^1, x^2)} \right), \tag{3.29}$$

$$0 = \frac{dx^2}{dt} - \frac{\partial(K, H)}{\partial(x^3, x^1)} - \partial_3 x^2 \left(\frac{dx^3}{dt} - \frac{\partial(K, H)}{\partial(x^1, x^2)} \right) - \partial_1 x^2 \left(\frac{dx^1}{dt} - \frac{\partial(K, H)}{\partial(x^2, x^3)} \right). \tag{3.30}$$

Evidently, then, providing that

$$0 \neq \det \begin{pmatrix} 1 & -\partial_2 x^1 & -\partial_3 x^1 \\ -\partial_1 x^2 & 1 & -\partial_3 x^2 \\ -\partial_1 x^3 & -\partial_2 x^3 & 1 \end{pmatrix} = 1 - \partial_2 x^1 \partial_3 x^2 \partial_1 x^3 - \partial_3 x^1 \partial_2 x^3 \partial_1 x^2$$
$$- \partial_2 x^1 \partial_1 x^2 - \partial_3 x^1 \partial_1 x^3 - \partial_3 x^2 \partial_2 x^3,$$

the Nambu equations of motion $\dot{x}^i = \frac{1}{2}\epsilon^{ijk} \frac{\partial(K,H)}{\partial(x^j,x^j)}$ must hold. The determinant condition is satisfied in general, since we have the degrees of freedom of three *arbitrary* functions $x^1(x^2, x^3, 0) = f(x^2, x^3)$, $x^2(x^3, x^1, 0) = g(x^3, x^1)$ and $x^3(x^1, x^2, 0) = h(x^1, x^2)$ as initial conditions for the *general* solutions of our partial differential equations. Clearly, if the initial surfaces are appropriately chosen, the intersection point is uniquely determined. However, the uniqueness is not an absolute necessity for the present argument provided that the distinctness (or isolation) of each intersection is satisfied. Rather, cases with multiple intersection points would suggest itself a new intriguing possibility for describing many body systems, though we do not pursue such a direction further in the present exposition.

It should be noted also that for each choice of a single and *fixed* base space, (x^1, x^2), (x^2, x^3) or (x^3, x^1), the corresponding Eqs. (3.28), (3.29), or (3.30), respectively, holds independently of the other cases, under each associated partial differential equation. Therefore, in each case, any two among the three equations of motion automatically guarantee the validity of the remaining one.

So far, we have discussed the Hamilton–Jacobi type theories for Nambu dynamics only in the case of $n = 3$. The basic ideas of the foregoing discussions can be applied straightforwardly to higher dimensions. But for the sake of conciseness, we refrain from pursuing such technical directions.

Exercise 3.2 : Here it is perhaps instructive as a further exercise to give a similar treatment of the conventional Hamilton equations of motion as above, since the geometrical characterization of the equations of motion using intersections of moving surfaces is certainly a new notion, which has not been mentioned before to the author's knowledge.

For notational brevity, we only treat the simplest case of 2-dimensional phase space (q, p). First let $p = p(q, t)$ with q being the base-space coordinate. By defining $\underset{p}{H} \equiv H(p(q, t), q)$, we have an identity

$$\partial_q \underset{p}{H} = \partial_q H + \partial_q p \partial_p H. \tag{3.31}$$

Requiring the Hamilton equations of motion , $\dot{p} = -\partial_q H, \dot{q} = \partial_p H$ for the identity $\dot{p} = \partial_t p + \partial_q p \dot{q}$, we derive $-\partial_q H = \partial_t p + \partial_q p \partial_p H$. Using (3.31), this gives a partial differential equation for $p(q, t)$,

$$\partial_t p = -\partial_q \underset{p}{H}. \tag{3.32}$$

Similarly, by interchanging the role of q and p, we have a partial differential equation for $q = q(p, t)$ with p now being the base-space coordinate,

$$\partial_t q = \partial_p \underset{q}{H}, \tag{3.33}$$

where $\underset{q}{H} \equiv H(q(p, t), t)$. The functions $p(q, t)$ and $q(p, t)$ describe a pair of time-dependent one-dimensional curves in the phase space (p, q), whose intersection gives a point $(p(t), q(t))$, evolving in accordance with the Hamilton equations of motion (as *ordinary* differential equations) by its construction. Note that these partial differential equations are equivalent to the vanishing condition for the two-form $\alpha^{(2)} = dp \wedge dq - dH \wedge dt \to 0$ under the projection $dp \to \partial_q p dq + \partial_t p dt$, $H \to \underset{p}{H}$ or $dq \to \partial_p q dp + \partial_t q dt$, $H \to \underset{q}{H}$, respectively. The counterpart of this property for Nambu dynamics will be discussed in the next subsection.

Conversely, suppose we are given the above two partial differential Eqs. (3.32) and (3.33). Then using the identities $\dot{p} = \partial_t p + \partial_q p \dot{q}$ and $\dot{q} = \partial_t q + \partial_p q \dot{p}$ for their solutions $p(q,t)$ and $q(p,t)$, respectively, we derive

$$0 = -\dot{p} - \underset{p}{\partial_q H} + \partial_q p \dot{q} = -\dot{p} - \partial_q H + \partial_q p(\dot{q} - \partial_p H),$$
$$0 = -\dot{q} + \underset{q}{\partial_p H} + \partial_p q \dot{p} = -\dot{q} + \partial_p H + \partial_p q(\dot{p} + \partial_q H).$$

The Hamilton equations of motion immediately follow, provided

$$\det \begin{pmatrix} 1 & -\partial_q p \\ -\partial_p q & 1 \end{pmatrix} \neq 0.$$

This is justified for the same reason as mentioned in the previous exercise: the partial differential Eqs. (3.32) and (3.33) allow two arbitrary functions $p(q,0) = f(q)$ and $q(p,0) = g(p)$ as the initial conditions for their general solutions.

As a concrete example, let us consider the simplest case of a free particle, $H = p^2/2$. The partial differential equations for $p = p(q,t)$ and $q = q(p,t)$ are $\partial_t p = -p\partial_q p$, $\partial_t q = p$. The general solution of the second equation is obviously $q = pt + g(p)$ with an arbitrary functions $g(p)$. On the other hand, the general solution $p = f(q,t)$ of the first equation is given implicitly by solving $pt - q = h(p)$, $h(p)$ being another arbitrary function independent of $g(p)$: as a check, we confirm that the partial derivatives of $pt - h(p) = q$ with respect to t and q yield

$$\partial_t p(t - \partial_p h) + p = 0, \qquad \partial_q p(t - \partial_p h) = 1 \qquad \rightarrow \qquad \partial_t p = -p\partial_q p.$$

At $t = 0$, we must have $-q = h(f(q,0))$ or $f(q,0) = h^{-1}(-q)$ which shows that arbitrariness of the function $h(p)$ represents the initial condition. The same can be said for $g(p)$. For arbitrary t, the condition of intersection of two curves described by $q - pt = g(p)$ and $q - pt = -h(p)$, respectively, is obviously $g(p(t)) = -h(p(t))$. By choosing these two functions $h(p)$ and $g(p)$ appropriately which are independent of each other, we can assume that the intersection condition is satisfied only at a *unique* value of $p = p_0$ at the intersection of two level-curves corresponding to them. It then follows that $p(t)$ describing the intersection must necessarily be a constant $p(t) = p_0$, and $q(t) = p_0 t + g(p_0)$, which obeys the free equations $\dot{p} = 0$, $\dot{q} = p$ of motion with initial conditions $q(0) = q_0$, $p(0) = p_0$ satisfying $q_0 = g(p_0)$, as it should. Since $g(p)$ is an arbitrary function, q_0 and p_0 can be varied independently.

In the figure below, we illustrate the situation when both $g(p)$ and $h(p)$ are chosen to be linear in p for simplicity, showing the configurations of intersecting level-lines at two different times (Fig. 3.3):

Extension of the foregoing arguments to general $2n$-dimensional phase space is not difficult: the equations of motion are obtained by considering the intersection of two n-dimensional hyper-surfaces represented by $p_i = p_i(q,t)$ and $q_i = q_i(p,t)$.

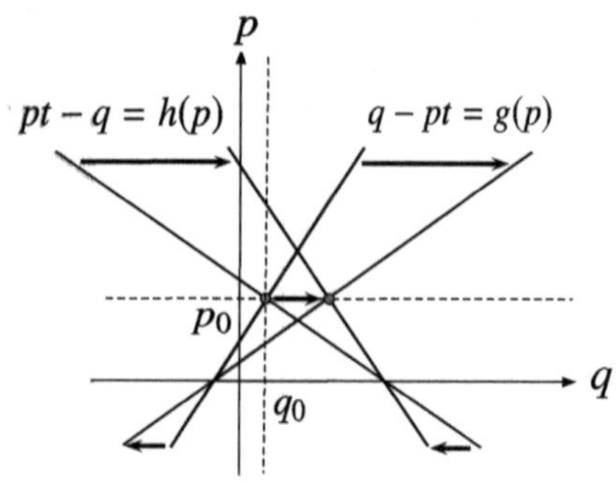

Fig. 3.3 The solution of the free-equations of motion as the intersection of two lines

3.4.3 Generalized Hamilton–Jacobi Equations

We notice that the partial differential Eq. (3.32) appearing in the above exercise is equivalent to the usual Hamilton–Jacobi equation: in fact, by setting $p(q,t) = \partial_q S(q,t)$, it reduces to

$$\partial_t S = -\underset{p}{H} = -H(q, \partial_q S).$$

Similarly, the partial differential Eqs. (3.25), (3.26) and (3.27) for Nambu dynamics, can be rewritten such that they become more akin to the usual Hamilton–Jacobi equation. Let us take (3.25) for definiteness, focusing our consideration to the case with base space (x^1, x^2) from now on. If we make a projection of the 2-form $\omega^{(2)}$ onto the base space-time,

$$\omega^{(2)}\big|_{(x^1,x^2,t)} = x^3(x^1, x^2, t)dx^1 \wedge dx^2 - \underset{3}{K}d\underset{3}{H} \wedge dt$$

then, (3.25) is actually equivalent to the vanishing condition

$$\begin{aligned} 0 = \omega^{(3)}\big|_{(x^1,x^2,t)} &= d\omega^{(2)}\big|_{(x^1,x^2,t)} \\ &= \partial_t x^3 dx^1 \wedge dx^2 \wedge dt - (\partial_1 \underset{3}{K} \partial_2 \underset{3}{H} - \partial_2 \underset{3}{K} \partial_1 \underset{3}{H})dx^1 \wedge dx^2 \wedge dt. \end{aligned} \tag{3.34}$$

This requires, by Poincaré's lemma, with some 1-form $S^{(1)} = S_1 dx^1 + S_2 dx^2 + S_0 dt$,

$$\begin{aligned} \omega^{(2)}\big|_{(x^1,x^2,t)} &= dS^{(1)} \\ &= (\partial_1 S_2 - \partial_2 S_1)dx^1 \wedge dx^2 - (\partial_t S_1 - \partial_1 S_0)dx^1 \wedge dt - (\partial_t S_2 - \partial_2 S_0)dx^2 \wedge dt. \end{aligned}$$

Thus we get

$$x^3 = \partial_1 S_2 - \partial_2 S_1, \quad \underset{3}{K} \partial_1 \underset{3}{H} = \partial_t S_1 - \partial_1 S_0, \quad \underset{3}{K} \partial_2 \underset{3}{H} = \partial_t S_2 - \partial_2 S_0,$$

giving the following set of partial differential equations in terms of the components fields of $S^{(1)}$,

$$\left.\begin{array}{ll}\partial_t S_i = \underset{3}{K}\,\partial_i \underset{3}{H} + \partial_i S_0, & (i = 1, 2),\\ \underset{3}{K} = K(x^1, x^2, \partial_1 S_2 - \partial_2 S_1), & \underset{3}{H} = H(x^1, x^2, \partial_1 S_2 - \partial_2 S_1),\end{array}\right\} \tag{3.35}$$

which are equivalent to (3.25) by construction. It is also to be noted that under the N-gauge transformation discussed in Sect. 2.2, $(K, H) \to (K', H')$ satisfying $\frac{\partial(K', H')}{\partial(K, H)} = 1$, we have

$$\underset{3}{K}'\partial_i \underset{3}{H}' + \partial_i S_0 = \underset{3}{K}\,\partial_i \underset{3}{H} + \partial_i \underset{3}{F} + \partial_i S_0,$$

where $\underset{3}{F} = F(\underset{3}{H}, \underset{3}{H}')$ with $F = F(H, H')$ being the generating function (see Sect. 2.2),

$$\frac{\partial F}{\partial H} = -K, \quad \frac{\partial F}{\partial H'} = K'.$$

This shows that the N-gauge invariance is kept maintained, since we can recover the same set of equations for (K', H') by redefining $S_0 \to S_0' = S_0 - F$. There emerges also another independent gauge symmetry for the S-vector under $S_i \to S_i + \partial_i \lambda$, $S_0 \to S_0 + \partial_t \lambda$, where λ is an arbitrary scalar function, which we call the 'S-gauge symmetry'.

We call (3.35) the *generalized Hamilton–Jacobi equation*. Comparing this result with the ordinary Hamilton–Jacobi equation, a single action function, 0-form $S(q, t)$, of the latter is now replaced by the 1-form $S^{(1)}(x^1, x^2, t)$ and the role of conjugate momentum vector $p_i = \partial_i S$ is played by a single function $x^3(x^1, x^2, t) = \partial_1 S_2 - \partial_2 S_1$, the 'rotation' or 'vorticity' of a vector field (S_1, S_2). In that sense, we may call our fibre bundles, such as $(x^1, x^2, x^3(x^1, x^2, t))$, the '*vorticity bundles*', in contrast to the *cotangent bundle* such as $(x^i, \pi_i(x, t))$, emerging in the Hamilton–Jacobi treatment of the universal action integral given in the previous section.

Now, the problem remaining is to investigate to what extent various well-known properties of conventional Hamilton–Jacobi theory can be extended to Nambu dynamics with the above generalized Hamilton–Jacobi equation. We shall focus on the most crucial problem of whether and how the general solutions of the Nambu equations of motion are extracted by imposing suitable conditions on the *complete solutions* of the generalized Hamilton–Jacobi equations in analogy with the Jacobi condition.

Remember that, by contrast, a new geometrical interpretation of the Nambu equations of motion given in the previous subsections presupposes the *general solutions* of (3.25)–(3.27), satisfying initial conditions associated with the appropriate choices of three arbitrary functions. Note also that the usual Jacobi condition is associated with a finite canonical transformation sending the Hamiltonian to zero (see Chap.

1). Our treatment in the following is more direct: we will provide two avenues, both of which allow us, in different ways, to circumvent dealing directly with finite generalized nonical transformations which are somewhat problematical intrinsically as we have discussed in Sect. 2.5.3.

(1) *Generalized Jacobi conditions I: a special case of 'axial gauge'*

We first study a special case, assuming that one of K or H, say H is independent of x^3, i.e. $\partial_3 H = 0$ or $\underset{3}{H} = H$. Due to the Clebsch form (2.9) of the gauge field A^i associated with X^i, this is an analog of the 'axial' gauge $A_3 = 0$ familiar in electromagnetism. However, it should be noted that, when we try to make the N-gauge transformation from a generic (K, H) to (K', H') such that $\partial_3 H' = 0$, this is possible only for a restricted class of Hamiltonians (K, H) for which the ratio of $\partial_3 K \partial_1 H - \partial_1 K \partial_3 H = \partial_3 K' \partial_1 H'$ and $\partial_3 K \partial_2 H - \partial_2 K \partial_3 H = \partial_3 K' \partial_2 H'$, being equal to $\partial_1 H'/\partial_2 H'$, is independent of x^3. This restriction arises because the Clebsch form is only a special case of vector potential in the sense that it cannot accommodate the whole physical degrees of freedom of the vector potential, as we have stressed in Sect. 2.2, in contrast to the situation of the conventional axial gauge in classical electrodynamics.

The condition $\partial_3 H = 0$ also implies $\partial_t \underset{3}{H} = 0$, since the dependence on time enters only through $x^3 = x^3(x^1, x^2, t)$. Let us also choose the gauge $S_0 = 0$ with respect to the S-gauge symmetry, and redefine $S_i = -S\partial_i H + g_i$, $(i = 1, 2)$ by introducing a function $S = S(x^1, x^2, t)$ that satisfies $\partial_t S = -\underset{3}{K}$, and a vector function g_i, the generalized Hamilton–Jacobi equation reduces to $\partial_t g_i = 0$. We thus have

$$x^3(x^1, x^2, t) = \partial_1 S_2 - \partial_2 S_1 = \partial_1 H \partial_2 S - \partial_2 H \partial_1 S + \partial_1 g_2 - \partial_2 g_1.$$

Since g_i is independent of time t, it can be brought into the form $g_i = \epsilon_{ij}\partial_j g$ satisfying $\partial_i g_i = 0$ with a time-independent scalar function g using the residual time-independent S-gauge transformation. Then, g_i can be absorbed into S by making a further redefinition $S \to S + f$ where f is independent of time and determined by the condition $f\partial_i H = g_i = \epsilon_{ij}\partial_j g$, yielding the equation for determining f,

$$d_H f = \triangle g, \quad \triangle \equiv \partial_i \partial_i, \quad d_H \equiv \partial_1 H \partial_2 - \partial_2 H \partial_1.$$

Thus we conclude that the generalized Hamilton–Jacobi equation is simplified,

$$x^3 = d_H S, \quad \partial_t S = -\underset{3}{K}. \tag{3.36}$$

Note that the single-component 'momentum'-vorticity x^3 is not a plain derivative of S, but is a 'curved' derivative depending on H and corresponding to an infinitesimal rotation $\delta_H x^i = -\epsilon^{ij}\partial_j H$ of the base coordinates x^i: by definition we have $d_H H = 0$ identically. Hence the infinitesimal rotation $\delta_H x^i$ preserves the value of H. In this sense, $\underset{3}{K}$ is effectively the Hamiltonian in the dynamics on the configuration space (x^1, x^2), while H plays only a kinematical role in this particular case.

Now suppose we have a 'complete solution' $S = S(x^1, x^2, t; Q_1, Q_2)$ for (3.36) involving two arbitrary constants Q_1 and Q_2. Since the equation involves x^i-derivatives only through d_H preserving H, we can choose one of the integration constants, say Q_2, to be the value of H itself. Then, in analogy with the ordinary Jacobi condition, let us impose

$$\frac{\partial S}{\partial Q_1} = Q_3 \tag{3.37}$$

with Q_3 being the third constant which, if our procedure is successful, would supply, together with (Q_1, Q_2), three integration constants to be required for giving general solutions to the Nambu equations of motion. We demand that this condition supplemented by $H = Q_2$ enable us to solve (x^1, x^2) as functions of time. Solvability is ensured when these conditions are independent of each other. That is the case when the left-hand side of (3.37) is not invariant under the action of d_H, namely,

$$\frac{\partial^2 S}{\partial x^1 \partial Q_1}\partial_2 H - \frac{\partial^2 S}{\partial x^2 \partial Q_1}\partial_1 H \neq 0, \tag{3.38}$$

which is the counterpart to the condition (1.13) in conventional Hamilton–Jacobi theory. By taking the time derivative of the conditions $H = Q_2$ and (3.37), we obtain, respectively,

$$\partial_1 H \frac{dx^1}{dt} + \partial_2 H \frac{dx^2}{dt} = 0, \tag{3.39}$$

$$\frac{\partial^2 S}{\partial Q_1 \partial t} + \frac{\partial^2 S}{\partial Q_1 \partial x^1}\frac{dx^1}{dt} + \frac{\partial^2 S}{\partial Q_1 \partial x^2}\frac{dx^2}{dt} = 0. \tag{3.40}$$

On the other hand, the generalized Hamilton–Jacobi Eq. (3.36) gives

$$\frac{\partial^2 S}{\partial Q_1 \partial t} = -\left(\partial_1 H \frac{\partial^2 S}{\partial Q_1 \partial x^2} - \partial_2 H \frac{\partial^2 S}{\partial Q_1 \partial x^1}\right)\partial_3 K, \tag{3.41}$$

recalling the fact that the dependence of K on Q_1 only resides through $x^3(x^1, x^2, t) = \partial_1 S_2 - \partial_2 S_1$. Combining (3.40) and (3.41), we get

$$\left(\frac{dx^1}{dt} + \partial_2 H \partial_3 K\right)\frac{\partial^2 S}{\partial Q_1 \partial x^1} + \left(\frac{dx^2}{dt} - \partial_1 H \partial_3 K\right)\frac{\partial^2 S}{\partial Q_1 \partial x^2} = 0.$$

Furthermore, (3.39) is equivalently written

$$\left(\frac{dx^1}{dt} + \partial_2 H \partial_3 K\right)\partial_1 H + \left(\frac{dx^2}{dt} - \partial_1 H \partial_3 K\right)\partial_2 H = 0.$$

Then, due to the condition (3.38), the last two equations immediately yield

$$\frac{dx^1}{dt} = -\partial_2 H \partial_3 K = \frac{\partial(K, H)}{\partial(x^2, x^3)}, \qquad \frac{dx^2}{dt} = \partial_1 H \partial_3 K = \frac{\partial(K, H)}{\partial(x^3, x^1)},$$

which are the first and second, respectively, of the Nambu equations of motion under the condition $\partial_3 H = 0$. Then, the third equation automatically holds because of the identity (3.28).

(2) *Generalized Jacobi conditions II: a 'secondary' dynamical fibration*

We turn now to the general case without requiring any restriction on the Hamiltonians K and H. Instead, in analogy with the conventional Hamilton–Jacobi theory in which we often study its solutions by setting the Hamiltonian to be a constant, we set $\underset{3}{K} = E$ with a constant E for studying solutions to the generalized HJ Eq. (3.35), $\partial_t S_i - \partial_i S_0 = E \partial_i \underset{3}{H}$. By making a redefinition $S_0 \to S_0 - E \underset{3}{H}$, this can be reduced to $\partial_t S_i - \partial_i S_0 = 0$. Furthermore, by using S-gauge transformation we can impose a gauge condition, say, $S_0 = 0$. Then the equations are trivially solved as $S_i = g_i(x^1, x^2)$ with a time-independent vector function g_i. We now have $x^3 = \partial_1 g_2 - \partial_2 g_1 = x^3(x^1, x^2; E)$, with the constraint

$$E = \underset{3}{K} = K(x^1, x^2, x^3(x^1, x^2; E)). \tag{3.42}$$

Now since $\underset{3}{H}$ remains active, we expect that there must be a natural procedure in which $\underset{3}{H}$ plays the role of the Hamiltonian governing the dynamics of the base space (x^1, x^2) itself. Comparing with the previous case (1), the dynamical role of H and K is thus interchanged. For its concrete realization, it is legitimate to introduce a further fibration, '*secondary* dynamical fibration', of the 2-dimensional base space itself, $(x^1, x^2) \to (x^1, x^2(x^1, t))$ that would enable us to recover time dependence.

We follow the previous procedure in the case of two-dimensional base space by generalizing it to the 'lower' case with one-dimensional base space. Namely, we start with the identity,

$$\frac{dx^2}{dt} = \partial_t x^2 + \partial_1 x^2 \frac{dx^1}{dt}, \tag{3.43}$$

being valid by definition. Using (3.42), we have also

$$0 = \partial_i \underset{3}{K} = \partial_i K + \partial_3 K \partial_i x^3, \quad 1 = \frac{\partial x^3}{\partial E} \partial_3 K. \tag{3.44}$$

Then, it follows from the first equation that

$$\partial_i \underset{3}{H} = \partial_i H + \partial_3 H \partial_i x^3 = \frac{1}{\partial_3 K}(\partial_3 K \partial_i H - \partial_i K \partial_3 H), \tag{3.45}$$

which allows us to rewrite the Nambu equations of motion for x^1 and x^2 as

$$\frac{dx^1}{dt} = \partial_2 K \partial_3 H - \partial_3 K \partial_2 H = -\partial_3 K \partial_2 \underset{3}{H},$$
$$\frac{dx^2}{dt} = \partial_3 K \partial_1 H - \partial_1 K \partial_3 H = \partial_3 K \partial_1 \underset{3}{H}.$$

Combining these results with the identity (3.43), we obtain a partial differential equation for $x^2(x^1, t)$,

$$\partial_t x^2 = \partial_3 K (\partial_1 \underset{3}{H} + \partial_1 x^2 \partial_2 \underset{3}{H}) = \partial_3 K \partial_1 \underset{23}{H}, \tag{3.46}$$

where $\underset{23}{H}(x^1, t) \equiv \underset{3}{H}\big(x^1, x^2(x^1, t)\big)$.

Now we show that the partial differential Eq. (3.46) is interpreted as the vanishing condition for the following closed 2-form on (x^1, x^2, t),

$$\hat{\omega}^{(2)} \equiv E\left(\frac{\partial x^3}{\partial E} dx^1 \wedge dx^2 - d\underset{3}{H} \wedge dt\right),$$

which is related to the previous 2-form $\omega^{(2)}|_{(x^1,x^2,t)} = x^3(x^1, x^2, t)dx^1 \wedge dx^2 - \underset{3}{K} d\underset{3}{H} \wedge dt$, discussed in the previous subsection, by making a replacement $x^3 \to E\partial x^3/\partial E$, $\underset{3}{K} \to E$. Indeed, after projection to the base space (x^1, t) of the secondary dynamic fibration $x^2 = x^2(x^1, t)$, the $\hat{\omega}^{(2)}$ reduces, using the second equation of (3.44), to

$$\hat{\omega}^{(2)}|_{(x^1,t)} = E\left(\frac{\partial x^3}{\partial E}\partial_t x^2 - \partial_1 \underset{23}{H}\right)dx^1 \wedge dt = E\left(\frac{1}{\partial_3 K}\partial_t x^2 - \partial_1 \underset{23}{H}\right)dx^1 \wedge dt,$$

whose vanishing condition coincides with (3.46) as promised.

On the other hand, by expressing $\hat{\omega}^{(2)}$ in an exact form, we have $\hat{\omega}^{(2)} = d\hat{\omega}^{(1)}$ and $\hat{\omega}^{(1)} \equiv E(p_1 dx^1 - \underset{3}{H} dt)$, where p_1 must satisfy $\partial_2 p_1 = -1/\partial_3 K$, thus

$$p_1(x^1, x^2) = -\int^{x^2} \frac{ds}{\partial_3 K\big(x^1, s, x^3(x^1, s; E)\big)}. \tag{3.47}$$

The vanishing condition of $\hat{\omega}^{(2)}\big|_{(x^1,t)}$ is then equivalently formulated as the requirement that $\hat{\omega}^{(1)}$ takes an exact form with some 0-form, say, $E\hat{S}(x^1, t)$,

$$\hat{\omega}^{(1)}\big|_{(x^1,t)} = Ed\hat{S} = E(\partial_1 \hat{S} dx^1 + \partial_t \hat{S} dt),$$

after the second dynamic fibration. This yields the desired secondary HJ equation,

$$\partial_t \hat{S} = -\underset{23}{H}, \quad p_1 = \partial_1 \hat{S}. \tag{3.48}$$

Our task is now to show that the converse is also true: namely, we have to derive the Nambu equations of motion from the above secondary HJ equation for $\hat{S}(x_1, t)$. Since the latter takes exactly the same form as the ordinary HJ equation, a complete solution must have one new integration constant denoted Q_1 in addition to E, we adopt the Jacobi condition in an ordinary way as we have reviewed in the first chapter of this book,

$$\frac{\partial \hat{S}}{\partial Q_1} = -P, \tag{3.49}$$

with P being a constant independent of (Q_1, E). Consequently, we have a set of three integration constants (Q_1, P, E), being required for ensuring general solutions for the Nambu equations of motion. This condition allows us to solve x^1 providing

$$\frac{\partial^2 \hat{S}}{\partial Q_1 \partial x^1} \neq 0. \tag{3.50}$$

Taking derivatives of the above condition with respect to time and also a derivative of $\underset{23}{H}$ with respect to Q_1, we have

$$0 = \frac{d}{dt}\frac{\partial \hat{S}}{\partial Q_1} = \frac{\partial^2 \hat{S}}{\partial Q_1 \partial t} + \frac{\partial^2 \hat{S}}{\partial Q_1 \partial x^1}\frac{dx^1}{dt} = -\frac{\partial}{\partial Q_1}\underset{23}{H} + \frac{\partial^2 \hat{S}}{\partial Q_1 \partial x^1}\frac{dx^1}{dt},$$
$$\frac{\partial}{\partial Q_1}\underset{23}{H} = \partial_2 \underset{3}{H}\frac{\partial x^2}{\partial Q_1} = \partial_2 \underset{3}{H}\frac{\partial x^2}{\partial p_1}\frac{\partial p_1}{\partial Q_1} = -\frac{\partial^2 \hat{S}}{\partial Q_1 \partial x^1}\partial_2 \underset{3}{H}\partial_3 K,$$

where use has been made of (3.48) and (3.47). Then using (3.50) and (3.45), we obtain the first component of the Nambu equations of motion,

$$\frac{dx^1}{dt} = -\partial_2 \underset{3}{H}\partial_3 K = \partial_2 K \partial_3 H - \partial_3 K \partial_2 H.$$

The second component immediately follows by putting this result to the right-hand side of the identity (3.43),

$$\frac{dx^2}{dt} = \partial_t x^2 + \partial_1 x^2 \frac{dx^1}{dt} = \partial_3 K(\partial_1 \underset{3}{H} + \partial_1 x^2 \partial_2 \underset{3}{H}) - \partial_1 x^2 \partial_2 \underset{3}{H}\partial_3 K$$
$$= \partial_3 K \partial_1 \underset{3}{H} = \partial_3 K \partial_1 H - \partial_1 K \partial_3 H.$$

The last component then follows from the identity (3.28) established in the previous subsection. Alternatively, we can use the constraint $K = E$ of the present case,

$$0 = \frac{dE}{dt} = \partial_1 K \frac{dx^1}{dt} + \partial_2 K \frac{dx^2}{dt} + \partial_3 K \frac{dx^3}{dt},$$

which gives

$$\frac{dx^3}{dt} = -\frac{1}{\partial_3 K}\left(\partial_1 K \frac{dx^1}{dt} + \partial_2 K \frac{dx^2}{dt}\right) = \partial_1 K \partial_2 H - \partial_2 K \partial_1 H.$$

Example 3.2 (Euler top in terms of generalized Hamilton–Jacobi theory): Using the angular momenta L_i to be the generalized canonical coordinates $x^i = L_i$ with the Nambu bracket $\{x^i, x^j, x^k\} = \epsilon^{ijk}$, we have

$$K = \frac{1}{2}((x^1)^2 + (x^2)^2 + (x^3)),$$
$$H = \frac{1}{2}\left(\frac{(x^1)^2}{I_1} + \frac{(x^2)^2}{I_2} + \frac{(x^3)^2}{I_3}\right).$$

This model fits in the special case (1) discussed above: by a simple linear N-gauge transformation we can redefine H such that $\partial_3 H = 0$:

$$K \to K, \quad H - \frac{K}{I_3} \to H = \frac{1}{2}\left(\alpha (x^1)^2 + \beta (x^2)^2\right)$$

with $\alpha = \frac{I_3 - I_1}{I_3 I_1}$ and $\beta = \frac{I_3 - I_2}{I_3 I_2}$. For definiteness, we assume $I_3 \geq I_1$, $I_3 \geq I_2$, $I_1 \geq I_2$, so that $\beta \geq \alpha \geq 0$.

The reduced generalized HJ Eq. (3.36) with the resulting new H function is then written as

$$\partial_t S = \underset{3}{K} = \frac{1}{2}((x^1)^2 + (x^2)^2 + (x^3)^2),$$
$$x^3 = \partial_1 H \partial_2 S - \partial_2 H \partial_1 S = \alpha x^1 \partial_2 S - \beta x^2 \partial_1 S.$$

Since $H =$ constant defines an ellipse, it is convenient to change the coordinates (x^1, x^2) to elliptic coordinates (u, v) with $v = H$,

$$x^1 = \left(\frac{2v}{\alpha}\right)^{1/2} \operatorname{sn} u, \quad x^2 = \left(\frac{2v}{\beta}\right)^{1/2} \operatorname{cn} u,$$

using Jacobi's elliptic functions satisfying

$$\operatorname{sn}^2 u + \operatorname{cn}^2 u = 1, \quad k^2 \operatorname{sn}^2 u + \operatorname{dn}^2 u = 1$$
$$\operatorname{sn}' u = \operatorname{cn} u \operatorname{dn} u, \quad \operatorname{cn}' u = -\operatorname{sn} u \operatorname{dn} u, \quad \operatorname{dn}' u = -k^2 \operatorname{sn} u \operatorname{cn} u,$$

where $'$ denotes differentiation with respect to u. Note that, for notational brevity, we suppressed the dependence on the modulus parameter k of the elliptic functions $\mathrm{sn}(u, k)$, $\mathrm{cn}(u, k)$ and $\mathrm{dn}(u, k)$; the value of k will be determined later. Remember that the function $\mathrm{sn}\, u$ is odd and doubly-periodic with the 'fundamental' periods $(u \to u + 4T_1, u \to u + 2iT_2)$ and is analytic except pole singularities at the points congruent to iT_2 or to $2T_1 + iT_2$; T_1 and T_2 are real for $0 < k^2 < 1$, given by complete elliptic integrals of the first kind:

$$T_1(k) \equiv \int_0^1 \frac{ds}{\sqrt{(1-s^2)(1-k^2s^2)}} = \frac{\pi}{2}\left[1 + \frac{1}{4}k^2 + \cdots\right], \quad T_2 \equiv T_1(\sqrt{1-k^2}).$$

In the limit $k \to 0$, $\mathrm{sn}\, u$ reduces to $\sin u$. Similarly, $\mathrm{cn}\, u$ and $\mathrm{dn}\, u$ are even, periodic with the fundamental periods $(u \to u + 4T_1, u \to u + 2T_1 + iT_2)$ and $(u \to u + 2T_1, u \to u + 4iT_2)$, and reduce to $\cos u$ and 1 at $k = 0$, respectively.

Taking into account the coordinate transformation $(x^1, x^2) \to (u, v)$, x^3 is

$$x^3 = -\frac{(\alpha\beta)^{1/2}}{\mathrm{dn}\, u}\partial_u S.$$

As in the usual treatment of the conventional HJ equation, setting $S = -Et + \bar{S}(x^1, x^2)$, (i.e. $K = E$) to eliminate the dependence on time, we have

$$\frac{\alpha\beta}{2\mathrm{dn}^2 u}(\partial_u \bar{S})^2 = E - \frac{v(\beta-\alpha)}{\alpha\beta}\mathrm{sn}^2 u - \frac{v}{\beta}.$$

This result is simplified by choosing the modulus parameter to be $k^2 = \frac{v(\beta-\alpha)}{\alpha\beta\bar{E}}$, $\bar{E} \equiv E - \frac{v}{\beta}$, so that the right-hand side becomes $\bar{E}(1 - k^2\mathrm{sn}^2 u) = \bar{E}\mathrm{dn}^2 u$. To keep everything real, we restrict ourselves to the case $0 \le k^2 < 1$, which amounts to the condition $E/v = K/H > 1/\alpha$. The case $K/H < 1/\alpha$ can be treated by changing the initial ansatz appropriately. Note that we can assume $\bar{E}$ to be positive, since, if we go back to the original definition of K and H,

$$\bar{E} = K - H/\beta = \frac{1}{2\beta}\left[(x^1)^2(\beta-\alpha) + \beta(x^3)^2\right] \ge 0.$$

It should also be mentioned that, with this choice of the parameter k, the limit $k = 0$ corresponds to the case of a symmetrical top with $I_1 = I_2$.

We can now express $\bar{S}$ as

$$\bar{S} = \frac{(2\alpha\beta\bar{E})^{1/2}}{\alpha\beta}\mathcal{E}(u; k),$$

where

$$\mathcal{E}(u;k) \equiv \int^{u} \mathrm{dn}^2 u\, du = \int_0^{\mathrm{sn}\, u} \left(\frac{1-k^2 s^2}{1-s^2}\right)^{1/2} ds$$

is known as the *Jacobi's epsilon function* or the fundamental elliptic integral of the second kind, obeying the differential equation

$$\frac{d\mathcal{E}}{du} = \mathrm{dn}^2 u = \mathrm{cn}\, u\, \mathrm{dn}\, u \frac{\mathrm{dn}\, u}{\mathrm{cn}\, u} = \left(\frac{1-k^2\mathrm{sn}^2 u}{1-\mathrm{sn}^2 u}\right)^{1/2} \mathrm{sn}'\, u$$

with the initial condition $\mathcal{E}(0;k) = 0$. This also leads to

$$x^3 = -\sqrt{2\bar{E}}\, \mathrm{dn}\, u.$$

In terms of the original coordinates, we have

$$S(x^1, x^2, t) = -Et + \left(\frac{2\left(E - \frac{v}{\beta}\right)}{\alpha\beta}\right)^{1/2} \int_0^{x^1/\sqrt{(x^1)^2 + \frac{\beta}{\alpha}(x^2)^2}} \left(\frac{1-k^2 s^2}{1-s^2}\right)^{1/2} ds,$$

which is a complete solution involving two integration constants, E and $v = H$.

Let us finally check whether this solution yields the general solution of the Nambu equations of motion. The Jacobi condition is taken to be

$$\frac{\partial S}{\partial E} = \text{constant},$$

being supplemented with $\frac{dv}{dt}$=0, for fixed base space-time coordinates (x^1, x^2, t). We compute the total time derivative of this condition, and the result expressed for $\bar{S}$ is

$$\frac{d}{dt}\left(\frac{\partial \bar{S}}{\partial E}\right) = \frac{du}{dt}\partial_u\left(\frac{\partial \bar{S}}{\partial E}\right) = 1. \tag{3.51}$$

Noting that $\mathcal{E}$ depends on E only through k^2, we have

$$\frac{\partial \bar{S}}{\partial E} = (2\alpha\beta\bar{E})^{-1/2}\left(\mathcal{E} - 2k^2\frac{\partial \mathcal{E}}{\partial k^2}\right), \quad \frac{\partial \mathcal{E}}{\partial k^2} = -\frac{u}{2} + \frac{1}{2}\int_0^{\mathrm{sn}\, u} dx \frac{\sqrt{1-x^2}}{\sqrt{1-k^2x^2}},$$

$$\frac{d}{dt}\frac{\partial \mathcal{E}}{\partial k^2} = -\frac{1}{2}\mathrm{sn}^2 u\frac{du}{dt} = -\frac{1}{2k^2}(1-\mathrm{dn}^2 u)\frac{du}{dt}.$$

Using these results and $\frac{d}{dt}\mathcal{E}(u) = \frac{du}{dt}\mathrm{dn}^2 u$, we find that

$$\frac{du}{dt} = \sqrt{2\alpha\beta\bar{E}}.$$

Hence, we can set $u = \sqrt{2\alpha\beta\bar{E}}t$, determining the coordinates explicitly as the periodic functions of time t with the period $4T_1(k)/\sqrt{2\alpha\beta\bar{E}}$ or $2T_1(k)/\sqrt{2\alpha\beta\bar{E}}$ for (x^1, x^2) and for x^3, respectively. It is easy to check the equations of motion, e.g.,

$$\frac{dx^3}{dt} = -2\sqrt{\alpha\beta}\bar{E}\mathrm{dn}'u = 2\sqrt{\alpha\beta}\bar{E}k^2\mathrm{sn}\,u\mathrm{cn}\,u = \frac{I_1 - I_2}{I_1 I_2}x^1x^2.$$

It seems justifiable to say that, comparing these results with those in conventional Hamiltonian formalism in which the Euler angles are used as canonical coordinates together with their momentum conjugates, the present formalism has greater simplicity and elegance in employing directly the components of angular momentum as canonical variables.

Chapter 4
Bibliographical Remarks

We give remarks on the literature for Nambu dynamics and related matters. As stressed in the Preface, our list will be quite subjective and selective.

For the present exposition, the following three papers constitute main original sources. First of all, Nambu's original paper is

[1] Y. Nambu, "Generalized Hamiltonian Dynamics", Phys. Rev. **D7**, 2405 (1973).

The whole development described in the present monograph germinated from this work. The 3-form $\omega^{(3)}$ examined in detail in Chaps. 2 and 3 was introduced in:

[2] F. B. Estabrook, "Comments on Generalized Hamiltonian Dynamics", Phys. Rev. **D8**, 2740 (1973).

The so-called fundamental identity was discovered in:

[3] L. Takhtajan, "On Foundation of the Generalized Nambu Mechanics", Comm. Math. Phys. **160**, 295 (1994).

This work gave new impetus and foundations for studying Nambu dynamics further; e.g., an action integral on the basis of the 2-form $\omega^{(2)}$ was discussed in this reference.

Our formulation of the *generalized* variational principles in Chap. 3 is, however, quite different from the last reference, in giving a more direct and straightforward derivation of the Nambu equations of motion through the projection (or pull-back) $\omega^{(3)}\big|_{M_3}$. Main difference lies in the choice of boundary conditions in treating the integral of $\omega^{(3)}$ and $\omega^{(2)}$ over M_3 and ∂M_3, respectively.

It should also be pointed out that the N-gauge transformations on which a special emphasis is placed as a crucial symmetry characterizing the generalized Hamilton-structure of Nambu dynamics in the present exposition have rarely been treated in the literature. Similarly rather sparse in the literature is the Hamilton–Jacobi-type formulation of Nambu dynamics. Nambu himself did not touch on this subject in his original paper. In reference [2], the Hamilton–Jacobi theory for Nambu dynamics with its connection with Schrödinger-type quantization was briefly mentioned, but

T. Yoneya, *Introduction to Nambu's Generalized Hamiltonian Dynamics*,
SpringerBriefs in Mathematical Physics 55,
https://doi.org/10.1007/978-981-95-7030-0_4

not pursued to any detail. The generalized Hamilton–Jacobi theories described in Chap. 3 are based essentially on the present author's relatively recent work in:

[4] T. Yoneya, "Generalized Hamilton–Jacobi Theory of Nambu Mechanics", Prog. Theor. Exp. Phys. **2017**, 023A01 (2017).

In Sect. 3.4 of the present exposition, a new geometrical picture in which the equations of motions are interpreted as the intersection of *moving* cross-sections with different choices of the base spaces in dynamical fibration is presented.

We have not proceeded to the problem of quantization in the present exposition. The author believes that exploring classical theory in-depth would naturally inspire the serious reader to advance his or her interest toward important open questions of quantization. One of the early attempts toward quantization from an extended viewpoint of *deformation quantization* is:

[5] G. Ditto, M. Flato, D. Steinheimer and L. Takhtajan, "Deformation Quantization and Nambu Mechanics", Comm. Math. Phys. **183**, 1 (1997).

A different approach in the framework of certain extended matrix-type algebras using multi-indices objects, inspired by some development in string theory, was given in:

[6] H. Awata, M. Li, D. Minic and T. Yoneya, "On the Quantization of Nambu Brackets", J. High Energy Phys. **0102**, 013 (2001).

For further related attempts, see, among others,

[7] T. Curtright and C. Zachos, "Classical and Quantum Nambu Mechanics", Phys. Rev. **D68**, 085001 (2003),

[8] Y. Kawamura, "Cubic Matrix, Nambu Mechanics and Beyond", Prog. Theor. Phys. **109**, 153 (2003),

and references therein. In connection with the possibility of matrix-type quantization, it is interesting that the triple commutator (1.24) mentioned in Chap. 1 had been briefly treated by E. Cartan in association with his definition of 'trivector' , much earlier than Nambu's paper [1]:

[9] Élie Cartan, "The Theory of Spinors" (Hermann, Paris, 1966; first appeared in French in 1937, and Dover edition published in 1981).

On the other hand, a wave-mechanical viewpoint on quantization was analyzed in detail in the reference [4] on the basis of generalized Hamilton–Jacobi equations, some aspects of which are in fact closely related with the discussion given in Sect. 2.4 of the present exposition about the generalized Poisson bracket. As mentioned in this reference, the author's idea of the generalized Hamilton–Jacobi theory with arbitrary dynamical fibrations was actually inspired by relatively unknown but precious works by Einstein published more than a century ago:

[10] A. Einstein, "Zum Quantenanzatz von Sommerfeld und Epstein", Köglich Pr. Akad. der Wissenschaften, Situngzberichte, 606 (1917) ; "Eine Ableitung des Thorems von Jacobi", Deut. Phys. Phys. Gesselfshaft 19, 606 (1917). English translation in *The Collected Papers of Albert Einstein* (Princeton University Press, 1977, Vol. 6).

In these works, he attempted to formulate the semi-classical quantum conditions in a coordinate-independent fashion, giving also a new ("free of surprising tricks of the trade") derivation of Hamilton–Jacobi equations as a by-product. These papers may be regarded as a precursor to Wave Mechanics.

It should also be noted that possible application of Nambu dynamics to statistical mechanics, which was certainly among Nambu's main motivations, has been scarcely the focus of serious study in the past. Indeed, such attempts are destined to suffer with an intrinsic difficulty of a kind different from the one arising in the quantization problem, since the Nambu equations of motion do not easily allow interactions. An approach toward interactions and statistical mechanics of Nambu dynamics will be given in a separate publication by the present author, starting with the Hamilton–Jacobi theory associated with our universal action principle.

More recently, Nambu dynamics has been receiving attention in diverse fields including fluid physics, plasma physics, and condensed matter physics. In principle, any fields in which vorticity plays key roles in dynamics would be able to enjoy fruitful applications of the basic concept of Nambu dynamics. The readers interested in such directions may find the following collection of papers useful:

[11] "Recent development of Nambu mechanics in physical systems of micro to macro scales: part I and II" (edited by Y. Fukumoto), Prog. Theor. Exp. Phys. **2021**,12C101–12C106 (2021); *ibid* **2024**, 03A101–03A104 (2014),

in which the researchers with different backgrounds contributed original and review papers on various topics related to Nambu dynamics. The readers who wish to glimpse the recent status of Nambu dynamics are recommended to consult some of these contributions. For instance, if the readers are interested in the possible connections of Nambu dynamics with string theory (or 'M-theory'), please refer to the present author's contribution (12C101) in this reference, in addition to [4, 6] which also contain further information on the related literature.

For general references about standard classical mechanics, the following comprehensive treatise and a review article from modern standpoints are recommended:

[12] V. I. Arnold, "Mathematical Methods of Classical Mechanics" (Graduate texts in Mathematics, Springer-Verlag, New York, 2nd edition, 1989),

[13] H. A. Kastrup, "Canonical Theories of Lagrangian Dynamical Systems in Physics", Phys. Reports 101, Nos. 1 and 2, 1–167 (North-Holland, Amsterdam, 1983).

The following books specialized to standard variational principles (with good historical and philosophical accounts in the first, and, in the second, written from a more general mathematical viewpoint) are also worthy of reference:

[14] C. Lanczos, "The Variational Principles of Mechanics" (Dover edition, 1986; originally published by University of Tronto Press, 1970).

[15] C. Carathéodory, "Calculus of Variations and Partial Differential Equations of the First Order" (Chelsea Publishing Company, New York, 1989, originally published by Holden-Day, Inc.,1965).

As a matter of course, in ordinary Hamiltonian dynamics, the time coordinate t has a special privilege compared with spatial coordinates. Nambu dynamics extended this feature to an extreme limit, because it seems to be wholly out of question to include Lorentz transformation in the framework of Nambu dynamics. However, we have to remember that an opposite direction of the extension of the Hamiltonian formalism is also quite important and indispensable: As to such a generalization of the standard Hamiltonian formalism aiming at the application to general relativity theory where all of space-time coordinates including time are required to be treated equivalently almost by definition, I would like to mention Dirac's fundamental work,

[16] P. A. M. Dirac, "Generalized Hamiltonian Dynamics", Can. Journ. Math. 2, 129 (1950). See also, "Lectures on Quantum Mechanics", New York, Belfer Graduate School of Science (1964) (Dover Edition, published in 2001).

In this work, he laid a foundation of generalized Hamiltonian dynamics which is applicable to a variety of dynamical systems with constraints, having decisive influences on later developments in quantizing string theory as well as general relativity.

Now, tracing back the historical origins of Nambu dynamics, let me mention Jacobi's extremely interesting series of lectures:

[17] C. G. J. Jacobi, "Vorlesungen über Dynamik" (University of Königsberg, 1842–1843, edited by A. Clebsch; English version, published by Hindustrian Book Agency, India, 2009),

which I could reach only after submitting the first version of manuscript of this book for refereeing; in particular, the Chapter 10 of this reference with the title "Principle of the Last Multiplier" is a precursor to Nambu dynamics, as we have touched on briefly in Remark 2.1. Actually, this finding proved my former anticipation "It would be no surprise if we could find the same Nambu equations of motion in some old literature written even a century ago" (see, e.g., 12C101 in [11]) to be true.

The historical origin of Nambu dynamics in connection with hydrodynamics is another subject which is beyond the scope of the present monograph. As a general reference on hydrodynamics, we recommend the following famous classic:

[18] H. Lamb, "Hydrodynamics", (Dover edition, 1945; originally published by the Cambridge Univ. Press, 6th edition, 1932).

Clebsch transformation of the hydrodynamical equations was succinctly explained in this treatise (pp. 248–249).

Historically, Clebsch transformation was introduced in the context of hydrodynamics in the second of the following two seminal papers:

[19] A. Clebsch, "Über eine allgemeine Transformation der hydrodynamischen Gleichhungen", Journal für die reine und angewandte Mathematik 54, 293 (1857); "Über die Integration der hydrodynamichen Gleighhugen", *ibid.* 56, 1 (1859).

The first paper (1857) took up Jacobi's work mentioned above which was done within the framework of particle (or solid) mechanics, applying it to hydrodynamical equations, under the assumption that the velocity field u_i takes the Jacobi form, automatically satisfying $0 = \partial_i u_i$ without any multiplier. On the other hand, in the second paper (1859), he set the velocity field $\dot{x}_i = u_i(x, t)$ in the form $u_i = \partial_i \varphi + m \partial_i \psi$ with 3 functions (φ, m, ψ) (in the case of 3 dimensions for simplicity), the second term being the 'Clebsch form'. Because of this particular restriction, this work has little relevance to Nambu dynamics. Namely, in the language of Sect. 2.2, the velocity field is identified directly with the vector potential A_i under the gauge condition $\partial_i A_i = 0$. By contrast, the Nambu equations of motion are instead, $\dot{x}_i = \epsilon_{ijk}\partial_j u_k = \epsilon_{ijk}\partial_j m \partial_k \psi$, which are independent of φ. However, from the viewpoint of hydrodynamics *per se*, its importance lies in the discovery that the pair of fields (m, ψ) plays the role of canonical variables for the Hamiltonian formulation of Euler's hydrodynamical equations of motion. For more details on these works, we recommend the reader to consult

[20] G. Grimberg and E. Tassi, "Comments on Clebsch's 1857 and 1859 papers on using Hamiltonian methods in hydrodynamics", The European Physical Journal H 47, article number 17 (2021),

and the references therein.

In more recent times, the Clebsch form for the gauge field played some role in an almost forgotten series of old works by Dirac:

[21] P. A. M. Dirac, "A New Classical Theory of Electors. I, II, and III", Proc. R. Soc. London, A209, 291 (1951); *ibid.* A212, 330 (1952); *ibid.* A291, 438 (1954).

In these works, he tried to develop a new classical and hydrodynamical formulation for electrons treating a "continuous stream of electricity rather than the motion of point charges", aiming ultimately at quantum electrodynamics completely free of ultraviolet divergences. In the first of these references, he studied gauge potential with a special gauge condition $A^\mu A_\mu =$ constant and gave a direct derivation of the Hamilton–Jacobi equation for an electron *without* relying on the equations of motion for the electron. Interestingly enough, Nambu arrived at the same equation much later, apparently being unaware of the Dirac's works when writing this paper:

[22] Y. Nambu, "Quantum Electrodynamics in Nonlinear Gauge", Prog. Theor. Phys. Suppl., E68, 190 (1968).

Nambu's motivation was to discuss a simple model of spontaneous breakdown of Lorentz invariance: he was influenced by Heisenberg's nonlinear unified field theory where in fact electromagnetism had been interpreted as a consequence of spontaneous broken Lorentz symmetry.

Dirac noticed also that the current associated with his gauge field obeying the HJ equation was irrotational and introduced, in the end, the vorticity of Clebsch's form. He could not succeed in attaining his final goal, and abandoned this and similar attempts within a few years, but proceeded later to a pioneering attempt toward a new theory of the electron:

[23] P. A. M. Dirac, "An extensible model of the electron", Proc. R. Soc. London, A268, 57 (1962),

in which he propounded a spherical-membrane model of the electron with the action being defined as an integral over the $(2+1)$-dimensional world volume that can be expressed using the square of the *Jacobian* (therefore of the *Nambu bracket* in $2+1$ dimensions) associated with the projection (3.4) ($k=3$). That arises geometrically from the induced metric of the world volume embedded in the flat Minkowski space-time. Starting around the late 1990s, the Dirac paper [23] combined with another pioneering (and much earlier) work on a non-linear theory of electromagnetism by Born and Infeld,

[24] M. Born and L. Infeld, "Foundations of the new field theory", Proc. Roy. Soc. London, A144, 425 (1934),

began to influence string theory in formulating an effective low-energy theory for the so-called 'D-branes' with *dynamical* extendedness of various dimensions. In fact, our work [6] was an example of the outcomes of such developments. It is to be noted in general that the privileged role of time in Nambu dynamics can be compatible with Lorentz invariance if 'time' in the sense of Nambu dynamics is reinterpreted as the Lorentz-invariant evolution parameter (or *proper time*) which can be intrinsically embedded in the world volumes of these extended objects. It is often possible also to utilize the Nambu-type equations of motion to describe the flows of symmetry transformations instead of dynamical flows themselves. That is the case for relativistic theories of extended objects. For a review of such approaches, see 12C101 in [11] and references therein.

In connection with string theory, an interesting attempt by Nambu to utilize a Clebsch-type representation in treating the 2-dimensional world sheet of strings in the spirit of Hamilton–Jacobi theory should also be mentioned:

[25] Y. Nambu, "Hamilton–Jacobi Formalism for Strings", Phys. Lett. 92B, 327 (1980); see also his earlier works, "Strings, Vortices, and Gauge Fields", reported in 'Quark Confinement and Field Theory', Proc. 1976 Conf. Univ. Rochester, John Wiley & Sons, Inc., 1977); "Monopoles, Strings, and Instantons", in Ann. New York Acad. Sci. 294, 74 (1977), in which it was mentioned that a part of the field strength around a monopole can be expressed in a form of Clebsch's transformation.

In this work he gave a certain generalization of the conventional Hamiltonian–Jacobi formalism on the basis of the so-called Schild action for the relativistic string:

[26] A. Schild, "Classical Null Strings", Phys. Rev. D16, 1722 (1977).

The Pfaffian 1-form for a particle is generalized to a 2-form, $p_{ij}dq^i \wedge dq^j - H d\sigma \wedge d\tau$, for a string and, as a consequence, Hamilton–Jacobi equation takes the form:

$$\sum_m \frac{\partial(S_m, T_m)}{\partial(\sigma, \tau)} + H = 0,$$

where the Hamiltonian, $H = H(p_{ij}, q^i, q^j)$, is a function of the generalized momenta $p_{ij} = \frac{\partial(S_m,T_m)}{\partial(q_i,q_j)}$ and generalized coordinates q^i (essentially, string coordinates, $x^\mu(\sigma, \tau)$, in terms of the conventional notation of string theory), and the set of functions (S_m, T_m) replaces the role of Hamilton's principal function S in the ordinary HJ equation $\partial_t S + H = 0$. However, it is to be noticed that no mention of [1] was made in [25], despite the appearance of the Clebsch transformation. This is understandable firstly because it seems that, in 1973, he was not aware of the connection of his original work [1] with hydrodynamics, particularly, with the Clebsch's transformation. Remember that he had never mentioned any possibility of connecting his equations of motion in [1] to Hamilton–Jacobi theory, as we stressed before. Another reason is perhaps that Nambu's motivation in [25] was solely to treat the world-sheet coordinates (σ, τ) of a string on an equal footing still with the *single* Hamiltonian H as above, appearing in the dynamical part $-Hd\sigma \wedge d\tau$ of his 2-form in a standard (*non-Clebsch*) form, in the context of traditional Hamilton–Jacobi theory.

By contrast, the dynamical part of the 2-form $\omega^{(2)}$ in Nambu dynamics in the sense of the present exposition has the Clebsch form $-KdH \wedge dt$ with two independent Hamiltonian functions (K, H). As our discussion in Sect. 3.4.3 clearly shows, the generalized Hamilton–Jacobi theory on the basis of $\omega^{(2)}$, in which the conventional scalar S-function is replaced by a vector S-field (S_1, S_2, S_0), does not require any additional physical parameter like σ other than time t for the base space of dynamical variables x^i. Of course, this is more than natural since in Nambu dynamics we are dealing with dynamics of a particle without any physical extension.

In fact, as pointed out in [13], the final result of [25] can be regarded as a special case (namely, the string coordinates $x^\mu(\sigma, \tau)$ as the fields on the two-dimensional *base* space (σ, τ)) of a general formalism which can be classified as a '*relativistic*' Hamilton–Jacobi theory (known as 'DWHJ theory') for field theory on the base space-times of general dimensions. The DWHJ theory had been developed in the 1930s mainly by Carathéodory, DeDonder and Weyl (see [13] for the literature).

Also, a quite different reformulation of the Schild action, which relates the nonstandard canonical structure exhibited in the Schild action to space-time noncommutativity as the characteristic short-distance structure of string dynamics, was given by the present author:

[27] T. Yoneya, "Schild Action and Space-Time Uncertainty Principle in String Theory", Prog. Theor. Phys. 97, 949 (1997); "String Theory and the Space-Time Uncertainty Principle, *ibid.* 103, 1081 (2000). At the writing of these papers, the author was not aware of Nambu's paper [25], and only mentioned briefly, in the second reference, a possibility of connecting the results with [1]. See also "Space-Time Uncertainty and Noncommutativity in String Theory", p. 305, in *Strings MM* (Proc. of the 2000 Int. Superstring Conf., World Scientific, eds. M. J. Duff et al., 2001).

Finally, in the present exposition, differential forms are constructed and utilized in a rather intuitive fashion from a physicist's viewpoint as an important tool for developing Nambu dynamics in general dimensions. The readers who wish to pursue differential forms and their applications further from more general and rigorous mathematical standpoints may find the following treatises useful:

[28] H. Flanders, "Differential Forms with Applications to the Physical Sciences" (Academic Press Inc., New York, 1963),

[29] R. Bott and L. W. Tu, "Differential Forms in Algebraic Topology" (Graduate texts in Mathematics, Springer-Verlag, New York, 1982).

Index

T. Yoneya, *Introduction to Nambu's Generalized Hamiltonian Dynamics*, SpringerBriefs in Mathematical Physics 55,
https://doi.org/10.1007/978-981-95-7030-0

MIX
Papier aus verantwortungsvollen Quellen
Paper from responsible sources
FSC® C105338

If you have any concerns about our products,
you can contact us on
ProductSafety@springernature.com

In case Publisher is established outside the EU,
the EU authorized representative is:
Springer Nature Customer Service Center GmbH
Europaplatz 3, 69115 Heidelberg, Germany

Printed by Libri Plureos GmbH
in Hamburg, Germany